GW01453133

# Monitoring for Drug Safety

*In memory of James Crooks
and Franz Gross*

SECOND EDITION

# Monitoring for Drug Safety

Editor
**William H. W. INMAN**

Assistant Editor
**Elaine P. Gill**

**MTP PRESS LIMITED**
a member of the KLUWER ACADEMIC PUBLISHERS GROUP
LANCASTER / BOSTON / THE HAGUE / DORDRECHT

Published in the UK and Europe by
MTP Press Limited
Falcon House
Lancaster, England

**British Library Cataloguing in Publication Data**
Monitoring for drug safety.—2nd ed.
1. Drug utilization
I. Inman, W. H. W.
615'.7 RM301

ISBN 0–85200–721–3

Published in the USA by
MTP Press
A division of Kluwer Boston Inc.
190 Old Derby Street
Hingham, MA 02043, USA

**Library of Congress Cataloging-in-Publication Data**
Monitoring for drug safety.
Bibliography: p.
Includes index.
1. Drugs—Side effects—Reporting. 2. Drugs—Testing. 3. Drugs—Law and legislation. 4. Pharmacy—Information services. I. Inman, W.H.W. (William Howard Wallace), 1929–
RM302.5.M66 1985 363.1'94 85–21707

ISBN 0–85200–721–3


Vantage Photosetting Co Ltd, Eastleigh and London
Printed in Great Britain by Butler & Tanner Ltd, Frome and London

# Contents

## SECTION 5: COMMUNICATIONS

# Preface to the Second Edition

The first edition of *Monitoring for Drug Safety* was assembled in 1979, some 3 years after its Editor had conceived the need for a new and independently based national drug monitoring system, complementary to the voluntary reporting system (yellow card scheme) that had been established 16 years earlier in the United Kingdom as a response to the thalidomide tragedy. To a considerable extent the book was inspired by the lack of a comprehensive account of the numerous attempts that had been made in many countries to establish methods for identifying and measuring the risks and benefits of drug therapy. It highlighted many of the deficiencies in current monitoring methods and some of the practical problems which the new system, based on the Drug Surveillance Research Unit in Southampton, would attempt to overcome. This compilation of expertise was invaluable in the subsequent development of Prescription-Event Monitoring (PEM) which is described in detail in Chapter 15. Sadly, PEM is probably the only entirely novel monitoring scheme to have been developed anywhere in the world during the last 5 years. Nevertheless many of the authors have been able to report significant technical progress in their monitoring schemes, and I believe that this work is the largest and most comprehensive collection of authoritative opinion ever assembled under one cover. 74 authors from 17 countries in Europe, North America, the Far East and Australasia have contributed to it.

Several new chapters have been added to this second edition and some old ones have been replaced or omitted. It was not possible, for example, to update Doctor Davies' excellent compilation of information sources; to do so would require a book by itself. Finland and Spain are welcome new contributors. New material has been included by many of the authors of the first edition and by 21 new authors.

While planning and developing a very detailed protocol for the first edition, I perceived my role to be that of critic and commentator as well as Editor. This is reflected in the five commentaries that link the various sections of the work, in which I have expressed personal views which do not invariably agree with those of individual chapter authors. Readers should also appreciate that the views expressed by all the authorities are also personal and do not necessarily reflect the official policies of the organizations many of them represent.

No attempt has been made in this present edition to reproduce the many different kinds of forms that are used in monitoring schemes. This is because they are frequently revised and because it would be necessary to photo-reduce them for reproduction, leading to problems of legibility. All the authors will be pleased to supply original copies of the latest forms available in their centres. Their addresses will be found in the 'About the Authors' section.

Since the first edition, two pioneers in drug safety, James Crooks and Franz Gross have died and this book is dedicated to their memory. Although not an author, James Crooks inspired the Aberdeen/Dundee system described by Doctor Moir (Chapter 18) and his tireless efforts as an adviser to WHO and the Committee on the Safety of Drugs will never be forgotten. Franz Gross' experience in industry and academic pharmacology and his extraordinary skills in communication had a catalytic effect on the early development of post-marketing surveillance and his contribuition to the first edition has been retained in the second. Readers should reflect that with few notable exceptions, the authors include the majority of people throughout the world who are experts in this very specialized field. About one in five have dedicated much of their professional lives to it. Pharmacoepidemiologists are a rare species and it is to be hoped that this comprehensive collection of papers will stimulate interest and lead to an injection of new blood.

Finally I must record my very special thanks to Elaine Gill, my Assistant Editor, without whose help a second edition would not have been attempted and to my secretary Barbara Hunt and her predecessor, Nadine Dingley, and to the staff of the Drug Surveillance Research Unit who processed most of the data incorporated in Chapter 15. Once again, I would like to thank the Editor of *Methods of Information in Medicine* for permission to reproduce Professor Finney's timeless article on statistical logic.

# About the authors

**Dr A. M. Adelstein,** MD, DPH, was Chief Medical Statistician to the Office of Population Censuses and Surveys (General Register Office). He was a regular contributor to *Health Trends* and has worked closely with the Committee on Safety of Medicines, especially in connection with the 'epidemic' of asthma deaths of the 1960s, which were associated with aerosol bronchodilators. Between 1981 and 1984 he was Visiting Professor at the London School of Hygiene and Tropical Medicine, where he is a Fellow of the Cancer Research Campaign (Chapter 33).

*Address:* London School of Hygiene and Tropical Medicine, Department of Medical Statistics and Epidemiology, Keppel Street (Gower Street), London WC1E 7HT.

**Dr G. Ansell,** MD, FRCP, FRCR, is Consultant Radiologist at Whiston Hospital, and Lecturer in Radiodiagnosis at Liverpool University. He has published numerous papers on adverse reactions to contrast media, and his special interest in this field has led him to develop a national system for collecting reports of these reactions; he is an adviser to the Committee on Safety of Medicines. He is assisted in the preparation of Chapter 22 by **Mr M. C. K. Tweedie,** MSc, Senior Lecturer in Biostatistics, **Mr C. R. West,** MA, Statistical Assistant at the University Department of Medicine, and by **Professor D. A. Evans.**

*Address:* Whiston Hospital, Merseyside L35 5DR.

**Dr I. Borda,** FRCP(C), an honours graduate of the University of Budapest Medical School, moved to Canada in 1957. He was Associate Professor of Medicine at the University of Western Ontario and Head of the Gastroenterology Department St. Joseph's Hospital, London, Canada. He was one of the founding members of the Boston Collaborative Drug Surveillance Program. He is on the World Health Organization Expert Panel on drug related matters. Since 1980 he has been Head of Active Drug Surveillance and Consultant on Special Medical Projects at Ciba–Geigy Basle in Switzerland (Chapter 14). **Dr G. C. Berneker** graduated in Freiburg (BRD) and is Head of the Drug Monitoring Unit of the Medical Department at Ciba–Geigy's headquarters in Basle (Chapter 14).

*Address:* Medical Department, Ciba–Geigy, CH-4002, Basle, Switzerland.

**Dr G. C. Berneker** graduated in Freiburg (BRD) and is Head of the Drug Monitoring Unit of the Medical Department at Ciba–Geigy's headquarters in Basle (Chapter 14).

*Address:* Medical Department, Ciba–Geigy, CH-4002, Basle, Switzerland.

**Dr W. Bruinsma,** MD of Amsterdam and New York is a dermatological consultant for Governmental and pharmaceutical agencies. He is a member of the Dutch Committee on Adverse Reactions to Drugs, and has established the international *File of Adverse*

*Reactions to the Skin*, which now regularly publishes the *Guide to Drug Eruptions* (Chapter 24).

*Address:* De Zwaluw, PO Box 21, 1474 ZG Oosthuizen, The Netherlands.

**Dr D. R. Chambers,** MBBS, LlB, DObst, RCOG, qualified in Medicine in 1953 and was called to the Bar in 1965. A former Medical Director of Hoechst Pharmaceuticals he is now Her Majesty's Coroner for Inner North London, and is an honorary Senior Lecturer in Medical Law in the Department of Medicine, University College Hospital Medical School. He is a member of the Council of the Coroners Society of England and Wales and its Senior Vice-President. (Chapter 28).

*Address:* Coroner's Court, Camley Street, London NW1 0PP.

**Dr D. M. Coulter,** MB, ChB, DTM and H General Practitioner. Assistant to the Medical Assessor, NZ Medicines Adverse Reactions Committee. **Professor I. R. Edwards,** FRCP. Associate Professor of Clinical Pharmacology, University of Otago Medical School, Medical Assessor of the NZ Medicines Adverse Reactions Committee, and Honorary Director of the National Poisons Information Centre and the Medical Research Council's Toxicology Research Unit. **Professor E. G. McQueen,** FRCP, FRACP, is Emeritus Professor of Clinical Pharmacology at the University of Otago Medical School, formerly Medical Assessor of the New Zealand Committee on Adverse Drug Reactions (Chapter 9).

*Address:* Department of Pharmacology, University of Otago, PO Box 913, Dunedin, New Zealand.

**Dr B. W. Cromie,** FRCP[1], is Chairman of the Pharmaceutical Division of Hoechst UK Limited, a member of the Medicines Commission and a former Vice-President of the Association of British Pharmaceutical Industries (ABPI). He has lectured and published extensively on the problems facing the UK Pharmaceutical Industry and the effects of government interference. His co-author, **Mr M Slater**[2], is now Director of Regulatory Affairs in Biogen Medical Research, Geneva, where he retains his interest in the effects of international drug regulation on innovation and development. (Chapter 48).

*Addresses:* [1] Hoechst UK, Limited, Pharmaceutical Division, Hoechst House, Salisbury Road, Hounslow, Middlesex. TW4 6JH. [2] Biogen Medical Research, 25 Route des Acacias, 1211 Geneva 24.

**Professor V. W. M. Drury,** OBE, MB, ChB, FRCGP, is Professor of General Practice at the University of Birmingham. He is a past member of the Sub-Committee on Adverse Reactions of the Committee on Safety of Medicines and of the editorial board of *Prescribers' Journal*. Professor Drury is currently the Chairman of the Research Division of the Royal College of General Practitioners. He is also President Elect of the Royal College of General Practitioners (Chapter 42).

*Address:* Department of Medicine, Queen Elizabeth Hospital, Edgbaston, Birmingham B15 2TH.

**Professor J. W. Dundee,** MD, PhD, FFARCS, FRCP, is Professor of Anaesthetics at The Queen's University of Belfast. He is author of many papers on this subject. He is Past Dean of the Faculty of Anaesthetists of the Royal College of Surgeons in Ireland, and Past President of the Section of Anaesthetics of the Royal Society of Medicine. He is a member of the Board of Faculty of Anaesthetists of the Royal College of Surgeons of England, and a member of the Committee on Safety of Medicines (Chapter 21).

*Address:* 24 Old Coach Road, Belfast 9, Northern Ireland.

**Dr J. F. Dunne,** BSc, PhD, MBBS, formerly a Lecturer in therapeutics at the London Hospital and a Principal Medical Officer to the Committee on Safety of Medicines, joined the World Health Organization in Geneva as Senior Medical Officer in Pharmaceuticals. He has been especially concerned with the programme for international drug monitoring, and is now responsible for all aspects of the general pharmaceutical programmes with the WHO (Chapter 13).

*Address:* World Health Organization, 1211 Geneva 27, Switzerland.

**Professor D. J. Finney,** CBE, MA, ScD, FRS, FRSE, was a pupil of the late Sir Ronald Fisher, and later was senior assistant to Dr Frank Yates at Rothamsted Experimental Station from 1939 to 1945. He is a past-President of the Biometric Society and the Royal Statistical Society, and a past-Chairman of the Computer Board for Universities and Research Councils. Currently he is Professor of Statistics at the University of Edinburgh. He is the author of several books and about 200 papers. Professor Finney was a founder-member of the Sub-Committee on Adverse Reactions of the Committee on Safety of Drugs (now Committee on Safety of Medicines); he is internationally recognized as a contributor to the development of drug-monitoring in the United Kingdom, and through his long service as adviser to the WHO (Chapter 31).

*Address:* Department of Statistics, James Clerk Maxwell Building, The King's Buildings, Mayfield Road, Edinburgh EH9 3JZ.

**Professor C. M. Fletcher,** CBE, MD, FRCP. Formerly Director of the Medical Research Council's Pneumoconiosis Research Unit; is Emeritus Professor of Clinical Epidemiology in the University of London (formerly the Royal Postgraduate Medical School at the Hammersmith Hospital). He is a well-known authority on communications in medicine and a specialist in pulmonary diseases (Chapter 44).

*Address:* 24 West Square, London SE11 4SN.

**Dr M. G. Franzosi,** is Senior Investigator in the Lombardy Regional Centre for Drug Information and in charge of some of the continuing projects described in Chapter 6.

**Dr G. Tognoni,** MD, is Head of the Lombardy Regional Centre for Drug Information, and since 1976, of the Laboratory of Clinical Pharmacology at the Mario Negri Institute in Milan. He is the author of numerous works on drug metabolism and monitoring.

*Address:* Istituto di Ricerche Farmacologiche 'Mario Negri', 20157 Milano, via Eritrea 62, Italy.

**Professor F. T. Fraunfelder,** MD, is Professor and Chairman of the Department of Ophthalmology at the Oregon Health Sciences University. He has been responsible for development of the *Drug-induced Ocular Side-Effects Registry,* and is the author of over 100 publications, including a book, *Drug-induced Ocular Side-Effects and Drug Interactions* (Chapter 28).

*Address:* Department of Ophthalmology, 3181 S.W. Sam Jackson Park Road, Portland, Oregon 97201.

**Dr O. Gillie,** PhD, graduated from Edinburgh University specializing in genetics in 1965. He then worked at the National Institute for Medical Research at Mill Hill. Later he became interested in journalism and at various times worked for *Science Journal,* edited *General Practitioner* and finally became medical correspondent to *The Sunday Times.* He was nominated Specialist Writer of the year in 1977 (Chapter 45).

*Address:* 61 Dartmouth Park Road, London NW5.

The late **Professor Dr F. H. Gross** was Professor of Pharmacology at the University of Heidelberg from 1968. Formerly Head of the Medical Department of Ciba in Basle, he was a past-President of the International Society of Hypertension, Secretary General of the International Union of Pharmacology, and Managing Editor of the *European Journal of Pharmacology*. The holder of many international awards, he had an outstanding reputation as one of the most effective conference chairmen in the field of pharmacology (Chapter 47).

**Dr D. Haler,** MB, BS (Hons), LMSSA, DCP, FRCPath, was a founder Fellow of the Royal College of Pathologists and has had a long and distinguished career in pathology. He was a Coroner's Pathologist for the Inner London and South Division of the Greater London Council and for East and West Surrey. In 1977 he was the Sir Arthur Keith medallist of the Royal College of Surgeons. He retired in 1983 (Chapter 29).

*Address:* Holly Lodge, Oat Lands Chase, Weybridge, KT13 9SE.

**Dr E. L. Harris,** CB, FRCP, FRCP(E), FFCM, is Deputy Chief Medical Officer of the Department of Health and Social Security. Formerly he was the Medical Director of Abbott Laboratories (UK) and later Medical Assessor to the Committee on Safety of Medicines (Chapter 49).

*Address:* DHSS, Alexander Fleming House, Elephant and Castle, London SE1.

**Margaretha Helling-Borda**[1] has worked in the pharmaceutical industry in Sweden and the United States. Since 1968 she has worked at the World Health Organization initially in the WHO Centre for International Monitoring of Adverse Reactions, and is now a Senior Programme Officer in the WHO Action Programme on Essential Drugs. Her co-authors are **H. Mandahl**, Deputy-Director at the Department of Drugs, and **P. Manell**,[2] Chief Pharmaceutical Officer, Department of Drugs, Sweden. **Mr Manell** has developed the Swedish Drug Information System SWEDIS. The authors regularly advise governments in developing countries on matters of drug control and administration (Chapter 20).

*Addresses:*[1] Action Programme on Essential Drugs, World Health Organization, 1211 Geneva 27, Switzerland.[2] Department of Drugs, Box 607, S-751 25 Uppsala, Sweden.

**Dr A. Herxheimer,** MB, FRCP, is Senior Lecturer in Clinical Pharmacology and Therapeutics at Charing Cross and Westminster Medical School in London and Editor of *Drug and Therapeutics Bulletin*. He is Chairman of the Health Working Group of the International Organization of Consumers Unions at the Hague, and a Vice-President of the recently established College of Health (Chapter 46).

*Address:* Department of Clinical Pharmacology, Charing Cross Hospital, Fulham Palace Road, London W6 8RF.

**Mr R. M. Hogarth** wrote his chapter while holding a visiting appointment at the London Graduate School of Business Studies and has now moved to the Graduate School of Business, University of Chicago, USA, where he is a Professor of Behavioral Science and Director of the Center for Decision Research. (Chapter 35).

*Address:* University of Chicago, Graduate School of Business, 1101 East 58th Street, Chicago, Illinois 60637, USA.

**Dr J. Idänpään-Heikkilä,** MD Docent, is Chief Medical Officer for Pharmacology at the National Board of Health (Health Directorate of Finland) in Helsinki, Finland. Formerly he was assistant professor in pharmacology at the University of Oulu and in 1982–1983 was a visiting scientist at the Office of New Drug Evaluation, Food and Drug Administration, Rockville, Maryland, USA (Chapter 5).

*Address:* National Board of Health, Siltasaarenkatu 18, 00530 Helsinki, Finland.

**Mr N. Ikeda** is Director of the Office of Drug Induced Damage, Division of Planning, at the Bureau of Pharmaceutical Affairs at the Japanese Ministry of Health (Chapter 39).

*Address:* Japanese Ministry of Health, 1.2.2. Kasumigaseki, Chiyodaku, Tokyo, Japan.

**Professor W. H. W. Inman,** FRCP, FFCM qualified in Cambridge and was a founder member of the secretariat of the Committee on the Safety of Drugs (Dunlop Committee) from 1964. He was responsible for developing the UK 'Yellow Card' system for voluntary reporting of adverse reactions (Chapter 1). In 1980 he established the Drug Surveillance Research Unit (DSRU) within the Faculty of Medicine at the University of Southampton and developed a second national system known as Prescription-Event Monitoring (Chapter 15). In Chapter 1 his co-author is **Dr J. C. P. Weber,** MD, who has recently retired from his appointment as Senior Medical Officer in the Medicines Division of the Department of Health and Social Security, and as medical adviser on the Secretariat of the Committee of Safety of Medicines. He joined the Division in 1976 after a long career both in clinical medicine and as a consultant to the pharmaceutical industry, and has published many papers on clinical topics and the methodology of adverse drug reaction monitoring. In Chapter 15 his co-authors are **Mr N. S. B. Rawson,** MSc, FSS and **Dr L. V. Wilton** BSc, PhD who are both Senior Research Fellows at the D.S.R.U. **Mr Rawson** was previously the statistician responsible for the National Childhood Encephalopathy Study at The Middlesex Hospital Medical School, while **Dr Wilton** was previously a Senior Research Scientist with British American Tobacco Company. (Chapters 1 and 15).

*Address:* Drug Surveillance Research Unit, North Croft House, Winchester Road, Botley, Hampshire SO3 2BX.

**Dr Judith K. Jones,**[1] MD, PhD is Special Assistant to the Associate Director, Office of Epidemiology and Biometrics, Center for Drugs and Biologics, U.S. Food and Drug Administration formerly, Director, Division of Drug Experience, FDA and Clinical Associate Professor, Department of Community and Family Medicine, Georgetown University School of Medicine. **G. A. Faich,**[2] MD, MPH, Director, Office of Epidemiology and Biostatistics, Center for Drugs and Biologics, US Food and Drug Administration. **C. A. Anello,**[2] ScD., Deputy Director, Office of Epidemiology and Biostatistics, Center for Drugs and Biologics, US Food and Drug Administration (Chapter 12).

*Addresses:*[1] Division of Internal Medicine, Georgetown University Hospital, Gorman Building, 3800 Reservoir Road NW, Washington DC 20007, USA.[2] Office of Epidemiology, Room 15B43, HSN700, Center for Drugs and Biologics, Food and Drug Administration, 5600 Fishers Lane, Rockville, Maryland 20857, USA.

**Dr D. H. Keeling,** MSc, MB, BChir, FRCR is Consultant Physician in Nuclear Medicine in Plymouth. As a former Lecturer at the Institute of Nuclear Medicine, Middlesex Hospital, he developed a national system for monitoring adverse reactions to the agents used in this speciality, and is now the Medical Assessor for the Radiopharmaceutical Reporting Scheme (Chapter 23)

*Address:* Nuclear Medicine Department, Freedom Fields, Plymouth PL4 7JJ.

**Professor G. S. McL. Kellaway,** MD, FRCP, FRACP, is Associate Professor in Clinical Pharmacology and Therapeutics at the Auckland School of Medicine. He is Chairman of the New Zealand Medicines Adverse Reaction Committee and several other committees, a member of the Medicines Assessment Advisory Committee to the Ministry of Health and Chief Consulting Editor of *Drugs* (Chapter 41).

*Address:* Department of Pharmacology, University of Auckland School of Medicine, Private Bag, Auckland, New Zealand.

**Dr K. H. Kimbel** is the Secretary-General and member of the Board of the German Drug Commission since 1972. Born in 1924, he qualified after the second world war, specializing in internal medicine and pharmacology. From 1955 to 1972 he held various experimental and clinical research positions in the pharmaceutical industry on both sides of the Atlantic and in Japan (Chapter 4).

*Address:* Medicines Commission of the German Medical Profession, PO Box 410125, 5000 Cologne 41, West Germany.

**Mr H. Komiya** is Director of the Pharmaceuticals and Chemicals Safety Division of the Pharmaceutical Affairs Bureau of the Ministry of Health and Welfare in Japan (Chapter 7).

*Address:* Pharmaceutical Affairs Bureau, Ministry of Health and Welfare, 2–2, 1-chome, Kasumigaseki, Chiyoda-Ku, Tokyo 100, Japan.

**Profesor J. -R. Laporte,** MD, is Professor of Clinical Pharmacology and Therapeutics at the Autonomous Univesity of Barcelona (AUB). He is a member of the Spanish Committee on Adverse Drug Reactions, and Chairman of the Spanish National Centre Collaborating in the WHO International Programme for Drug Monitoring. He is the author of numerous papers on various pharmacology topics (Chapter 11).

*Address:* Divisió de Farmacologia Clínica Unitat Docent de la Facultat de Medicina Universitat Autònoma de Barcelona Ciutat Sanitària de la Vall d'Hebron. P. Vall d'Hebron, s. n. Barcelona - 32/35 Spain.

**Professor D. H. Lawson,** MD, FRCPEd, is Consultant Physician at the Royal Infirmary, Glasgow, Visiting Professor in the School of Pharmaceutical Sciences at the University of Strathclyde and Visiting Consultant at the Boston Collaborative Drug Surveillance Program, Boston University. He has been a member of the Committee on Review of Medicines since 1979. He has a special interest in developing clinical pharmacology services in the Glasgow area. He is the author of more than 130 papers on various medical topics (Chapter 17).

*Address:* Department of Clinical Pharmacology, Royal Infirmary, Glasgow G4 0SF.

**Mr H. Lester** is Senior Partner at Lester, Schwab, Katz & Dwyer, Attorneys-at-Law in New York. He is a Lecturer for several Bar Associations, and a member or chairman of numerous committees; at various times he has been President of the Brooklyn–Manhattan Trial Lawyers Association, President of the Trial Lawyers Section of the New York State Bar Association and President of the Federation of Insurance Counsel. He is assisted by **Mr A. Fudim** who is a partner in the firm, a member of the New York and Californian Bars and of the Food and Drug Section of the New York State Bar Association (Chapter 38).

*Address:* Lester, Schwab, Katz & Dwyer, 120 Broadway, 38th Floor, New York, NY10271, USA.

**Dr S. P. Lock,** MB, BChir, FRCP, was appointed Assistant Editor of the *British Medical Journal* in 1964 and has been Editor since 1975. From 1966 to 1974 he was medical correspondent to the BBC Overseas Service. His books include *Better Medical Writing, Family Health Guide* and *Medical Risks of Life*, and he has run many courses in several countries on the subject of medical writing (Chapter 51).

*Address:* BMA House, Tavistock Square, London WC1.

**Dr J. I. Mann,** DM, PhD, is a Lecturer in Epidemiology at the Department of Social and Community Medicine at the University of Oxford and a graduate of the Univerities of

Oxford and Cape Town. Much of his most recent work has been devoted to the study of various aspects of the safety of oral contraceptives, including a study of their role in myocardial infarction, in collaboration with the staff of the Committee on Safety of Medicines (Chapter 33).

*Address:* Department of Community Medicine and General Practice. Gibson Laboratory Building, Radcliffe Infirmary, Oxford OX2 6HE.

**Dr J. Marks,** MD, FRCP, FRCPath, Formerly University Assistant Pathologist at Cambridge, later Medical and subsequently Managing Director of Roche Products Ltd, is now Fellow, Tutor and Director of Medical Studies at Girton College, Cambridge. He is currently mainly concerned with experimental therapeutics and has a wide range of interests in the field of drug development (Chapter 50).

*Address:* Girton College, Cambridge CB3 0JG.

**Dr M. L. Mashford,** FRACP, is the Reader in Clinical Pharmacology in the University of Melbourne. He is a member of the Australian Drug Evaluation Committee and Chairman of the Adverse Drug Reactions Advisory Committee (Chapter 2).

*Address:* St Vincent's Hospital, Fitzroy, 3065, Australia.

**Dr R. H. B. Meyboom** studied medicine at the University of Leyden. Since 1973 he has been in charge of the Netherlands Centre for Monitoring Adverse Reactions to Drugs of the Ministry of Welfare, Public Health and Culture (Chapter 8).

*Address:* PO Box 439, 2260 AK Leidschendam, Netherlands.

**Dr Dorothy C. Moir,** MD, MFCM, is Community Medicine Specialist with the Grampian Board of Health, and Clinical Senior Lecturer in Community Medicine at the University of Aberdeen. Since 1966 she has been involved in developing the Medicines Evaluation and Monitoring Group which, in collaboration with a similar group in Dundee, has investigated the problems of prescribing and adverse drug reactions in hospitals (Chapter 18).

*Address:* Medicines Evaluation and Monitoring Group, Aberdeen Royal Infirmary, Foresterhill, Aberdeen AB9 2ZB.

**M. L. Morse** is president of Health Information Designs, Inc. He is a clinical pharmacist with graduate training in drug epidemiology and computer science. Since 1978 he has been the project director of the FDA-Medicaid PMS project, and currently directs PMS projects for the FDA, university collaborators and the pharmaceutical industry. He has a faculty appointment as a clinical instructor in drug epidemiology, Georgetown University School of Medicine. **Dr A. A. Le Roy** is co-founder of Health Information Designs, Inc. and co-developer of COMPASS. **Dr B. L. Strom** is co-director of the Clinical Epidemiology Unit of the University of Pennsylvania School of Medicine, and the principal academic investigator for COMPASS (Chapter 16).

*Address:* Health Information Design, 1616 North Fort Meyer Drive, Suite 1420, Arlington, VA 22209, USA.

**Dr E. Napke,** BSc, MD, DPH, is Chief of the Product Related Disease Division, and is known internationally for his unique 'pigeon-hole' system for monitoring adverse drug reactions. His Division is unusual in that one small unit monitors chemical products adverse effects (drugs, cosmetics, vaccines, foods) on humans and animals ranging from overt poisoning to adverse reactions and lack of effect (Chapter 3).

*Address:* Tunney's Pasture, Ottawa, Ontario, K1A OL2, Canada.

**Dr A. Pedersen,** MD, PhD is head of Department of Cardiology, Copenhagen County Hospital, DK-2600 Glostrup, Denmark. Along with clinical work and teaching in Internal Medicine and Cardiology, he has participated in different activities within Clinical Pharmacology, Under National Board of Health, Chairman of Board of Adverse Drug Reactions from 1968, member of Registration Board 1958–76, member of the Board evaluating economic subsidies to medicine 1961–69, editor of the section of drug information in the Danish medical journal (Ugeskrift for Læger) 1966–72, co-author of the official drug catalogues (Lægeforeningens Medicinfortegnelse, Lægemiddelkataloget) from 1962, author of some books and several articles within the field.

*Address:* Danish National Health Service, Board on Adverse Reactions to Drugs, 378, Fredeikssundvej, DK-2700 Brønshøj, Denmark.

**Mr J. W. Poston,** BPharm, MPS, was appointed to the first lectureship in Clinical and Social Pharmacy in the UK in 1976 at the Welsh School of Pharmacy in Cardiff. Prior to this he worked in the Clinical Department of the Wellcome Foundation and at the Queen Elizabeth Hospital, Birmingham with a special interest in drug-prescribing and information systems. His co-author, **Professor P. A. Parish,** MD, MRCS, MFCM, FRCGP, is the Director of the Medicines Research Unit in Cardiff, and Professor of Clinical Pharmacy at the Welsh School of Pharmacy. He has written and lectured extensively on the factors which influence prescribing (Chapter 43).

*Address:* The Welsh School of Pharmacy, UWIST, PO Box 13, Cardiff CF1 3XF.

**Professor D. L. Sackett,** MD, MSc, is Professor of Clinical Epidemiology, Biostatistics and Medicine at McMaster University, with major research interests in the diagnostic and management processes in medicine and in clinical research methodology. His co-authors are **Dr R. B. Haynes,** MD, PhD, FRCP, **Professor M. Gent** and **Mr D. W. Taylor,** MA, all of whom share a common interest in clinical trials (Chapter 34).

*Address:* Department of Clinical Epidemiology and Biostatistics, McMaster University, 1200 Main Street West, Hamilton, Ontario L8N 3Z5, Canada.

**Professor J. S. Scott,** MD, FRCS, FRCOG, is Professor of Obstetrics and Gynaecology at the University of Leeds. Until 1977 he was a member of the Committee on Safety of Medicines. He is a former member of the Council of the Royal College of Obstetricians and Gynaecologists and Chairman of its Scientific Advisory and Pathology Committee; Chairman of the Medical Research Council's Ovarian Cancer Study Group; and the Royal College's Sims Black Professor 1979 (Chapter 26).

*Address:* Department of Obstetrics and Gynaecology, University of Leeds, Clarendon Wing, Leeds LS2 9NS.

**Mr K. G. Siehr,** MCL, Dr iuris has been a research associate with the Max-Planck-Institute for Foreign and Private International Law in Hamburg since 1968. Since 1980 he has also been a Lecturer in Law (Privatdozen) at the University of Zurich (Chapter 37).

*Address:* Max-Planck-Institute, Mittelweg 187, 2000 Hamburg 13, West Germany.

**Professor D. C. G. Skegg,** BMedSc, MB, ChB, DPhil, graduated in New Zealand, and was a Rhodes Scholar at Balliol College before becoming a lecturer in epidemiology in the Department of the Regius Professor of Medicine at Oxford. He was appointed to the Chair of Preventive and Social Medicine at the University of Otago in 1980. Much of his research has been in the field of drug epidemiology (Chapter 19).

*Address:* Department of Preventive and Social Medicine, University of Otago Medical School, Dunedin, New Zealand.

**Professor R. W. Smithells,** FRCP, FRCPE, DCH, established the Registry of congenital abnormalities while Lecturer in Paediatrics at Liverpool University. He is now Professor of Paediatrics and Child Health at the University of Leeds and was a member of the Committee on the Review of Medicines from 1975 to 1979 (Chapter 27).

*Address:* Department of Paediatrics and Child Health, D Floor, Clarendon Wing, Leeds General Infirmary, Belmont Grove, Leeds L52 9NS.

**Mr J. D. Spink,** qualified as a pharmacist in 1946 and started his career in general practice pharmacy. He joined the Wellcome Foundation in 1950. He was appointed Assistant Company Secretary in 1960 and became Regulatory Controller in 1976. Mr Spink is a past chairman of the ABPI Regulatory Committee, and is now a member of its Product Liability Committee and Specialist Legal Group. He was Honorary Treasurer of the Research Defence Society from 1975 to 1983 (Chapter 40).

*Address:* The Wellcome Foundation Limited, The Wellcome Building, 183 Euston Road, London NW1 2BP.

**Professor J. Venulet,** is Head of Intensive Surveillance, Drug Moinitoring, Medical Department, Pharmaceuticals Division, Ciba–Geigy, Ltd Basle, (Switzerland). He was responsible for the World Health Organization's International Drug Monitoring Project during the first 7 years of its existence. Before joining Ciba–Geigy he was 'Professor invité' of clinical pharmacology at the Geneva University (Chapter 36).

*Address:* Ciba-Geigy Ag, CH-4002 Basle, Switzerland.

**Dr G. N. Volans** qualified in medicine at the University of Newcastle upon Tyne were he also gained an Honours Degreee in Physiology and Biochemistry. After a series of appointments in general medicine and nephrology in Nottingham and Newcastle upon Tyne, he obtained a Migraine Trust Research Fellowship in Clinical Pharmacology at St Bartholomew's Hospital in London. He was later appointed lecturer in Clinical Pharmacology at that hospital where he remained until joining the Poisons Unit as Consultant Clinical Pharmacologist and Deputy Director in 1975. He became Director of the Poisons Unit in October 1980 (Chapter 30).

*Address:* Poisons Unit, New Cross Hospital, Avonley Road, London SE14 5ER.

**Dr B-E. Wiholm,** PhD was trained in internal medicine and clinical pharmacology at Karolinska Institutet, Huddinge Hospital where he holds a research fellowship. Since 1982 he has been acting professor in clinical pharmacology and head of the Adverse Drug Reactions Section of the Department of Drugs, National Board of Health and Welfare and as such Secretary of the Swedish Adverse Drug Reactions Advisory Committee. (Chapter 10). **C. F. Borchgrevink,** has been Professor of General Practice at the University of Oslo since 1969. He is chairman of the Norwegian Adverse Drug Reactions Advisory Committee.

*Address:* Socialstyrelsen, Läkemedelsavdelningen, Box 607 S-751 25 Uppsala, Sweden.

# Section 1:
# Post-marketing Surveillance in the General Population

# Editor's Introduction and Commentary

## INTRODUCTION

Post-marketing surveillance (PMS) is a term that has often been used to describe techniques for detecting and measuring the incidence of adverse drug reactions (ADRs). Voluntary reporting schemes, such as the 'Yellow Card' system in the United Kingdom, are often excluded because they do not measure incidence. This exclusion is inappropriate, and in this book we have used PMS in its broadest sense to include all kinds of schemes for generating or testing hypotheses.

ADRs are usually defined as noxious and unintended events which occur when drugs are used for the purposes of treatment, prophylaxis or diagnosis at the normally recommended dose. Pharmacologists usually distinguish two types of drug effects. Type A effects are those which are due to exaggerated pharmacological actions or to interactions with other concurrent therapy. They are usually identified and evaluated before a new drug is marketed. Type A effects tend to be fairly common and are frequently dose-related. Many of them could be avoided by using doses which are appropriate to the individual patient. Hepatorenal failure, due to benoxaprofen, is a classic example of a Type A effect which could have been avoided by using lower doses in elderly patients. Its victims succumbed to poisoning rather than to ADRs.

Type B effects are sometimes described as 'idiosyncratic', they may be life-threatening, and they are generally unpredictable as far as an individual patient is concerned. Aplastic anaemia and Stevens–Johnson syndrome are examples. The more serious Type B reaction is usually too rare to be detected in most epidemiological studies. They are often published as anecdotes in the medical journals or reported to monitoring centres as suspected ADRs. Because of their rarity and the fact that there may well be alternative causes, Type B effects are extremely difficult to evaluate.

There is a third type of event which I have called a Type C reaction. This is not, at first sight, a true 'drug reaction', since it is often a commonly occurring disease such as diabetes or cancer. Thrombosis associated with oral contraceptives is a good example. We should emphasize 'associated with' rather than 'caused by' because, although epidemiological studies have shown that the incidence of thromboembolism is higher in women who use the Pill, it is never possible to prove that an individual patient developed thrombosis because she was taking the Pill. This classification reflects the various disciplines that must be involved in the investigation of ADRs. Type A reactions are largely the responsibility of the clinical pharmacologist. Type B and Type C reactions are studied by pharmacoepidemiologists whose first job is to determine *if* a problem exists and then, how frequently it occurs, and finally, how important it may be. When these questions have been answered, the problem may then be handed over to the pharmacologist who explores the *mechanism* of the ADRs. Sometimes they are reclassified. Type B or Type C reactions may turn out to be Type A reactions once their mechanism has been explained.

Clinical trials in a few hundred, or at most a few thousand patients, should detect most of the Type A effects, but they are usually too small to detect Type B or uncommon Type C effects. The size of the population which must be studied in order to allow events occurring at various frequency levels to be detected is discussed in more detail in later sections of this book. When considering very rare examples of a Type B event, a useful guide is the 'rule of three'. Supposing, for example, that the true frequency of a reaction which occurs only as a response to a drug and never spontaneously, is 1 in 10 000, we will be 95% certain of encountering one or more cases of this reaction if we studied at least 30 000 patients who had been exposed to it. If, on the other hand, the reaction was one that could occur spontaneously in unexposed patients, much larger populations would have to be compared. When a reaction is as rare as in this example, it is extremely unlikely that causality will ever be confirmed. The level of risk that can be measured is inversely related to the size of the population exposed to this risk. The smaller the risk (i.e. incidence), the larger the number of users that must be monitored.

It has often been suggested that greater safety could be achieved if drugs could be introduced onto the market more slowly. In practice, curbing the promotion of a new drug is no way to increase safety. The slower the rate of penetration of the market, the less likely it is that serious or unexpected side-effects will be identified, because alertness is linked to novelty. The benoxaprofen affair was attributed by many people to a manufacturer's promotional zeal. What killed patients, however, was not promotion but the fact that elderly patients were overdosed, presumably because the authorities failed to appreciate the significance of pharmacodynamic studies published by the manufacturers some 14 months before the drug was eventually removed from the market. In practice, the only way to increase safety is to monitor as many drug exposures as possible during the early market life of a new drug.

## VOLUNTARY REPORTING SYSTEMS

All the nations contributing to this book have established voluntary or 'spontaneous' reporting systems in order to identify drug safety problems. In most of the countries, the systems are operated by independent bodies who advise the regulatory authorities. The various chapters raise many important points which I shall attempt to identify, discuss and sometimes criticise in this editorial commentary.

Voluntary reporting can be applied from the moment a drug is first marketed, and is probably the only practicable way, short of total medical record linkage, in which ADRs and particularly the very rare ADRs can be detected. Unfortunately, as there is always considerable doubt about the completeness of reporting (the numerator), the number of patients who have been treated (the denominator), and the validity of individual reports, voluntary reporting cannot provide reliable estimates of the attributable incidence of ADRs. It is also enormously vulnerable to reporting bias resulting from publicity, and it must be regarded only as a means of providing *internal alerting signals* and not as a base for regulatory action. Many of the problems inherent in voluntary reporting can be overcome by Prescription-Event Monitoring (PEM) which is described in Chapter 15.

It is becoming increasingly doubtful whether monitoring can be conducted effectively within the regulatory agencies. Monitoring is a scientific activity in which conclusions or opinions may be right or wrong. Scientists can change their minds if new evidence suggests that their early conclusions were wrong, but civil servants whose advice may have resulted in ministerial action are only rarely permitted to admit that a decision (for example, action to ban the use of a drug) may have been wrong. However, a more important reason why monitoring should be conducted by independent institutions or individuals who are not involved in regulatory activity, is that only in these situations can political or media pressure to release incompletely evaluated data, such as lists of alleged ADRs, be resisted for as long as it may be necessary to complete investigations, consult with colleagues and arrive at a balanced appraisal of the data.

The first chapter describes voluntary reporting in the United Kingdom (the Yellow Card system). Its future will remain uncertain until the full effects of recently introduced legislation on data-protection are revealed. The new legislation provides for right of access to personal information held on computers, one of the few exceptions being medical information collected *for the purposes of medical research*. Clearly, if patients had access to yellow cards, doctors would stop sending them, because each yellow card contains a written admission or opinion that something may have gone wrong as a result of the doctor's treatment. It is important that monitoring of ADRs should continue, and it is essential that the use of confidential reports for research purposes should be clearly defined. It must be established whether or not routine collection for regulatory purposes can be regarded as research. The new law becomes effective in 1985, and it is vital that these questions should be resolved as a matter of great urgency. If necessary, rather than risk the loss of the system, responsibility for collecting and assessing yellow cards should be transferred to an independent non-regulatory research institution.

Chapters 2–12 describe the monitoring systems in countries other than the United Kingdom. This edition includes, for the first time, contributions from Finland and Spain. The chapters are arranged alphabetically and not in order of size or merit.

The Australian Drug Evaluation Committee (Chapter 2) is independent of the Department of Health, but the Minister is committed to accepting its advice. For practical purposes, the arrangement is similar to that in the United Kingdom where the Minister usually agrees with the advice of the CSM.

Dr Mashford notes an interesting contrast between the two countries. In Australia, the rule that drug companies should report all ADRs during the first 3 years of a product's marketed life has been generally unproductive of reports. A similar rule applies in the United Kingdom, and this is complied with by the manufacturers, accounting for 16% of the total input of reports of ADRs to the CSM. Dr Mashford has stressed that although voluntary reporting cannot produce reliable estimates of incidence, scrutiny of the reports 'with knowledge and imagination' can give considerable insight into ADR problems. He notes that some 10% of the reports are followed up, a figure which resembles the proportion of reports followed up by the CSM in the United Kingdom in the 1960s and 1970s, but not perhaps in the 1980s when drugs have been removed from the market long before follow-up by medical field workers could have been completed.

Follow-up is essential if false conclusions are to be avoided. This is particularly true when large numbers of reports have followed publicity in the medical or lay press – the so-called 'band wagon' effect. Once one case has been reported in a journal, other cases will be reported as suspected ADRs. Unless these are thoroughly investigated, they are quite likely to be attributed to a drug incorrectly.

It is interesting to note that in Canada (Chapter 3), *lack of effect* is considered to be a adverse drug reaction, on the grounds that the patient may be harmed by being deprived of more effective treatment. This is clearly an issue of great importance. Even with the most effective drugs, it is likely that perhaps one third of patients will not respond to treatment for a variety of reasons. If all these cases were reported routinely, they could greatly overload the monitoring system. We are, however, reminded that the study of efficacy is just as important as the study of safety. The great majority of drugs are remarkably safe, but many are not particularly effective.

In the Federal Republic of Germany (Chapter 4), there are striking differences between the pattern of ADRs reported during the period 1967–1976, which were quoted in the first edition of this book and those reported in 1983. If we consider the 30 most frequently reported ADRs, we find, for example, 'circulatory failure' in second place in the

1967/76 list and in 17th place in the 1983 list. 'Drug dependence' was not listed in 1967/76 but is top of the list in 1983. 'Drug abuse', also unlisted in 1967/76, lies in fourth place in 1983. In contrast, 'anaphylactic shock' is in tenth place in both lists. Dramatic swings such as these almost always result from extensive publicity. In the late 1960s, in the United Kingdom, for example, the Adverse Reactions Register was greatly distorted by reports of thromboembolism among women using oral contraceptives. In 1974, reports of conjunctivitis and psoriasiform rashes attributed to practolol again distorted the picture, and in 1982, a similar distortion occurred when there were many hundreds of reports of photosensitivity associated with benoxaprofen.

Listings of this type may be misleading and, as a general rule, computer printouts of ADR registers have only limited uses. They do not reflect the true pattern of ADRs which occur under 'real life' conditions. On the other hand, the distorted picture that results from biased reporting may effectively draw attention to a problem that might otherwise have been overlooked. Their greatest value is to serve as a reference directory, leading to the records of patients which may be worth following up.

The population of Finland (Chapter 5) is slightly less than five million, and the number of patients likely to be exposed to any one drug is smaller than in many countries with less well-developed monitoring systems. This must impose some limitation on the power of the Finnish system to detect rare ADRs. Nevertheless, their ability to compare the frequency of events associated with different drugs, diagnoses, age groups and so on, must be an enormous advantage, since drug risks will be seen in their true perspective in comparison with other day-to-day risks and, most important, with the much greater risks of the diseases for which drugs are used.

The sad state of drug monitoring policy in Italy is reported in Chapter 6. A WHO regional monitoring centre, staffed by eight physicians, received only 205 reports during its first year. Attempts are being made to improve the monitoring arrangements, and it is hoped that the obvious enthusiasm of workers in Milan will be eventually rewarded by the emergence of more effective monitoring in this country.

In Japan (Chapter 7), spontaneous ADR reporting of prescribed drugs is largely concentrated on 'monitoring hospitals' and, although arrangements for collecting reports are complex and well organized, the total number of reports during some 15 years (1968–1982) has only been about 7000, in spite of the increase in the number of participating hospitals from 192 at the start of the programme to 1001 in 1982. The author stresses that confidentiality is strict, and he mentions that doctors may be fearful of litigation. This could account for the low rate of reporting. A pharmacy based scheme is also in operation for drugs sold over the counter and, under a new law introduced in 1979, manufacturers are now required to submit ADR reports. It remains to be seen what results these additional sources of data will provide.

The contributions from the Netherlands (Chapter 8) and New

Zealand (Chapter 9) both illustrate the high quality of assessment that can be achieved by experienced and sophisticated drug monitoring centres working in a country with a comparatively small population, provided very close contact can be achieved with reporting physicians. These chapters reveal several advantages of separation from regulatory activities. Perhaps the greatest advantage is the time available for meticulous investigation of case reports. The Dutch experience with triazolam is of exceptional interest. Although triazolam was used in several countries, including the United Kingdom, it appears that an epidemic of bizarre psychosensory disturbances had occurred in Holland. Critics, of whom the Editor was one, suspected that the number of reports might have been heavily inflated as a result of the TV appearance of a well-known Dutch psychiatrist. There had been very few similar reports in other countries with good monitoring arrangements. Dr Meyboom persisted with his enquiries, however, and it was eventually shown beyond all reasonable doubt that the signal his system had generated in the Netherlands was valid. The pharmacological mechanisms involved in this phenomenon were subtle. The absence of a corresponding signal in the United Kingdom could have been because the tablet strength was only half that used in the Netherlands.

In an attempt to enhance voluntary reporting, the New Zealand monitoring centre introduced an 'Intensive Medicines Monitoring Program' (IMP) in 1977. Doctors were encouraged to report all adverse events, whether or not they were considered to be drug reactions. IMP had been applied to 14 different drugs at the time of writing, and it is interesting to note that the pattern of events has changed in a way that was very similar to that which was noted in the United Kingdom in 1976, when the reporting rates suddenly doubled for a different reason. The sudden increase in the United Kingdom was almost certainly a response to a suggestion by Mr Sidney Cardy, that a slip of paper should be inserted into each prescription pad reminding doctors of the importance of reporting ADRs. The total number of reports doubled quite suddenly and has remained at a higher level for nearly a decade. It is noteworthy that the number of fatal reactions reported has not increased. In New Zealand, the proportion of conditions classified as severe fell from 42% to 14% for those drugs subjected to IMP. These results in two countries suggest that increasing the reporting does not necessarily being more adverse reactions to light, and that reporting may well be more complete than has often been thought. Certainly, this is borne out by early experience with Prescription-Event Monitoring (Chapter 15) in the comparatively small range of drugs studied so far.

A second arm of the New Zealand IMP was a scheme in which pharmacists identified cohorts of patients receiving certain drugs. Working from a register of patients for whom these drugs had been dispensed, questionnaires are then sent to doctors. The scheme closely resembles Prescription-Event Monitoring although the number of patients using new drugs is likely to be much smaller because the population of New Zealand is so much smaller than England.

It is sad to note that, even though they are justifiably proud of their dissociation from regulatory activities, Dr Coulter and colleagues have been compelled after 20 years to substitute 'Medicines' for 'Drugs' in the title of their committee. Hopefully, 'Adverse Medicines Reactions (AMRs)' will not generally displace the 'ADRs' which have served us so well for decades.

In the United Kingdom, the passage of the Medicines Act of 1968 had many consequences, the least important of which was the change of title from Committee on Safety of Drugs to Committee on Safety of Medicines (see Chapter 1). The staff needed to administer the Medicines Act is more than ten times larger than was required to operate the very effective voluntary system that it replaced. There are long delays in the introduction of new drugs, some of which could deny patients more beneficial treatment, and there have been huge increases in the cost of satisfying the regulations which are passed on to tax-payers as many-fold increases in the cost of drugs supplied through the NHS. The Medicines Act did not prevent the practolol tragedy, the 'Opren' affair or many lesser incidents.

In Chapter 10, the very similar arrangements in three Scandinavian countries are compared and contrasted. Norwegian doctors and dentists have been obliged by law to report fatal or life-threatening ADRs since 1973, and new or unexpected ADRs of a less serious nature since 1979. A similar scheme was introduced in Sweden in 1975, but in Denmark, although reporting is encouraged, it is not a legal requirement. It seems that the changes in the law in two of the three countries have not made any material differences to the number of ADRs actually reported. It is difficult to see how such a law could be enforced, since it is almost always impossible to attribute causality to an individual case report. If such measures were introduced to England, it is quite likely that they would be counter-productive. Doctors would see them as yet another restriction of their freedom to practise medicine.

Various local surveys in Scandinavia have suggested that the proportion of ADRs reported to the national centres is very small, in the order of perhaps 5%. It is interesting, however, that for certain classes of serious events, the reporting rate is possibly much greater, even reaching 100% for fatal thromboembolism associated with the use of oral contraceptives. This again is evidence that the reporting of serious ADRs may well be more complete than has been thought.

In Spain (Chapter 11), drug monitoring is a welcome recent development. The scheme for voluntary reporting has been modelled on the UK system, and employs Spanish and Catalan versions of the CSM's Yellow Card. It is hoped that the enthusiasm of the initiators of this scheme will be reflected by an equally enthusiastic response from Spanish practitioners.

For many years, the Food and Drug Administration (FDA) in the

United States (Chapter 12) has played a vital co-ordinating role, and it has also been the funding agency for a number of major independent projects. The FDA has maintained an effective and credible ADR reporting system, in spite of the inevitable pressures inherent in a vast bureaucracy and the unsettling effects of frequent changes of management. Judith Jones, Charles Anello, Alan Rossi, Arthur Ruskin and others have, over many years, contributed greatly to the development of effective monitoring in their own and in other countries, much to the credit of the FDA.

In addition to its in-house monitoring capability, the FDA has close links with many organizations which are able to supply epidemiological or drug utilization data. Fourteen different sources of such information are mentioned in the Chapter, and they represent a more varied assembly of facilities than are available in any other country.

The WHO system, described in Chapter 13, was established on the principle that even though inputs from individual national centres may be small, large international bases should generate signals earlier than would be possible in individual countries. Great care has to be taken when interpreting and reacting to these signals because action by one country can easily lead to pressures on the others to take action which might be inappropriate. It would be wrong, for example, to circulate warnings in the Third World about an increased risk of thrombosis associated with oral contraceptives when the background level of venous thrombosis is so low that even a 50 or 100 fold increase in relative risk would be neither detectable nor important compared to the risks of unwanted pregnancy. Such warnings could damage compliance with contraceptive advice.

Several of the senior advisers to the WHO expressed serious concern when it was moved to Sweden in 1978. The arrangement is unsatisfactory in many ways. The centre is separated from its top management and from many facilities that only the headquarters in Geneva can provide. Located near one of Europe's northernmost capitals, the Centre is comparatively inaccessible. The most valuable role of the WHO has been to act as a focal point for people to meet and understand each other's problems, and it is to be hoped that the centre will soon be relocated in its truly international setting.

Many of the larger pharmaceutical companies have established adverse reactions monitoring centres. The activities of one of them, Ciba-Geigy Ltd, are described in Chapter 14. An obvious limitation of company monitoring is that each company can only apply detailed monitoring to its own products. A number of companies have attempted various forms of 'monitored release'. They identify a population of patients who have been treated by doctors prepared to submit reports to the company. Post-marketing studies have sometimes been conducted at the request of the national regulatory authorities.

Company-managed studies have three major disadvantages. Firstly, they tend to be expensive, since a fee is usually paid to the doctor for each patient included in the study. Secondly, they are uncontrolled because competitors are unlikely to volunteer the use of one of their products for comparison. Thirdly, however carefully they are carried out, it is likely that there will be accusations of 'whitewashing' or studies may be seen to be promotional. Increasingly, manufacturers have come to appreciate the advantages of independent postmarketing studies by institutions separated from government and industry, but working in close collaboration with both.

In the appendix to Chapter 14, the authors review the controversy surrounding epidemiological studies which suggested that rauwolfia alkaloids might induce breast cancer. Such a finding would have important medico-legal and regulatory implications. The most outstanding feature of this affair was that the authors of some of the earlier studies were prepared to admit that their conclusions had probably been wrong. As we shall see later in this volume, pharmacoepidemiological studies are fraught with difficulties, not the least of which has been the bias caused by the massive publicity often given to the first tentative hypotheses. All too frequently they are not confirmed in subsequent studies. Typical examples of hypotheses that have been disproven by subsequent work are the suggestions that 'Debendox' ('Bendectin') and sex hormones, particularly the so-called hormonal pregnancy test, might be teratogenic. The overwhelming weight of evidence from numerous studies is against the possibility that either of these preparations might have caused birth defects.

# 1
# The United Kingdom

**W. H. W. INMAN and J. C. P. WEBER**

## INTRODUCTION

The thalidomide incident encouraged many governments to set up drug regulatory authorities or agencies (DRAs) and some, including the United Kingdom, established voluntary or spontaneous reporting systems (VRS) as the chief methods for detecting unexpected hazards. The practolol incident, some 14 years later, reminded us that these alone would not ensure that serious toxicity will always be detected and there was renewed interest in more sophisticated arrangements for post-marketing surveillance[1–4]. Much of this chapter is devoted to the 'yellow card system', which has been in operation in the United Kingdom for the past 20 years. Its main advantage is that doctors may use the system from the moment a drug is first marketed, and it is capable of detecting hazards which were not identified during the course of clinical trials even though such reactions may be extremely rare. The disadvantage is that the numerator (the number of adverse reactions) is always uncertain because the degree of under-reporting is usually not known and the denominator (number of patients treated) is also uncertain. For this reason, the yellow card system cannot determine the incidence of adverse reactions.

In 1980, a second national post-marketing surveillance scheme, known as Prescription-Event Monitoring (PEM), was developed by the Drug Surveillance Research Unit (DSRU) at the University of Southampton. In PEM, the numerator is not restricted to the events which doctors believe are the result of drug treatment, and the denominator is precisely defined as the number of patients who have been identified by means of prescriptions for the drug under surveillance. PEM is described in Chapter 15.

In 1978, Inman and Vessey attempted to define two types of voluntary reporting systems: *systematic* and *non-systematic*.[5] Prior to 1964, the only method of alerting doctors to the existence of a possible hazard was to send a paper or a letter to one or other of the medical journals. This form of the anecdotal reporting was described by Inman and Vessey as *non-systematic* voluntary reporting. It is non-systematic in the sense that the reports are not solicited and, whether or not they appear in the journals, depends on a decision by the individual editor. Systematic voluntary reporting, on the other hand, depends on the setting up of a central Register of Adverse Reactions (the 'yellow card system' in the UK). This combines the unpublished reports addressed directly to the Register with anecdotal reports which have appeared in the literature and are clearly identifiable as originating in the population covered by the Register, in this case the whole of the United Kingdom.

A voluntary reporting system has the following five objectives:

(1) To identify drug safety problems,
(2) To investigate causality,
(3) To establish incidence,
(4) To facilitate risk–benefit judgements,
(5) To inform prescribers and patients

This chapter describes the development and some of the achievements of the yellow card scheme in the United Kingdom and its limitations.

## DRUG SAFETY COMMITTEES

The Committee on the Safety of Drugs (CSD) was set up by the Health Ministers in 1964 with Sir Derrick Dunlop as its chairman. It was financed by the Departments of Health and was provided with a suite of offices and a small medical and administrative secretariat based in London. By the end of that year the professional staff comprised three doctors and two pharmacists. Collaboration with the CSD was voluntary; the pharmaceutical industry, through its trade associations, agreed to submit for approval, data on the chemistry and pharmacy, the results of animal experiments, and of subsequent human clinical trials of new drugs. Sub-committees on Toxicity, Clinical Trials and Adverse Reactions were established in order to assist the CSD with decisions about pre-clinical laboratory studies, clinical trial results and post-marketing surveillance. The lack of legal powers to enforce its decisions was no great disadvantage, but as the scale and complexity of the operation increased it was considered necessary to formulate regulations and to introduce a licensing system.

The Medicines Act of 1968 determined that the Health Ministers would establish a Licensing Authority to control the marketing and importation of medicinal products which were intended for human or veterinary use. A Medicines Commission was appointed to advise on policy and act as an appeals body. The CSD was reconstituted as the Committee on Safety of Medicines (CSM), and, with effect from September 1971, this Committee, which had substantially the same membership as the CSD, began to advise the Licensing Authority on the granting of clinical trial certificates and product licences for new drugs. Drugs which were already on the market (including those processed earlier by the CSD) were granted a temporary Product Licence of Right (PLR). Subsequently a separate Committee for the Review of Medicines (CRM) was established with the purpose of revising all PLRs over a period of several years. A further body, the Committee on Dental and Surgical Materials (CDSM) was established to process applications for materials other than drugs (e.g. contact lenses, intrauterine contraceptive devices). More details about the relations with other bodies are given by Dr Harris in chapter 49. Since this book is concerned mainly with the safety of licensed products, only the activities of the CSM with regard to monitoring adverse reactions will be further described. The same mechanism, however, is used to supply information to the CDSM. A detailed account of the procedures for licensing drugs will be found elsewhere.[6]

### Sub-Committee on Safety, Efficacy and Adverse Reactions (SEAR)

In January 1982 the Sub-Committee on Adverse Reactions was merged with the Sub-Committee on Toxicity, Clinical Trials and Therapeutic Efficacy to form a new committee, the Sub-Committee on Safety, Efficacy and Adverse Reactions (SEAR). Its membership includes six physicians, four clinical pharmacologists, a biochemist, a general practitioner, a pathologist, a pharmacologist, a psychiatrist, a statistician and a toxicologist. Advice on special problems such as those which may arise in anaesthesia, ophthalmology, paediatrics or other disciplines can readily be obtained by consultation outside the Sub-committee. The work of the Sub-committee is conducted by a staff of three doctors, a part-time pharmacist, an information scientist who reviews the medical literature, and appropriate clerical and administrative staff.

## REPORTING OF ADVERSE REACTIONS

### Confidentiality

The importance of confidentiality was recognized by the CSM from the outset.

On May 4th, 1964, Sir Derrick Dunlop, wrote to all doctors and dental surgeons requesting reports of 'any untoward condition in a patient which *might* be the result of drug treatment'. He announced the establishment of a *Register of Adverse Reactions* and enclosed a small supply of yellow business reply-paid postcards for reporting suspected reactions.

He undertook that '*all reports or replies that the Committee receive from doctors will be treated with complete professional confidence by the Committee and their staff. The Health Ministers have given an undertaking that the information supplied will never be used for disciplinary purposes or for enquiries about prescribing costs*'.

## Instructions for Reporting

It is difficult to define precisely what should be reported. Ideally, especially with new drugs, the Committee would wish to obtain information about *events* or *adversities* experienced by patients even when the reporter is uncertain about the exact role of the drug.[7] In practice, few doctors report unless they strongly suspect that a drug has been responsible for an ADR. Well-known minor reactions (e.g. rashes with ampicillin) need not be reported except for recently introduced products for which all events, however trivial, should be reported. Serious or unusual reactions should be reported with all drugs. Deliberately, no attempt has been made to lay down precise definitions of terms such as 'new', 'serious' or 'unexpected'. The motto should be 'When in doubt – report'[8]. As a guide to reporting, certain products are marked with an inverted black triangle in the *Monthly Index of Medical Specialities* (MIMS),[9] a booklet distributed to all doctors without charge each month and probably used more frequently as a source of prescribing information than any other publication.

## The 'yellow card'

The design of the yellow card has changed progressively over the years. Initially it did not include any instructions for reporters or request information about the indication for which a drug had been used. Later it became clear that doctors who troubled to report were usually prepared to give more details, so much so that the yellow card may provide a more complete and precise summary of the patient's condition at the time of the adverse event than is likely to be found elsewhere in hospital or practice notes. In 1971 a survey revealed that among a random selection of 50 yellow cards, all but one gave the route of administration, the date of starting treatment and the date of onset of the suspected reaction. In only two reports was the dose not recorded precisely. All 50 gave the indication for treatment. This result was felt to be generally satisfactory.

The most recent modification of the yellow card design has been to increase the size to A4 (210 × 297 mm) to permit the questions to be answered more fully. It also includes a heavily outlined box for entering the drug suspected of having caused the adverse reaction, and more space is provided for the doctor to request information from the Register of Adverse Reactions.

## Sources of input to the *Register of Adverse Reactions*

The main sources of nearly 40 000 reports received during the period July 1978–June 1982 is set out in Table 1. General practitioners were responsible for 71% of all reports and hospital doctors for most of the remainder. Less than one report in every 200 was derived from an article published in a medical journal describing a case which had not already been reported to the CSM before submission to the journal. The proportion of reports submitted by the drug industry sample is considerably larger (16%) than was usual before the Medicines Act became effective in 1971. Before this, the proportion was in the order of 5%.[10]. Many drug companies now use forms, similar to the standard yellow card, which are issued to them by the CSM.

**Table 1** Proportion of reports from various sources (%) registered during 4-year period ending June 30th, 1982

| | *General practitioner* | *Hospital consultant* | *Hospital junior* | *Others (e.g. coroner)* | *Total* |
|---|---|---|---|---|---|
| *Yellow card* | 60 | 2 | 13 | 3 | 78 |
| *Drug company* | 10 | 2 | 4 | — | 16 |
| *Letter* | 1 | 1 | — | 4 | 6 |
| *All sources* | 71 | 5 | 17 | 7 | 100 |

## Drugs most frequently suspected as a cause of an ADR

It is estimated that about 9500 licensed medicinal products (excluding homoeopathic medicines) were currently available on the United Kingdom market in 1984. About 4000 of these licences related to products on general sale. The prescribable medicines contained about 1100 active ingredients. The Data Sheet Compendium issued by the Association of the British Pharmaceutical Industry (ABPI) lists more than 2000 products containing about 900 different active ingredients, produced by 122 companies;[11] 53% of them contain more than one ingredient.

Forty-two drugs are listed in Table 2 which were mentioned, either as a possible cause of a suspected adverse reaction or as concurrent treatment, in more than 1000 reports registered between 1964 and 1984. Ten of the drugs are either exclusively or almost invariably combined in drug mixtures such as oral contraceptives or vaccines. The list includes 12 analgesics or non-steroidal anti-inflammatory drugs, six sex hormones, four β-blockers, four vaccines and 16 other drugs. Four of the drugs (benoxaprofen, practolol, phenylbutazone

**Table 2** *Drugs or components of drug mixtures mentioned in more than 1000 reports registered between 1964 and 1984*

| | Drug | Reports | | Drug | Reports |
|---|---|---|---|---|---|
| * | Ethinyloestradiol | 6752 | | Oxprenolol | 1684 |
| * | Norethisterone | 5098 | | Diazepam | 1677 |
| * | Tetanus vaccine | 4106 | | Ampicillin | 1671 |
| | Benoxaprofen | 4001 | | Hydrochlorothiazide | 1611 |
| | Cimetidine | 3764 | | Naproxen | 1601 |
| | Mestranol | 3732 | * | Ethynodiol | 1569 |
| * | Diphtheria vaccine | 3565 | | Acetylsalicylic acid | 1466 |
| | Indomethacin | 3541 | | Frusemide | 1451 |
| † | Cotrimoxazole | 3180 | | Lynoestrenol | 1295 |
| | Fenbufen | 2684 | | Measles vaccine | 1274 |
| * | Paracetamol | 2544 | | Amitriptyline | 1229 |
| | Propranolol | 2614 | | Feprazone | 1223 |
| | Practolol | 2454 | | Metoclopramide | 1213 |
| | Norgestrel | 2086 | | Mianserin | 1210 |
| | Phenylbutazone | 2060 | | Nalidixic acid | 1159 |
| | Atenolol | 2045 | * | Dextropropoxyphene | 1152 |
| | Piroxicam | 2044 | | Amiloridine | 1141 |
| * | Pertussis vaccine | 1989 | | Amoxycillin | 1060 |
| | Nifedipine | 1824 | | Diclofenac | 1032 |
| | Methyldopa | 1818 | | Cyclopenthiazide | 1030 |
| | Ibuprofen | 1729 | | Carbamazepine | 1029 |

* Drugs almost always combined with others in this list
† Cotrimoxazole is a mixture of trimethoprim and sulphamethoxazole

and feprazone) are no longer available for use in general practice.

Figure 1 illustrates part of a page from a monitoring print-out. The print-out covers a period of 3 months but is repeated every 2 weeks, so that every fortnight some reactions will disappear at the bottom of the list and others appear at the top. The numbers 1–6 at the left hand side of the adverse reaction indicate periods of 2 weeks. The list includes a 'culpability' code of index in terms of A (probable), B (possible), C (unlikely) to be drug related. The code D is used if the reaction is unassessable, and U if it has not been assessed (e.g. all reactions before the date of introduction of this system.) Deaths are indicated as 01 – probably due to the reactions, 02 – unlikely and 03 – possibly. The age and sex of the patient is listed, and also the registration number of the report for easy isolation if needed. This print-out provides an excellent means of continuous surveillance.

The Register should be interpreted with great caution and scepticism. Its main use is as a means of determining if further searches for information would be worthwhile. Finney,[7] has warned against the dangers of confusing tabulations of ADR data which superficially resemble those produced in scientific experiments such as clinical trials. References to problems with 'feedback' will be made later in this chapter in the section dealing with dissemination of information.

```
F16   COMMITTEE ON SAFETY OF MEDICINES   DATE 15/12/82  PAGE 62


  TIMEBAND - LAST 12 WEEKS
SUS.DRUG  FTNIGHT  MOST IMPORTANT REACTION   CI DTH SEX  AGE  REGNO

DEBRISOQUINE
239050

               3 RASH                        A       F    61  111451
          TOTAL REPORTS FOR ABOVE DRUG   = 1

          TOTAL REPORTS IN 1981          = 0
          TOTAL REPORTS IN 1982 TO DATE  = 4

GUANETHIDINE
230010

               4 GLAUCOMA                    C       F    51  110061
           TOTAL REPORTS FOR ABOVE DRUG  = 1

           TOTAL REPORTS IN 1981         = 2
           TOTAL REPORTS IN 1982 TO DATE = 2

HYDRALLAZINE
238010

            1 ARTHROPATHY                    A       F    38  112951
            1 GOITRE                         B       F    43  112228
            1 VOMITING                       A       F    41  112227
            2 IMPOTENCE                      D       M    NK  111888
            2 LACRIMAL GLAND DISORDER        B       F    48  112028
            2 URINARY RETENTION              B       M    73  112226
            3 COORDINATION ABNORMAL          A       M    41  110077
            3 FLATULENCE                     A       M    57  107068
            3 NEUROPATHY                     A       M    62  109162
            3 PSYCHOSIS                      A       M    62  105275
            3 RASH PSORIAFORM                B       M    45  108506
            4 ARTHRITIS                      A       M    60  110063
            4 LE SYNDROME                    A       F    61  110068
            4 LE SYNDROME                    B       M    43  110065
            4 RASH PURPURIC                  B       F    71  111461
            4 THROMBOCYTOPENIA               C       F    63  110771
            4 VASCULITIS                     A       F    61  109528
            5 ARTHRALGIA                     A       F    45  109518
            5 STOMATITIS ULCERATIVE          A       F    77  109510
            6 ARTHRITIS                      A       F    58  109090
            6 HEPATIC CIRRHOSIS              A   01  M    69  109022
            6 MYALGIA                        A       F    63  106926
           TOTAL REPORTS FOR ABOVE DRUG  = 22

           TOTAL REPORTS IN 1981         = 19
           TOTAL REPORTS IN 1982 TO DATE = 66
```

**Figure 1** Page from CSM's 'F16' printout

## ADRs most frequently reported

Table 3 shows some of the organ systems most frequently involved in

**Table 3** Proportion of reports of suspected ADRs affecting certain organ-classes (%) during 4-year period ending June 30th 1982 (based on approximately 29 000 reports)

| *System organ class* | *% of all reports registered* |
|---|---|
| Skin and appendages | 38 |
| Central and peripheral nervous | 18 |
| Gastrointestinal | 17 |
| Cardiovascular | 10 |
| Psychiatric | 9 |
| Haematologic | 5 |
| Ophthalmic | 4 |
| Female reproductive | 4 |
| Hepatic | 3 |
| Metabolic | 3 |
| Respiratory | 3 |
| Musculoskeletal | 2 |
| Urinary | 2 |
| Endocrine | 2 |
| Other systems | 15 |

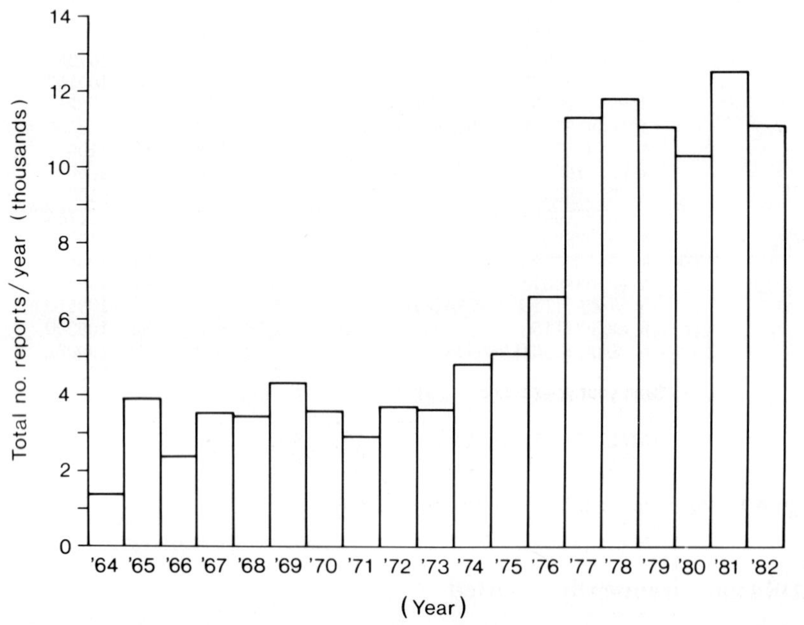


**Figure 2** Total number of reports of suspected ADRs received by the CSM between 1964 and 1982

suspected ADRs. Considerable care is needed with interpretation because not only may more than one drug have been involved, but the response to it may have involved more than one organ system.

## Variations in the rate of reporting

For many years the rate of reporting, first to the CSD and later to the CSM, remained very stable (Figure 2). From 1976, however, there was a profound and apparently consistent increase in the rate of reporting on yellow cards. The reasons for this have not been completely explained. Possible factors include increasing concern about drug safety following the practolol incident, or the introduction of new leaflets in the 'Current Problems' series.[12] Perhaps the most likely explanation, however, was the introduction of prescription pads (FP 10) containing a slip of yellow paper (Figure 3) reminding doctors

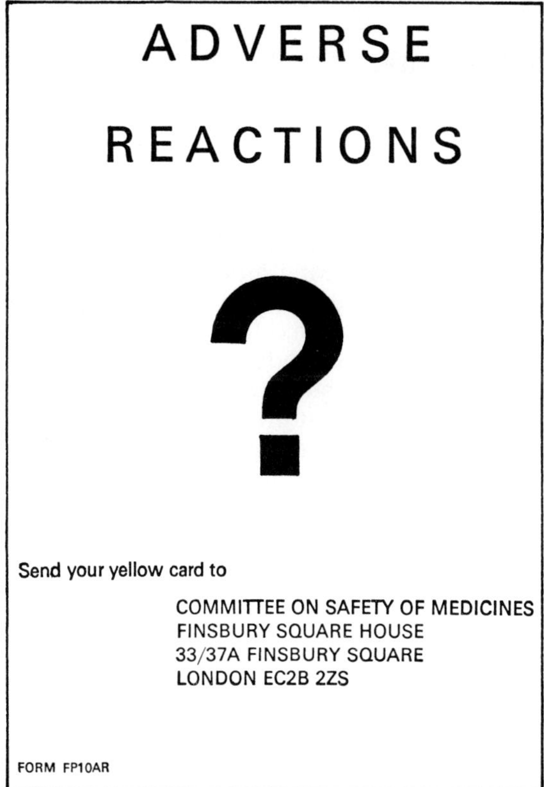
ADVERSE

REACTIONS

?

Send your yellow card to

COMMITTEE ON SAFETY OF MEDICINES
FINSBURY SQUARE HOUSE
33/37A FINSBURY SQUARE
LONDON EC2B 2ZS

FORM FP10AR

**Figure 3** Prescription pad insert (printed in yellow) used to remind prescribers of the need to report adverse reactions

to report reactions. General practitioners use many pads of prescriptions each month, and this reinforcement may well have contributed greatly to the increase. The innovation was the result of a suggestion by the officer in charge of ADR coding for 15 years, Mr Sidney Cardy.

### Data processing

A detailed description of the procedures for automatic data processing (ADP) would be inappropriate in this chapter. The procedure is changing as ADP is developed, and the CSM are always willing to assist other centres requiring help with the design of their own ADR monitoring system.

The CSM now has a mini-computer system and is currently experimenting with an 'electronic yellow card system' originally developed by Squibb Ltd, which links general practitioners' microcomputers by means of the telephone system with the CSM's mini-computer.

## IDENTIFYING HAZARDS

### Generating hypotheses

The input of voluntary reports is scrutinized by the monitoring staff at case-conferences which are held each week. Scrutiny by several staff members working together is much more productive of new hypotheses than by individuals working alone on their share of the input. Equipped with various cumulative tabulations, those attending the conference can exchange ideas, explore 'hunches', and make the best possible use of each other's individual expertise. Great importance is attached to consensus decision-making.[13] Although signals may be generated by the computer, most problems identified by VRS are first brought to the Committee's attention as a result of this initial human scrutiny.

As well as direct signals from VRS or from doctors who enquire about suspected hazards, the CSM investigates hypotheses which have been raised elsewhere, for example in medical publications. It was noted on page 17 that only one in every 200 reports originated in a published article; this does not, however, fairly represent the importance of this source of information, because many case reports submitted for publication in UK journals are first sent in draft to the CSM and are therefore included in the 6.1% of input to the register listed in Table 1 under the heading of 'Correspondence'. A great advantage in this type of communication is that many of these cases are already well documented by the time they reach the CSM. On the other hand, a serious disadvantage is that there may be considerable delay while individual physicians collect a group of cases and convince themselves that there is sufficient evidence of causal relationship to justify a publication.

Experience has shown that three situations are most likely to produce a new hypothesis. The reports may appear to describe events which are *relatively more numerous* than would be expected in the population of patients suffering from the disease under treatment; or they may describe *serious events*; or the events themselves may be of an *unusual* nature. Occasionally two or all three of these apply at the same time.

Although the primary denominator (the number of patients being treated) is often unknown, it may be possible to obtain a secondary denominator (e.g. estimate of drug sales) and decide that the number of reports received is unexpectedly large. Transient jaundice associated with the use of the estolate of erythromycin was a good example. In 1973 all but one of 41 reports described jaundice following the use of the estolate of erythromycin, yet other forms such as the stearate, ethylsuccinate or lactobionate, accounted for more than half the total sales of this antibiotic. A recent study described in chapter 15 suggests that this was an artefact due to selective reporting of jaundice associated with the estolate. Much smaller numbers of serious reactions may alert the monitoring centre, but there is no 'threshold' for suspicion that the drug may be dangerous. A single report of suspected mercurial poisoning led to the abandonment of a proprietary preparation as a treatment for nappy-rash. Seven reports of anaphylaxis with a desensitizing vaccine led to withdrawal of a batch of the vaccine.

Signals derived from unusual events included, for example, the bizarre central nervous effects of nalidixic acid and the sudden deaths of previously healthy young women using oral contraceptives. Had VRS been operating at the time of the thalidomide incident it is probable that the Committee would have received all three types of signals – large numbers of serious and unusual events. Some simple techniques which identify problems that would not immediately be apparent by simple scrutiny of the reports will now be described in some detail.

## ADR profiles

When the patterns of ADRs produced by chemically similar drugs are compared, they are often found to be similar. Sometimes, however, one drug appears to produce a *relatively* larger proportion of reports of a particular reaction. If the number of reports of each class of reaction is calculated as a percentage of all the reports received for the drug, a histogram describing its *profile of reactions* can easily be constructed. It should be noted that for this procedure we need not know the denominator since we are seeking only relative differences in proportions and not differences in the incidence of ADRs.

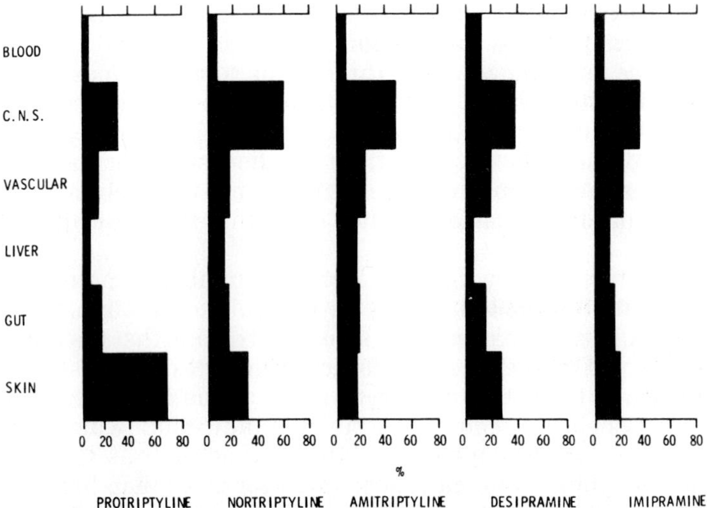


**Figure 4** Adverse reaction profiles of five tricyclic antidepressant drugs, showing a large relative excess of reports of skin reactions to protriptyline

Figure 4 shows the profiles for five tricyclic antidepressant drugs. Four are almost identical but there is a large relative excess of skin reactions associated with protriptyline. This suggested that a *skin-reaction profile* should be constructed showing the proportions of individual skin reactions. Figure 5 shows that the great majority of skin reactions attributed to protriptyline were cases of photosensitivity, which appears to be very rare when compared with the other members of the group. It is easy to see how this type of signalling could be performed by a computer, and one of the Committee's programs

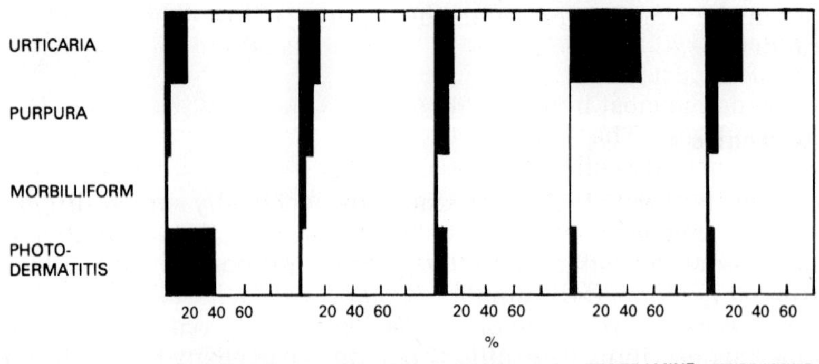


**Figure 5** Skin reaction profiles of tricyclic antidepressants showing that relative excess of skin reactions was due to reports of photosensitivity.

compares individual drug profiles with a *group profile*; each type of reaction to each drug is considered in turn and a signal is generated when the proportion of the reports of that reaction linked with one member of the group exceeds the proportion in the whole group by a predetermined amount.

The main advantage of profile analysis is that it is capable of generating useful signals in situations in which the incidence of reactions is unknown or denominators cannot be obtained.

## Use of sales or prescription estimates

Reasonably accurate estimates of the secondary denominators are available in the United Kingdom for all drugs prescribed by general practitioners. They are based on a random sample of prescriptions processed by the Prescription Pricing Authority (PPA). In certain cases, knowing the dose that is most commonly used, it is possible to calculate the probable extent of patient-exposure. With long-term treatments this may be conveniently expressed in terms of *patient-years* of treatment. It is not uncommon, for example, to find that the average prescription is for about 90 tablets, equivalent to 1 month's supply of a drug for use at a daily dose of three tablets. Less frequently, with drugs used mainly for short-term treatment, e.g. an antibiotic, it will be found that each prescription corresponds to an average course of treatment for one patient. In such circumstances the PPA estimate is equivalent to the primary denominator – the number of patients actually treated.

Although the *absolute incidence* of ADRs cannot be measured by VRS because the events are usually under-reported to an unknown extent, some information can be derived from an estimate of the *reported incidence* which gives some indication of the lower limit of risk in using the drug. Even more valuable can be a comparison of the reported incidences of ADRs when several similar drugs have been introduced to the market at about the same time, and when no biases are detected which account for selective reporting of ADRs to one or other of the drugs.

Perhaps the most important example was related to the use of oral contraceptives. The drug-utilization statistics were provided by Intercontinental Medical Statistics Ltd (IMS). In the 1960s, before oral contraceptives were generally available on Health Service prescription, IMS estimates facilitated a discovery that may have played a major role in the safer use of oral contraceptives.

In June 1966, before the CSD were able to demonstrate for the first time (in August) that there was a significant relationship between oral contraceptives and certain forms of thromboembolic disease, it was noticed that there were relatively more notifications of thromboembolism linked with oral contraceptives containing mestranol than with those containing ethinyloestradiol.[15] The IMS estimates, however, showed that the sales of such products were almost equal (52% and 48% of the market, respectively). It seemed reasonable to assume that doctors would be unlikely to report ADRs more frequently because a mestranol-containing product had been prescribed. The numbers of reports that had been sent to the Committee over a 2-year period are shown in Table 4. The market data suggested that the ratio between mestranol and ethinyloestradiol (the M/E ratio) should have been 1.1 if there was no difference in their possible thrombogenic effects. With fatal venous thromboembolism the ratio of reports was 3.1 and with non-fatal venous thromboembolism (mainly deep venous thrombosis in the legs) the ratio was 1.6. In the small group of cases of cerebral thrombosis the ratios of fatal and non-fatal disease were 2.0 and 2.6, respectively. With myocardial infarction there was no difference. Analyses of reports of all other types of reaction showed only minor differences, and the M/E ratio for all reactions except those shown in Table 4 was 1.1, exactly what would be expected from the sales figures.

**Table 4** Observed and expected numbers of reports of certain types of thromboembolic disease reported between September 1964 and August 1966.

| *Reaction* | *Mestranol* | | *Ethinyloestradiol* | | *Ratio* |
|---|---|---|---|---|---|
| | *Observed* | *Expected* | *Observed* | *Expected* | *M/E** |
| Venous thromboembolism | | | | | |
| Fatal | 28 | 19.2 | 9 | 17.8 | 3.1 |
| Non fatal | 354 | 298.0 | 219 | 270.0 | 1.6 |
| Cerebral thromboembolism | | | | | |
| Fatal | 6 | 4.7 | 3 | 4.3 | 2.0 |
| Non fatal | 37 | 26.5 | 14 | 24.5 | 2.6 |
| Myocardial infarction | | | | | |
| Fatal | 11 | 12.0 | 12 | 11.0 | 0.9 |
| Non fatal | 17 | 17.2 | 16 | 15.8 | 1.1 |

*M/E ratio of sales during this period 1.1

Thus far, the analysis of the reports had shown an unexpected excess of thromboembolism in patients taking mestranol. Was this simply due to the fact that larger doses of mestranol were generally used or was mestranol more thrombogenic? Before August 1966, although there had been several anecdotal accounts of thromboembolism in the medical literature, no studies had demonstrated a significant relationship. By chance this same month, sufficient evidence from the Committee's own case-control study was available to show, for fatal pulmonary embolism, a statistically significant relationship with oral contraceptives. It was hoped, when the study was completed, that the

M/E phenomenon would be explained. This study included most women dying from thromboembolism in 1966, at which time between half and three-quarters of a million women were believed to be using oral contraceptives. When completed, however, although there was a significant relationship with the use of oral contraceptives, the 34 women whose brand of oral contraceptive preparation was clearly identified did not show a disproportionate number of users of mestranol.[16]

The question remained unresolved for 3 years, by which time there had been more than 1300 reports of thromboembolism. In 1969 it became clear that the total dose rather than the possible differences between two oestrogens was the critical factor.[17] The view that, because mestranol was a weaker oestrogen in terms of its ability to inhibit ovulation in animals it was also likely to be less thrombogenic, had been misleading.

This analysis of the reports derived from the yellow cards illustrates an important and quite sophisticated use of VRS data. It also demonstrates the value of international collaboration. Comparable data were obtained from the Danish and Swedish DRAs. Using sales data from each country to calculate the expected proportion of cases of thromboembolism, the relative risks of using oral contraceptive preparations containing various doses of oestrogen were estimated. In Table 5 the estimates for the relative risks of various doses of the two oestrogens is shown for the three countries. In Sweden and Denmark no preparations containing 50 μg of mestranol or 100 μg of ethinyloes-

**Table 5** Comparison of relative risks of various dose-levels of oestrogen for different diagnoses. (Values based on less than 10 reports in italics)

| *Oestrogen* | *Mestranol* (Dose in μg) | | | | *Ethinyloestradiol* (Dose in μg) | | *No. of* reports |
|---|---|---|---|---|---|---|---|
| | 150 | 100 | 75–80 | 50 | 100 | 50 | |
| Venous thromboembolism | | | | | | | |
| United Kingdom | 2.4 | 1.6 | 1.2 | 1.5 | 2.5 | 1.0 | 780 |
| Sweden | *7.3* | 1.6 | 1.4 | — | — | 1.0 | 183 |
| Denmark | *3.4* | 1.6 | *0.9* | — | — | 1.0 | 122 |
| Cerebral thrombosis | | | | | | | |
| United Kingdom only | *3.9* | 1.4 | *0.8* | *0.6* | — | 1.0 | 79 |
| Coronary thrombosis | | | | | | | |
| United Kingdom only | *3.0* | 1.4 | *0.3* | *1.3* | *2.1* | 1.0 | 61 |

Data from Inman *et al.*[17]

tradiol had been mentioned in reports of suspected ADRs and some dose-levels were represented by less than ten reports. It can be seen that there is a trend towards a greater risk with the larger doses of oestrogen. An attempt was also made to examine the possible effects of the various progestogens. There were 18 different combination products containing various doses of six progestogens and the two oestrogens. A direct comparison of various doses of progestogen combined with a fixed dose of oestrogen was only possible, however, for four combinations of norethisterone acetate with 50 μg of ethinyloestradiol. At doses of the former of 4 μg, 3 μg, 2.5 μg and 1 μg, the ratio between observed and expected number of reports was 0.63, 0.78, 0.55 and 0.80, respectively. No trend which might suggest either a protective or a synergistic effect was apparent.

It is important to recognize that, once publicity had been given to these findings and the high-dose preparations, for the most part withdrawn from the oral contraceptive market early in 1970, further comparisons were no longer possible. In recent years new preparations containing doses of oestrogen of 30 μg or less have been introduced, but it is very unlikely that reporting is sufficiently unbiased to make further research of this nature worthwhile.

Various attempts were made to correlate morbidity and mortality trends with the oestrogen content of oral contraceptives[18,19]. There has been no large-scale increase in spite of the rapid growth of oral contraceptive sales in the United Kingdom, and it may be reasonable to suggest that this analysis of relatively crude VRS data has contributed in an important way to the safety of oral contraceptive drugs which are now being used by many millions of women throughout the world.

## In-depth study of ADR reports

So far we have seen how simple techniques such as profile-analysis, or the use of sales estimates, may enhance the rather crude data derived from VRS. Occasionally it may be possible to identify sub-populations of patients within a single drug file who appear to be at greater risk either because of their age, the presence of concurrent illness, the administration of other drugs or the use of certain doses of the suspect drug. All ADR reports deserve as much detailed study as resources allow, and the following example illustrates the value of such 'in-depth' study.

For many years there has been suspicion that halothane is an occasional cause of post-operative hepatitis; moreover, it has been suggested that repeated exposure at short intervals may increase the risk. The fact that reports of post-operative jaundice are sent to the Committee is therefore to be expected and is of little consequence in itself. They are few in number in relation to the enormous extent to which this anaesthetic agent is used, and the small reported incidence of jaundice would certainly not deter anaesthetists from using this

**Table 6** Effect of number and timing of exposure to halothane on the mean interval between the last exposure and the onset of jaundice. (Number of cases in which onset or exposure was known precisely shown in parentheses)

| No of exposures | No. of cases of jaundice | *Time between last exposure and onset of jaundice (days)* | |
|---|---|---|---|
| | | *Interval between last two exposures more than 28 days* | *Interval between last two exposures less than 28 days* |
| 1 | 46 | — | 11.4 (46) |
| 2 | 86 | 10.5 (19) | 5.6 (67) |
| 3 | 51 | 7.4 (11) | 4.6 (40) |
| 4 + | 25 | 5.5 (8) | 3.4 (17) |

valuable agent. A careful study of the temporal relationship between exposure, the onset of jaundice and its outcome[20, 21] has, without necessarily producing proof of causal relationship in individual patients, greatly strengthened the evidence for 'halothane-hepatitis' and identified as a high-risk group patients who are exposed more than once within a period of a few weeks. The essential finding in this investigation is that as the total number of past exposures increases, the interval between the most recent exposure and the onset of jaundice decreases. When more than one exposure occurs within a 28-day period, the interval is especially short and may, in some cases, be less than 24 h. The effect of increasing the number of exposures to halothane and reducing the time between them is shown in Table 6. The mean time of onset of jaundice in a patient who had never been exposed to halothane previously was 11.4 days. Where two or more exposures had been given and the interval between the last two exposures exceeded 28 days, jaundice developed after 10.5–5.5 days depending on the number of previous exposures. Where the last two exposures had been less than 28 days apart, the jaundice developed 5.6–3.4 days after the last exposure. These findings led the Committee to recommend that where possible, in situations where a series of anaesthetics were required, halothane should be reserved for the one procedure where its advantages would be greatest. This announcement led to boisterous exchanges between anaesthetists and the Committee, which are discussed in Chapter 49.

## ESTABLISH CAUSALITY

### General considerations

A constant difficulty for the pharmacoepidemiologist is that of distinguishing drug-induced from spontaneous disease and eliminating alternative causes for the suspected ADR. Many recognized ADRs are indistinguishable, clinically, pathologically or biochemically from conditions which can occur spontaneously. There is no way, for example, in which venous thrombosis which may have been induced by oral contraceptives can be distinguished in an individual patient from thrombosis in a non-user. Many drug rashes resemble those produced by non-drug allergens such as shellfish or household chemicals. Convulsions, headache or psychic changes can all be produced by drugs or can occur for a variety of other reasons. Congenital defects may be related to the use of anti-convulsants or to the epilepsy that is being treated.

When an event which is normally rare is found to be associated with the use of a drug in a high proportion of cases, the probability may be high that it has been caused by it, but pharmacoepidemiological techniques beyond the scope of this chapter may be required to confirm causality. If, however, a rare event occurs within a few minutes or hours of the administration of a drug, and especially if this happens several times after different courses of treatment (re-challenge), such studies may be unnecessary.

In assessing ADRs Karch and Lasagna[22] use the following criteria (which have been adapted here as a series of questions):

(1) Does the event follow a reasonable temporal sequence following administration of the drug?
(2) Does the event follow a known response-pattern to the suspect drug?
(3) Does the condition improve when the drug is stopped (de-challenge)?
(4) Does the condition recur if the drug is restarted (rechallenge)?
(5) Can the events reasonably be explained by the known characteristics of the patient's disease or by other forms of treatment?

**Table 7** Criteria for assessing causality

| *Assessment of causality* | *Definite* | *Probable* | *Possible* | *Conditional* |
|---|---|---|---|---|
| (1) Reasonable temporal sequence | Yes | Yes | Yes | Yes |
| (2) Known response-pattern to drug | Yes | Yes | Yes | No |
| (3) Reaction improved on dechallenge | Yes | Yes | Yes or No | Yes or No |
| (4) Reaction returns on rechallenge | Yes | ? | ? | ? |
| (5) Alternative explanation for reaction | No | No | Yes | No |

Adapted from Karch and Lasagna[22]

Reactions can be assessed as *definite, probable, possible, conditional* or *doubtful* (see Table 7).

Doubtful reactions are those which do not meet the above criteria. A 'conditional' classification allows for reclassification at a later date. The answers to question No. 4 are usually not obtained because it is unethical to rechallenge a patient who has already experienced an ADR.

There are several other criteria which can be useful. For example, if the event was not a known response to the suspect drug, but was a known response to another drug that was chemically related to it, this might lead the assessor towards a 'probable' classification. The identification of an unusual combination of several events associated with the drug in the same patient may also lead to this verdict. A combination of ocular, skin and visual changes afer practolol is a good example.

## Validation of reports

The response to an ADR signal may be regarded as an 'early-warning' and VRS is often referred to as an 'early warning system'. It is important, however, to recognize that until such signals have been validated, they must be regarded as *internal early warnings*. Only rarely is it necessary for the monitoring centre to issue an immediate public warning. Premature disclosure can be harmful not only to the reputation of a valuable drug, but also to the profession's confidence in the monitoring system and the people who run it. Reporting bias resulting from publicity can easily produce false signals. Where the total number of reports is small, a single doctor can easily generate a signal and his report of suspected ADRs could be misleading and even positively harmful if made public. Scientists have a duty to report their findings, but much human suffering has been caused by premature or ill-informed dissemination of their preliminary observations by the popular press.

It is equally undesirable to delay warnings until there is scientific certainty of causality. To do so may expose thousands of patients to avoidable risk. It is therefore essential that signals are investigated as soon as possible and the Committee has recruited a team of approximately 200 medically-qualified field workers who interview reporting physicians or others concerned with the patient's care. The questions that are asked depend on the nature of the drug and the suspected ADR, but should always include the following:

(1) Has an alternative explanation been found for the ADR?
(2) Were other drugs administered that were not mentioned in the original report?
(3) Is the doctor satisfied that the suspect drug was actually taken by the patient?

(4) Have the same or related drugs been taken before and with what effects?
(5) What further developments have there been since the report was made?
(6) What other details were omitted in the original report (e.g. dose and duration of treatment, medical or family history, indication for drug, etc.)?
(7) Has the doctor encountered other cases with similar ADRs.

There are numerous examples of reports which are modified or rejected after follow-up. Suspected drug-induced jaundice has been found to be due to carcinoma of the pancreas; reactions to new β-blocking drugs have been related to previously administered practolol; patients have admitted that they have not taken the drug, or took a different dose; rechallenge reactions have been confirmed; initially trivial reactions have been found, after interviewing the doctor, to have been fatal.

It is easy for a doctor reporting an ADR to overlook treatment with another drug, possibly prescribed by another doctor. For example, a consultant reporting thrombocytopenia with a new drug may not be aware that the patient was receiving a sulphonamide mixture given by a general practitioner for a minor infection. The follow-up investigation should, if possible, always include enquiries about the use of over-the-counter or 'handbag' medicines. The consensus of a large group of experts who met in Washington in 1970 was that on average one VRS report in four was a 'false positive'.[23]

Alternatives to interviewing include attempts to answer these questions in correspondence or to rely on the routine acknowledgement which is sent in response to each report and which requests the doctor to submit a second report if the patient's status changes.

**Table 8** Probability of causal relationships between drug and reaction, before and after follow-up

| *Assessment* | | | |
|---|---|---|---|
| *Initial* | | *Final* | |
| Probable | 68 | Probable | 61 |
| | | Possible | 6 |
| | | Unlikely | 1 |
| Possible | 14 | Probable | 2 |
| | | Possible | 6 |
| | | Unlikely | 6 |
| TOTAL | 82 | | 82 |

Sometimes the centre will rely on follow-up by physicians employed by a drug company.

In order to test the validity of VRS, a random sample of reports was followed up in 1972 using two methods.[24] Eighty-two of the original sample of 100 reports were successfully evaluated. These included 17 fatal, 26 serious and 39 moderately severe or minor ADRs. 78% of the reports were assessed to be probably, 13% possibly and 9% unlikely to be drug-related using criteria similar to those of Karch and Lasagna. Modifications to the initial assessment are shown in Table 8. Seven of the 68 reports initially rated probable were 'down-graded' as a result of follow-up. Of 14 initially rated possible, 2 were 'up-graded' to probable and 6 were rated unlikely after follow-up. Of those followed up by interview, useful information was obtained in 41 cases (72%) and of those followed up only by correspondence, useful information was obtained in 10 cases (60%). The total amount and quality of the information obtained by interview, however, was much greater than these proportions suggest. The overall picture suggested that considerable confidence could be placed in the reports sent to the Committee at the time.

It is generally unwise to depend on unvalidated reports if any action to publicize dangers or to modify manufacturers' literature is intended. Of the methods available, personal interview is to be preferred as the main means of validation. Clearly, however, the choice of method has to take cost into account. If there are very large numbers of similar reports it may be decided to follow up a sample by interview and the remainder by postal questionnaire.

## ESTIMATING INCIDENCE

Study of published reports of hospital investigations show incidences of ADRs ranging from 2% to 25%, suggesting differences in the methods of data collection and the criteria used for defining ADRs rather than real differences in toxicity. A Department of Health, Education and Welfare task force estimated that one hospital bed in seven in the United States was occupied by a patient with an ADR at a projected cost to the nation of $300 000 000 per annum, but such extrapolations, whether based on fact or guesswork, are usually misleading and are potentially harmful. They taken no account of the benefits of treatment.

For VRS to produce estimates for the absolute incidence of adverse reactions we would require three reliable sets of data. Firstly, we would need to know the natural incidence of the events (background); secondly, the number of patients treated (denominator) and thirdly, we would need to be sure that all events, or a known proportion of them, had been reported (numerator).

In practice, none of these data are easily obtained but two of the characteristics of VRS data may be exploited to good effect. Firstly, an estimate of the *reported incidence* of an adverse event may, as we have already seen, provide a useful indication of the likely *lower limit of incidence*. Secondly, comparison of the reported incidence with several drugs used for the same indication may, with suitable safeguards, be useful in making decisions about individual products. Sometimes, when the events are very rare in the untreated population but appear to be fairly frequent among those receiving a drug, the background incidence may be ignored. We have seen how the denominator may be obtained from prescription data. If we could find some means of estimating the level of reporting it might be possible to derive a rough estimate of the actual incidence by extrapolating from the reported incidence. One method would be to identify a random sample of doctors who prescribe the drug, ask them how many patients they had treated, how many had developed a reaction and how many they have reported (the answer to the last question could be checked against the *Register of Adverse Reactions*). This approach would only be useful if the drug was very infrequently prescribed and the doctor's recall was good. A second method would be to refer back to clinical trial records, but this would be unlikely to be helpful if the reaction was rare. A third method would be to identify a group of patients suffering from a particular disease for which the drug might be used, to interview their doctors, determine how many had received the suspect drug or other related drugs, and how many had developed complications.

If the reaction is a condition which is entered on registers such as those for deaths or cancer, it may be possible to investigate such patients to determine the number who were exposed to drugs. This technique has been used by the CSM on several occasions.[16,25,26a,b] Using a combination of these approaches it was possible to estimate the incidence of fatal aplastic anaemia due to phenylbutazone (PBZ) and oxyphenbutazone (OXZ). For many years the Committee had been concerned about the high frequency of reports of fatal blood dyscrasias with these two drugs. Over a 10-year period 513 deaths had been reported. Approximately half were notified on copies of the draft death entries supplied by the Office of Population Censuses and Surveys (POCS), the remainder on yellow cards, reports from the manufacturers or in other ways. It was suspected that other unreported deaths were likely to have occurred and that these might be located among the death certificates that did not mention one of these drugs. It was therefore decided to carry out an epidemiological survey of these deaths.[25]

No fewer than five sources of information were used for this study:

(1) Reports to the Committee (including death entries mentioning PBZ or OXZ).
(2) Death certificates mentioning aplastic anaemia or agranulocytosis but not citing a drug as a cause of these conditions.
(3) A large sample of prescriptions for PBZ and OXZ extracted by

hand from a random sample of doctors' 'bundles' supplied by the Pricing Bureaux.

(4) Details of prescribing practice supplied by Intercontinental Medical Statistics Ltd (IMS).

(5) General practitioner prescription estimates for the whole of England and Wales, supplied by the PPA.

During a 1-year period there had been five reports to the Committee of fatal aplastic anaemia which were assessed to be probably due to PBZ or OXZ. Using death certificates, 269 from a total of 376 deaths were successfully followed up. Among these were 83 cases in which a drug was assessed to be a probable cause of the blood dyscrasia (excluding cytotoxic drugs used to treat malignant disease). Included among the 83 there were 39 deaths attributable to PBZ or OXZ. These drugs had also been used in a number of other cases in which the assessment of causality was rated possible or unlikely.

The doses that had been taken by the patients who died were compared with those recorded in the replies to a questionnaire returned by 137 doctors identified from their prescriptions, and were found to be very similar, the average daily dose for either drug being 300 mg. This enabled the total duration of patient-exposure to be calculated. Finally, the proportion of new patients starting treatment, and the proportion who were on maintenance therapy, was determined. This enabled the prescription estimates to be interpreted in such a way that two estimates of death-rate could be calculated, one expressed in 'patient-years' of treatment and the other as the actual number of patients exposed. It was now possible to calculate the incidence of fatal aplastic anaemia on the basis of the five cases notified directly to the Committee plus the 39 deaths that had not been reported during the same 12-month period. These estimates are shown in Table 9. When calculated only on the basis of the total number of prescriptions and the knowledge of the average daily dose (the only method normally available to the Committee) the estimates of 16.6 and 40.0 per 100 000 patient-years of treatment with PBZ and OXZ, respectively were somewhat alarming figures which might have led to

**Table 9** Estimates of mortality due to aplastic anaemia in England and Wales during the year ending September 30th, 1975

| | *Phenylbutazone* | *Oxyphenbutazone* |
|---|---|---|
| No. of prescriptions | 3 070 000 | 505 000 |
| Estimated No. of 'patient-years' of exposure | 192 000 | 30 000 |
| Estimated No. of patients actually treated | 1 440 000 | 318 000 |
| Death-rate per 100 000 'patient-years' | 16.6 | 40.0 |
| Death-rate per 100 000 patients treated | 2.2 | 3.8 |

a decision to curb the use of these drugs on the grounds that the risk was unacceptable. However, it was established that the majority of patients were only treated for a comparatively short period, many receiving only a single prescription and some taking only enough tablets for 1 or 2 weeks' treatment. The actual number of patients receiving these drugs was thus very large and the risk of death of 2.2 and 3.8 per 100 000 patients who started treatment with PBZ or OXZ respectively was considered to be by no means unacceptable for drugs which have proved their efficacy in the treatment of a large number of painful conditions.

One further analysis is worthy of mention. When the risks of PBZ were calculated separately for men and women in different age-groups it was found that the risk for men under the age of 65 was only 0.5 per 100 000. For men over 65 it was 1.3. For women the corresponding figures were 1.2 and 6.5 respectively. The excess in elderly women could not be accounted for by their greater use of these drugs and confirmed other findings[27] which have suggested that elderly women are an especially high-risk group. PBZ and OXZ accounted for about one-third of all drug-induced deaths from aplastic anaemia (excluding cancer chemotherapy). The anti-bacterial mixture of sulphamethoxazole and trimethoprim (cotrimoxazole) was thought to have been responsible for 13 of only 17 deaths from agranulocytosis which usually occurred after only a few weeks of treatment. A study on similar lines might produce estimates for mortality rate for this mixture, though it is likely to be many times less than the risk with PBZ or OXZ because of the enormous number of patients who are treated.

## UNDER-REPORTING

Although bias may result from the reporting of events which are not drug-induced, experience over many years has shown that under-reporting of adverse reactions is in practice the most important bias.

We have already discussed blood dyscrasias, where only 5 of 44 (11%) of deaths in which PBZ or OXZ had probably been responsible, had been reported independently to the Committee. In Sweden[28] it has been estimated that one-third of major adverse reactions are reported, but in the United Kingdom the evidence points to a much lower general rate except where there has been extensive publicity.

During the Committee's study of fatal thromboembolism in 1966/7,[16] 53 general practitioners were interviewed who had been aware that their patient was taking oral contraceptives when she died. Only two of these doctors, however, reported the death to the Committee prior to the special investigation. Another six were notified by consultants, bringing the total report rate to about 15%. There is, of course, no evidence that any of the deaths that were reported were actually caused by the pill.

In the mid-1960s an 'epidemic' occurred in the United Kingdom in which an excess of 3500 deaths from asthma were attributed to excessive use of pressurized aerosols. Only six doctors considered the possibility that these deaths were related to treatment and reported about a dozen of these deaths.[29].

Perhaps the most striking example of under-reporting occurred with practolol. Only a single case of conjunctivitis associated with the drug was reported during the first 4 years after practolol had been marketed. Once the association between the drug and serious eye reactions was recognized[30] nearly 200 cases with eye signs were notified within a few weeks. It is now known that several thousand reactions, many of which antedated this publication, had been caused by practolol; moreover some serious reactions have appeared long after the drug had been stopped.

There are many reasons why ADRs are under-reported. Broadly speaking they fall into two groups: either doctors fail to recognize the events as ADRs or they fail to report those they do recognize. Frequently they fail to recognize a drug effect because they are unable to distinguish it from a spontaneous event, or they may even be unaware that a drug has been given. The more common an event, the less likely is a doctor to consider the possibility that treatment may have caused it. The patient's 'drug-hstory' may be incompletely recorded or he may have purchased drugs 'over the counter' from a pharmacy, a supermarket or a vending machine. A patient may be perfectly aware that the trouble is due to treatment prescribed by one doctor, but may not report this to a second doctor because of a feeling of loyalty to the first. Hyperchondriacs develop many trivial or imaginary symptoms which may obscure important manifestations of an ADR.

Some doctors are not prepared to co-operate with a governmental DRA, or they may require payment for reports, or fear that confidentiality may be breached or that their treatment may be criticized. Some of the more important reasons for failure to report a reaction to be drug-induced have been described as the 'seven deadly sins'.[31] These are:

(1) *Complacency*, the mistaken belief that only safe drugs are allowed on the market.
(2) *Fear* of involvement in litigation, a lesser problem perhaps in the United Kingdom than in the USA.
(3) *Guilt* because harm to the patient has been caused by the treatment the doctor has prescribed.
(4) *Ambition* to collect and publish a personal series of cases, a common human failing that may lead to serious delays in recognition of a hazard.
(5) *Ignorance* of the requirements for reporting, perhaps as a result of failure in communication between the reporting centre and the professions.

(6) *Diffidence* about reporting mere suspicions which might perhaps lead to ridicule.
(7) And finally, *lethargy* – an amalgam of procrastination, lack of interest or 'time', inability to find a report-card and other excuses.

## THE USE OF VITAL STATISTICS

A more detailed account of the use which may be made of vital statistics can be found in Chapter 33. Information obtained from registers of deaths, cancer, congenital abnormalities, the Hospital In-Patient Enquiry and the Hospital Activity Analysis and various epidemiological surveys may provide base-line estimates for the frequency of events. If the lower limit of incidence of an ADR, using VRS reports as numerator and sales or prescription estimates as denominator, is found to be greatly in excess of this base-line incidence (remembering that the base-line incidence will include a proportion of patients treated with the suspected drug), it may be reasonable to assume that the drug is causally related to the reaction. Clearly if there is a serious reporting bias it may be impossible to reach any conclusions. When the event is fairly common (e.g. coronary thrombosis, hypertension, carcinoma of the breast) it is unlikely that any investigation short of a case-control study will help.

The overall annual incidence of death from aplastic anaemia (excluding cases associated with malignancy) is about 0.6 per 100 000 per year. If allowance is made for the fact that this includes drug-induced cases, the base-line incidence for 'spontaneous' aplastic anaemia would be about 0.3 per 100 000 or about one-seventh of the incidence estimated for PBZ. This suggests, in this example, that this complication should always be carefully considered by prescribers, but that it is not one which should necessarily be a deterrent to prescribing.

National vital statistics are frequently used by the monitoring centre as an aid to assessment of the possible importance of VRS reports. It is particularly important, for example, to know the incidence of various forms of cancer or congenital abnormalities. Occasionally doctors report cases of cancer in women taking sex-hormones, or congenital abnormalities when a woman has taken anti-histamines in early pregnancy. Even allowing for probable under-reporting it is reassuring to them and their patients to know that these reports account for only a small fraction of the *expected incidence* in the untreated population.

In 1965, it was noted that the total number of reports of fatal pulmonary embolism in women using oral contraceptives sent to the Committee was about the same as the number that would be expected in the general population.[15] If all deaths had been reported it would have been possible to reassure women that there was probably no special hazard. Lack of confidence in the assumption that reporting was complete, however, gave impetus to the study that was set up the following year which demonstrated for the first time a significant association between the Pill and fatal pulmonary and cerebral thromboembolism.[16]

Trends in the incidence of many diseases should be carefully monitored. A sudden increase in cancer, hepatic or renal failure or cardiovascular disease might coincide with the introduction of a new drug. Examples of situations in which this method of surveillance has actually signalled a new problem are, however, quite rare. Perhaps the best is the observation of an increase in asthma mortality which coincided with the introduction of pressurized aerosol bronchodilators.[32, 39]

## RISK-BENEFIT JUDGEMENTS

This is dealt with extensively by Hogarth in Chapter 35. The balance of risk and benefit is invariably the subject of much debate at meetings of the CSM and of discussions with manufacturers and clinicians. If a drug is found to have appreciable dangers, and offers no special therapeutic advantages over a related product, it may be withdrawn (e.g. phenacetin, amidopyrine). If it is effective in the treatment of a life-threatening or lethal disease, a level of toxicity which would be quite unacceptable in other circumstances may be tolerated (e.g. cancer chemotherapeutic agents). At an equivalent level of toxicity, a drug with less efficacy may be withdrawn (e.g. sequential oral contraceptives). Even in the absence of proof that adverse events are drug-related, the CSM may recommend their withdrawal if an alternative agent is available (e.g. high-dose oral contraceptives). A special case was the withdrawal of hormonal pregnancy diagnosis tests; although the evidence that they may cause congenital abnormalities was weak and based on a small number of inconclusive case-control studies and although the association was not found in several large prospective studies, these products were withdrawn for use as pregnancy tests because satisfactory non-invasive methods of diagnosing pregnancy were available.[33]

Risk-benefit judgements are complex, especially when objective information is imperfect or lacking. Irresponsible reporting by the lay press frequently leads to political pressure to restrict or ban drugs. Decisions which are scientifically resonable may not be publicly acceptable. Fear of cancer or damage to children is probably the greatest source of such pressures. The continued use of many valuable drugs must depend on the ability of the monitoring and regulatory agency to withstand criticism. Their policy on the whole is to warn about dangers rather than ban drugs because of them. Thalidomide should not be used by women of childbearing age or for prolonged periods by elderly patients who might develop a neuropathy, but it could still find a place in the treatment of other classes of patient.

Practolol, in spite of its dangers and the medico-legal risk of prescribing it, could still be useful for selected patients with bronchospasm. Supposing there was a drug which could be used to treat a disease that was invariably fatal, but which unfortunately caused cancer within 10 years in half the patients who received it, yet preserved the lives of the remainder for the full 10 years; those who valued life and cared little for the manner of their inevitable death might choose to accept a risk even of this magnitude. Fortunately no such drug exists, but useful drugs may be withdrawn for inadequate reasons. An extraordinary and illogical concern is shown by patients who may be at a risk of death of one in 10 000 if they take a drug for some serious condition, yet who will willingly submit themselves to a surgical operation with a mortality exceeding 1%.

Unfortunately litigation and compensation loom increasingly large in the minds of decision-makers and may, if they lack confidence, lead them to pass unnecessarily harsh judgements on the fate of a drug. A hasty official warning may deter doctors from prescribing for fear that, in the light of the warning, they may be vulnerable in legal proceedings. There can be few factors so destructive of the human spirit as the hope of compensation, for once an injury has been associated with a drug, there is no way in which the sufferer will be convinced that the cause of the injury *in his case* is anything other than the drug.

Against this background, the monitoring agency should decide *on scientific grounds alone* how great is the risk and how much risk is acceptable. It then has to make an entirely different set of judgements about that action that should be taken and how best to pass its scientific assessment on to the profession and the public. In making this second type of decision it is important to remember that most members of the CSM are physicians who are themselves actively engaged in various branches of medical practice. This enables them to consider each problem through the eyes of a doctor at the bedside, and with the added advantage of access to information which is not readily available to most of their colleagues.

Whether or not a clinician will choose the most appropriate treatment depends on his ability to predict the outcome of withholding treatment on the one hand or selecting a medicine from the large range currently available on the other. This in turn depends on the extent of his knowledge of the relative benefits and the relative risks of these medicines. Since his personal experience is limited he has to rely very largely on the experience of others, which is conveyed partly through his reading the results of clinical trials demonstrating the efficacy of new treatments (mostly sponsored by drug manufacturers) and, increasingly, by studying the information supplied by drug safety advisory bodies of various kinds. Prominent among the latter are the monitoring groups attached to drug regulatory agencies (DRAs). Frequently the guidance he obtains in these ways is unbalanced. Efficacy is comparatively easy to measure, since controlled prospective studies in comparatively small numbers of patients are readily arranged. Safety, on the other hand, is usually difficult to assess because it depends on observations made in very large populations of patients treated in 'uncontrolled' circumstances, on the ability of clinicians to distinguish drug-induced from spontaneous disease and to report their observations, and on the ability of the monitoring centre to interpret them correctly and make the right decisions not only on what advice to give but on how to give it. The clinician at the bedside may ask himself – is the disease lethal, self-limiting or preventable? – will treatment be worse than the disease? – how much risk is justified to shorten the course of a self-limiting condition? – is the cost of the treatment acceptable? The DRA has to make these decisions at 'community' level. For example, are the social advantages of oral contraception worth the risk that four or five children in some families may lose their mother? Should a child who is at no risk of dying of whooping-cough be subjected to the risk of vaccination in order to decrease the chances that his younger sibling will suffer from the disease? Short-term risks with drug A may exceed those with drug B, but the long-term risks of A may have been measured and found to be low, while the long-term risks of B may be unknown.

For a DRA to retain its credibility it has to be seen to be free from political or commercial interest. Although the Licensing Authority has legal powers to withdraw drugs, it would be very rare for a decision of this kind to be made without reference to the CSM. The latter is held in high regard by the profession and the public who can be confident that its decisions are impartial.

## INFORMATION (FEEDBACK)

No entirely satisfactory mechanism for informing the professions about decisions on drug hazards has even been found. 'Decisions about decisions' are difficult because of the unpredictable response of the professions and the news media. Clearly it is the duty of the CSM to disseminate relevant information, but whatever its decision about how to do it there are always critics. Some will accuse the CSM of undue delay in issuing a warning, others will regard the same warning as scaremongering; some want more detail, others demand the barest essentials; some claim they never receive warnings while others complain of waste of taxpayers' money. More sinister are the complaints that the CSM's attempts to inform doctors for the benefit of their patients, place doctors in a difficult legal position and may interfere with their freedom to practise medicine. Infrequent warnings may have too great an impact; too frequent warnings may have little effect. Nearly always the media emphasize the dangers and ignore the benefits.

In the United Kingdom there is no regular 'house journal' comparable to the adverse-reaction booklets published by some DRAs, but nine distinct vehicles for feedback are regularly used:

(1) An adverse-reactions information service.
(2) The *Register of Adverse Reactions*.
(3) Manufacturers' literature.
(4) Letters to medical journals.
(5) 'Dear Doctor' letters.
(6) Scientific papers.
(7) The 'Current Problems' series.
(8) The 'Adverse Reactions' series.
(9) CSM Update.

In roughly ascending order, these tend to have progressively greater impact on the news media. Indeed, all but the first three almost invariably provoke some response, though this may be modified by the subject matter; oral contraceptives, for example, always evoke more interest than announcements about analgestics or antibiotics.

### (1) Adverse reactions information service

A considerable effort is made by the secretariat of the CSM to provide an individual service. Each doctor who reports a suspected reaction or enquiries about them receives an up-to-date computer print-out which lists all the reactions to the relevant drug that have previously been reported.

Whenever possible, the medical assessors will provide more detailed abstracts of case histories or general opinions based on their experience of monitoring. Clearly the main constraint is the limited time and the small number of staff available to deal with enquiries. This type of feedback occupies a considerable proportion of medical staff time, but it does much to foster good relations with the profession and to maintain the input of reports.

### (2) The Register of Adverse Reactions

Periodically the CSM issues a complete print-out of reports.

At various times, copies of the Register have been lodged in each main hospital pharmacy, all schools of medicine and pharmacology and overseas monitoring agencies.

### (3) Manufacturers' literature

Whenever necessary, the CSM will recommend to the Licensing Authority that the manufacturers' literature, and particularly the data sheets for its products, should be modified to bring them in line with current knowledge about side-effects. In almost all cases manufacturers will make the necessary revisions without compulsion. No data are available on the proportion of doctors who regularly refer to the data sheet, and to ensure that they are appraised of new warnings or contraindications, one or other of the following vehicles may be used to get the message across.

### (4) Letters to the medical journals

These may originate from the manufacturers or the CSM or from independent clinicians, frequently at the suggestion of the Committee. The 'low-key' publication of anecdotal reports of adverse reactions, provided they are well-authenticated, is an important method by which information is disseminated. It rarely excites the interest of the news media, yet it serves to alert at least the doctors who regularly read a medical journal and provides a stimulus to further reporting. There is, of course, a danger that anecdotal reports will become part of the 'folklore' of adverse reactions and will continue to be referred to in the literature long after causality has been discounted. Correspondents to journals have a duty to correct their reports if alternative explanations for the alleged reaction are subsequently found. Editors should provide space for such corrections.

### (5) 'Dear Doctor' letters

These may be circulated by manufacturers or by the CSM, generally utilizing a commercial mailing agency to achieve the greatest possible coverage of the medical, dental or pharmaceutical professions. They are sometimes taken up by the press, but do not usually produce public alarm. This method of feedback is perhaps the most effective for transmitting detailed information, for example, about dosage instructions. It has also been used to warn the professions about the results of laboratory work (e.g. animal carcinogenicity studies) which the CSM considers the profession should be aware of, without necessarily recommending that the drug should not be used.

### (6) Scientific papers

A small number of scientific papers have been published by members of the secretariat and of the CSM, in addition to numerous papers on monitoring techniques, especially those relating to the VRS. The former provide a permanent reference source to some of the more important epidemiological work of the Committee, or the results of special analyses of spontaneous reports.[16,17,20,25,26a,b,27] Sometimes the CSM also issues a brief statement timed to precede these publications by a few days, in the hope that clinicians will read the detailed account as soon as it appears.

### (7) The 'Current Problems' series

This is a comparatively new venture. 'Current Problems', provides another form of fairly low-key communication. As its title implies, is intended to draw the profession's attention to safety hazards which appear to be important, yet have not been sufficiently investigated to justify firm recommendations. The material presented may vary from suspected reactions of unconfirmed causality to those of proved causality whose incidence is unknown. At the time of writing, thirteen editions have been distributed.

### (8) The 'Adverse Reactions' series

Some early editions of this series contained material which might now be included in 'Current Problems'. Some of the pamphlets have been reminders of known hazards and one described the reporting mechanism.[8] There can be little doubt of their effectiveness. A pamphlet drawing attention to the possible dangers of pressurized aerosols in asthma[35] in June 1967 appears to have marked the start of a profound fall in the excessive mortality among asthmatics, which had amounted to an 'epidemic' that claimed several thousand lives.[29] On average, about one death attributable to chloramphenicol was reported each month until the CSD published a reminder that it should be used only for certain limited indications.[38] From January 1967, when the pamphlet was published, to the present time only one death due to treatment in the UK has been reported – a possible saving of some 130 lives. A mere ten minutes was spent drafting this pamphlet, which was accepted for publication by the CSD almost without modification.

### (9) CSM Update

Recently, the CSM has begun a regular monthly column – the CSM Update – in the *British Medical Journal*. It is written by the members of staff of the CSM and sets out to explain and discuss the Committee's activities.

## CONCLUSIONS

This chapter has reviewed the VRS, which has been operating in the UK since 1964, in the hope that the details of its design will be useful in countries which are still developing systems for post-marketing surveillance, and that some of the techiques evolved over the years to make the most of relatively unsophisticated data will be generally helpful. Our VRS owes much to three facilities that may not yet be available in the majority of countries. First, and most important, is the ability to follow up and validate the reports with the help of medically-qualified field investigators. Next is the availability of drug-utilization statistics through the National Health Service and commercial sources. Finally, we have the advantage of highly-developed registers for death, cancer and congenital abnormalities, and the Hospital In-Patient Enquiry, from which are derived vital statistics which may be used to study disease trends in relation to drug use, and which also enable patients to be identified for in-depth study. Above all, the Committee responsible for VRS commands the respect and co-operation of the medical professions and the pharmaceutical industry.

VRS has detected a number of new safety problems and has also enabled some long-recognized dangers to be better understood. After 20 years of continuous monitoring experience, most drugs currently marketed may be deemed to be reasonably safe; only a small number have fallen by the wayside. VRS has failed to detect some problems, notably practolol, but such cases are probably rare, and we should not over-react to them. Recently, VRS in the UK has been supplemented by a second national scheme known as Prescription Event Monitoring. This is described in Chapter 15. There is also a pressing need for more data on efficacy, for however well we identify and quantify their dangers, the profession must be provided with objective information on the benefits of the drugs they prescribe.

We have seen how 'signals' are generated and interpreted and how seemingly unsophisticated material may be 'teased' or otherwise manipulated to yield important clues to safer drug use, such as the reduction of oestrogen in oral contraceptives or avoidance of too-frequent exposure to halothane. Automatic data-processing is an essential adjunct to monitoring and needs to be developed further, but it will never be a complete substitute for human scrutiny of the reports.

Drug-monitoring demands patience, determination and confidence and there are surprisingly few people throughout the world with experience in this field. It is essential that the conditions under which drug-surveillance is conducted are attractive enough to ensure a steady flow of new recruits. It is easy to enforce the removal of a suspicious drug. It may require considerable courage to allow a dangerous but useful drug to remain, in the face of firm and sometimes hostile pressures from the public and the media. Concern about thalidomide, reinforced by publicity surrounding other drugs such as oral contraceptives or vaccines and, more recently, by practolol, has made increasing demands on the surveillance team. With progressively greater difficulty over the years, they resist the erosion of their most valuable asset – time to detect and investigate ADRs.

Finally, we have examined various methods by which information may be released to the professions and the public. Frequently the CSM finds itself in a 'no-win' situation. Whatever decision it may make on the balance of risks and benefit, or on the dangers of delaying a warning while scientific certainty is sought, or issuing an early warning which may alarm patients, it is usually criticized by some. But the Committee does not work merely to protect itself; however tough the running, the race is only won when safety has been established and patients are successfully treated with the most effective drugs available.

## References


1. Inman, W. H. W. (1977). Recorded release. In F. H. Gross and W. H. W. Inman (eds). *Drug Monitoring*, pp. 65–78. (London: Academic Press)
2. Dollery, C. T. and Rawlins, M. D. (1977). Monitoring adverse reactions to drugs. *Br. Med. J.*, **1**, 96
3. Lawson, D. H. and Henry, D. A. (1977). Monitoring adverse reactions to new drugs: 'restricted release' or 'monitored release'? *Br. Med. J.*, **1**, 691
4. Wilson, A. B. (1977). Post-marketing surveillance of adverse reactions to new medicines. *Br. Med. J.*, **2**, 1001
5. Inman, W. H. W. and Vessey, M. P. (1978). In A. E. Bennett (ed.), *Recent Advances in Community Medicine*, pp. 215–230 (London: Churchill Livingstone)
6. Cuthbert, M. F., Griffin, J. P. and Inman, W. H. W. (1978). In W. M. Wardell (ed.). *Controlling the Use of Therapeutic Drugs*, pp. 99–134. (Washington DC: American Enterprise Institute for Public Policy Research)
7. Finney, D. J. (1978). Statistical aspects of monitoring systems. In M. Gent and I. Shigamatsu (eds.). *Epidemiological Issues in Reported Drug-induced Illnesses S.M.O.N. and Other Examples*. Honolulu, 1976. (Hamilton, Ontario: McMaster University Library Press)
8. Committee on Safety of Drugs (1968). *When in Doubt – Report*. 'Adverse Reactions' series, No. 7
9. *Monthly Index of Medical Specialities* (MIMS). (London: Haymarket Publishing Ltd)
10. Inman, W. H. W. (1972). Monitoring by voluntary reporting at national level. In D. J. Richards and R. K. Rondel (eds.). *Adverse Drug Reactions*, pp. 86–102. (London: Churchill Livingstone)
11. Association of the British Pharmaceutical Industry (1978). *Data Sheet Compendium*. (London: Pharmind Publications Ltd)
12. Committee on Safety of Medicines. 'Current Problems' series HMSO
13. Inman, W. H. W. (1977). Detection and investigation of adverse drug reactions. In D. M. Davies (ed.). *Textbook of Adverse Drug Reactions*, pp. 41–53. (Oxford University Press)
14. Committee on Safety of Medicines (1973). *Jaundice and erythromycin estolate*. 'Adverse Reactions' series, No. 10
15. Inman, W. H. W. (1970). Role of drug-reaction monitoring in the investigation of thromboembolism and 'The Pill'. *Br. Med. Bull.*, **26**(3), 248
16. Inman, W. H. W. and Vessey, M. P. (1968). Investigation of deaths from pulmonary, coronary and cerebral thrombosis and embolism in women of childbearing age. *Br. Med. J.*, **2**, 193
17. Inman, W. H. W., Vessey, M. P., Westerholm, B. and Engelund, A. (1970). Thromboembolic disease and the steroidal content of oral contraceptives. *Br. Med. J.*, **2**, 203
18. Inman, W. H. W. (1972). Monitoring adverse reactions to contraceptive agents. 'Clin. Proc. 1st Internat. Planned Parenthood Fed. South-East Asia and Oceania Regional Med. and Sci. Congr., Sydney, 14–18 Aug. 1972', pp. 155–161. (*Aust & N.Z. Obstet. & Gynaecol.*)
19. Vessey, M. P. and Inman, W. H. W. (1973). Speculations about mortality trends from venous thromboembolic disease in England and Wales and their relation to the pattern of oral contraceptive usage. *J. Obstet. Gynaecol. Br. Commonw.*, **80**(6), 562

20. Inman, W. H. W. and Mushin, W. W. (1974). Jaundice after repeated exposure to halothane: an analysis of reports to the Committee on Safety of Medicines. *Br. Med. J.*, **1,** 5
21. Inman, W. H. W. and Mushin, W. W. (1978). Jaundice after halothane; a further report. *Br. Med. J.*, **2,** 1455
22. Karch, F. E. and Lasagna, L. (1976). Evaluating adverse drug reactions. *Adverse Drug Reaction Bulletin*, **59,** 204
23. Report of the International Conference on Adverse Reactions Reporting Systems, October 22–23 1970. (Washington, DC: National Academy of Sciences)
24. Inman, W. H. W. and Price Evans, D. A. (1972). Evaluation of spontaneous reports of adverse reactions to drugs. *Br. Med. J.*, **3,** 746
25. Inman, W. H. W. (1977). Study of fatal bone marrow depression with special reference to phenylbutazone and oxyphenbutazone. *Br. Med. J.*, **1,** 1500
26a. Mann, J. I. and Inman, W. H. W. (1975). Oral contraceptives and death from myocardial infarction. *Br. Med. J.*, **2,** 245
26b. Mann, J. I., Inman, W. H. W. and Thorogood, M. (1976). Oral contraceptive use in older women and fatal myocardial infarction. *Br. Med. J.*, **2,** 445
27. Fowler, P. D. (1976). Marrow toxicity of pyrazoles. *Ann. Rheum. Dis.*, **26,** 344
28. Böttiger, L. E. and Westerholm, B. (1973). Drug-induced blood dyscrasias in Sweden. *Br. Med. J.*, **3,** 339
29. Inman, W. H. W. and Adelstein, A. M. (1969). Rise and fall of asthma mortality in England and Wales in relation to use of pressurised aerosols. *Lancet*, **2,** 279.
30. Wright, P. (1974). Skin reactions to practolol. *Br. Med. J.*, **2,** 560
31. Inman, W. H. W. (1978). Detection and investigation of drug safety problems. In M. Gent and I. Shigamatsu (eds.). *Epidemiological Issues in Reported Drug-induced Illnesses*. Honolulu, 1976. (Hamilton, Ontario: McMaster University Library Press)
32. Doll, R., Speizer, F., Heaf, P. and Strang, L. (1967). Increased deaths from asthma. *Br. Med. J.*, **1,** 756
33. Committee on Safety of Medicines (1975). *Hormonal Pregnancy Tests; a Possible Association with Congenital Abnormalities*. 'Adverse Reactions' series, No. 13
34. Committee on Safety of Medicines (1976). *Register of Adverse Reactions*. (London: Department of Health and Social Security)
35. Committee on Safety of Drugs (1967). *Aerosols in Asthma Vaccines*. 'Adverse Reactions' series, No. 5
36. Committee on Safety of Drugs (1967). *Chloramphenicol*. 'Adverse Reactions' series, No. 4
39. Greenberg, M. J. (1965). *Lancet*, **2,** 104.

# 2
# Australia

**M. L. MASHFORD**

---

## INTRODUCTION

In the wake of thalidomide an expert committee was established in 1963 to advise the Minister for Health on the safety and efficacy of drugs; this was termed the Australian Drug Evaluation Committee (ADEC). It was and has remained an independent body and, within its terms of reference, the Act of the Australian parliament under which it operates commits the Minister to accept its advice. The secretariat is provided by the Department of Health and all negotiations with the drug industry are conducted by departmental officers, but ADEC is, formally, the arbiter in all matters of drug regulation. In 1964, ADEC invited members of the medical and dental professions to report suspected adverse drug reactions (ADRs). Support for the scheme was immediate but modest; however by 1969 a monthly average of 90 reports was being received. In 1970, ADEC set up a sub-committee to supervise the operation of this voluntary reporting scheme and other matters relating to ADRs. The Adverse Drug Reactions Advisory Committee (ADRAC), so formed, currently comprises two clinical pharmacologists, four physicians in private practice and a medically qualified secretary from the staff of the Department of Health. It enjoys considerable freedom of action but reports to and acts through ADEC which, as mentioned above, is the body formally responsible for regulatory decisions. Actions decided upon by ADRAC are undertaken by the staff of the Department of Health. Funds for committee meetings, data-processing, publications and warnings of emergent problems, are drawn from the budget of the Department of Health, and the Committee has no independent resources. Thus it can suggest actions, but their funding is, as it probably should be, ultimately in political hands. Although minor expenditures are readily approved, this does limit the likelihood that new ventures of any size can go forward.

## REPORTING ADVERSE DRUG REACTIONS (ADRs)

Reports are now sought from members of the medical, dental and pharmaceutical professions, and public hospitals are encouraged to submit discharge summaries of patients in whom an ADR has been suspected. It is a condition of release of new drugs that all ADRs are reported by the sponsoring company for 3 years, but this rule is not enforced and has been quite unproductive.

The vexed question of what to report has not been clearly resolved. The extreme options are either to solicit reports of any or all adverse events thought to be due to drugs or to seek a restricted category such as fatal reactions or those occurring with recently released drugs. It has been ADRAC policy for several years to take the former approach. It is realized that only a small fraction of possibly drug-related events will be reported by even the most zealous supporter. A report from a physician may be prompted by the unfamiliarity of the ADR, its influence on the course of the patient's illness or the reporter's satisfaction in a diagnostic coup. However, it can be assumed that the event engaged the reporter's interest. This does give a sounding of what seems to be important to reporters, and thus what is likely to be interesting and instructive to their colleagues. The insights thus obtained are of use in guiding the choice of educational material for dissemination.

These considerations do not, in general, apply when the reporter is a pharmacist. Some reports are received from pharmacists in community practice, but the number is not very large. However, a considerable proportion of reporting from hospitals is undertaken by pharmacists enjoying varying degrees of collaboration with medical staff. These reports have seemed to differ in nature from those made by doctors, there being more detailed information about the drugs, but it is often difficult to get a 'feeling' for the clinical situation being described. An analysis of the content of reports has recently been made and preliminary results do not appear to detect any objective difference to support the committee's impression.

## PROCESSING THE REPORTS

Each report is examined on receipt by the secretariat staff. In approximately 10% of cases further information is requested; the rest are coded for storage and processing. Data stored are those required by the WHO International Centre together with details of investigations and the results of various classifications of the reaction.

The latter are concerned with the type of reaction, the body system involved and the probability of the reaction being drug-related. The last of these classifications is potentially the most useful but is beset by deserts of vast uncertainty. A simple hierarchy is adopted ranging from *definite* through *probable* and *possible* to *unlikely*; in addition, a general list is maintained which retains reports considered not to refer to drug-related events. The rules for classification are concerned only with the individual report, and for this purpose previous knowledge of the relationship of drug and event are not considered. This avoids the 'bandwagon effect' when suspicion is voiced about a drug. This is likely to occur when the suspect event is common in the absence of the drug; thus a strong suggestion that a drug is hepatotoxic receives apparent confirmation from each occurrence of hepatitis among patients receiving that drug. The situation of a collection agency is quite different from that of the clinician who must take action on unconfirmed suspicion in the management of the patient; in contrast, the agency should ensure that it does not contribute to suspicion of a drug from flawed evidence.

The designation *certain* is reserved for circumstances in which there has been a positive response to rechallenge, a temporal or spatial relationship between drug and event which leaves no substantial doubt, for example, 'end of the needle' or injection-site responses, or when objective evidence, such as *in vitro* studies, confirms the suspicion. If the event bears a convincing temporal relationship to drug administration, and is not explicable by alternative mechanisms, the association is regarded as *probable*; this designation is not acceptable if other treatment has been given concurrently with stopping the drug, e.g. steroids for arthralgia. Most reports lack the strength of association necessary for these two categories and are termed *possible*; this always applies when two or more agents are given concurrently unless subsequent negative rechallenge with one of them rules it out as the sole cause. This approach gives few suspected reactions regarded as *certain* (7%) or *probable* (21%) but correspondingly increases the significance of such appellations.

All reports receive an acknowledgement of their contribution in the form of a card or a letter. Reports are scanned by members of ADRAC and discussed at the regular meetings if the suspected reaction was fatal, unusual, involved a new drug or was otherwise worthy of note. This produces much-sifted clinical material of interest and educational value. The total experience is published from time to time in the form of a cumulative summary, by drug, of suspected reactions using the trade name given in the report. Each report may relate to more than one drug and may mention several symptoms and signs. The latter are termed *manifestations*. The entry for a particular drug will give the total number of reports and list the manifestations with a probability assigned to each.

## OUTPUT OF THE SYSTEM

The output of ADRAC activities and the spontaneous monitoring programme may be divided into two categories:

(1) Educational material, and

(2) New information.
These are both of great importance and both must be taken into account in evaluating ADRAC's success.

## Educational output

This begins with direct feedback to the reporter. Other channels used include publication of actual case histories and brief comments, which appear in medical publications and also in the small Adverse Drug Reaction Bulletin mailed to all medical practitioners and dentists, and to pharmacists on request, the distribution of which has recently been resumed. Cases are selected to make particular points and are kept brief and uncomplicated. There is also a policy of publishing analyses of holdings on specific matters such as hypertension with sympathomimetic amines, immediate reactions with measles vaccine,[1] and agranulocytosis with mianserin[2] and with mebhydrolin.[3] From time to time the complete holdings of the registry are produced as a cumulative list. This includes all reactions which have been received since the initiation of the scheme.

Apart from information directed at reporters other material is produced from the data base. Members of the pharmaceutical industry may, on request, receive a quarterly summary of reports in which identifying details of patient and reporter are suppressed; this service appears to have been considered helpful. Where questions arise in the minds of the members of the pharmaceutical company staff, attempts are made to answer queries within the capacity of the secretariat.

A more recent approach has been to use the material in an attempt to produce awareness of adverse drug reactions in a wider audience. A film entitled *The New Epidemic* has been produced, in which seven case histories from the data base have been dramatized as vignettes accompanied by suitable commentary of an explanatory nature, but with a minor hortatory element. This has been widely used with audiences of medical practitioners, pharmacists and medical students as the basis of a general discussion of adverse drug reactions, the necessity to constantly be aware of their possible occurrence and to participate in the spontaneous monitoring programme. Showings of the film are associated with distribution of a booklet, also known as *The New Epidemic* which describes in detail the background of spontaneous monitoring and presents the actual case histories from the film together with approximately 100 other case histories and comments divided into groups to illustrate particular points.

## New information

Expectations from such a monitoring system must be realistic. It is clear to ADRAC that the voluntary reporting scheme is not a data gathering tool capable of yielding valid estimates of the incidence of ADRs. The low but unknown reporting rate and variability in what is reported make the numerator used to calculate any incidence quite unreliable. In addition to this, only indirect estimates of drug exposure are available. The yield can only be qualitative or at best semi-quantitative. Despite this, ADRAC sees it as the cornerstone of the national programme to control the problem of ADRs, and the imperfections of the basic input to the system do not prevent unexpected insights coming from the data base if it is scrutinized with knowledge and imagination. Two examples where new information accrued, show different aspects of the operation of the system. The tetracyclic anti-depressant mianserin was released on the Australian market in mid-1979 and within 18 months, during which time sales had been comparatively small, four patients who developed severe disturbances in their polymorphonuclear neutrophil count were reported to ADRAC. Subsequent events have supported the association although the true frequency is still unknown.[2] The example of mebhydrolin illustrates that relationships which are obscured by concomitant therapy in individual reports may emerge from pooled data. Scrutiny of drugs associated with white blood cell disorders revealed a disproportionate frequency of mebhydrolin use. This anti-histamine was not the suspected drug in any of the cases, but the frequency of its association in comparison with other more commonly used anti-histamines was striking.[3] This association was also evident when sought in the data collection of at least one other national centre.

## ADVANTAGES AND LIMITATIONS OF THE SYSTEM

Within limits, therefore, the spontaneous monitoring programme is an excellent means of generating hypotheses covering the occurrence of adverse drug reactions. The great weakness, well illustrated in the case of mianserin, is the inability to test hypotheses so produced.

Virtually all significant reactions are detected by astute clinicians; confirmation of a causal relationship may require a more quantitative approach, but that usually comes later. A corollary is that a heightened awareness of ADRs among the medical and allied professions is the best way to encourage their detection. The provision of a simple channel for reporting suspicions gives a means for the interested and conscientious practitioner to follow up a clinical intuition, and to have it subjected to a screening process. Prompt feedback of material such as details of similar events held in the registry, literature references or simply the result of the assessment of the report, frequently stimulate the reporter to become a regular contributor. The value of this type of feedback in stimulating reporting has been clearly demonstrated in the Australian context. Issue of the cumulative report is always followed by a marked increase in reports received. From November 1974 to June 1975 ADRAC published a monthly *Adverse Drug*

*Reaction Bulletin* containing abstracts of articles dealing with timely or important subjects related to local experience. Each issue dealt briefly with four to six subjects presented on one single folded sheet – to facilitate reading and digestion before consignment to the waste-paper basket. The quadrupling of the reporting rate by practitioners over this period suggests that the bulletin was widely read. More recently, coincident with the wide circulation of the film *The New Epidemic* and other efforts to promote response, there has been a marked increase in reporting levels. It is a reasonable assumption that this implies an increased interest in the question of ADRs.

ADRAC accepts that the voluntary reporting scheme cannot yield acceptable epidemiological data, but has been impressed by its ability to respond quite rapidly to a suggestion that a problem exists. There was a prompt response to news of the practolol syndrome and the occurrence of infected abortions with the intrauterine device, the 'Dalkon Shield.' The latter case was instructive; the first information on the matter was aired in July 1974, and an alerting letter sent to all medical practioners in October. By the end of 1974 there were 67 reports which confirmed that this complication was indeed occurring in Australia, but it was evident that the 'Dalkon Shield' was not the only intrauterine device involved. On the other hand, a warning letter at that same time relating to the suggested relationship of reserpine to breast cancer produced very little response. This is a far from perfect test of the responsiveness of the system since a carcinogenic effect would be much less immediate and impressive, and this example should not be pressed too far.

A more recent example was the rapid identification of a syndrome associated with vaccination for measles. A reaction occurring after a week or more is very common and represents an attenuated infection, but a report in the *Medical Journal of Australia* of reactions occurring within 30 minutes of injection in three children triggered many more reports in the system and thereby the rapid characterization of the clinical phenomenon.[1]

Another role for the system is as a clearing house to encourage further study of a suspected ADR. This is exemplified in the case of bismuth toxicity. In 1972, twelve reports were received by ADRAC from a lay association of patients with colostomies or ileostomies. They referred to mental deterioration in individuals using bismuth subgallate to firm and deodorize bowel contents. These were followed up and the reality of the syndrome was established. Contact was also made with several neurologists who had observed similar cases. As a result this entirely new syndrome of bismuth toxicity[4–6] was documented and has since been confirmed elsewhere.[7] Similar activity was undertaken to clarify the complex issues surrounding erythromycin estolate jaundice, and this resulted in the partial withdrawal of this drug from the Australian market in 1974. Subsequently, doubt has been cast on this decision,[8] but the almost complete absence of reports linking jaundice to other forms of erythromycin since the regulatory action, suggests that in Australia the estolate form of the antibiotic was a cause of cholestasis. During 1973 ADRAC gathered more than 20 cases of SMON (subacute myelo-optic neuropathy) associated with clioquinol use, and this was, at the time, the most substantial body of such cases outside Japan.[9]

The activity of several small intensive monitoring schemes are integrated into the overall ADRAC system. Reports are also received from what might be called *extensive monitoring* programmes in which hospital pharmacists usually play a key role by attempting to record as many as possible of the ADRs occurring in the hospital. Reports originating from this source are identified in storage, in order that their unbalancing effect on the data base can be allowed for.

## ADDITIONAL APPROACHES

ADRAC is attempting to supplement the extant spontaneous monitoring programme, and in particular to establish methods of testing hypotheses generated by it or arising from other sources.

In a society which could be run on experimental lines it would be possible to obtain all the information required to characterize a drug's toxic potential, but few of us would want to live in such a society, even as the research director. We, therefore, have to be content with partial information. Drug surveillance in the real world must obtain as much information as possible within the framework of competing demands for resources and of competing demands for privacy and protection of individual rights. Any conceivable programme will be fair game for criticism because on the one hand it is too elaborate, expensive and intrusive or on the other because it doesn't go far enough. Furthermore the compromise position taken up in one society may be very different from that deemed feasible in another. In the long term view, questions of drug surveillance become just part of a wide range of programmes which require some basic re-ordering of society. In view of the low probability that such changes will arise to meet the needs of drug surveillance, ADRAC has chosen one of the least complex options.

Monitored release of a drug, which has been attempted in several instances, can be regarded as having two essential parts which are separable both conceptually and in practice. The first is to define an enumerated population exposed to the drug. The second is to acquire information on events occurring in that population.

The assembly and retention of a list of patients exposed to a drug is relatively cheap and could be applied to many entities. Acquisition of information about them is costly and would be wasteful of resources, since in most instances little information would be found. The availability of a flagged population for study only if the need arises conforms to the principle that resources should be kept in reserve to cope with really significant problems rather than squandered by deploying them too widely.

A *recorded use* programme of this type may be likened to an insurance policy; for relatively small expenditure one buys the ability to respond subsequently to a serious challenge whether it is a suspected drug catastrophe or the more commonplace crumpled mudguard. This strategy also permits the response to be graded to match the seriousness of the challenge.

There are various ways of assembling such a list. It need not include all exposed individuals, but there should be no bias operating to determine entry, that is in effect, the sampling procedure. There is no generally applicable method and each society needs to examine the structures within it to decide what is best for it. Inman is able to utilize the Prescription Pricing Authority, but in Australia access to scripts presented for reimbursement is forbidden by the current law, although that could perhaps be changed if there were to be sufficient support for the proposal. More fundamental defects are the decreasing number of drugs covered due to government health policies, and the period which usually intervenes between marketing of the drug and acceptance for public subsidy. Various other points could be chosen to tap into the target population, for instance at the level of the prescriber or the dispenser. A pilot scheme based on the last of these has been completed with reasonable success.

In 1981–1982, a 12 month study was undertaken in Victoria with three specific aims. These were first to obtain demographic details on a sample of patients treated with cimetidine or with sodium valproate, using information supplied by pharmacists: second to check the completeness of reporting by pharmacists of patients for whom they dispensed cimetidine or valproate and finally to obtain suitable control groups.

The study demonstrated that such a scheme of recording drug use by pharmacist's reporting is feasible. The number of patients accumulated suggested that a widely based scheme could produce lists of suitable size within a reasonable period, but there was some indication that the extremes of age were under-represented. At the conclusion of the study a Workshop involving representatives of the medical and pharmaceutical organizations, the pharmaceutical industry and consumer groups, supported the study. It emerged from the discussion that concern for confidentiality was a major issue, and that there are unresolved problems concerned with the need for consent by the patient to being listed. The legal requirements of consent and confidentiality probably vary from country to country.

Such a programme by no means fills all the needs in Post-marketing Surveillance and for it to begin to contribute to reasonable safeguards, the methods of producing alerts to possible problems must be maintained at a high pitch. The single most important factor is a high level of awareness amongst doctors, dentists, pharmacists and the consuming public as well, that drugs can cause problems.

## References

1. McEwen, J. (1983). Early-onset reactions after measles vaccination – further Australian reports. *Med. J. Austr.*, **2,** 503–5
2. Adverse Drug Reactions Advisory Committee (1980). Mianserin – a possible cause of neutropenia and agranulocytosis. *Med. J. Austr.*, **2,** 673–4
3. McEwen, J. and Strickland, W. J. (1982). Mebhydrolin napadisylate – a possible cause of reversible agranulocytosis and neutropenia. *Med. J. Austr.*, **2,** 523–5
4. Lowe, D. J. (1974). Adverse effects of bismuth subgallate. A further report from the Australian Drug Evaluation Committee. *Med. J. Austr.*, **2,** 664
5. Burns, R., Thomas, D. W. and Barron, V. J. (1974). Reversible encephalopathy possibly associated with bismuth subgallate ingestion. *Br. Med. J.*, **1,** 220
6. Morgan, F. P. and Billings, J. J. (1974). Is this subgallate poisoning? *Med. J. Austr.*, **2,** 662
7. Loiseau, P., Henry, P., Jallon, P. and Legroux, M. (1976). Encephalophathies myocloniques iatrogenes aux sels de bismuth. *J. Neurol. Sci.*, **27,** 133
8. Inman, W. H. W. and Rawson, N. S. B. (1983). Erythromycin estolate and jaundice. *Br. Med. J.*, **286,** 1954–5
9. Report from the Australian Drug Evaluation Committee. (1972). Subacute myelo-optic neuropathy and the halogenated hydroxyquinolines. *Austr. Fam. Phys.*, **1,** 106

# 3
# Canada

E. NAPKE

## INTRODUCTION

Canada has promoted drug safety and efficacy for many years by regulatory means through the Food and Drug Act and Regulations, Narcotic Control Act and Regulations and, until 1977, the Proprietary and Patent Medicines Act. In 1965, the Federal Drug Adverse Reaction Reporting Program, a voluntary monitoring programme, was initiated.

In order to comprehend the monitoring of drug safety in Canada, the regulatory and voluntary monitoring programme must be seen concomitantly. This combination of regulatory and voluntary approach to the problem of drug safety will give not only an overall view of 'monitoring' in Canada but should indicate that some of the differences in the voluntary programmes from country to country are mainly due to the different regulations in each country.

In Canada a drug is defined by the Food and Drug Act as any substance or mixture of substances manufactured, sold or represented for use in (a) the diagnosis, treatment, mitigation, or prevention of a disease, disorder, abnormal physical state, or the symptoms thereof, in man or animal; (b) restoring, correcting or modifying organic function in man or animal; or (c) disinfections in premises in which food is manufactured, prepared or kept, or the the control of vermin in such premises.

## THE REGULATORY PROGRAMME

The Food and Drug Act and Regulations have provisions for both premarketing and post-marketing monitoring of drugs. Both the regulatory and voluntary programmes for monitoring for drug safety are part of the Health Protection Branch of the Department of Health and Welfare.

A brief description of some of the various regulatory aspects of pre-marketing monitoring for drug safety is necessary in order to understand the post-marketing monitoring for drug safety and how it fits into the whole picture of monitoring for drug safety. Public, academic, media, professional and governmental attitudes are the 'ingredients' or 'seasonings' in each country that finally determine how monitoring will function in the nation. These attitudes concerning drug monitoring for safety vary from country to country and thus, in addition to the regulations, contribute to the differences in monitoring for drug safety.

There is a continuous interplay between the pre-marketing and post-marketing process in monitoring for drug safety. Information and experience gathered in one process or the other is exchanged so that the 'monitoring stance' is always in a state of flux. Monitoring for drug safety includes research, establishing and maintaining the production and product standards as well as the monitoring of the effects or lack of effects of drugs by studies in humans and animals.

## HEALTH PROTECTION BRANCH

The Health Protection Branch's monitoring for drug safety organization is as follows: Food Directorate, Drugs Directorate, Environmental Health Directorate, Laboratory Centre for Disease Control (LCDC), and Field Operations Directorate (see Figure 1). A condensed description of this organization taken from the Health Protection Branch publication Dispatch No. 36 1975–76 is as follows.

> The Health Protection Branch's primary purposes are: to protect Canadians from harmful (foods), drugs, cosmetics, medical devices, and radiation-emitting devices; to control fraudulent practices concerning drugs and medical devices; to determine the possible adverse effects of environmental factors on health; to investigate the causes and cures of communicable and non-communicable diseases; to collect and distribute data on the health and disease status of Canadians; and to engage in informational activities, research and funding of community projects intended to prevent harmful use of alcohol, tobacco, illicit drugs and to remedy the consequence of such use.

### Food Directorate

> The Food Directorate is responsible for branch programmes relating to wholesomeness, nutritional quality, chemical and biological hazards in the food supply, and for programmes relating to the nutritional status of Canadians. It conducts research on nutrition, food composition, food additives, pesticides, veterinary drugs and environmental contaminants in foods; updates and promulgates food standards and regulations; and evaluates submissions from food manufacturers.

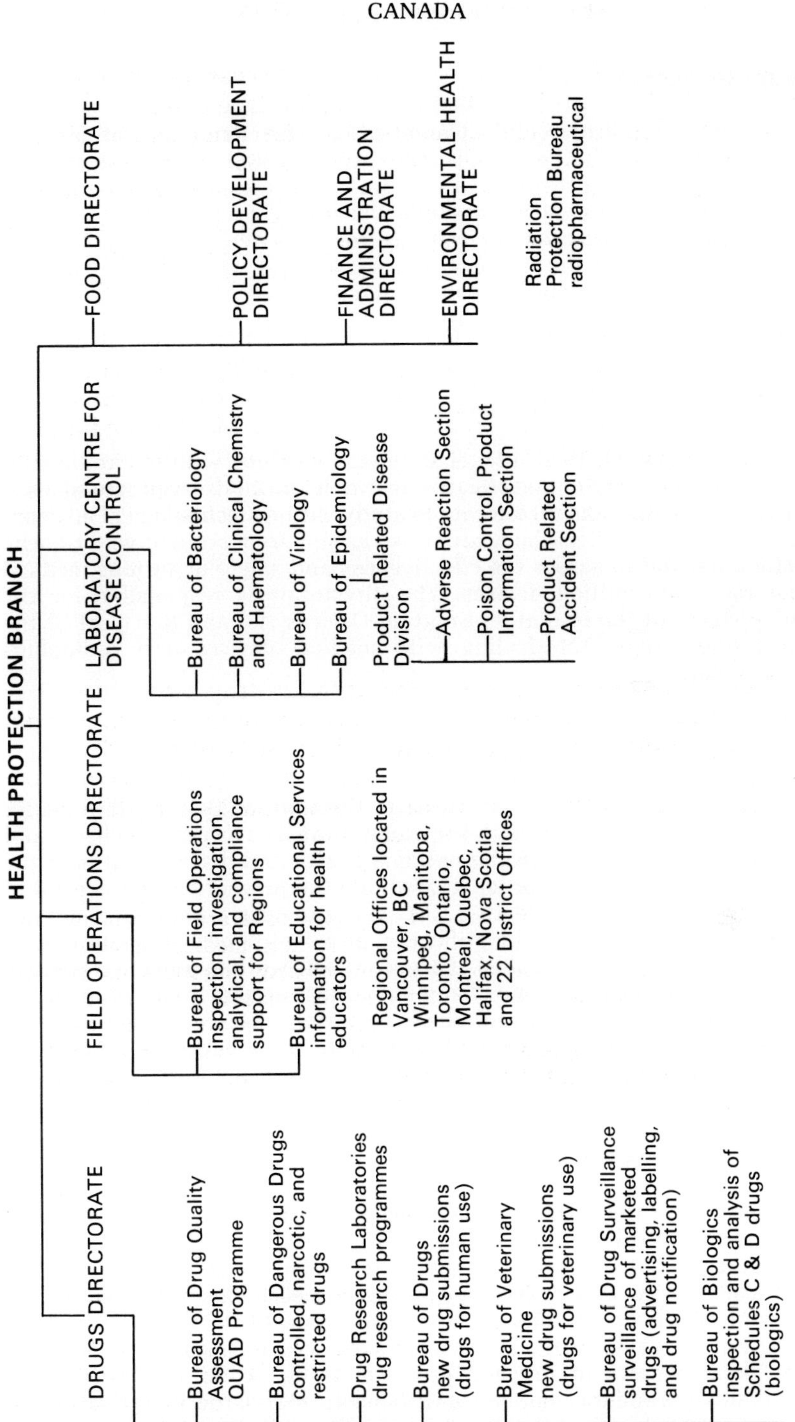


**Figure 1** Chart reflecting the drug organization of the Health Protection Branch

### Drugs Directorate

Through the application of the Narcotic Control Act and Regulations, and those portions of the Food and Drugs Act and Regulations referring to drugs and cosmetics, the Drugs Directorate is responsible for programmes relating to the safety, purity and effectiveness of drugs on the Canadian market and for programmes relating to the safety of cosmetics. The directorate monitors the manufacture, marketing, distribution, and advertising of drugs, and engages in continual research on drug quality, toxicity, pharmacology and bioavailability.

### Environmental Health Directorate

The Environmental Health Directorate is concerned with environmental safety. A wide range of investigative research and advisory programmes is carried out within the directorate to study various technological environments which can affect the health risks arising from air- and water-borne pollutants, and to assess the effectiveness and safety of various medical and radiation-emitting devices. The directorate is responsible for the enforcement of the Radiation-Emitting Devices Act and that part of the Food and Drugs Act dealing with medical devices and radiopharmaceuticals.

### Laboratory Centre for Disease Control

The Laboratory Centre for Disease Control (LCDC) is the health surveillance arm of the Health Protection Branch. The centre collects and distributes information on the national health and disease status of the Canadian population in order to facilitate the prevention and control of disease, disability, and death. LCDC also provides a national reference laboratory service for the identification and control of disease-producing bacteria, viruses and parasites. It also conducts work to provide corrective information to meet new and changing hazards arising from technological and sociological stresses and the accelerating rate of change in these stresses. The *Product Related Diseases Division* is part of the Bureau of Epidemiology which is within the Laboratory Centre for Disease Control.

### Field Operations Directorate

The Field Operations Directorate is responsible for the reduction of health hazards, to which the public may be exposed through the importation, manufacture, advertisement or sale of marketed foods, drugs, cosmetics, medical devices and radiation-emitting devices. This is accomplished through regulatory actions such as: inspections of the premises of food, drug and cosmetic manufacturers, importers, distributors and retailers; analytical surveys of finished products to check for the presence of contaminants and for compliance with federal standards; investigations of consumer product complaints; and enforcement actions.

Within the directorate, Education Services explain branch activities and interprets branch policy to the public and acts as the liaison between consumers and the Health Protection Branch. Through this two-way avenue of communication, HPB is made aware of consumer health concerns and is able to keep Canadians up-to-date on what the Health Protection Branch is doing for them (see Figure 1).

From the above, it is obvious that the Canadian regulations for monitoring for drug safety are very extensive and cover various aspects of the development, manufacturing, storage, sales and claims of a drug product.

## THE VOLUNTARY PROGRAMME

Prior to 1965, there was no official organization specifically created to which physicians could report their suspicions concerning drugs after marketing. This clinical area of concern led to the development of the Federal Voluntary Drug Adverse Reaction Reporting Program (DARRP) in 1965.

The regulatory drug laws did not have provisions for direct feedback from the health practitioners once a product is marketed, although there are regulations for other methods for monitoring drug safety after marketing. The Federal government, after studying the situation in Canada and other countries, decided that voluntary reporting by practitioners was a necessary factor in drug safety monitoring. In 1965, voluntary reporting of suspected drug adverse reactions was initiated by the Federal government with the support of the medical and paramedical health associations.

The following programme concepts are presented to give insight on the functioning of the programme.

### Definition of an adverse drug reaction (ADR)*

Our definition of an ADR is: lack of action or action that is not of therapeutic, diagnostic or prophylactic benefit to the patient. If the product is not effective then the patient is harmed because of the time lost from effective medication. Lack of effect may also result because of drug-food, drug-drug, or other interactions.

### Monitoring for trends in suspected ADRs

The monitoring for drug safety consists of the continuous monitoring, collecting and coordinating of data from research, manufacturing, distribution and usage of a drug. One aspect of this monitoring for drug safety is the monitoring of suspected and proven ADR data.

*Editor's footnote: The author would prefer 'DAR' (Drug Adverse Reactions). The more usual 'ADR' has been retained for the sake of uniformity throughout this book, and to facilitate indexing.

In the monitoring of suspected ADRs, we generally watch for trends which suggest that there may be a problem with a specific product or family of products. The total process of trend analysis, investigation, research, conferring with experts, resulting in advice to one of the regulatory bodies, is called an 'alerting process'. The advice with the supporting data is called an 'alert'. Generally speaking, an 'alert' may be generated from within the Drug Adverse Reaction Reporting Program or any of the other monitoring groups for drug safety in the Health Protection Branch. Data from appropriate sources are collected and reviewed by the professional staff of the DARRP; a decision is made as to whether more data or research is needed, or whether there is enough information to support an 'alert' on the product. Included in the data is the examination of regional, national and international similarities and differences in adverse reaction per product and per active ingredient. The alert is then sent to the appropriate regulatory officers. Up to this point the 'alert' is an *internal* procedure of the Health Protection Branch. The regulatory officers, using the 'alert' and other important data at their disposal, decide on what the next step will be; i.e. further investigation; consultation with professional groups, industry; drug brochure changes or withdrawal of the product from the market. An 'alert' could develop from one report to the programme, although in the vast majority of 'alerts' the initiation of an alert is based on a much wider informational and epidemiological data base.

From the beginning of the programme, the system has been 'product'-orientated. Data are steadily accumulating in the literature which indicate that there are efficacy and adverse reaction differences between some products having the same active ingredients.

At present in the literature almost all adverse reactions which occur with a drug product have been assigned to that product's active ingredient. Thus, for example, adverse effects resulting from 'colouring matter' or other excipients in drugs may inadvertently be ascribed to the active ingredient of the product.

'Hindsight' knowledge (experience) has shown that sometimes even slight changes in the salt of a product will give a different adverse effects profile, e.g. erythromycin estolates and stearates. Simply stated, by being product-orientated one can more easily determine whether the reaction is due to the product composition or only to the active ingredient. The failure to recognize the effects of the excipients of a drug product should raise concern about the level of validity of current tables in the literature linking drugs (active ingredients) and adverse reactions.

Since most of the reports sent to the adverse reaction reporting programme are reports of effects or adverse reactions suspected to be due to a drug, the Canadian centre does not evaluate the diagnosis. The rationale for this is that the physician at the bedside is in a better position to make the diagnosis than others far removed from the case. Hence the reports are *not* classified or evaluated as probable, possible, etc. since the reporter in submitting his opinion or diagnosis may not have given all the information on which the diagnosis was based. In addition, there may be a tendency to downgrade unusual or unexpected types of reports. In a voluntary programme, to go back to the originator of the report to obtain the details on the case may be self-defeating. The reporter responds less to a burdensome form or requests for answers to multiple questions for updating the file; especially if the product in question is not in an 'alert status'. The reports are received and acknowledged with or without 'feedback'. If a product is in an 'alert' status, the reporter may be contacted for more information. Although the reports are not evaluated as to possible, probable reactions etc., the reports are colour-coded as to seriousness of reaction, death, unusual reaction, rechallenge etc.

We request that *all* reactions to all new and old drugs should be reported. We do not expect to receive anywhere near 100% compliance. One wonders whether the 'practolol' story would have evolved more quickly had physicians been impressed with reporting all events including rashes.

Unfortunately, there has developed in the literature a check-list or laundry list of signs and symptoms of adverse reaction to specific drugs rather than concepts of diseases or syndromes. The recognition of adverse reactions is a medical problem and forms part of the differential diagnoses in each case or patient.

The Canadian Drug Adverse Reaction Reporting Program is linked within the division to other adverse reaction reporting programmes, i.e. Poison Control Program, the Veterinary Drug Adverse Reaction Program, Food Adverse Reaction Program, Cosmetic Adverse Reaction Program. These programmes complement each other. The Veterinary Drug Adverse Reactions Program often gives some interesting leads, since quite often the drugs used in veterinary medicine are also used in human medicine.

### Reporting forms

Reporting forms were developed to best suit each of the various sources of reporting: A short form for physicians, a long form for hospitals and a special form for specialists. Reports are accepted from physicians, pharmacists, nurses, veterinarians, government agencies, manufacturers and consumers. Consumers are encouraged to have their reports confirmed by their respective physicians. These forms are printed in English and French.

## DOUBLE MONITORING SYSTEM

The reports are monitored via two major methods

(1) a computer system, and
(2) a pigeon-hole system

Both systems are primarily 'Trade Name' orientated with appropriate methods for 'Generic' analysis.

### The computer system

The system is described in a general sense in Chapter 20. In addition, there is an on-line interactive system. All and various combinations of the information elements of the case reports can be retrieved. A variety of computer programs have been developed for monitoring, feedback, statistics, etc. Canada was one of the first countries to input information on tape to the WHO program.

### The pigeon-hole system

The pigeon-hole system is an open file system of the original reports (see Figure 2). Each report has been colour tagged as to severity, unusualness of reaction, death, congenital anomaly, cancer, etc. When appropriate, one or more colour tags are attached to the report in such a position to be easily seen when the report is in its respective pigeon-hole. The visual impact of the contents of a pigeon-hole; the colour tags, number of reports, time indicators and so on, stimulates the monitor(s) to investigate the situation. (Invariably, visiting professionals and non-professionals will reach instinctively for one or other pigeon-hole to survey the contents.)

Locating and retrieval of reports is made easy by a locating directory, listing products, diseases, etc., in alphabetical order against the appropriate pigeon-hole number.

This is a very simple and inexpensive system for monitoring for drug safety, disease or other subjects. The system can be used at any level of activity; from the national level to the individual practitioner level. Any number of monitors can use it at the same time. There is no line-up or dependence on other experts' time for computer services.

The system is ideal for those centres and circumstances in which computer facilities are not available. In point of fact, even if there is the possibility of a computer facility, one should start with a system similar to a pigeon-hole system to get a feel for the area of drug adverse reaction monitoring and drug safety. The combination of systems is ideal for monitoring.

It should be noted that continual surveillance of drug poisoning, veterinary drug adverse reactions, plays an important role in drug safety surveillance.

## CURRENT ACTIONS

The Drug Adverse Reaction Reporting Program alerts are based on the

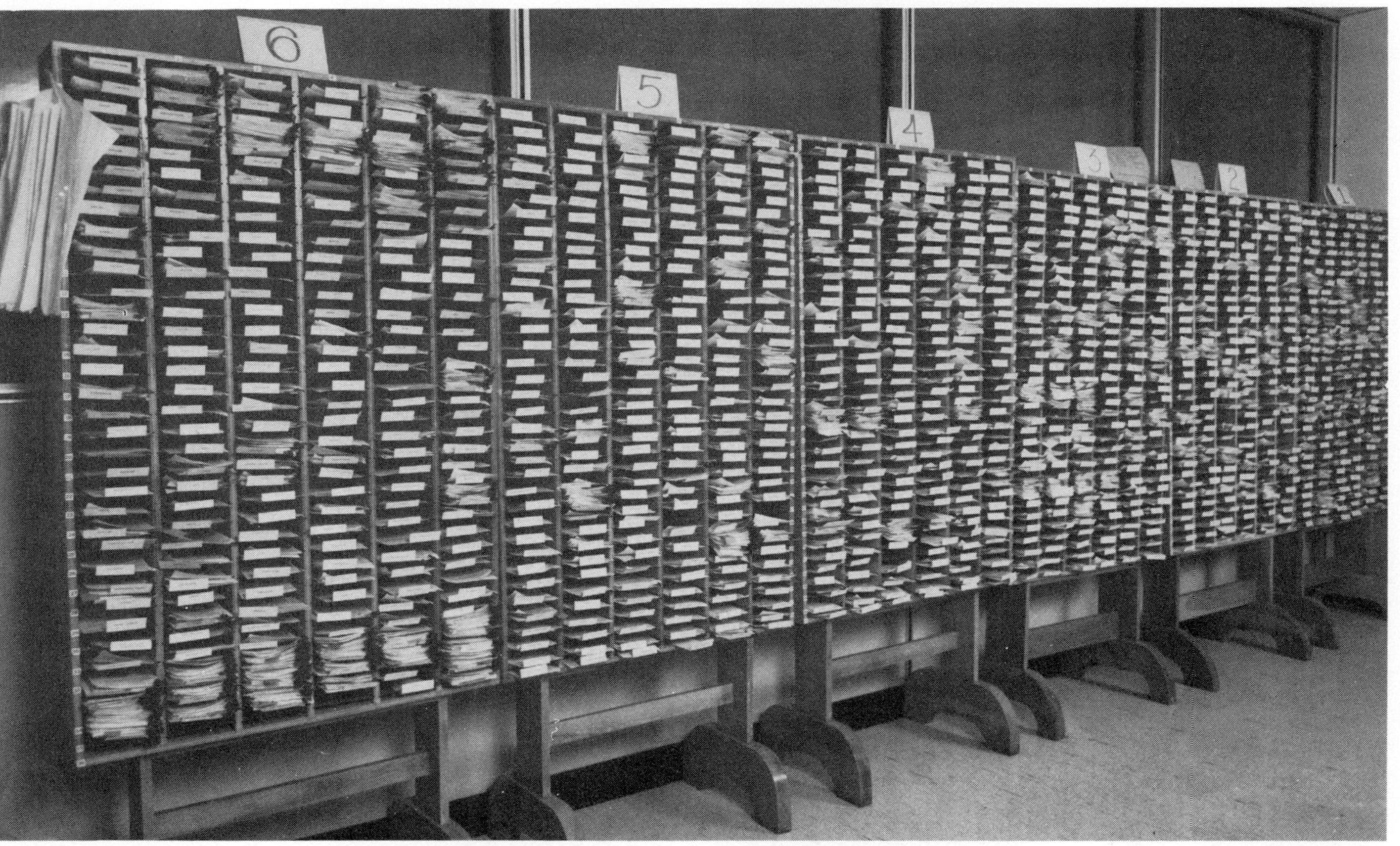


**Figure 2** The pigeon-hole system. In this open file system, each report is colour tagged according to severity, unusualness of reaction, death, etc. The visual impact of the contents of a pigeon-hole, the colour tags and numbers of reports, stimulates the monitor to investigate the situation

reports involving Canadians. Drug safety problems described in other countries will trigger a review of the Canadian data, while bearing in mind differences between countries in genetics, medical practice, disease and food.

Table 1 shows some of the alerts sent to the respective regulatory agency and some of the subsequent action(s) taken.

## DEMOGRAPHIC AND DRUG ADVERSE REACTION REPORTING DATA

The population of Canda is about 24 000 000, with approximately 30 000 practising physicians. The drug adverse reaction programme's professional staff consists of one pharmacist and half-time of one physician. In 1983 the total number of reports of suspected drug adverse reactions case reports was 7000, including approximately 200 from the manufacturer.

## NEW APPROACHES

Adverse reactions to drugs are medical problems. Organized medicine has not collectively faced the problem of drug adverse reaction monitoring. In Canada this is being addressed. One provincial medical association and several national specialist associations have formed monitoring programmes, the individual reports of these programmes are sent to the Federal DARRP. The Federal programme computerizes the data and 'feedback' to the appropriate body for their information and action. In addition, we are reactivating our 'excipients' and 'additives' file with appropriate cross linkage, since a number of adverse effects are due to these ingredients alone or in the company of the 'active ingredients'.

**Table 1** Some of the alerts sent to regulatory agencies since 1965

| *Drugs* | *Problem area* | *Action taken* |
|---|---|---|
| Enteric Coated KCl | small intestine ulceration | removal from the market |
| Halothane | hepatotoxicity | (1) Dear Doctor Letter<br>(2) article in Rx Bulletin* |
| Procainamide | lupus erythematosus syndrome | warning in package insert |
| Methoxyflurane | nephrotoxicity | article in Rx bulletin |
| Methoxyflurane + Tetracycline | nephrotoxicity | article in Rx bulletin |
| Erythromycin estolate | hepatotoxicity | article in Rx bulletin |
| Clindamycin | pseudomembranous colitis | 'Dear Doctor letter' from the manufacturer |
| Lincomycin | pseudomembranous colitis | 'Dear Doctor letter' from the manufacturer |
| NPH Insulin | change in onset and duration of action | lots involved recalled |
| Cerumenex | severe allergic reaction | package insert for consumer's information prepared by manufacturer and reviewed within DARRP |
| Minocycline | vestibular reaction | product monograph |
| Nitrofurantoin | pulmonary reaction<br>peripheral neuropathy | article in Rx bulletin |
| Methysergide | fibrosis | article in Rx bulletin |
| Diphenidol | hallucination | promotion of product to physicians stopped |
| Spironolactone | gynecomastia | modification of product monograph |
| Phenformin | lactic acidosis | removal from the market |
| Alcohol | fetal alcohol syndrome | article in *Canadian Medical Association Journal* |
| Oral contraceptive | thrombophlebitis | (1) 'Oral Contraceptive Advisory Committee'<br>(2) product monograph revised |
| Liquid high protein diet products | sudden deaths | (1) press release<br>(2) warning on labels of the products |
| 'Feldene' | gastrointestinal bleeding<br>death in the very elderly | pending |
| Excipients and additives | hidden drug product adverse reaction | publication of article 'excipients and additives; hidden hazards in drug products and in drug substitution' |

* The Rx Bulletin was a HPB publication mailed to all physicians and pharmacists in Canada

# 4
# The Federal Republic of Germany

K. H. KIMBEL

## REGULATORY STATUS OF THE VOLUNTARY REPORTING SYSTEM (VRS)

The first federal law governing the manufacture and distribution of medicines in the FRG became effective in 1961. Except that it prohibited the marketing of drugs which 'are liable, if used for the intended purpose, to exert noxious effects beyond those deemed acceptable according to the knowledge of medical science and not being the consequence of the peculiar circumstances of the individual case', nothing in the law provided for the systematic collection of reports of adverse drug reactions (ADRs). Almost 10 years passed before an advisory committee to the Ministry of Youth, Family and Health (*Beirat 'Arzneimittelsicherheit'*) drafted a plan to 'coordinate necessary measures and ways of distributing information about suspected adverse drug reactions'. This was issued in August 1970. It provided for collaboration between the (private) Drug Commission, the (federal) National Health Institute (*Bundesgesundheitsamt*), the State Health authorities and the manufacturers in the collection and evaluation of reports of ADRs. This worked smoothly, deriving its efficiency mostly from the scientific prestige of the members of the Drug Commission. This, and the success of the VRS, was also the main reason why the new German Medicines Act of 1976 (which became effective on January 1st, 1978) determined that the National Institute of Health should be fully responsible for the centralized documentation and evaluation of all drug risks and the coordination of protective measures, while leaving the collection and scientific interpretation of the data to the professional organizations. The Drug Commission of the Medical Profession served as a model for analogous commissions for dental surgeons, veterinarians, pharmacists and paramedical therapists (*Heilpraktiker*). All these commissions were required by regulation to issue recommendations on the proper use of drugs. The relationships between the various bodies are shown in Figure 1.

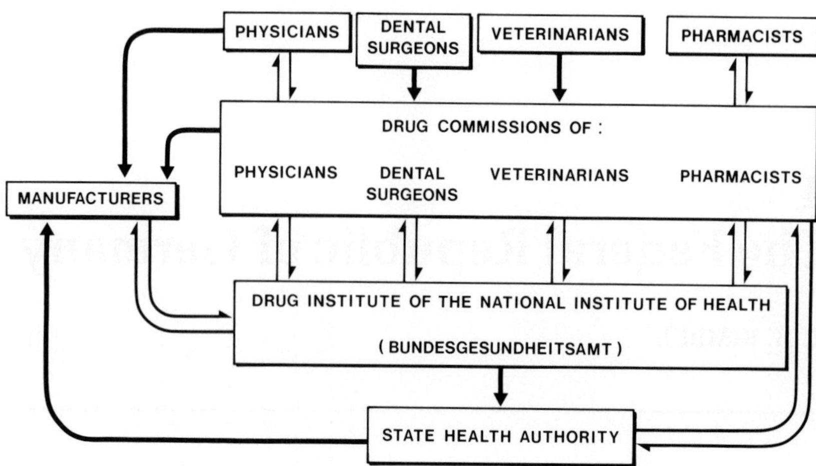


**Figure 1** Flow chart of ADR reporting and ensuing executive measures

## DEVELOPMENT OF VRS

The 'Drug Commission of the German Congress (now Society) of Internal Medicine' was established in 1911. One of its aims was the elimination of 'therapeutically useless and even noxious drugs'. The necessity for a systematic VRS was fully recognized 50 years later. Meanwhile in 1950 the Drug Commission expanded its services to specialists in internal medicine to become the official body representing the whole profession. As early as 1956 it had collected information on the adverse effects of Thorium-X, appetite-suppressants, and abuse of opiate antitussives. In 1958 the Drug Commission called on all physicians to report all ADRs to the Drug Commission, but it required a whole day devoted to 'Side effects of modern therapy' at the 1961 meeting of the German Society for Internal Medicine, and the thalidomide tragedy, to get things moving. The first report forms were published in 1963 and from modest beginnings German physicians eventually reach second place among the 23 nations participating with the WHO's international drug monitoring centre (Figure 2).

## DEMOGRAPHIC AND DRUG-USAGE DATA

The population of the FRG as of 30th December 1984 was 61 354 000. There were 152 158 active physicians, giving one physician for every 403 inhabitants. There is one GP per 4264 inhabitants, and one physician in private practice per 958 inhabitants. There is one specialist in internal medicine for every 3266 patients, and one hospital physician per 834 patients. More than 90% of the population are members of the Public Health Insurance Scheme (*Gesetzliche*

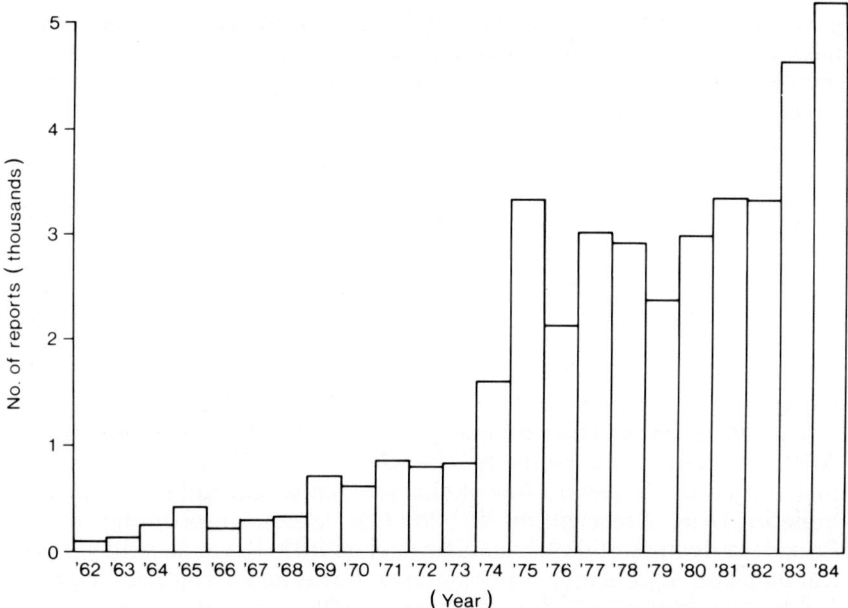


**Figure 2** Number of reports satisfying WHO requirements entered into FRG's ADR data bank

*Krankenkassen*) and its equivalents (*Ersatzkassen*), the remainder being privately insured or reimbursed in part by their employer. In 1984, 70 000 physicians were under contract to the Public Health Insurance System through their organization (*Kassenärztliche Vereinigung*). During this year, the Public Health Insurance System spent over 14 billion DM on drugs for ambulatory patients; drug costs in hospitals are included in a flat rate paid per patient-day. The system absorbs two-thirds of pharmacy sales, about 20% of these sales account for self-medication and the remainder for private prescriptions or non-reimbursed items such as contraceptives. Drug consumption seems to be similar to that of other developed countries, but the number of products may be greater than in most – no fewer than 130 000 are currently registered with the *Bundesgesundheitsamt*, the regulatory agency. If different presentations of the same drug and the vast number of borderline drugs (e.g. mineral waters) are taken into account, this number can be reduced to about 30 000. This multiplicity of products is not conducive to the identification or prevention of ADRs.

## MOTIVATING DOCTORS TO PARTICIPATE IN VRS

Traditionally, German doctors believe they should regulate their own professional affairs, including drug therapy, before turning to the government for help. A professional organization has to persuade its members that the additional burden of paperwork, such as that involved in VRS, is necessary and useful. From the start, the Drug Commission had not only to 'sell' the system to the busy physician (especially the general practitioner), they had also to give something in return for their co-operation. The medical staff acknowledge each report individually, advise the physician on prevention or mitigation of ADRs and give personal attention to many enquiries about ADRs that are not associated with a case-report. Files of data are maintained for most of the drugs marketed in the FRG in addition to ADR information from the world literature using e.g. *Medlars, Excerpta Medica*, the FDA services, Clin-Alert and the API's 'micropharm II' microfiche system. In this way information is available for physicians who could not possibly maintain comprehensive files of the own.

The Drug Commission regularly informs the profession about new ADRs in their statements in the *Deutsches Ärzteblatt*, which is distributed to all doctors free of charge each week, and issues its own bulletin *Drug Prescription in Practice* (*Arzneiverordnung in der Praxis*) to doctors and pharmacists each month. Every second year the Commission also issues a pocketbook formulary *Drug Prescriptions* (Arzneiverordnungen). Regular lists of ADRs are not issued because drug companies who co-operate actively by collecting reports on their own drugs would be placed at a disadvantage to their competitors who may even dissuade physicians from reporting.

Since 1981 all new and severe ADRs are discussed at monthly meetings of a special advisory committee, consisting of experts from all theoretical and clinical disciplines involved. The resolutions form the basis for warnings and information to the profession and are made known to the regulatory agency.

## ANALYSIS OF REPORTING OF ADRs

The participation of physicians in large and medium-sized cities (the total number of doctors is known for those with a 1- or 2-digit zip code) varies widely from 0.6% to 25%. A map showing the variations of reporting density is of value in deciding priorities for promotional activities such as lectures and postgraduate educational programmes.

Table 1 divides reporting physicians into specialities in hospital and private practice. Although there were about 50 000 specialists in hospital and private practice as compared to 26 000 general practitioners (as of January 1st, 1977), it is encouraging that more of the latter report ADRs. Specialists in internal medicine in hospital and private practice ranked second. In the remaining specialities the distribution reflects the relative importance of drug use fairly well. It seems remarkable that there are twice as many reporting physicians in private practice as in hospitals or clinics considering their numbers are equal (52 690 and 52 587 respectively). This may in part be due to

**Table 1** Reporting physicians according to speciality and location as of July 1976.

| | *Clinic or hospital* | *Private practice* | *Total* |
|---|---|---|---|
| General practice | — | 1051 | 1051 |
| Internal medicine | 553 | 358 | 911 |
| Paediatrics | 89 | 81 | 170 |
| Neurology and psychiatry | 57 | 40 | 97 |
| Anaesthesiology | 68 | — | 68 |
| Obstetrics and gynaecology | 28 | 57 | 85 |
| Surgery | 48 | 24 | 72 |
| Dermatology | 18 | 49 | 67 |
| Urology | 19 | 17 | 36 |
| Otorhinolaryngology | 9 | 43 | 52 |
| Radiology | 13 | 17 | 30 |
| Orthopaedics | 4 | 28 | 32 |
| Ophthalmology | 11 | 20 | 31 |
| Chest diseases | 5 | 16 | 21 |
| Totals | 922 | 1801 | 2723 |

the fact that in some hospitals reporting is delegated to one responsible physician.

Table 2 shows the distribution of individual case-reports among the various disciplines. Again general practitioners rank first, while the number of reports correlates fairly well with the numbers of other specialists, exceptions being internal medicine and surgery where the rate is influenced by routine reporting during the course of some special studies.

**Table 2** Annual number of reports according to disciplines (1967–76)

| | *In hospital* | *In Private practice* | *Total* |
|---|---|---|---|
| General practice | — | 1547 | 1547 |
| Internal medicine | 1045 | 629 | 1674 |
| Paediatrics | 184 | 141 | 325 |
| Neurology and psychiatry | 99 | 46 | 145 |
| Anaesthesiology | 103 | — | 103 |
| Surgery | 125 | 29 | 154 |
| Dermatology | 39 | 135 | 174 |
| Gynaecology | 34 | 78 | 112 |
| Urology | 59 | 20 | 79 |
| Otorhinolaryngology | 12 | 74 | 86 |
| Radiology | 17 | 19 | 36 |
| Orthopaedics | 5 | 38 | 43 |
| Ophthalmology | 12 | 26 | 38 |
| Chest diseases | 9 | 17 | 26 |
| Totals | 1743 | 2799 | 4542 |

**Table 3** Annual Number of reports per reporting physician (1967–76)

| | *In hospital* | *In private practice* |
|---|---|---|
| General practice | — | 1.5 |
| Internal medicine | 3.81 | 1.75 |
| Paediatrics | 2.06 | 1.7 |
| Neurology and psychiatry | 1.73 | 1.15 |
| Anaesthesiology | 1.5 | — |
| Surgery | 2.6 | 3.75 |
| Dermatology | 2.16 | 2.75 |
| Gynaecology | 1.2 | 1.36 |
| Urology | 3.1 | 1.17 |
| Otorhinolaryngology | 1.3 | 1.72 |
| Radiology | 1.3 | 2.7 |
| Orthopaedics | 1.25 | 1.6 |
| Ophthalmology | 1.1 | 1.3 |
| Chest diseases | 1.8 | 1.3 |

Table 3 shows the average number of reports by each type of reporting physician, and reveals that the workload over a 10-year period is rather small.

## ANALYSIS OF THE ADRs

Table 4 shows the principal drug entities involved in ADRs. From 1967 to 1976 penicillins ranked first. The fact that plasma substitutes ranked next may be explained by almost complete reporting of these then new anaphylactic reactions. The same may be true for radio-opaque media whose ADR level was closely watched by the principal manufacturer. The high rank of the cardiac glycosides may be due to their small dose-range, while that of co-trimoxazole may be simply the result of enormous sales. BCG vaccine caused many cases of lymphadenitis when a change of strain was made during its production. Almost all aescin cases occurred after intravenous injection, mostly in surgical patients.

In 1983, the spectrum of drugs involved in ADRs differed from that of 10 years earlier. The only survivors among the first 20 were diazepam and BCG vaccine. Almost all leading drugs in 1983 had yet to be marketed in the early 1970s. The NSAID boom is reflected in the two leaders and two more new compounds. The almost identical ranking of BCG vaccine indicates that the problem has still not been solved in 1985, despite the continuing demand for BCG vaccination.

Table 5 shows the most frequently reported ADRs. It is not

**Table 4** A comparison of the drugs most frequently associated with ADR reports (1967–76 and 1983)

| Drug or drug group | Number of reports (1967–1976) | Drug or drug group | Number of reports (1983) |
|---|---|---|---|
| Penicillins | 418 | Piroxicam | 199 |
| Dextran preparations | 264 | Carprofen | 179 |
| Amidotrizoate | 231 | Tetanus vaccine | 115 |
| Nitrofurantoin preparations | 231 | Hepatitis B vaccine | 96 |
| | | Indomethacin | 93 |
| Digitalis preparations | 215 | Haloperidol | 93 |
| Co-trimoxazole | 203 | **Diazepam** | 86 |
| Spironolactone | 193 | Isoxicam | 84 |
| Ioglycamate | 181 | Diclofenac | 82 |
| D-penicillamine | 173 | **BCG vaccine** | 71 |
| **Benzodiazepines** | 153 | Lorazepam | 66 |
| **BCG vaccine** | 135 | Buprenorphine | 65 |
| Tetracyclines | 120 | Cimetidine | 60 |
| Propranidid | 109 | Ketoconazole | 57 |
| Phenprocoumon | 101 | Bromazepam | 55 |
| Aescin | 99 | Ranitidine | 54 |
| Verapamil | 94 | Zomepirac | 53 |
| Cephalosporins | 94 | Tromantadin | 50 |
| Oral contraceptives | 93 | Orgotein | 49 |
| Sulphonylureas | 84 | Diphtheria–tetanus vaccine | 48 |
| Chloramphenicol | 81 | | |

surprising that hypersensitivity reactions head the list. Lethal ADRs account for nearly 4%. We should refrain from making a more detailed interpretation of the frequency of reports on individual drugs or ADRs because VRS reports are very poor indicators of true frequency. Relatively complete reporting, e.g. of vaccine or radio-opaque media incidents, may seriously distort the general pattern. VRS reports serve mainly to produce hypotheses which may be rejected or confirmed by prospective controlled studies. Eight years later, the distribution of ADR symptoms had changed considerably. Drug dependence (mostly appetite suppressants, barbiturate combinations and benzodiazepines) topped the list. Hypersensitivity reactions came next, severe anaphylaxis maintaining about the same rank compared with 1967–76. Trivial ADRs such as vomiting and nausea were reported less frequently, perhaps due to our request to report only new or serious ADRs.

Unfortunately, we have not yet evaluated our material for the consequences of ADRs, except those which are fatal. In future we hope to report the proportion requiring hospital or out-patient care, or those in which an ADR prolonged hospitalization.

**Table 5** A comparison of the ADRs most frequently reported – 1967–76 vs 1983. (Using WHO ADR terminology)

| *Reaction* | *Number of reports (1967–76)* | *Reaction* | *Number of reports (1983)* |
|---|---|---|---|
| Rash, erythematous | 697 | Drug dependence | 346 |
| Circulatory failure | 576 | Rash | 234 |
| Pruritus | 499 | Injection site reaction | 233 |
| Vomiting | 478 | Fever | 208 |
| Nausea | 476 | Drug abuse | 183 |
| Dyspnoea | 448 | Dermatitis contact | 165 |
| Urticaria | 424 | Urticaria | 151 |
| Fever | 348 | Allergic reaction | 145 |
| Fatal ADRs | 340 | Pruritus | 140 |
| Anaphylactic shock | 331 | Anaphylactoid reaction | 124 |
| Rash, maculopapular | 257 | Anaphylactic shock | 119 |
| Hypotension | 254 | Vomiting | 105 |
| Flushing | 230 | Rigors | 105 |
| Tachycardia | 225 | Abdominal pain | 103 |
| Cyanosis | 196 | Hepatic function abnormal | 88 |
| Abdominal pain | 195 | Nausea | 79 |
| Coma | 191 | Circulatory failure | 77 |
| Diarrhoea | 183 | Rash, erythematous | 77 |
| Paraesthesia | 174 | Lymphadenopathy | 76 |
| Rigors | 172 | Vertigo | 74 |
| Headache | 171 | Headache | 70 |
| Rash | 162 | Photosensitivity reaction | 66 |
| Cardiac arrest | 161 | Alopecia | 61 |
| Oedema of the face | 155 | Death | 59 |
| Somnolence | 149 | Dyspnoea | 52 |
| Angioedema | 142 | Bronchospasm | 50 |
| Dizziness | 137 | Skin necrosis | 49 |
| Purpura | 137 | Thrombocytopenia | 49 |
| Sweating | 127 | Angioedema | 48 |
| Apnoea | 122 | Extrapyramidal disorders | 48 |

## EVALUATION OF REPORTS

All the reports are discussed at daily meetings of the medical staff of the Commission's secretariat. They are checked against similar events already reported and those described in the literature or reference sources already mentioned in the section on motivation. Doubtful cases are referred to the appropriate Commission members requesting expert opinions. Attempts are made to obtain additional data, mostly by telephone. Some pharmaceutical houses assist with these enquiries. One or other of the 120 members of the Commission often arrange to have the patient examined at a university clinic or municipal hospital. We are reluctant to decide finally on the causal relationship between a drug and an event, except where a rechallenge was possible and positive. Reports of identical events from separately located and independent sources may strengthen suspicion, but the ultimate decision must be left to a controlled study. Print-outs of ADRs are distributed confidentially only to members of the Commission to avoid discriminating against a valuable drug by an as-yet-unconfirmed suspicion. On one occasion the publication of a Table similar to Table 5, but giving trade-names, led one pharmaceutical manufacturer to seek permission to make thousands of reprints for distribution by their representatives (a reminder of how easily such data may be misused for competitive purposes).

## ACTION FOLLOWING EVALUATION OF ADRs

VRS would be only of limited value if the release of data was restricted only to those ADRs in which causality had been proven beyond doubt. It is necessary to alert the profession, and for the regulatory authorities to take preventive measures, as soon as possible before certainty is reached. One of the most difficult and demanding tasks for the members of the advisory body of a VRS is to decide when the profession should be warned in order to protect the public and when the regulatory agency should be advised to consider restrictive measures. Since 1958 the Drug Commission has issued statements, mostly to alert the profession to new or increasingly frequent ADRs. Statements by the Drug Commission are now published after consultation with the Federal authorities, but the former has full responsibility. All executive measures on the other hand, fall within the authority of the federal and state institutions, the National Institute of Health (*Bundesgesundheitsamt*) and State Health Ministries (*Landesgesundheitsministerien*). After notification of a drug risk the representatives of the Drug Commissions, manufacturers, government officials and experts will be invited to *ad hoc* conferences, and there are also routine meetings when general problems are discussed.

## NEED FOR COMPLEMENTARY INVESTIGATIONS

VRS, as we have already seen, may not give firm evidence of new or increasingly frequent ADRs. Since intensive hospital monitoring systems are rarely of help in proving causality or estimating frequency at such an early stage, decisions with far-reaching consequences often have to be made by the authorities on the basis of a few chance observations and the opinions of their expert advisers. It speaks well for their farsightedness and objectivity that nearly all their decisions in the drug field have been proved to be right. However, since this cannot always be relied on, the Drug Commission proposed, in 1973, to establish an 'epidemiological fire-brigade'. A permanent office would maintain data on drug usage where product-orientated intensive monitoring could be established on an *ad hoc* and temporary basis. This could be in a municipal hospital, outpatient clinic, homes for the aged or groups of general practices. Populations of patients who were at risk to the suspect drug could be identified and placed under surveillance. Control populations could similarly be organized. Despite the obvious interests of the manufacturers, however, the Commission has not yet been successful in securing their co-operation. Thus no serious attempts have been made by industry or a regulatory agency to develop a post-marketing surveillance system beyond voluntary reporting.

## FUNDING AND DATA-PROCESSING

A rough estimate of the cost of VRS in the FRG is \$20 (DM 60) per report – less than \$1 per licensed physician in the country. The Drug Commission is financed about equally by the Federal Chamber of Physicians (*Bundesärztekammer*), which all physicians are obliged to belong to through the State Chambers, and the Association of Public Health Insurance Physicians (*Kassenärztliche Bundesvereinigung*) representing all physicians participating in the care of the publicly insured. There are no contributions from government or industry.

One experienced medical officer responsible for ADR monitoring, and a further two physicians and one pharmacist of the medical secretariat contribute their experience. A university-trained archivist is head of documentation, assisted by a file-keeper and a central typing office. The permanent staff can rely on the advice of 40 active and 80 corresponding members of the Commission, representing all the medical disciplines.

Initially the computing centre of the Max-Planck Institute in Göttingen provided data-processing facilities. Later, the WHO coding system was adopted and the data were sent to the Research Centre for International Monitoring for Adverse Reactions to Drugs in Geneva. With the help of the German Cancer Research Centre in Heidelberg, the Commission also established its own data-bank which is now maintained and upgraded at the computing centre of the KBV in Cologne. The secretariat also keeps close contact with those intensive hospital monitoring programmes run by members of the Commission in Berlin, Bochum, Heidelberg and Munich.

### Bibliography

Anon. (1985) Spontanerfassung unerwünschter Arzneimittelwirkungen–Eigeninitiative der Ärzte-. *Dtsch Ärztebl.*, **82,** 592–3

Homann, G. (1973). Die Erfassung und Vermeidung von Arzneimittelschäden. *Internist*, **14,** 19

Homann, G. (1973). Wirksamkeit und Sicherheit von Arzneimitteln. *Arzneim-Forsch.*, **25,** 1220

Kimbel, K. H. (1976). Monitoring adverse drug reactions: spontaneous reporting – possibilities, problems and responsibility: national monitoring centres. *5th European Symposium on Clinical Pharmacological Evaluation in Drug Control*, WHO, Deidesheim. October 26th–29th, 1976

Kimbel, K. H., Ehlers, J. and Kimbel, U. (1977). Spontanerfassung unerwünschter Arzneimittelwirkungen in der Bundesrepublik. *Münch. Med. Wochenschr.*, **119,** 841

Kimbel, K. H. (1978). Drug monitoring: why care? In M. N. G. Dukes (ed.). *Side Effects of Drugs Annual*, No. 2 (Amsterdam–Oxford Excerpta Medica)

Köhler, C. and Kimbel, K. H. (1978). Spontaneous monitoring data processing and information feedback to the physician. *Conference on Computer Aid to Drug Therapy and to Drug Monitoring*. IFIP TC4. Berne: March 6th–10th, 1978

Ochsenfahrt, H., Meyer und Heyde, M. (1981). Spontanberichte uber unerwünschte Arzneimittelwirkungen in den Jahren 1978 u. 1979, *Fortschr. Med.*, **99,** 1753–8

Mathias, B., Kimbel, K. H., Ochsenfahrt (1983). Sichere Verordnung durch Erfahrungsaustausch, *Dtsch. Ärztebl.*, **80,** 36–41

# 5
# Finland

J. IDÄNPÄÄN-HEIKKILÄ

---

## INTRODUCTION

Finland is the easternmost of the five Nordic Countries. Its population at the end of 1984 was 4.9 million and there were about 11 000 physicians giving approximately one physician per 445 inhabitants.

There are five nationwide computerized health surveillance registries in Finland. The main goal of these registries has been to collect data for general health surveillance in the country, and to provide information for the further planning and development of the national health care system. During the past 10 years the purpose of these registries has been extended to drug safety.

When the medical records are used for drug safety studies prescriptions of cases and controls are linked with records of events such as hospital admissions, hospital discharges, birth defects, diagnosed cancer, etc., depending on the aim and goals of the study. The linkage is possible because every citizen has a single individual identification code (social security number) in all records and data sources.

The linkage of existing records does not usually require special facilites for data collection. In fact the 'raw data' are notified by physicians to the data bank as a routine part of the daily work on patients' medical records.

The advantages and disadvantages of these health surveillance registries in conducting drug safety studies has been discussed elsewhere.[1] In this chapter I shall describe these registries and give some examples of how they have been utilized for drug safety purposes in Finland.

## HEALTH SURVEILLANCE REGISTRIES AND THEIR DATA COLLECTION

### Finnish Register of Congenital Malformations

Since 1963, notification of all congenital malformations detected in liveborn and stillborn children has been compulsory in Finland. For every child with a defect, a control child without a defect, born immediately before the 'case' child in the same maternity welfare district is selected (time–area matched pairs). The register is sent copies of both mothers' records, including data on pregnancy, delivery, malformations and drug use. In each case these forms are filled in by a physician at the maternity hospital and supplemented by detailed antenatal records from maternal health service centres which cover the whole country. In 1964 about 98% and in 1978 almost 100% of the pregnant women in Finland were examined, usually before end of the first trimester, in these 1300 local centres which operate on a communal basis. The data recorded include all drugs prescribed, together with any others, such as OTCs, known to have been used during pregnancy. These records are further supplemented by structured interviews with the mothers after delivery.

The data collection for this register is effective due to the well-organized and functional maternity welfare centre system in Finland. The maternal memory bias is largely avoided because most of the information on drug use is collected prospectively during the mother's antenatal visits. (Table 1).

The notifications serve statistical purposes such as monitoring the incidence, trends, geographical distribution and seasonal variations of malformations. In addition, they are used as the material for a 'matched pair' register for continuous detailed analysis concerning the causes of malformations such as infections, vaccinations, special working conditions, toxic environmental agents and drugs. The 20 years cumulative experience with the congenital malformation register in Finland were recently reviewed by Saxen.[2]

### The Finnish Cancer Registry

Since 1953 all cases of cancer in Finland have been reported to the Finnish Cancer Registry. All hospitals, pathological and cytological laboratories and physicians are requested to report to the Registry any new cancer case that comes to their attention. This reporting became compulsory in 1961. The Registry receives a copy of every death certificate, in which there is a mention of cancer. In addition, annual checks are made against the Registry files of all death certificates issued in the country. Accordingly, apart from cancer deaths, the Registry acquires information on the deaths of cancer patients attributable to causes other than cancer.

**Table 1** The informants and data content linking possibilities of the Finnish Health Surveillance Registries

| *Register* | *Informants* | *Reported cases/year* | *Cumulative number of cases in data bank* | *Linkage* to other registries possible* |
|---|---|---|---|---|
| Cancer Registry | hospitals<br>doctors<br>pathology laboratories<br>Central Statistical Office<br>(death certificates) | 15 000 – 17 000 | 350 000 | yes |
| Congenital malformation register | hospitals<br>doctors | 600 cases<br>600 matched controls | 30 000 | yes for mother |
| Register of persons entitled to free drugs | pharmacies<br>doctors | 60 000 | 800 000 | yes |
| Hospital discharge register | hospitals<br>doctors | 750 000 | 14 million | yes |
| Register of adverse reaction to drugs | doctors<br>(HDs and GPs) | 500–800 | 7000 | yes |

*By using a single individual identification code (social security number).

Based on multiple information sources for each case the data collection of this Registry is exceptionally complete.

About 15 000–17 000 new cases of cancer are registered each year (Table 1). The data contained in this Registry are routinely used to monitor the national and regional incidences of various forms of cancer, and to screen the outcome of patients with specified cancers. The Registry has been used to measure the effects of health education campaigns, such as anti-smoking programmes, on the frequency of cancer. The Registry has also been used to monitor drug safety as described below.

## Hospital Discharge Register

Whenever a patient is discharged from a Finnish hospital, a notification form is filled in by the doctor and sent to the National Board of Health. This notification card includes, among other things, the main diagnosis and two other diagnoses and the type of treatment given.[1] In its final form the data on the magnetic tapes can be linked with the original hospital record by the patient's social security number. The data bank collects annually about 750 000 hospital discharges with 13 million patient days (Table 1). The information in this register can be linked with any of the above health registers by the identification system described earlier. In addition, the Register gives an easy access to the original hospital records of the individual patients if necessary.

This register is a useful tool for studying factors behind diseases which can be caused by adverse drug reactions, such as agranulocytosis, liver disorders, anaphylaxis, digitalis intoxications, etc. The information available in the original patient records is the most important one for such studies if the data are adequately recorded by the doctor. The design of this Register and its data collection has been discussed elsewhere.[1]

## Register of Persons Entitled to Free Drugs

Since 1966 the National Health Insurance System in Finland has fully refunded the drug treatment of 47 severe chronic diseases such as heart failure, hypertension, diabetes, epilepsy and cancer. Concomitantly, a national register of persons entitled to free drugs was established. The register contains copies of doctors' prescriptions as well as the so-called B-certificate.[4] The right to free drug treatment is granted by a local social insurance committee after its medical adviser has inspected the physician's B-certificate. This is a standard form in which the patient's own doctor certifies the presence of the chronic condition in question. It also contains information on the patient's occupation, a brief history, the drugs used and the physician's clinical findings. Over 99% of persons who have been granted the right to free drugs take advantage of it.[4] The personal identification number is also used in this Register. Some 60 000 cases are reported annually and the cumulative number of cases in the data bank is close to 800 000 (Table 1).

## Register of Adverse Reactions to Drugs

The register for spontaneous notification of adverse reactions to drugs (ADRs) was established in Finland in 1966.[3] By using the social security number of the reported case, a record linkage is possible between the ADR data and data in other registries.

Based on the national drug consumption statistics at the National Board of Health an approximated number of users can be calculated for each drug. If a new, unexpected and severe ADR occurs we have been able to estimate the rate of exposure to the suspected drug. These data have enabled us to get rough incidence figures for some new

ADRs, although it is understandable that under-reporting of ADRs may further complicate this kind of evaluation.

## USE OF HEALTH SURVEILLANCE REGISTRIES TO MONITOR DRUGS

### Cancer Registry

A typical application of Medical Record Linkage was the testing of the hypothesis suggested by previous studies that treatment with rauwolfia derivatives may increase the risk of breast cancer.[4] Linkage between two nationwide registries, Cancer Registry and Register of Persons Entitled to Free Drugs, identified patients with and without breast cancer who had received drugs for hypertension. The relative risks from the use of rauwolfia, methyldopa and any other synthetic antihypertensives or diuretics used as antihypertensives ranged between 0.9 and 1.11. Thus, there was not a consistent drug-specific association between rauwolfia-use and breast cancer in hypertensive patients.

In 1976–77 PUVA treatment (oral psoralen plus long-wave ultraviolet light) was introduced in many countries as a new and effective treatment for psoriasis. Some preliminary findings suggested that certain groups of psoriatics may develop skin cancer during or after PUVA.[5] Therefore in 1979 we began a long-term study to monitor the safety of PUVA treatment.

Using the Hospital Discharge Register and Cancer Registry two groups were isolated: psoriatics treated with PUVA and psoriatics treated with other regimens. Since then the incidence of skin carcinomas has been intensively monitored in these two groups as well as in an age-matched group of general population. Our preliminary findings suggest that if patients with a history of earlier skin carcinomas are excluded from PUVA treatment, the number of skin cancers in PUVA-treated psoriatics does not exceed the expected incidence in the normal Finnish population.[6,7]

Härö linked the data in the Cancer Registry with the Finnish vaccination index to study the leukaemia risk in tuberculin-negative (BCG vaccinated), tuberculin positive (naturally T.B. infected) and in non-participants (those whose TB status is unknown in the Finnish Vaccination Index). His results suggested that BCG vaccinated and naturally T.B. infected persons had a considerably diminished risk of developing leukaemia compared to the non-participants many of whom have not been infected or vaccinated.[8]

### Malformation Register

In 1972 McBride suggested that there may be an association between imipramine use in early pregnancy and abnormal fetal development.[9]

The report was alarming, and prompted us to review in the space of a few weeks nearly 3000 maternal pairs in the files of the Finnish Register on Congenital Malformations. Three cases among study mothers had taken imipramine while none were found in the control group.[10] The finding was somewhat inconclusive due to the small number of cases, but it demonstrated that our data could be rapidly used to check a hypothesis launched elsewhere.

There has been one joint study with the Drug Epidemiology Unit at Boston University Medical Center in the USA. The data from a case/control study in the Finnish Register and the data from a prospective cohort study in USA were evaluated to study an association between birth defects and anticonvulsants/parental epilepsy.[11] In conclusion, the Finnish and American findings taken together confirmed that treated maternal epilepsy was associated with an increased incidence of malformations. In both studies, cleft palate anomalies were present in excess.

In 1975, Safra and Oakley reported directly to our Register that their preliminary findings seem to show that diazepam may cause congenital malformations.[12] The matter was urgently investigated in our files and an association between the intake of diazepam in early pregnancy and cleft palate in neonates was observed.[13] The sample was, however, small and further studies are required.

The use of oral contraceptives prior to or during pregnancy has been found to be teratogenic in some studies.[2] An analysis of 3002 maternal pairs taken from the matched-pair register from the years 1967–1976 (Table 2) gave no support to the hypothesis that contraceptives may induce birth defects.[14]

Most Finns go to sauna at least once a week. Sauna causes a short-term hyperthermia which has been suggested as being associated with an elevated risk of anencephaly and other CNS defects in the newborn.[2] These claims have met considerable scepticism in the Finnish scientific community. Saxen has studied the question in depth with the malformation register and concluded that the mild, short-term hyperthermia induced by the Finnish sauna should not be considered hazardous to the embryo.[15]

The Finns are among the heaviest coffee drinkers in the world. The

**Table 2** Analysis of discordant pairs according to the use of oral contraceptives (OC) among mothers of malformed children and their matched pairs[14]

| *Cases* | *Controls* | |
|---|---|---|
| | *No OC* | *With OC* |
| No OC | 2219 | 461 |
| with OC | 439 | 153 |

(Savolainen *et al.*, 1981)

**Table 3** Relative risk that can be excluded for heavy coffee drinking ($\geqslant$4 cups per day) during early pregnancy[16] (Assuming $\alpha = \beta = 0.05$ or $\alpha = \beta = 0.01$)

| *Birth defect* | *Odds ratio* | |
|---|---|---|
| | *0.05* | *0.01* |
| CNS defects | 3.0 | 4.1 |
| Oral clefts | 2.1 | 2.7 |
| Skeletal defects | 2.2 | 2.8 |
| Cardiovascular defects | 2.5 | 3.4 |
| Total | 1.6 | 1.8 |

(Kurppa *et al.*, 1982)

preliminary results from a study in the Malformation Register[16] do not support the claims that extensive consumption of coffee during pregnancy could be harmful to the fetus (Table 3).

Several other studies from the Finnish Malformation Register were recently reviewed by Saxen.[2]

## ADR Register

The spontaneous ADR reporting system, drug consumption data and the national morbidity/mortality statistics were used to verify the actual risk of fatal agranulocytosis with clozapine (Leponex). This promising anti-psychotic drug was introduced in Finland in January 1975. Five months later the first fatal case of agranulocytosis was reported to the ADR Register. Within 7 weeks seven cases of neutropaenia and ten additional cases of agranulocytosis (eight of them fatal) were reported. The risk of agranulocytosis among patients receiving clozapine was estimated to be 0.5–0.7% on the basis of drug utilization data.[1,17] The number of fatal cases of agranulocytosis induced by clozapine in 6 months was the same as the total number of all fatal agranulocytosis cases discovered annually in the country. The risks of clozapine were considered unacceptable and the drug was withdrawn from the market.[17]

A new tetracyclic antidepressant, mianserin, was introduced in Finland in 1979. The data accompanying the new drug application for marketing approval did not reveal any pattern of haematological disorders. Since 1980 there have been an increasing number of reports of blood dyscrasias to the ADR Register[18] and by the end of 1984 14 cases (two of them fatal) had been discovered (Table 4). Based on the ADR Register and drug consumption data the estimated annual frequency of mianserin associated agranulocytosis/neutropenia has been about 1/7000. Since 1980 over 50 cases of neutropenia/agranulocytosis with mianserin have been reported to ADR registries in other countries.[18]

**Table 4** Blood dyscrasias (agranulocytosis, granulocytopenia and leukopenia) associated with the use of mianserin in Finland, 1980–1984

| *Year* | *No. of reported cases in ADR Register* | *Annual incidence in users of mianserin* |
|---|---|---|
| 1980 | 1 | 1/5000 |
| 1981 | 2 | 1/5300 |
| 1982 | 3 | 1/6000 |
| 1983 | 3 | 1/5800 |
| 1984 | 5 | 1/7000 |

Levamisole seems to have an immunostimulant action, and it has been studied as an adjunct to conventional antineoplastic therapies in different types of cancer.[19] Among 174 patients with advanced breast cancer there were 17 reported cases of agranulocytosis in Finland.[20] According to other published data, levamisole-associated agranulocytosis seemed to be exceptionally common in the Finnish study population. Among some 2600 patients treated in clinical trials in various countries with levamisole there were 38 patients who developed agranulocytosis.

It is still unclear why the Finns so often develop agranulocytosis when exposed to drugs which seem comparatively safe in other populations.

Seven cases of pleurisy accompanied by effusion, pleural thickening and pulmonary infiltrates were reported in association with a high dose bromocriptine (Parlodel) treatment for Parkinson's disease in 1980. The drug consumption data showed that only 123 patients with Parkinson's disease had been exposed to such high doses of bromocriptine.[21] The discoveries initiated further studies to assess the relationship of the reactions to therapy.

There are several other drug safety dilemmas in which we have used the data from the ADR Register, the Hospital Discharge Register and the national drug consumption statistics. Examples of these are nitrofurantoin-induced eosinophilic lung reactions,[22] lactic acidosis occurring in diabetics treated with biguanides[23] and oesophageal ulcers caused by emepronium bromide tablets.[24]

## CONCLUSIONS

Health surveillance registries and medical record linking systems provide data which can be used for the detection of serious drug-induced illnesses. In addition, they can be used for the rapid testing of hypotheses, whether generated from within the surveillance systems itself or from other sources such as from animal experiments, clinical observations, anecdotal reports or adverse drug reaction registries.

## References


1. Idänpään-Heikkilä, J. (1977). Population monitoring: Medical record linkage for drug safety surveillance. In Gross, F. H. and Inman, W. H. W. (eds.) *Drug Monitoring*. pp. 17–26. (London/New York: Academic Press)
2. Saxen, L. (1983). Twenty years of study of the etiology of congenital malformations in Finland. In Kalter, H. (ed.) *Issues and Reviews in Teratology*, Vol. 1, pp. 73–110. (New York: Plenum Publishing Corp)
3. Idänpään-Heikkilä, J. (1982). Spontaneous notification. In Auriche, M., Burke, J., and Duchier, J. (eds.) *Drug Safety, Progress and Controversies*, pp. 73–82. (Pergamon Press)
4. Aromaa, A., Hakama, M., Hakulinen, T., Saxen, E., Teppo, L. and Idänpään-Heikkilä, J. (1976). Breast cancer and use of rauwolfia and other antihypertensive agents in hypertensive patients: A nationwide case-control study in Finland. *Int. J. Cancer*, **18**, 727
5. Stern, R. S., *et al.* (1979). Risk of cutaneous carcinoma in patients treated with oral methoxsalen photochemotherapy for psoriasis. *N. Engl. J. Med.*, **300**, 809
6. Lassus, A., Reunala, T., Idänpään-Heikkilä, J., Juvakoski, T. and Salo, O. (1981). PUVA treatment and skin cancer: A follow-up study. *Acta Dermat.*, **61**, 141
7. Eskelinen, A., Halme, K., Lassus, A. and Idänpään-Heikkilä, J. (1984). Risk of cutaneous carcinoma in psoriatic patients treated with PUVA. *Photodermatology* (in press)
8. Härö, A. S. (1983). Mass BCG vaccination, tuberculosis infection and leukemia risk. Register linkage study of long-term effects. In Crispen, R. G. (ed.) *Cancer: Etiology and Prevention*. pp. 419–433 (Amsterdam: Elsevier)
9. McBride, W. G. (1972). Limb deformities associated with iminodibenzyl hydrochloride. *Med. J. Austr.*, **1**, 492
10. Idänpään-Heikkilä, J. and Saxen, L. (1973). Possible teratogenicity of combination imipramine-antihistamine. *Lancet*, **2**, 282
11. Shapiro, S. *et al.* (1976). Anticonvulsants and parental epilepsy in the development of birth defects. *Lancet*, **1**, 272
12. Safra, M. J. and Oakley, G. P. (1975). Association between cleft lip with or without cleft palate and prenatal exposure to diazepam. *Lancet*, **2**, 478
13. Saxen, I. and Saxen, L. (1975). Association between maternal intake of diazepam and oral clefts. *Lancet*, **2**, 498
14. Savolainen, E., Saksela, E. and Saxen, L. (1981). Teratogenic hazards of oral contraceptives analyzed in a national Malformation Register. *Am. J. Obstet. Gynecol.*, **140**, 521
15. Saxen, L. *et al.* (1982). Sauna and congenital defects. *Teratology*, **25**, 309
16. Kurppa, K. *et al.* (1982). Coffee consumption during pregnancy. *N. Engl. J. Med.*, **306**, 1548
17. Idänpään-Heikkilä, J. *et al* (1977). Agranulocytosis during treatment with clozapine. *Eur. J. Clin. Pharmacol.*, **10**, 1
18. Idänpään-Heikkilä, J. (1985). Experience with international post-marketing surveillance of new drugs – some recent discoveries. In *Proceedings of the Drug Information Association Meeting*, June 1984, San Diego (In press)
19. Amery, W. K. and Butterworth, B. S. (1983). The dosage regimen on levamisole in cancer: Is it related to efficacy and safety? *Int. J. Immunopharmacol.*, **5**, 1
20. Teerenhovi, L., Heinonen, E., Gröhn, P., Klefström, P., Mehtonen, M. and Tilikainen, A. (1978). High frequency of agranulocytosis in breast-cancer patients treated with levamisole. *Lancet*, **2**, 151

21. Rinne, U. K. (1981). Pleuropulmonary changes during long-term bromocriptine treatment for Parkinson's disease. *Lancet*, **1**, 4
22. Sovijärvi, A. R. A., Lemola, M., Stenius, B. and Idänpään-Heikkilä, J. (1977). Nitrofurantoin-induced acute, subacute and chronic pulmonary reactions. *Scand. J. Resp. Dis.*, **58**, 41
23. Korhonen, T., Idänpään-Heikkilä, J. and Aro, A. (1978). Biguanide induced lactic acidosis in Finland. *Eur. J. Clin. Pharmacol.*, **15**, 407
24. Puhakka, H. J. (1978). Drug-induced corrosive injury of the oesophagus. *J. Laryngol. Otolaryngol.*, **92**, 927

# 6
# Italy

M. G. FRANZOSI and G. TOGNONI

## INTRODUCTION

The situation in Italy, in the field of drug evaluation and control, is one of a permanent polarization between the maintenance of the status quo – apparently the main objective of the central regulatory authority, and the launching of 'peripheral' initiatives by Regional Health Authorities, research groups and with the recent recruitment of representative organizations of general practitioners.[1–3]. Inevitably drug monitoring, which is at the centre of the process of drug evaluation and marketing, reflects this split.

This rather depressing situation was the main theme of this chapter in the first edition of this book. Since 1980, there have been a number of changes with respect to legislation on drug monitoring and related research. Some of the developments are outlined here.

## THE CENTRAL POLICY

The present central drug policy is unsatisfactory. No real skills or resources are available for drug evaluation during any phase of experimentation, registration, marketing approval, surveillance, advertising or withdrawal. Promising trends have been developed by the Regional Health Authorities, where a new, positive attitude towards drug control has been encouraged by the wide application of hospital formularies. These initiatives have been reluctantly recognized, in principle, by the government, but in practice they have been thwarted, and on a national scale, the National Health Service (NHS) drug policy has failed to ensure coherence between legislation and action.

The procedure for the approval of new drugs is strict, at least from the legal aspect. The practical application, however, is largely unsatisfactory. Mixtures of drugs and useless products are readily approved, while new molecules of potential or proven importance wait for months before trials can start. General guidelines for drug trials have never been set down, resulting in low-quality planning and research. When the Commission for drug trials was established in Lombardy, up to 85% of proposals had to be rejected on technical and sometimes ethical grounds during the first year. Prospects for the future are no better, if publication of the *Therapeutic Formulary* for the NHS and the new arrangements for drug information are taken as indicators. Criteria which largely depend on market conditions and on industry's vested interests have over-ridden pharmacological principles and health needs in guiding the selection of drugs to be included in categories of totally (i.e. essential), partially, or non-reimbursable drugs.[4]

This state of affairs at central levels fits the medical tradition in Italy, where teaching about the iatrogenic potential of drugs has always been ignored, if not positively denied. To quote only one well-known example: no chloramphenicol-induced aplastic anaemia was admitted to have occurred in Italy, until a publication reporting three fatal cases[5] made the long-held belief in the Italian population's 'genetic resistance' untenable.

Drug surveillance has been the topic of specific attention and legislative intervention by the State drug authorities (curiously enough with no reference to the WHO-National Centre described below). In the process of implementing the law instituting the NHS, the establishment of an efficient network for collecting data on drug effects was given high priority. The Government's response to this need fully reflects the defects in official understanding and planning. The text speaks for itself:

> The Ministry of Health will send doctors, through the local health authorities, supplies of cards prepared as per the model attached to the present law, on which to collect data on drug use.
>
> Doctors, in the context of their cooperation as required by existing legislation on the institution of NHS, will complete a card every time they encounter toxic, secondary or otherwise unexpected adverse reactions, either local or systemic, consequent to or at any rate related to the use of drugs. The firms holding permission to deal commercially in medicinal specialities are expected to collect these cards from doctors, using their detailmen (representatives) if necessary. Doctors may also send copies of the cards directly to the Ministry of Health, General Management of the Pharmaceutical Services.[6]

The strong criticism raised both by the content of the law and the way it was prepared and published (the term 'clandestine' has been used to define the procedure, and nobody could find a more appropriate one) resulted in the matter being put on ice. It was revived again some 18 months later. The long sleep does not seem to have been beneficial since drug monitoring is the only topic to have been literally untouched during the purely formal revision of the law.[7] In fact no concrete measures have been taken by the State to support the initiative, or at least to give it an appearance of reality.

## CURRENT REALITY AND EMERGING TRENDS

Why should a discussion of drug monitoring in Italy be of any interest in the light of the 'negative' information given so far? In our view, drug monitoring already has a place in Italy, and is likely to gain momentum if some leads, now in their formative stage, start to mature.

### The WHO monitoring scheme

A regional WHO monitoring centre was established in Ancona, Italy in September 1975, with a staff of eight physicians. A total of only 205 reports were received during the first year of activity. No qualitative analysis of data has been made available up to now. A booklet was issued containing a list of adverse effects collected over 3 years, cross-referenced with drugs and apparatus, but it gives no key to the origin, amount, or levels of validity of the reports.[8] This initiative has had little general impact among the medical profession, at least as far as making the philosophy and habit of drug monitoring more widely known and practised.

Since this report came out in 1980, no further reports have been published, although occasional summaries of clinically relevant notifications are circulated to the mailing list of the Italian edition of the *Adverse Drug Reactions Bulletin*.[9]

### Post-marketing surveillance

Because of the Government's formal requirements (see above), and, more importantly, because of the interest shown by a few groups working within the pharmaceutical industry, some recent theoretical and practical work has been done in the field of non-steroidal anti-inflammatory agents and of beta-blockers[10–12]. Some professional groups have also taken the initiative in performing post-marketing exercises.[13] The drugs chosen (e.g. carnitine) and the schemes adopted cannot be considered satisfactory, but this is at least a promising sign of the medical profession's readiness to take an active part in PMS programmes.

### Drug utilization studies and monitoring of drug prescriptions

Drug utilization studies offer a basis for problem-orientated investigations, including the assessment of prevalence or incidence of side-effects within defined populations.[14] This line of research has developed into more formal programmes outlined in Table 1. The activities which have been approved and incorporated into the National Research Council's 5-year plan are summarized.

A further promising activity is the development of a Drug Informa-

**Table 1**

| *Areas of interest* | *Protocol method* | *Population observed* |
|---|---|---|
| Prevalence of side-effects of anticonvulsant drugs | intensive surveillance of patients coming to the attention of various levels of health care | 52 hospital ambulatories |
| Patterns of drug use in pregnancy | interviews with women at parturition to be repeated every 3 years | 10% of the whole population of participating wards, for a total of ~5000 women |
| Monitoring of therapeutic strategies applied to post-infarct patients | integrated surveillance through hospital ambulatory records and GP involvement | ~3000 patients from 40 hospitals |
| Medical events associated with therapeutic interventions in ICU | *ad hoc* monitoring of prevalence in index-day | 35 ICUs |
| Psychotropic drug use in areas with different nursing facilities | monitoring medical records and assessment of the autonomy of a sample of the treated population, with specific attention to the elderly | 4500 patients, 25 in acute wards; 15 therapeutic communities; 40 long-term homes |

tion System for Local Health Authorities (*Sistema Informativo Farmaci – Unità Sanitaria Locale*: SIF–USL). Prescriptions provide administrative data for reimbursements to pharmacies (cf. the Prescription Pricing Authority (PPA) in England.[15] A system has been developed whereby prescriptions are translated into their generic names for further processing in terms of defined daily doses (DDDs), and for linkage with basic data identifying the prescribing doctor and the receiving patient.

The SIF–USL, developed on a research basis by two groups of pharmacologists and clinical pharmacists, is now adopted in several health areas, and will regularly provide 'denominator' or index cohorts of patients exposed to the various drugs. Newcomers in the market are obviously automatically flagged to provide a quick profile of the population's exposure, which for the first time will be available in detail for well defined territories and populations, outside the traditionally 'confidential' market surveys.

### Case-control studies

A cohort and case-control study on oral contraceptive associated risks, which were quoted as promising experiences in this chapter, in the first edition, have failed, as the majority of those physicians who had enthusiastically agreed to be part of the studies and who had gone through the pilot phase did not comply with the study protocols. Much has been learnt from such negative results, however, in terms of motivation strategies and organization.[16] A clear preference of case-control approach has been noted, and this has been intensively applied in order to create a permanent network of hospitals and other health care systems according to the model proposed by the Drug Epidemiology Unit.[17] Female hormone-related pathologies or disorders have been the primary object of interest.[18–20] The Italian arm of a continuing international study on agranulocytosis and aplastic anaemia[21] has recently closed its recruitment, and has now become a part of a case-control surveillance scheme, focussing on major acute events such as gastrointestinal haemorrhages, hepatic failure and acute renal insufficiency, as well as blood dyscrasias. A project is under way to provide a permanent network of nursing schools where problem-orientated interviewing of cases and controls is a routine part of the curriculum, cutting costs while at the same time spreading knowledge and awareness of this epidemiological technique.

## CONCLUSIONS

Despite the precarious standards of the national policy, the view that drug monitoring is important seems to be gaining ground in Italy. Besides the above mentioned case-control surveillance scheme, there has been the somewhat surprising success of very large scale clinical trials and of the prospective surveillance of cohorts of at risk populations such as the elderly treated for hypertension. Such studies have been able to recruit several thousand patients over a period of a few months[23] and is a hint at the potential of this sector within the medical profession (see Table 1 for other strategies and continuing projects). It is not being over-optimistic to say that drug monitoring is becoming one of the fastest moving sectors of epidemiology in Italy.

## References

1. Tognoni, G., Bellantuono, C., Colombo, F., Farina, M. L., Ferrario, L., Franzosi, M. G., Mancini, M. and Mandelli, M. (1978). Drug utilization strategies within regional programs on drug control and evaluation. In Duchêne-Marullaz, P. (ed.) *Advances in Pharmacology and Therapeutics*, (Clinical Pharmacology, vol. 6) pp. 101–12. (Oxford: Pergamon Press)
2. Franzosi, M. G., Colombo, F., Fiorica, E. and Tognoni, G. (1982). Drug information as seen from a Regional Drug Information Centre. In Ostino, G., Martini, N. and van der Kleijn (eds.) *Progress in Clinical Pharmacy IV*. pp. 115–22. (Amsterdam: Elsevier/North-Holland)
3. Editorial. (1982). Italy. Continuing education and research in general practice. *Lancet*, **2**, 653
4. Ministero della Sanità. (1978–1980–1983). Decreto 26 agosto 1978. Decreto 19 marzo 1980. Decreto 25 maggio 1983. *Gazzetta Ufficiale della Repubblica Italiana*
5. Masera, G., Uderzo, C., Brecher, A. and Tognoni, G. (1976). Il cloramfenicolo oggi. *Prospett. Pediatr.*, **22**, 245–55
6. Ministero della Sanità. (1981). Decreto 23 giugno 1981. Disciplina della attività di informazione scientifica sui farmaci. *Gazzetta Ufficiale della Repubblica Italiana*, No. 180, 2-7-1981
7. Ministero della Sanità. (1982). Decreto 23 novembre 1982. Disposizioni integrative e modificative del decreto ministeriale 23 guigno 1981, recante disciplina dell'attività di informazione scientifica sui farmaci. *Gazzetta Ufficiale della Repubblica Italiana*, No. 333, 3-12-1982
8. Centro Nazionale ITA-OMS di Farmacovigilanza. (1975–1978). Segnalazioni di reazioni avverse associate all'uso dei farmaci. No. 1
9. Notiziario del Centro Nazionale ITA-OMS di Farmacovigilanza. (1980–1983). *Adverse Drug Reaction Bull.* (edizione italiana): no. 15, 6/80, p. 60; no. 22, 8/81, p. 88; no. 32, 4/83, p. 128
10. Emanueli, A. and Sacchetti, G. (1981). Post-marketing surveillance methodology as applied in a Pharmaceutical Medical Department. *4th International Meeting of Pharmaceutical Physicians*. Paris, April, 27–30
11. Emanueli, A. and Viaro, D. (1982). Post-marketing surveillance: preliminary results with a non-steroidal anti-inflammatory drug. *International Meeting on Side-effects of Anti-inflammatory Analgesic Drugs*. Verona, September, 13–15
12. Maistrello, I. and Rigamonti, G. (1983). Adverse drug reactions: an algorithm for the follow-up of the findings of diagnostic procedures. *2nd World Conference on Clinical Pharmacology and Therapeutics*, Washington, DC, July 31–August 5, 1983 (Abstract no. 169, p. 30)
13. ANCE (1981). Come giudicare gli effetti collaterali dei farmaci. *Il Medico d'Italia*, Suppl. to no. 37–8
14. Tognoni, G., Liberati, A., Pellò, L., Sasanelli, F. and Spagnoli, A. (1983). Drug utilization studies and epidemiology. *Rev. d'Epidemiol. Santé Publ.*, **31**, 59–71
15. Andreani, A., Colombo, F., Fiorica, E., Mandelli, M., Mosconi, P., Tognoni, G., Bozzini, L. and Martini, N. (1983). SIF–USL: A drug information system for administrative and epidemiological use. In Fernandez Perez de Talens, A.,

Luzzana, M. and Palumbo, M. (eds.) *Health Information System: The Italian Approach.* pp. 61–4 (MEDINFO 83 Special Session X3)

16. Pello, L., Begher, C., Mancini, M., Tognoni, G. and Crosignani, P. G. (1982). Risultati di 'non risultati'? Il caso di una ricerca epidemiologica sui contraccettivi orali. *Medicina, Riv. EMI,* **2,** 200–2
17. Slone, D., Shapiro, S. and Miettinen, O. S. (1977). Case-control surveillance of serious illnesses attributable to ambulatory drug use. In Colombo, F., Shapiro, S., Slone, D. and Tognoni, G. (eds.) *Epidemiological Evaluation of Drugs.* pp. 59–77 (Amsterdam: Elsevier/North-Holland)
18. Franceschi, S., La Vecchia, C., Helmich, S. P., Mangioni, C. and Tognoni, G. (1982). Risk factors for epithelial ovarian cancer in Italy. *Am. J. Epidemiol.,* **115,** 714
19. La Vecchia, C., Liberati, A. and Franceschi, S. (1982). Non-contraceptive estrogen use and the occurrence of ovarian cancer. *J. Nat. Cancer Inst.,* **69,** 1207
20. La Vecchia, C., Franceschi, S., Gallus, G., Decarli, D., Colombo, E., Liberati, A. and Tognoni, G. (1982). Prognostic features of endometrial cancer in estrogen users and obese women. *Am. J. Obstet. Gynecol.,* **144,** 387–90
21. International Agranulocytosis and Aplastic Anemia Study. (1983). The design of a study of the drug etiology of agranulocytosis and aplastic anemia. *Eur. J. Clin. Pharmacol.,* **24,** 833–6
22. Shapiro, S. (1984). Agranulocytosis and pyrazolone. *Lancet,* **1,** 451–2
23. Tognoni, G., Franzosi, M. G. (1984). Tra sperimentazione clinica ed epidemiologia: sovrapposizioni, confini, ricerca. In Tognoni, G., Laporte, J. R. (eds). *Epidemiologia del Farmaco.* pp. 157–69. (Roma: Il Pensiero Scientifico Editore)

# 7
# Japan

H. KOMIYA

## INTRODUCTION

In Japan, there has been an increasing awareness of the importance of post-marketing surveillance (PMS), not only by the government, but also in the pharmaceutical industry and among academic institutions and health professionals.

PMS by the Japanese government was given a big boost when the 1979 revision of the Pharmaceutical Affairs Law introduced the 'Re-examination System for New Drugs' and other provisions. This amendment was intended to ensure the quality, efficacy and safety of drugs.

The Japanese System for Collection and Dissemination of ADR Information is shown in Figure 1.

The main routes for collection of ADR information under this scheme are: the National Drug Monitoring System (prescription drugs-oriented), the National Pharmacy Monitoring System (over-the-counter drugs-oriented), the Re-examination System for New Drugs, and ADR reporting from the industry.

The data collected via these routes are carefully examined by the ADR subcommittees in the Central Pharmaceutical Affairs Council for possible causal relationships between a drug and an event, severity of an event, and reversibility of ADR signs or symptoms. Depending on the contents of the advisory report from the subcommittee, rapid, pertinent administrative action is taken.

Furthermore, the manufacturer (or importer) of the drug involved is instructed to pass on the information without delay to the medical profession by way of package inserts, 'Dear Doctor' letters, etc. At the same time, the Ministry of Health and Welfare (MHW) also transmits the information and administrative action to the monitoring hospitals (addressed also to their dispensary departments) and reporting doctors by means of the bulletin entitled *Adverse Drug Reaction Information* (on prescription drugs). The ADR information is also

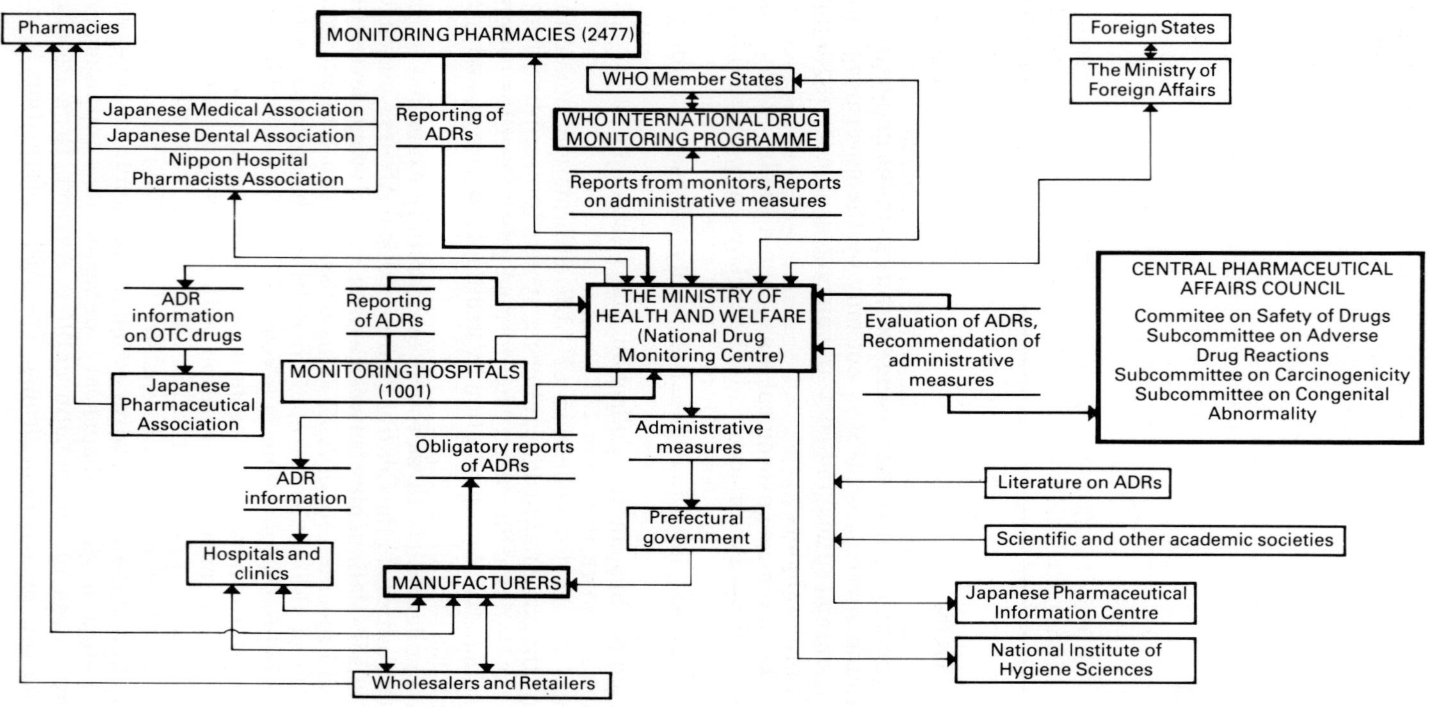


**Figure 1** System for collection and dissemination of adverse drug reaction information.

published in various medical and pharmaceutical periodicals for broader dissemination of ADR information. For over-the-counter (OTC) drugs, the bulletin entitled *Pharmacy Drug Monitoring* serves the same purpose. Moreover, as shown in Figure 1, the MHW is constantly exchanging ADR information with WHO and governments of foreign countries as well as with the Japanese Medical Association, prefectural governments, and National Institute of Hygiene Sciences.

## THE NATIONAL DRUG MONITORING SYSTEM

The National Drug Monitoring system was inaugurated in Japan in 1967 as a voluntary reporting system. This system has been operated by the Japanese government, with its centre located in the Pharmaceuticals and Chemicals Safety Division of the Pharmaceutical Affairs Bureau of the MHW. At its inception, a total of 192 national and university hospitals were designated as 'monitoring hospitals'. Since then, the number of reporting hospitals has steadily increased, until by August, 1982 a total of 1001 hospitals, comprising 101 national hospitals, 138 university hospitals, 345 public hospitals and 417 other hospitals, were on the MHW's roster of monitoring hospitals. All these hospitals have been asked to report ADRs to the National Drug Monitoring Centre. The reporting of ADRs is not a legal obligation but doctors who encounter ADRs are expected to report them to the Centre.

The primary purpose of this system is to alert the medical profession to ADRs which are either 'novel' or serious, and to take pertinent action towards ensuring drug safety as quickly as possible.

### ADRs – what should be reported

The following types of adverse reactions should be reported to the National Drug Monitoring Centre.

(1) Undesirable reactions to drugs which were not foreseen at the time of treatment by the usual administration schedule (dosage and route).
(2) Undesirable reactions which are serious or abnormal.
(3) Other undesirable reactions which the doctors consider important or worth reporting.

### Reporting form

In the monitoring hospitals, doctors may use one of two different reporting forms which are provided by the Centre. Form 1 is a 14-item brief, pre-paid, envelope-type reporting form, whilst Form 2 is for more detailed reporting. Any reporting doctor is rewarded for each report by a small sum of cash and also receives a free 2-year subscription to *ADR Information*.

## Trend in ADR reporting

The number of ADR reports submitted annually to MHW from the monitoring hospitals is shown in Table 1. It can be seen that the number has been steadily increasing, and since 1981 has reached about 800 per year.

**Table 1** Number of adverse reaction reports submitted from monitoring hospitals, 1966–1983

| *Fiscal year* | *No. of reports* | *Fiscal year* | *No. of reports* |
|---|---|---|---|
| 1966 | 3 | 1976 | 416 |
| 1967 | 44 | 1977 | 456 |
| 1968 | 595 | 1978 | 530 |
| 1969 | 293 | 1979 | 712 |
| 1970 | 200 | 1980 | 669 |
| 1971 | 338 | 1981 | 816 |
| 1972 | 271 | 1982 | 822 |
| 1973 | 360 | 1983 | 766 |
| 1974 | 285 | | |
| 1975 | 336 | *Total* | 7912 |

Table 2 shows these ADR reports classified into pharmacotherapeutic categories. Antibiotics top the list of the drugs involved, followed by CNS (central nervous system) drugs and synthetic chemotherapeutic drugs. The drugs mentioned most often in the ADR reports during 1980 and 1983 tended to be those which are used most frequently, for example antibiotics such as amoxicillin, cefalexin; antipyretic–analgesic–anti-inflammatory drugs such as indomethacin, mefenamic acid, piroxicam and topical drugs such as betamethasone oxalate. Of the reported adverse reactions, dermatological symptoms such as skin rash and pruritus were the most frequent, accounting for approximately 30–40%, followed by gastrointestinal symptoms such as nausea, abdominal pain and diarrhoea, and blood disorders such as leukocytopenia and anaemia.

Some of the ADR reports pointed to the possible hazards of several ADRs then unknown in Japan, while others provided at least *prima facie* evidence of some ADRs which had not been expected in view of experience with other drugs of the same category.

These reports led to the immediate institution of counter measures including revision of 'Precautions' in the package inserts, distribution

**Table 2** Adverse reaction reports by pharmacotherapeutic category of drugs, 1967–1983

| | *Fiscal year* | | | | |
|---|---|---|---|---|---|
| | *1967–74* | *1975–77* | *1978–80* | *1981–83* | *Total* |
| Number of reports | 2389 | 1208 | 1911 | 2404 | 7912 |
| Number of suspected drugs | 2635 | 1343 | 2159 | 2885 | 9022 |
| *Category* | *Adverse reactions* | | | | |
| Antibiotics | 817 (31.0%) | 362 (27.0%) | 551 (25.5%) | 725 (25.1%) | 2455 (27.2%) |
| CNS drugs | 356 (13.5%) | 258 19.2%) | 385 (17.8%) | 570 (19.8%) | 1569 (17.4%) |
| Drugs for dermatological application | 263 (10.0%) | 219 (16.3%) | 235 (10.9%) | 301 (10.4%) | 1018 (11.3%) |
| Chemotherapeutic drugs | 273 (10.4%) | 82 (6.1%) | 113 (5.2%) | 119 (4.1%) | 587 (6.5%) |
| Cardiovascular drugs | 146 (5.5%) | 119 (8.9%) | 192 (8.9%) | 271 (9.4%) | 728 (8.1%) |
| Miscellaneous drugs | 780 (29.6%) | 303 (22.6%) | 683 (31.6%) | 899 (31.2%) | 2665 (29.5%) |

of 'Dear Doctor' letters, intensive surveillance by the industry and so on.

## Follow-up of ADR reports

When additional information, such as a more detailed case history, outcome or laboratory test results, is considered to be necessary for an accurate interpretation of the event, the request is made to the reporting physician by letter or telephone.

When case reports are too few to permit a positive judgement on the causal relation between the drug and the ADR, we ask all monitoring hospitals to report, once a year, all the adverse reactions they encounter with certain designated drugs, regardless of whether these drugs are new or of long standing.

## Confidentiality

The identity of the patient, reporting doctor and monitoring hospital is held in strict confidence. As in other countries, doctors are very concerned about the possibility that their reports might be used in a charge of negligence against them or as evidence in lawsuits. The rationale is that doctors should not be exposed to public censure or involved in litigations on account of their co-operating with the Centre.

We guarantee that we will use ADR reports only for drug safety measures and never for other purposes. Should it be felt necessary to pass on any individual case report, we delete the names of the patient, the reporting doctor and the monitoring hospital, and cover up all other details which might otherwise reveal their identities.

## ADR reports from manufacturers and 'Re-examination System for New Drugs'

The MHW's request that drug manufacturers report ADRs relating to their products has been in effect since 1976. The 1979 amendment to the Pharmaceutical Affairs Law made the reporting legally binding.

Under the new law, for new drugs, the manufacturers are under the legal obligation to submit information each year on the use of their drugs, ADRs and the results of surveys, usually for 6 years, following approval of manufacture. The information is reported on the form 'Report on Investigation of Adverse Reactions and Other Results of Use of New Drugs'.

Manufacturers should be expected to collect about 10 000 drug experience reports in the first 2–3 years after approval, and compare the data with those obtained during the pre-marketing phase. They should then continue the surveillance with emphasis on some specific hypothesis or hypotheses generated by the above procedure.

Re-examination usually takes place after 6 years of marketing experience with a particular drug. Applications for re-examination are submitted to the MHW, and sufficient evidence of safety and efficacy must be presented before clearance is given.

In addition to the above requirements and measures, and regardless of whether the drugs are new or not, all the manufacturers are required to report new or serious ADRs, and to pass on important research reports relating to their products to the MHW within 30 days from the date they first become known to them.

## The Pharmacy Drug Monitoring System

The Pharmacy Drug Monitoring system was instituted in 1978 for a systematic monitoring of mild ADRs due to OTC drugs, with the participation of 2477 pharmacies designated by the MHW among some 33 000 pharmacies in Japan.

Pharmacists in the monitoring pharmacies are required to inform the MHW twice a year of any ADRs which they suspect are due to OTC drugs, and all the cases reported by consumers.

The Ministry passes on the reports annually, with its comments, to the monitoring pharmacies by way of the bulletin *Pharmacy Drug Monitoring*. These reports are also published elsewhere for the benefit of all pharmacists.

# 8
# The Netherlands

**R. H. B. MEYBOOM**

## INTRODUCTION

The population of the Netherlands is approximately 14 million. The total number of medical doctors, is approximately 28 900. There are 5700 general practitioners and 10 300 specialists (mostly hospital-based). There are 1600 doctors employed in social medicine in addition to those already included in the GP and specialist figures. The remaining 12 300 doctors includes hospital trainees. There are about 5300 dentists. There are about 1500 pharmacists (excluding pharmacists working in pharmaceutical companies but including 92 hospital pharmacists. There are 1133 pharmacies. In addition, about 1000 general practitioners provide independent pharmaceutical services.

The Netherlands do not have a national health service comparable to that of the United Kingdom, but the majority of people (70%) are compulsory members of one of the several health insurance funds which are all affiliated.

Since 1963, an independent Drug Regulatory Committee has been operating a licensing system. As in the United Kingdom, all drugs on the market before this time were automatically given a provisional license. A number of drugs are still being reviewed.

There are about 3500 different brands of medicine, but the actual number of compounds and mixtures is no more than 2000.

## THE NETHERLANDS CENTRE FOR MONITORING OF ADVERSE REACTIONS TO DRUGS

A nationwide voluntary reporting scheme was started in the Netherlands in 1963, and this developed into the present Netherlands Centre for Monitoring of Adverse Reactions to Drugs (NARD). The NARD is a subunit of the Central Drug Inspectorate of the Ministry of Welfare, Public Health and Culture. It has a permanent staff of three medical officers.

The NARD has the support of an advisory committee for the interpretation of data and for decision-making as regards the appropriate actions to be taken. The NARD and its advisory committee are independent of the drug licensing committee, although there is close collaboration between them.

NARD's objectives are:

(1) The early detection of hitherto unknown adverse reactions to drugs,
(2) The assessment of the practical significance of adverse drug effects,
(3) The dissemination of information on drug hazards, and
(4) The initiation of in-depth studies and the development of improved methods for drug safety monitoring.

Up to the present time, the case reporting scheme, which is not compulsory, has been the main source of information on ADRs in the Netherlands. In the past few years the annual number of case reports has increased from 500 to 1000. Sixty percent of the reports come from general practitioners and 40% from hospital doctors. Occasionally, reports are received from dentists, pharmacists or the drug industry.

The case reports are confidential: not only with regard to the identities of the patients and the reporting doctors, but also the suspected drug-adverse reaction associations. It is the Committee's responsibility to advise on the disclosure and publication of the reported data. The decision-making process involved is a scientific and medical ethical issue.

For a national voluntary reporting scheme there is an optimal reporting rate which depends on factors such as the size of the population, the number of physicians, the number of drugs and drug combinations marketed and the size of the centre's medical staff and processing capacity. Below the optimum, the system will be unreliable, whereas the receipt of a very large number of reports could overwhelm the system so that the material would not be used to its best advantage. The optimum reporting number in the Netherlands appears to be in the range of about 4000 cases a year.

High priority is given to evaluating and following up the individual case report. After checking the authenticity of a report, the reaction is assessed in the light of previous knowledge, e.g. published data, file reports and information from the WHO Collaborating Centre for International Drug Monitoring. Frequently, additional information is required, and it may be necessary to retrieve the report at a later stage in order to identify an underlying disease which may have become apparent in the meantime. For this purpose the patient's name or identification code is essential.

Special attention is given to the likelihood of a causal relationship between drug and suspected reaction. This assessment is based mainly on the association in time (including 'dechallenge' and 'rechallenge') and sometimes place, knowledge of the drug, clinical or pathological characteristics of the phenomenon and the exclusion of alternatives. The relative importance of these criteria may differ considerably. Reactions may in this context be divided into: contact reactions, immediate reactions, immuno-allergic reactions, pharmacological effects, malignant or congenital disorders.

For internal use, the case reports are classified into one of the following categories of likelihood of causality:

(1) *Not classified*: incomplete or conflicting data. A malignancy or malformation is only classified when there are very special reasons to suspect the drug.

(2) *Unlikely (but not excluded)*: time relation seems inappropriate; another cause more likely (but not proven).

(3) *Possible (meaning not impossible)*, when the time relation is appropriate: a trivial event which may be a coincidence; an objective event which is unknown or is inexplicable as a reaction to the suspected drug; an immunologic reaction to a rarely sensitizing drug; another drug or cause is equally suspected; as (4) but with fewer details.

(4) *Plausible*: consistent with a reaction to suspected drug; good reasons for assuming causality but no proof; no likely alternative; a contact reaction; an immediate reaction; an objective or characteristic event and known or explicable as a reaction to the drug; an immunologic reaction to a frequently sensitizing drug or a characteristic reaction to the drug; a subjective event with positive rechallenge; as (5) but with fewer details.

(5) *Convincing*: well-documented case, all evidence implicates the drug, outcome as expected, alternatives ruled out; an objective event, convincing rechallenge; an objective event, known or explicable reaction to the drug.

The main aim is to differentiate between the unlikely or the uncertain reports on the one hand ((1), (2) and (3) above), and the reliable case reports on the other ((4) and (5)). On average, the full assessment of a case report takes about 2 hours. Although it is envisaged that a computer will be used in the near future, at present the reports are processed by hand using the WHO terminologies.

Since reporting is entirely voluntary, there are limits to the extent to which inquiries can be made without irritating doctors and discouraging them from continued reporting.

We encourage the reporting of any suspected complication of a relatively new drug and all the serious suspected reactions to other drugs, but this is not a rigid guideline. If a doctor considers a case sufficiently important to report it, then we believe it is worthy of our attention.

## RESULTS AND FEED-BACK

Despite its many shortcomings, experience in our country shows that spontaneous monitoring can provide useful information.

The dilemma of the early warning principle is that one wishes to provide information on new reactions as early as possible, while ensuring that the generation of a false alarm or the dissemination of unbalanced information is prevented. Some countries, including the Netherlands have reservations about the public use of the data, while in others data on reported suspected reactions are readily available – for example in Australia.

In the Netherlands, the NARD reports at monthly intervals to the drug registration authority so that the necessary regulatory actions can be taken. In the case of new or serious reactions, the medical and pharmaceutical professions are informed on an *ad hoc* basis by direct mailing or by publications in the *Netherlands Medical Journal*, in the governmental *Drug Bulletin* or other journals, or in the *Side Effects of Drugs* series.

Examples in which the case reporting scheme has provided early information on adverse reactions are listed below:

| | |
|---|---|
| Glafenine | anaphylactic shock;[1] hepatitis[2] |
| Benzydamine | visual and psychic effects[3] |
| Azapropazone | photodermatitis |
| Lorazepam | withdrawal reactions[4] |
| Aprindine | agranulocytosis[5] |
| Metrizamide | aseptic meningitis[6] |
| Triazolam | hyperaesthetic psychosis; amnesia |
| Nomifensine | fever; hepatitis[7] |
| Camazepam | rash |
| Cimetidine | interstitial nephritis[8] |
| Ticlopidine | agranulocytosis; thrombocytopenia[9] |
| Valproic acid | adult hyperammonaemia[10] |
| Ketoconazole | hepatitis;[11] anaphylactic reactions[12] |
| Mianserin | thrombocytopenia[13] |
| Pinaverium-bromide | oesophagitis[14] |

A number of drug–drug interactions have also been traced at an early stage:

*Azopropazone*: potentiates coumarin anticoagulants (1973)[15]

*Anticonvulsants*: cause reduction in efficacy of oral contraceptives (1974)[16]

*Vitamin K-containing dietary products*, e.g. ('Modifast'): cause inhibition of anticoagulants – and increased coumarin effect after stopping the diet (1982)[17]

*Flurbiprofen*: potentiates coumarin anticoagulants (1982)[18]

*Griseofulvin*: causes reduction in efficacy of oral contraceptives.[58]

The azapropazone-coumarin interaction was 'rediscovered' 4 years later in the English literature.[20,21]

Sometimes new adverse effects come to light which are caused by drugs which have been in use for many years. The case reporting scheme may also be of value in this situation, as is illustrated by the following examples:

| | |
|---|---|
| Phenprocoumon | hepatitis[22] |
| Tetracycline | oesophageal damage[23] |
| Salazosulphapyridine | infertility |
| Nitrofurantoin | parotitis[24] |
| Nalidixic acid | thrombocytopenia[25] |
| Spironolactone | agranulocytosis[26] |

Sometimes, adverse reactions appear to be forgotten. The reporting scheme can help to refresh our memory. It has, for example, reminded us that ergotamine can cause superficial phlebitis, and that methyldopa can cause pancreatitis.[27]

For many drugs there are no accurate data on the frequency of adverse reactions. Moreover, quantitative data may refer to obsolete studies in foreign countries or to selected groups of patients and are therefore of limited value.

In the absence of more precise estimates, the case reporting scheme may provide a useful guide to the practical importance of the adverse reactions to certain drugs, and may identify the most important causes of specific types of reactions. For example, among 90 case reports of suspected drug-induced granulocytopenia, pyrazolone derivatives were involved in 42 cases, of which 20 were accounted for by noramidopyrinemethanesulphonate (dipyrone). Cytostatic drugs were not included.[28]

On another occasion, 84 out of 116 reports of anaphylactic reactions over a 28-month period referred to analgesics, of which 66 (57%) could be accounted for by one drug alone: glafenine.

## THE 'TRIAZOLAM SYNDROME'

The Dutch experience with triazolam attracted international attention. The first countries to register this potent and very short-acting hypnotic drug were Belgium (March 1977) and the Netherlands (November 1977). From January 1978, triazolam was vigorously promoted in the Netherlands as a safe, first-choice hypnotic, and was soon being used by a large number of people.[29] By July 1979 the NARD had received about 30 reports on triazolam, some describing serious reactions, others referring to rather unusual perceptive complaints. One of the reporting doctors, Dr C. van der Kroef, interviewed several of his patients during a popular television programme.

In order to assess the nature of the problem, the NARD sent a letter to doctors asking for reports of reactions to triazolam. As a result, within several weeks we had received approximately 1100 case reports from more than 700 physicians, exceeding the number of reports on all other drugs in that year.

Characteristic symptoms included: paraestesiae, photophobia, pains and hyperacusis, other sensory disturbances, anxiety, depression, unreality, depersonalization, paranoia and amnesia.

Since triazolam had at that time only very recently been introduced in most countries, little information on the drug was available from these sources. (In some countries the drug has still not been approved, for example in Sweden and Australia and in the United States it was not approved until November 1982.) Because of the strong suspicion of serious toxicity, the Dutch product license was suspended, and since the new conditions for registration imposed by the Medicines Committee were not accepted by the manufacturer, the license was terminated.

The essence of the debate is whether triazolam differs significantly from other benzodiazepines with respect to side effects. As early as 1976, Kales *et al.* described the occurrence of remarkable nightly episodes in two out of seven patients taking 0.5 mg triazolam.[29] One patient arose during the night to prepare lunch for her children, but had no recollection of this activity in the morning. The second patient experienced a gallbladder attack during a night in a sleep laboratory, but in spite of the considerable pain and emotional stress experienced during the attack, had no memory of it the next day.

In Canada, one of the few other countries with early experience of triazolam, the approved product information for 1978 already listed several of the symptoms which were reported in our country. These included restlessness, irritability, taste alterations, burning eyes, visual disturbances, tinnitus, palpitations, impaired co-ordination, confusion, depression and hallucinations. A special warning about anterograde amnesia was also given.

As well as Van der Kroef,[30] Einarson,[31] Einarson and Yoder,[32] Trappler and Bezeredi,[33] Mostert[34] and Rudnick[35] have reported serious reactions after triazolam. Case reports to the drug authorities in Denmark,[36] the United Kingdom,[37] and Canada,[38] although fewer in number, also show a pattern for triazolam which differs from benzodiazepines with a long half-life, and recent experiences in the United States[39] and in France[40] are reminiscent of the reports in the Netherlands.

Van der Kroef has reviewed 56 patients and presented a decription of the 'triazolam syndrome.[41] In addition, the results have been published of an analysis of data on 356 such patients.[42]

An interesting hypothesis later emerged from two British studies. Petursson and Lader reported on 16 benzodiazepine-dependent subjects in whom the drug was gradually withdrawn.[43] During the withdrawal period, these patients experienced symptoms which are strikingly similar to those already described for triazolam. In another study, Tyrer and co-workers also observed triazolam-like experiences in a series of patients after withdrawal of lorazepam or diazepam.[44]

Recently, work by Ashton has confirmed these studies.[45] She has given a masterly description of the characteristics and the severity of the benzodiazepine withdrawal syndrome, and has pointed out that the symptoms may develop in patients still taking the drug (tolerance).

Morgan and Oswald demonstrated increased daytime anxiety in patients on triazolam as compared with the long-acting loprazolam.[47] Scharf and Jacoby found significant withdrawal anxiety and feelings of panic on stopping the short-acting lorazepam.[48] Serious withdrawal reactions to benzodiazepines, especially the short-acting ones, have been described by several other authors.[48,49,50]

The evidence now available indicates that besides the pharmacological addiction to benzodiazepines, there appears to be a benzodiazepine withdrawal syndrome which is characterized by emotional and perceptive hypersensitivity, insomnia[51] and sometimes delirium and convulsions.[53] Anterograde amnesia is a well known benzodiazepine effect, which is therapeutically exploited for minor surgical interventions or pregnancy termination.[53] Although most experience has related to the intravenous use of diazepam, oral lorazepam[47] and flunitrazepam[54] have also been shown to cause amnesia.

Although in Canada a special warning about amnesia was included in the data sheet on triazolam, no reference to this side effect had been made in the Netherlands.

The occurrence of amnesia with triazolam has recently been confirmed by Shader and Greenblatt.[56] Periodical amnesia in Western life is a disturbing phenomenon, and one might even question whether amnesia is acceptable in a drug used for 'out-patient' treatment of insomnia.

It is noteworthy that in the United Kingdom triazolam is used in 0.125 mg and 0.25 mg tablets, and that the recommended dose for geriatric patients is only 0.125 mg, whereas in the Netherlands 0.5 and 1.0 mg tablets are most frequently used. Since benzodiazepine side effects are dose-related the two or four-fold difference in dosage may have accounted for the apparent differences between these two countries. A distinct difference between triazolam and other benzodiazepine hypnotics is its very short half-life of about 2 hours. With barbiturates and opiates, there is a direct relation between the severity of withdrawal symptoms and the shortness of the withdrawal time. Long-acting benzodiazepines on the other hand, by delaying and spreading the adaptation process mitigate the effects of withdrawal, as has been shown for rebound insomnia.

In summary, in 1979 a relatively large number of case reports were received on triazolam, describing unusual and often severe symptoms. Although the existence of a special problem with triazolam has been denied,[56] the occurrence of these reactions has been confirmed in several countries where triazolam has since been approved. Many questions regarding triazolam reactions can now be understood in the light of the recent recognition of a distinct benzodiazepine withdrawal syndrome. Presumably, the reactions to this strong but short-acting drug, develop as a result of the rapid and recurrent succession of strong benzodiazepine effects and subsequent withdrawal states. So far, the exact frequency of these reactions has remained uncertain. Presumably reactions are uncommon when low doses are used. It should, however, be emphasized that serious complications have been encountered in patients on 0.25 mg triazolam per 24 hours, and that in a number of cases the relationship with the drug may have been overlooked.

## COLLABORATION WITH OTHER INSTITUTIONS

Drug safety monitoring is not a separate science. It has strong links with clinical pharmacology on the one hand and general epidemiology on the other. Adverse effects frequently mimic natural diseases. The slow development of drug epidemiology in our country is considered to be a major drawback.

The NARD encourages the development of special registers: drug-induced eye disorders; skin reactions (Dr Bruinsma's 'skin reactions' – see Chapter 24); blood dyscrasias; congenital malformations; interactions with anticoagulants; and intensive monitoring of selected drugs of patients groups – for example antirheumatic drugs and drug use in pregnancy. So far, the results have not been very satisfactory.

The NARD participates in the WHO Collaborating Centre for International Drug Monitoring in Uppsala. This institute gives important support to our work, as is probably the case in other countries.[57] The NARD maintains a direct exchange of information with national agencies in many countries.

## LITERATURE

As many other centres will have experienced, maintaining a reliable, up-to-date literature information system is an arduous and never-ending task. Although much information can be obtained from reference books and commercial data bases, a national monitoring agency is expected to be well informed about data which cannot be found in these sources. The very new and the old literature present special problems. There is a considerable delay before new data are published, and there are good examples of old but pertinent data on adverse reactions which have simply disappeared from recent text books.

Relevant data on adverse reactions are published in very many medical, pharmaceutical and related journals, congress reports and books. Frequently, suspicions are first aroused in the correspondence sections of medical journals, hidden amongst a variety of unrelated topics.

The NARD screens some 70 periodicals for new information to follow trends and to recognize early pointers to new problems. The

Iowa Drug Information System is used in addition to current textbooks and our own index-card system, and computer searches can be made by the governmental library.

## RELATIONS WITH THE DRUG INDUSTRY

The NARD has no obligation to report to the industry, and there is no routine information of the drug firms. When reviewing a particular problem relating to ADRs, the knowledge and experience of scientists working in industrial research can be invaluable. Although considerable pressure is sometimes used by the drug firms to try to gain access to details of individual case reports, as a rule this information is refused because of their confidential nature. Information is usually limited to the type of the reaction and the number of reports and may only be used for internal purposes. Specific questions will be answered, although there may be a time problem.

## THE FUTURE

In the Netherlands, the following developments are envisaged. The NARD will disseminate the results of the reporting scheme more regularly in future, so that information will reach the prescribing doctor sooner. It is hoped that the number of case reports will increase and their quality improve.

It is our belief that intensive hospital monitoring is an important addition to 'voluntary reporting', and is very much needed in our country. The importance of the availability of drug utilization data is recognized. The possibility of using health insurance funds for this purpose is being studied. Fundamental research into the exact pathogenesis of adverse reactions, such as genetic differences and the development of specific immunological tests are expected to provide tools for the identification of patients at risk and the demonstration of the causative agents.

Finally, we are particularly interested in the various new methods which are now being developed or tested, such as prescription event monitoring (see Chapter 15). In this respect, it is hoped that changing attitudes and understanding may overcome the traditional obstacles, in particular the secrecy of drug use, which have seriously hindered the identification of those populations exposed to certain drugs, and of the assessment of the true frequencies of adverse reactions to drugs.

### References

1. Meyboom, R. H. B. (1976). Anafylaxie na het gebruik van glafenine. *Ned. T. Geneesk*, **120**, 926

2. Stricker, B. H. C. and Meyboom, R. H. B. (1979). Hepatitis bij gebruik van glafenine. *Pharm. Weekbl.*, **114,** 405
3. Meyboom, R. H. B. (1975). Merkwaardige verschijnselen tijdens het gebruik van benzydamine (Tantum). *Ned. T. Geneesk.*, **119,** 1044
4. Broek, G. P. L. A. van den. (1975). Temesta – addictie. *Med. Contact.*, **30,** 1458
5. Leeuwen, R. van and Meyboom, R. H. B. (1976). Agranulocytosis and aprindine. *Lancet*, **2,** 1137
6. Dukes, M. N. G. and Ansell, G. (1980). Radiological contrast media and radiopharmaceuticals. In Dukes, M. N. G. (ed.) *Meyler's Side Effects of Drugs*. pp. 749. (Amsterdam–Oxford–Princeton: Excerpta Medica)
7. Dankbaar, H. and Mudde, A. H. (1980). Koorts en leverfunctiestoornissen ten gevolge van nomifensine (Alival). *Ned. T. Geneesk.*, **124,** 2184
8. Stricker, B. H. C. and Reith, C. B. (1980). Ernstige nierfunctiestoornis tijdens gebruik van cimetidine (Tagamet). *Ned. T. Geneesk.*, **124,** 2183
9. Fraiture, W. H. de, Claas, F. H. J. and Meyboom, R. H. B. (1982). Bijwerkingen van ticlopidine; klinische waarneming en immunologisch onderzoek. *Ned. T. Geneesk.*, **126,** 1051
10. Stricker, B. H. C. (1982). Leverbeschadiging door valproïnezuur. *Ned. T. Geneesk.*, **126,** 2111
11. Dijke, C. P. H. van. (1983). Hepatitis tijdens gebruik van ketoconazol (Nizoral). *Ned. T. Geneesk.*, **127,** 339–41
12. Van Dijke, C. P. H., Veerman, F. R. and Haverkamp, H. C. (1983). Anaphylactic reactions to ketoconazole. *Br. Med. J.*, **287,** 1673–4
13. Stricker, B. H. C., Barendregt, J. N. M. and Class, F. H. J. (1985). Thrombocytopenia and leucopenia with mianserin-dependent antibodies. *Br. J. Clin. Pharmacol.*, **19,** 102–4
14. Stricker, B. H. C. (1983). Slokdarmbeschading door pinaverium-bromide. *Ned. T. Geneeskd.*, **127,** 603–4
15. Hoogslag, K. (1973). Interactie tussen Prolixan 300 en anticoagulantia. *Ned. T. Geneesk.*, **117,** 1103
16. Meyboom, R. H. B. (1974). Kunnen geneesmiddelen de betrouwbaarheid van 'de pil' beinvloeden? *Ned. T. Geneesk.*, **118,** 1767
17. Meyboom, R. H. B. (1982). Beinvloeding van antistolling door vermageringsproducten. *Tromnibus*, **10** (1), 3
18. Stricker, B. H. C. and Delhez, J. L. (1982). Interaction between flurbiprofen and coumarins. *Br. Med. J.*, **285,** 812
19. Powell-Jackson, P. R. (1977). Interaction between azapropazone and warfarin. *Br. Med. J.*, **1,** 1193
20. McElnay, J. C. and D'Arcy, P. F. (1977). Interaction between azapropazone and warfarin. *Br. Med. J.*, **2,** 773
21. Meyboom, R. H. B. (1976). Icterus door phenprocoumon. *Tromnibus*, **4** (1), 4
22. Meyboom, R. H. B. (1977). Slokdarmbeschadiging door doxycycline en tetracycline. *Ned. T. Geneesk.*, **121,** 1770
23. Meyboom, R. H. B., Gent, A. van and Zinkstok, D. J. (1982). Nitrofurantoin-induced parotitis. *Br. Med. J.*, **285,** 1049
24. Meyboom, R. H. B. (1984). Thrombocytopenia induced by nalidixic acid. *Br. Med. J.*, **289,** 962
25. Stricker, B. H. C. and Oei, T. T. (1984). Agranulocytosis caused by spironolactone. *Br. Med. J.*, **289,** 731
26. Heide, H. van der, Haaft, M. A. ten, and Stricker, B. H. C. (1981). Pancreatitis caused by methyldopa. *Br. Med. J.*, **282,** 1930
27. Zwaan, F. E. and Meyboom, R. H. B. (1979). Causes and consequences of bone marrow insufficiency in man. *Neth. J. Med.*, **22,** 99
28. Editorial. (1979). Halcion – Ontmaskering van een mythe. *Ned. T. Geneesk.*, **123,** 1653
29. Kales, A., Kales, J. D., Bixler, E. O., Scharf, M. B. and Russek, E. (1976). Hypnotic efficacy of triazolam: Sleep laboratory evaluation of intermediate term effectiveness. *J. Clin. Pharm.*, **16,** 399–406

30. Kroef, C. van der. (1979). Reactions to triazolam. *Lancet*, **2,** 526
31. Einarson, T. R. (1980). Hallucinations from triazolam. *Drug Intell. Clin. Pharm.*, **14,** 714
32. Einarson, T. R. and Yoder, E. S. (1982). Triazolam psychosis – a syndrome? *Drug Intell. Clin. Pharm.*, **16,** 330
33. Trappler, B. and Bezeredi, T. (1982). Triazolam intoxication. *CMA J.*, **126,** 893
34. Mostert, J. W. (1981). Die Halcion-affêre. *S. Afr. Med. J.*, **5,** 967 (27 June)
35. Rudnick, H. L. (1981). The Halcion affair. *S. Afr. Med. J.*, **60,** 378 (5 September)
36. Schou, J. (1980). Indberetninger af benzodiazepinbivirkninger. *Ugeskr. Laeg.*, **142,** 1695
37. Committee on Safety of Medicines, 1 Nine Elms Lane, London SW8 5NQ
38. Poison Control and Adverse Reactions Reporting Program Division, Health Protection Branch, Department of National Health and Welfare, Tunney's Pasture, Ottawa, Canada
39. Division of Drug Experience, National Centre for Drugs and Biologics, Food and Drug Administration, Rockville, MD 20857, USA
40. Comité Nationale de Pharmacovigilance, Centre Hopital Universitaire, 54037 Nancy, France
41. Kroef, C. van der. (1982). Het Halcion-syndroom – een iatrogene epdiemie in Nederland. *T. Alc. Drugs*, **8,** 156
42. Wijngaart, G. F. van de and Kleingeld, P. A. F. (1982). Statistische gegevens over de klachten van Halcion-gebruikers. *T. Alc. Drugs*, **8,** 163
43. Petursson, H. and Lader, M. H. (1981). Withdrawal from long term benzodiazepine treatment. *Br. Med. J.*, **283,** 643
44. Tyrer, P., Rutherford, D. and Huggett, T. (1981). Benzodiazepine withdrawal symptons and propranolol. *Lancet*, **1,** 520–2
45. Ashton, H. (1984). Benzodiazepine withdrawal: an unfinished story. *Br. Med. J.*, **288,** 1135–40
46. Morgan, K. and Oswald, I. (1982). Anxiety caused by a short life hypnotic. *Br. Med. J.*, **284,** 942
47. Scharf, M. B. and Jacoby, J. A. (1982) Lorazepam – efficacy, side effects, and rebound phenomena. **31,** 175–9
48. Stewart, R. B. and Salem, R. B. Springer, P. K. (1980). A case report of lorazepam withdrawal. *Am. J. Psych.*, **137,** 1113
49. Fuente, G. R. de la, Rosenbaum, A. H., Martin, H. R. and Niven, R. G. (1980). Lorazepam-related withdrawal seizures. *Mayo Clin. Proc.*, **55,** 190
50. Kahn, A., Joyce, P. and Jones, A. V. (1980) Benzodiazepine withdrawal syndrome. *NZ. Med. J.*, **92,** 94
51. Kales, A. Scharf, M. B. and Kales, J. (1978). Rebound insomnia: a new clinical syndrome. *Science*, **201,** 1039–41
52. Howe, J. G. (1980). Lorazepam withdrawal seizures. *Br. Med. J.*, **1,** 1163
53. Greenblatt, D. J. and Shader, R. I. (1974). *Benzodiazepines in Clinical Practice.* p. 204. (New York: Raven Press)
54. Mattila, M. A. K. and Larni, H. M. (1980). Flunitrazepam: a review of its pharmacological properties and therapeutic use. *Drugs*, **20,** 353–74
55. Shader, R. I. and Greenblatt, D. J. (1983). Triazolam and anterograde amnesia: all is not well in the Z-zone. *J. Clin. Psychofarmac.*, **3,** 273
56. Barclay, W. R., Curran, W. J., Greenblatt, D. J. *et al.* (1979). Behavioural reactions to triazolam. *Lancet*, **2,** 1018
57. Meyboom, R. H. B. (1977). Experiences with international collaboration. In Gross, F. H. and Inman W. H. W. (eds.) *Drug monitoring* p. 235 (London: Academic Press)
58. Van Dijke, C. P. H. and Weber, J. C. P. (1984). Interaction between oral contraceptives and griseofulvin. *Br. Med. J.*, **288,** 1125–6

# 9
# New Zealand

**D. M. COULTER, I. R. EDWARDS, and E. G. McQUEEN**

An agency for the surveillance of adverse medicine reactions was inaugurated in New Zealand in 1965. Amongst such agencies the New Zealand one is unusual in being effectively disassociated from the governmental Health Department and having no regulatory responsibility. It was set up under the joint auspices of the Royal Australasian College of Physicians, the Royal NZ College of General Practitioners, the NZ Dental Association and the Department of Pharmacology of the University of Otago Medical School. Each of these bodies is represented on the NZ Medicines Adverse Reactions Committee (MARC) which also has representation from the Department of Health and the NZ Accident Compensation Commission.

Responsibility for monitoring adverse medicine reactions rests with the Committee whose administrative office is closely associated with the Pharmacology Department of the University of Otago Medical School. The professional staff consists of the Medical Assessor, who is a member of the academic staff and acts in an honorary capacity to administer the affairs of the MARC Committee. He is assisted by two part-time medical officers and a small secretarial staff.

Finance is provided through the University of Otago by the Health Department. Computer services are provided by the University and the Health Department, data being entered via a terminal purchased under a grant from the WHO. Substantial assistance with programming and other aspects of data storage and retrieval are made available by the Department of Preventive and Social Medicine in the Medical School. Meetings of the Committee are held at approximately 4-month intervals in Wellington, the capital city of New Zealand, where the Health Department seconds additional secretarial staff for the Committee meetings.

The Committee has no executive function, but is advisory to the Minister of Health through its recommendations to the Director General of Health. It is the Committee's view that there are considerable advantages in being substantially independent of the regulatory authority. Appreciation by practitioners of this dissociation from regulatory activities enhances the degree of collaboration by the profession in adverse reaction reporting.

The activities of the MARC implemented through its administrative office will be discussed in this chapter. These have included the spontaneous medicine reaction reporting scheme, now in its 20th year, a scheme for post-marketing surveillance of certain selected new medicines, and, collaboratively with the Health Department, a nation-wide system for alerting to the medicine-reaction susceptibility of individuals. In addition, the Health Department conducts a programme for monitoring the incidence of fetal malformations, and this will be referred to.

## SPONTANEOUS MEDICINE REACTION REPORTING

The major activity of the MARC has been and remains the spontaneous reporting scheme. Reporting cards on which the return postage is pre-paid are regularly circulated to doctors (and senior medical students), dentists and pharmacists. These are designed to provide enough information to enable evaluation of minor or relatively straightforward reactions without further documentation. The Medical Assessor has the responsibility for processing the reports, their evaluation, coding and entry into the computer file. He also formulates appropriate comments based on the Centre's own data and its extensive store of information from other sources, particularly the WHO Collaborating Centre, and returns these comments, with a fresh reporting card, to the doctor, dentist or pharmacist concerned. Where additional data are required a follow-up form is sent for further documentation. Lists of reports are periodically forwarded to the WHO Collaborating Centre on magnetic tape.

Annual reports are published in the New Zealand medical, dental and pharmaceutical journals giving summaries of the year's reporting. A more comprehensive version is circulated to all medical practitioners, and lists of reactions are made available in full to Committee members, adverse reaction agencies elsewhere, hospital superintendents, pharmaceutical manufacturers and interested individuals or institutions. Where appropriate, additional bulletins are circulated on topics thought to require particular comment, these often being prepared by specialists in the relevant area at the request of the Committee. Occasional publications as articles or letters in medical journals also form part of the MARC output.

Currently some 800 case-reports are received per annum. Of these 60% are from GP's, 38% from hospital doctors and consultants and a handful from dentists and pharmacists. Although considerable effort has been expended in ensuring that pharmacists are given facilities for reporting, in fact very few reports have come from them. However, as indicated later, pharmacists have collaborated extensively in the NZ post-marketing surveillance scheme called the Intensive Medicines Monitoring Programme.

The reactions reported and the medicines associated therewith are of a closely comparable character to those reported from the United Kingdom, Western Europe and the United States. Non-steroidal anti-inflammatory medicines are consistently associated with the largest number of reactions, and of these many are severe, and some fatal. Reactions of a type not initially thought to be associated with this group of medicines, such as interstitial nephropathy, were brought to our attention through the spontaneous reporting scheme. Such cases continue to be reported. Anti-infective agents are next in number, and there are still occasional reports of a novel character such as agranulocytosis with tetracycline. Good collaboration by anaesthetists has drawn attention to the disconcerting frequency of severe immediate hypersensitivity reactions with intravenous anaesthetic agents and relaxants. Continued reporting of vascular occlusive lesions with oral contraceptives serves to maintain awareness of the responsibility involved in prescribing these hormones for healthy young women.

The office of the Medical Assessor also serves as a medicine information centre for enquiries about potential medicine reaction or interaction hazards. In addition, information is often given on pharmacological, particularly pharmacokinetic, problems of all kinds. The staff is also involved in undergraduate and postgraduate teaching, during which every opportunity is taken to emphasize responsibility to watch for adverse reactions. These activities serve, hopefully, to diminish the frequency of reactions and to contribute significantly to the safety and efficacy of medicine therapy in New Zealand.

## THE NEW ZEALAND POST-MARKETING SURVEILLANCE SCHEME

In early 1977 a scheme entitled 'The Intensified Adverse Drug Reaction Reporting Scheme', now entitled 'Intensive Medicines Monitoring Programme' (IMP) was instituted by the Department of Health in New Zealand to facilitate the early recognition of adverse reactions in the post-marketing phase of certain new medicines. Medicines are selected for monitoring because they are of a novel character, pharmacologically or chemically, or because they are related to medicines which have caused serious problems in the past. For the most part they are also intended for use on a widespread and/or chronic basis. Since its inception the scheme has been applied to 14 medicines (Table 1).

At the time of writing, the last five medicines were on the scheme plus tocainide and enalapril, both of which as yet have insignificant numbers of patients. Medicines in general have been retained on the

**Table 1** Monitored medicines, monitoring periods and patient cohorts in the New Zealand Intensive Medicines Monitoring Programme

| *Monitoring medicine* | *Monitoring commenced* | *Recording ended* | *Patient cohort* |
|---|---|---|---|
| Acebutolol | Apr/77 | Mar/80 | 1891 |
| Atenolol | Apr/77 | Mar/80 | 2656 |
| Metoprolol | Apr/77 | Mar/80 | 11086 |
| Perhexiline maleate | Apr/77 | Aug/81 | 3926 |
| Sodium valproate | Apr/77 | Mar/83 | 10447 |
| Cimetidine | Nov/77 | Aug/81 | 9190 |
| Labetalol | Nov/77 | Mar/80 | 2837 |
| Nifedipine | Oct/80 | Dec/84 | 9725 |
| Amiodarone | Jul/81 | continues | 1828 |
| Captopril | Jul/81 | continues | 3028 |
| Acyclovir | Jan/83 | continues | 375 |
| Mianserin | May/83 | continues | 3901 |

scheme for about 3 years to obtain as large a cohort as possible, although compliance in the spontaneous reporting of events has been observed to fall off after about 2 years.

The IMP has two aspects; firstly an intensified spontaneous 'event' reporting component which, it is hoped, may convey an enhanced alerting potential, and secondly a cohort recording provision whereby data identifying all patients receiving medicines on the IMP list are recorded. The scheme thus confers the opportunity for precise verification of postulated medicine-event associations.

## Intensified spontaneous reporting of adverse events

Doctors are exhorted to report all 'adverse events' befalling patients on the listed medicines whether recognizable as adverse medicine reactions (AMRs) or not. Such adverse events include death from any cause, deterioration in a pre-existing condition, any intercurrent illness, requirement for referral for specialist consultation, admission to hospital, changes in laboratory test results, possible medicine interactions and fetal malformations. Also to be reported would be accidents, involving motor vehicles or otherwise, which may have resulted from drowsiness, vertigo, syncope or interference with visual acuity possibly resulting from medicinal action. Suspected AMRs are of course also included as events.

Repeated reminders are circulated concerning the scheme together with the list of medicines currently included. A special Desk Reminder card, financed by the pharmaceutical firms involved, is periodically mailed to all doctors. Articles and editorials in medical journals,

Medical Association circulars as well as material published or circulated by the Medicines Adverse Reaction Committee are used to keep the profession's obligation to report events constantly before its members. All advertising material for the medicines involved must include reminders that they are on the Intensive Monitoring list. Pharmaceutical firm representatives undertake to remind practitioners of the inclusion of their products on the list.

A triennial distribution of the usual spontaneous reporting cards is made through the courtesy of the ADIS Press *New Ethicals Catalogue of Drugs* which is received by most doctors in New Zealand. Pharmaceutical firm representatives are expected to distribute additional report cards to doctors likely to be prescribing any of their firms' products which are on the scheme.

A comparison of 210 IMP events with 210 adverse reaction reports to non-IMP medicines received contemporaneously was carried out shortly after the IMP was started. This appeared to indicate that the IMP events were of an appreciably different character from the reactions being reported as such. The IMP series contained a lesser proportion of conditions classified as severe (14% as against 42%) and a higher proportion of questionable or unlikely sequelae (18% as against 7%).

## Patient cohort recording

This unique feature of the IMP is achieved through the collaboration of dispensing pharmacists who are asked to provide the office of the Medical Assessor, on forms supplied, with the patient's surname, first name, title (Mr, Mrs, Miss, child), date of birth and address each time they dispense a medicine on the IMP list. In addition they also enter the prescribing doctor's name and locality and the total daily dose of the medicine. the completed forms are forwarded to the Medical Assessor's office every 4 months and the information is stored on computer.

The length of time each of the monitored medicines has been on the scheme and the numbers of patients recorded as having received each medicine are listed in Table 1.

## Results achieved by the IMP

### *Cardioselective β-blockers*

The cardioselective β-blockers were the first medicines to be included in the scheme because of the concern felt that they might replicate the practolol experience. Labetalol was added a little later. The profiles of events reported during the 3 years they were on the scheme are shown in Figure 1. Also shown are the profiles for adverse reactions spontaneously reported for practolol during the 46 months it was

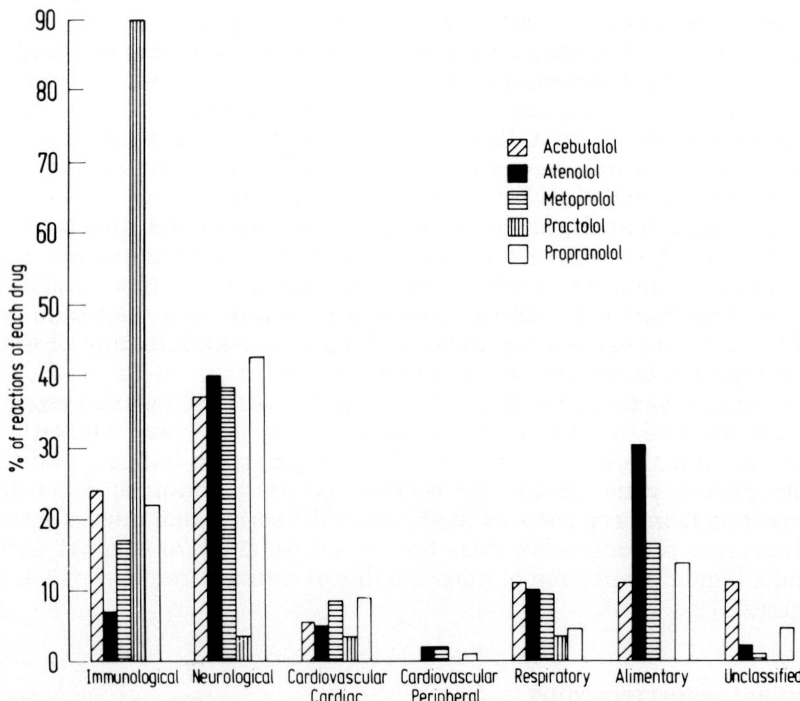


**Figure 1** Profile of events reported under the IMP with newer β-blocking medicines compared with New Zealand practolol and propranolol reactions

available in New Zealand, and for propranolol to 1982. The second generation medicines manifested a markedly different profile of 'events' from the reaction profile of practolol. The striking difference was in the absence of the massive preponderance of 'immunological' reactions to practolol. These were made up principally of skin rashes, cases of arthritis, medicine fever, etc. A relatively small proportion was contributed to by reactions recognizable in retrospect as components of the oculo-mucocutaneous syndrome. Possibly the unique set of complications of practolol resulted from a combination of potent immunogenic capacity and the fibrosis-promoting potential which is common to all β-blockers.[1,2] Although the profiles for the new medicines were closely comparable to those for propranolol, some aspects of their event profiles were rather unexpected, for example the occurrence of events related to the alimentary tract particularly with atenolol.

*Cimetidine, perhexiline, valproate, labetalol*

The period of monitoring of these medicines was as shown in Table 1. The events reported foreshadowed the adverse reaction pattern that subsequently emerged, although some of the events reported were of a character which at the time were scarcely to be anticipated with these medicines. For example, events involving the central nervous system were reported with cimetidine and with perhexiline, including papilloedema with the latter. Events involved the haemopoietic system with valproate and polydipsia was associated with labetalol. The availability of patient cohorts for these medicines prompted a series of studies which reflected the compliance by doctors with the IMP.

After the first year of the scheme it could be seen from the returns rendered by pharmacists dispensing IMP medicines, that about 25% of patients had stopped treatment with each of the seven medicines then being monitored. To identify the reasons for cessation, and in particular to ascertain whether or not this may have related to adverse effects, patients who appeared to have stopped taking perhexiline, valproate or labetalol were identified. The relevant 358 prescribing doctors were sent lists of those patients under their care and asked to complete a questionnaire concerning reasons for cessation. Replies were received from 289 of the doctors (81%). The findings are shown in Table 2.

**Table 2** Reasons for cessation of therapy

| | *Perhexiline* | | *Valproate* | | *Labetalol* | |
|---|---|---|---|---|---|---|
| | No. | (%) | No. | (%) | No. | (%) |
| Total known to have stopped* | 89 | | 52 | | 53 | |
| Condition improved | 26 | (29) | 6 | (12) | 2 | (4) |
| Change in treatment (no events) | 10 | (11) | 2 | (4) | 3 | (6) |
| Poor compliance | 4 | (4) | nil | | 7 | (13) |
| Poor therapeutic response | 9 | (10) | 28 | (54) | 13 | (25) |
| Death (as an event) | 22 | (25) | 8 | (15) | 5 | (9) |
| Adverse event (non-fatal) | 18 | (20) | 8 | (15) | 23 | (43) |

*Information was not available to the doctor contacted in 42 patients taking perhexiline, 52 taking valproate and 23 taking labetalol

During the period to which the above questionnaire related, there was a similar number of events with each of these medicines reported spontaneously. However, with few exceptions these were from different patients than those elicited by the questionnaire (Table 3).

The most disconcerting outcome of this questionnaire was the obvious failure of doctors to report fatalities as events amongst patients on IMP medicines. It was clear also that events other than death which were nevertheless of sufficient significance to warrant cessation of the medicine concerned were being poorly reported. Measures taken to improve reporting are referred to below.

**Table 3** Comparison of events spontaneously reported and events from questionnaires

| | Perhexiline | | Valproate | | Labetalol | |
|---|---|---|---|---|---|---|
| | Qu* | Sp† | Qu | Sp | Qu | Sp |
| Total | 46 | 39 | 18 | 15 | 35 | 46 |
| Deaths | 22 | 1 | 8 | nil | 5 | nil |
| Other events | 24 | 38 | 10 | 15 | 30 | 46 |

*Qu – questionnaires; †Sp – spontaneously reported

## *Cohort study of valproate toxicity*

The anticonvulsant medicine valproate is in extensive use for the management of epilepsy. During the late 1970s and 1980 a number of cases of severe hepatotoxicity were reported in the literature, mostly involving children, a high proportion of them terminating fatally. Two other associations, acute pancreatitis and hyperammonaemia with encephalopathy had also come under scrutiny. These events had led to questioning by some national authorities on the permissibility of the continued use of valproate. Valproate, therefore, seemed an appropriate context in which to assess the value of the cohort recording aspect of the NZ intensive monitoring programme. In 1980 an enquiry was directed to practitioners concerning each of the patients under their care for whom they had prescribed valproate. Specific questions were asked concerning clinical or laboratory evidence of hepatotoxicity, hyperammonaemia or pancreatitis.

A total of 1862 patients had been prescribed valproate. Satisfactory data for analysis were returned on 1800 of these (97%). The age distribution of the cohort was of the character that might have been expected for this medicine, with a mode in the 11–16 years age group. Dosage was most frequently in the 400–600 mg per day range.

The returns from the questionnaire elicited no cases of *clinical* hepatotoxicity apparently related to valproate, although two cases have been reported since. Liver function tests (AST and/or ALT, alkaline phosphatase in adults) were abnormal in 21 cases. There was no report of clinically recognizable toxic encephalopathy, and laboratory evidence of mild hyperammonaemia was reported in only 2 patients, although it was not tested for routinely.

A grossly obese mentally retarded male died after a complaint of abdominal pain, and was found at autopsy to have acute pancreatitis. Serum and urinary amylase were raised in three other patients who continued on treatment.

Although too small in number to enable statistically reliable estimates to be made of the frequency of these complications of valproate, the study gave reassurance concerning the relative infrequency of toxic hepatitis and of hyperammonaemic encephalopathy. It did, however, support the reality of an association with pancreatitis which, if the three cases of abnormal amylase levels are included, occurred more than 10 times as frequently in the cohort as might have been anticipated.

*Novel medicine-event associations with labetalol*

Adverse events concerning labetalol reported to the Medical Assessor at a relatively early stage had included five of scalp tingling, three of polyuria, one of polydipsia and one of polyuria and polydipsia. Scalp tingling was a known association with labetalol; polydipsia and polyuria had not previously been reported.

To assess the significance of the latter reports it was decided to send a questionnaire directly to patients receiving labetalol. A group of 300 patients was identified from the computer file. The prescribing doctor for each of these patients was contacted and asked whether he would have any objection to the forwarding of a questionnaire, a copy of which was enclosed, to the patients concerned. Scalp tingling was used as a marker event to assess validity of method. As a control medicine, metoprolol was chosen. A group of 300 patients on metoprolol was identified from the file and their doctors contacted.

In the questionnaire, patients were asked to tick boxes for 'tingling of the scalp', 'passing more urine than usual', 'an unusual degree of thirst' or 'none of the above symptoms'. Patients were informed that labetalol was the medicine under review and that the same questions were being put to patients on metoprolol for comparison. There were few objections to the direct approach to the patients, and retrospectively no doctor reported that receipt of the questionnaire had occasioned anxiety in their patients. The results are shown in Table 4.

By specific enquiry, change in diuretic therapy was ruled out as a factor in these results. The observation concerning thirst and labetalol had not been made previously. It presumably resulted from the α-blocking component of the action of labetalol. The possibly associated

**Table 4** Responses to questionnaires concerning frequency of symptoms with labetalol and metoprolol

| | *Labetalol* | *Metoprolol* | †*Significance* |
|---|---|---|---|
| Questionnaires sent | 293 | 300 | |
| Replies | 255(87*) | 231(77) | |
| Scalp tingling | 52( 2) | 17( 7) | $p < 0.001$ |
| Thirst | 38(15) | 19( 8) | $0.05 > p > 0.025$ |
| Polyuria | 63(25) | 44(19) | $0.27 > p > 0.1$ |

*Figures in brackets are percentages. † Student's *t*-test

polyuria may have resulted from increased fluid intake aimed at relieving the dryness of the mouth.

*Nifedipine, captopril*

The nifedipine cohort consisted at the time of writing of 9725 patients. The greatest proportion of the 291 events spontaneously reported with nifedipine involved the cardiovascular system, as might have been expected, and were related to its vasodilator effects. Flushing, hypotension and oedema, in some instances gross, were prominent amongst these. However, neurological and ocular symptoms were also reported, the latter appearing relatively more prominently in the profile of events than in that of adverse reactions to nifedipine that appears in the WHO Collaborating Centre file. Reports had been received of painful eyes in three patients and blurred vision in two.

The highest proportion of the 175 events reported spontaneously to date with captopril from a 3028 patient cohort was dermatological. However, a small but significant incidence of hypotension, CNS symptoms and renal deterioration emerged at a stage when these side effects of captopril were not generally known.

A study of the ocular symptoms related to nifedipine and referred to above was carried out utilizing the captopril cohort as a control.

*Methodology* – The study was undertaken by sending questionnaires to patients. Printouts of the patient cohorts for nifedipine and captopril were obtained, and the prescribing doctors were asked for permission to write to their patients. The patient questionnaires asked if eye problems had developed since commencing nifedipine or captopril. Patients were asked to tick boxes indicating any of the following: 'painful eyes', 'blurred vision', 'stinging eyes' and 'dry eyes'. They were also asked about the severity of the symptoms, 'How much does it bother you? Very little, a moderate amount or a lot?' They were told only one medicine was under suspicion, but not which one. The results are shown in Table 5.

**Table 5** Eye problems with nifedipine

| | *Nifedipine* | | *Captopril* | | **Significance* |
|---|---|---|---|---|---|
| | *No.* | *%* | *No.* | *%* | |
| Total patients | 757 | | 289 | | |
| Painful eyes | 107 | 14.1 | 26 | 9.0 | $p = 0.033$ |
| Stinging eyes | 71 | 9.4 | 19 | 6.6 | $p = 0.19$ |
| Blurred vision | 238 | 31.4 | 88 | 30.4 | $p = 0.81$ |
| Dry eyes | 42 | 5.5 | 17 | 5.9 | $p = 0.95$ |
| Painful + stinging eyes | 156 | 20.6 | 42 | 14.5 | $p = 0.031$ |

*Student's *t*-test

The significantly greater frequency of painful eyes with nifedipine suggests that the ocular pain or irritation results from a specific reaction to nifedipine. However, the pathogenesis of the symptoms has not as yet been determined.

During the course of this study a disparity was noticed between the proportion of deaths that had occurred in the two cohorts, although both medicines were being used for serious cardiovascular diseases. Death had occurred in 14.3% of patients on nifedipine and 25.7% of patients on captopril, the difference being highly significant. The composition of the groups was similar with about 60% in each being males. There was a higher proportion of males amongst those who had died since entering the cohort than in the whole cohort, and this was even higher for nifedipine (80%) than for captopril (70%). The mode for age in the two cohorts was a little higher for nifedipine than for captopril, and the same applied to those who had died. The average duration of treatment for the survivors was similar for each medicine (19.0 months for nifedipine, 19.5 for captopril), but data on the duration of exposure of patients who had died are not available. Major causes of death differed significantly. Of the nifedipine deaths 46.5% were from myocardial infarction as against 11.2% for captopril. Of the captopril deaths 30.6% were from congestive cardiac failure as against 3.1% for those on nifedipine. This difference, and the other differing feature in the deceased patients, presumably follow from the differences in the type of cardiovascular disease for which the two medicines are used.

### *Amiodarone*

From an amiodarone cohort of 1828 patients only 135 events have been spontaneously reported to the present time. Events involving the skin (25%) and eyes (14%) were most frequent, followed in other categories by neurological (13%), cardiovascular (8%), endocrine (8%) and alimentary (7%). However, a survey carried out through the prescribing doctors has presented a somewhat different picture. The two are compared in Table 6. Event recording survey forms were sent to all doctors recorded as having prescribed amiodarone. Most of these were specialist cardiologists, but a request was made for the name of each patient's general practitioner who in turn was sent a survey form. Doctors were asked to record all clinical events from the time amiodarone was started, whether or not they appeared to have any association with amiodarone. Returns were received from 149 (84%) of the doctors first contacted (some of whom were general practitioners) and 74 (67%) of second doctor contacts (all general practitioners) concerning 243 patients.

A total of 550 events was recorded. Cardiovascular events (22%) were most common, neurological (18%), alimentary (17%), skin (10%) and eye (7%).

The ratio of the survey reporting rate to the spontaneous rate was

**Table 6** Profiles of events for amiodarone in spontaneous reporting and the event recording survey

| | *Survey* | | *Spontaneous* | |
|---|---|---|---|---|
| | *No.* | *%* | *No.* | *%* |
| Cardiovascular | 114 | 21 | 11 | 8.2 |
| Neurological | 101 | 18 | 18 | 13.3 |
| Alimentary | 95 | 17 | 15 | 11.1 |
| Skin | 56 | 10 | 34 | 25.2 |
| Eyes | 40 | 7 | 19 | 14.1 |
| Respiratory | 32 | 6 | 9 | 6.7 |
| Endocrine/metabolic | 27 | 5 | 11 | 8.2 |
| Musculoskeletal | 25 | 5 | nil | |
| Urogenital | 20 | 4 | 3 | 2.2 |
| Accidents | 10 | 1.8 | nil | |
| Interactions | 7 | 1.3 | 5 | 3.7 |
| Haematological | 4 | 0.7 | nil | |
| Miscellaneous | 7 | 1.3 | nil | |
| Died | 12 | 2.2 | 10 | 7.4 |
| Total events | 550 | | 135 | |
| Total patients | 243 | | 1828 | |

Percentage figures are those of the total number of events

31:1. It is clear that spontaneous reporting does not present an accurate picture of the event profile, and that not more than about 3% of events are being reported spontaneously.

In the event recording survey, cardiovascular events were the most common, but most of these were clinical incidents expected in this group of patients and were probably not medicine related. Unexpectedly, this places the neurological group of events as the most important medicine-related events or reactions. A further survey has been undertaken to assess the frequency of neurological problems by requesting doctors to review their patients and record any neurological events. Replies were received concerning 392 patients and the incidence of neurological events is as follows: paraesthesiae 10.5%, definite peripheral neuropathy 1.3%, vertigo 7.7%, true ataxia 7.7%, tremor 5.4%, impaired intellect or confusion 5.1%, muscle weakness 4.6%, cerebrovascular accident (CVA) or transient ischaemic attack 2.3%, speech disorder 2.3%, and diplopia 2.8%. Most of these problems were minor. The more serious events (except for CVA) proved reversible on withdrawal of the medicine.

### *Acyclovir*

A different approach to monitoring is necessary for medicines used in the short term. The method for acyclovir, which is frequently administered for only 5 days, has been to send a reporting card to the prescribing doctor each time a prescription is recorded. Numbers of patients receiving acyclovir are small (375), but the following events have been recorded; two cases of temporary disturbance of renal function and one each of haematuria, proteinuria, abdominal discomfort, headache, ulceration of injection site and, from ocular treatment, two patients with a mild corneal irritation.

## Future accessibility of patients on IMP file

At the outset identifying data included only surnames, initials, titles (Mr, Mrs, Miss, child) and addresses. Even in the short term, difficulty was experienced in establishing patient identity. First names and birth date are now requested, and these data should make patient identification in the future more practical should there arise at any time in the future anxieties about long-term sequelae of monitored medicines, e.g. carcinogenesis.

## Duplicate prescription pad scheme

In order to improve both the accuracy of patient data and the event reporting rate, a pilot trial of a duplicate pad scheme has been introduced in one region with another similar region, continuing as at present, being used as a control. Both regions are receiving the same promotion. Doctors are supplied with duplicate pads. For private practitioners these are personalized with their name and address. For hospital doctors their designation and the hospital department is requested. Patient data requested includes title, full name, address and date of birth. In addition doctors are asked to indicate the presence or absence of any events by ticking either of two boxes. Duplicate prescription forms are used for all prescriptions written for patients on a monitored medicine, and both copies are given to the patient to take to a pharmacist. The pharmacist then returns the copy to this centre. If the doctor has indicated the presence of any events a reporting card complete with patient data, doctor's identification and name of medicine, is sent to the prescriber who is asked to record the events and return the card.

## Summary of intensive monitoring methods used

*Compilation of patient cohorts*

(1) Recording and return of prescription data by pharmacists,

(2) The use of duplicate prescription pads (under trial)

*Basic collection of data on events*

(1) Spontaneous event reporting,

(2) Event recording surveys,

(3) Sending reporting cards to doctors after each prescription,
(4) The use of duplicate pads (under trial).

*Special studies*
(1) Reasons for cessation of therapy. This provides information concerning deaths as well as other events,
(2) Specific enquiry of doctors (e.g. neurological events with amiodarone),
(3) Specific enquiry of patients with use of a control medicine (e.g. painful eyes with nifedipine).

To obtain a satisfactory rate of event reporting has been the most difficult problem. Spontaneous event reporting has achieved at the most a reporting rate of about 3% of the total events, though even this rate of reporting is higher than that for the standard reaction reporting scheme. Event recording surveys are a fruitful method, though are very laborious and make considerable demands on some doctors and the Centre staff. Recording the rate of event reporting should prove of value in assessing the effectiveness of event collection. For instance the event recording survey undertaken with captopril produced a recording rate of 2.2 events per patient year, and with amiodarone (243 patients) an overall rate of 2.5 events per patient year was achieved, increasing to 3.7 for patients when survey forms were received from both specialist and general practitioners. The use of duplicate prescription pads should prove to be less laborious and more cost effective.

## MEDICAL DANGER/WARNING SYSTEM

A majority of hospitals in New Zealand utilize a centrally based computer system which provides for a variety of administrative functions. Amongst these, the registration data for patients attending these hospitals, which includes a national patient number, allows for a brief record of any significant adverse reaction by an individual patient to be recorded. This information is subsequently available at any of the collaborating hospitals should the patient be readmitted to any of them. Additionally the MARC provides hard copy of the information for the patients' hospital notes and for the general practitioner's record. Furthermore, a letter is sent to the general practitioner suggesting that he discuss with the patient the advisability of registering with the privately administered Medic-Alert system, through whom warning bracelets and the like can be arranged.

Input to the system is from two sources, one being from the collaborating hospital who can record reactions through their terminals, and the other being the MARC who can input data based on reports to them, whether or not the patient has previously been in hospital.

Two levels of severity of reaction are recorded, the most serious being a 'Danger' which includes only life-threatening or potentially life-threatening reactions which have been directly observed by a qualified medical practitioner. These must be checked and approved by MARC. 'Warnings', on the other hand, include reactions that are not of immediate serious import, and which may have been reported rather than observed. Clearly these 'Warnings' do not carry the power of contraindication that 'Dangers' have and are not validated by the MARC.

In addition to the above, a small number of medical conditions which are likely to have a major impact on therapy are recorded as 'Dangers', such as atopy, inherited coagulopathies, diabetes and the like.

This system allows for adverse medicine reaction information to be used for the direct benefit of the patient.

## FETAL MALFORMATION SURVEILLANCE SCHEME

In spite of repeated representations to doctors, reporting of possible association between medicines and fetal malformations has remained very poor. This state of affairs would be intolerable if it were not for the New Zealand Health Department's fetal malformation recording system. The form for registration of births includes a requirement for observable malformations to be entered. The data are collated by the Statistics Division of the Health Department and presented at 3-monthly intervals to the appropriate bodies, including the MARC. Any apparent increase in malformations either generally over the whole country or in a specific area is investigated at the earliest opportunity by district Medical Officers of Health, who enquire from the mothers concerned about any possible association with medicines, pesticides, etc. in the appropriate period of pregnancy.

## References

1. McQueen, E. G. (1979). Sclerosing serositis after practolol. *New Zealand Committee on Adverse Drug Reactions Bulletin No. 3*
2. Ahmad, S. (1981). Sclerosing peritonitis and propranolol. *Chest*, **79**, 361–2

# 10
# The Scandinavian countries

**B.-E. WIHOLM, C. BORCHGREVINK and A. PEDERSEN**

## INTRODUCTION

In 1965 national monitoring centres for voluntary reporting were started as pilot projects in Norway and Sweden. Denmark followed in 1968. During the following years all centres became permanent. They are now established institutions within the drug control agencies (DRAs) and all participate in the WHO international monitoring system.

## ORGANIZATION AND REGULATORY STATUS

All three centres are part of the regulatory bodies of their respective countries, and are financed by their governments. During the pilot phase the reporting was voluntary, but official recommendations or regulations now state what should be reported. Since 1973 it has been compulsory for Norwegian doctors and dentists to report suspected fatal or life-threatening adverse drug reactions (ADRs). From 1979 reactions leading to serious sequelae and new or unexpected ADRs must also be reported. A similar explicit compulsory reporting scheme has been in force in Sweden since 1975. In Denmark reporting of the same ADRs is recommended but there is no legal obligation.

It should be noted that no medico-legal action has been taken to reinforce the compulsory reporting, but emphasis has been placed on information and feedback to the medical profession. In spite of these measures, in a postal enquiry 38% of Swedish doctors indicated that they were uncertain about what to report.

In the Scandinavian countries all reports come directly from the practising physicians and not via the pharmaceutical industry. The industry, however, sends reports based on their world-wide experience when relevant new experience is gained or requested.

## PROCEDURE, ASSESSMENT AND STORAGE OF REPORTS

As a rule ADRs are reported on a special form, specific for each country, but in accordance with the WHO form. Copies of medical records, etc are also accepted. The reports are treated confidentially. Medical officers make their primary assessment of the reports in Denmark and Sweden whereas in Norway this is made by pharmacists. All reports are classified according to the likelihood of a causal relationship between the suspected drug and adverse reaction. These categories vary between the countries. In Denmark reports are classifed as certain, probable, possible, or unclassified. Norway has only the three latter groups. In Sweden the classification was similar to that in Norway up to 1978 when for practical reasons probable and possible were merged into one group (code P) and unlikely and unassessable into another (code N). Information from the reports is stored in computers with on-line accessibility, and the material is sent to the WHO monitoring scheme on magnetic tapes four times a year. Advisory boards on ADRs assist the centres with the evaluation of reports, scientific studies of the material, resolutions and information. The advisory boards comprise between two and seven clinical specialists and, (in Denmark and Sweden), a representative from the pharmaceutical industry.

## FEEDBACK AND INFORMATION

Personal letters are sent in reply to the reporting physicians. Computer print-outs of the reports are regularly sent to the pharmaceutical industry in Norway and Sweden and upon request in Denmark. In Sweden and Norway these lists are also sent to other interested parties, e.g. hospital drug committees. In all countries copies of the reports and additional information (without the name of the patient and doctor) are sent to the manufacturer on request.

Analyses of the material with reviews or special alerts or warnings are regularly published. In Denmark this is done by frequent short letters in the national medical journal. In Norway feedback from the system is incorporated in the regular Bulletin from the Drug Control Agency and in the national medical journal. In Sweden a special ADR bulletin is published three times a year.

## RATE OF REPORTING

The annual number of reports has gradually increased in all three countries and the latest figures are presented in Table 1. Obviously the inherent problem of under-reporting also applies to the Nordic countries, although in Denmark and Sweden the number of reports in

**Table 1** Reports of ADRs in the Scandinavian countries

| *Year* | *Denmark* | *Norway* | *Sweden* |
|---|---|---|---|
| | *No. of reports (fatal cases)* | | |
| 1978 | 1943 (45) | 546 (28) | 2225 (42) |
| 1979 | 2060 (44) | 909 (18) | 2409 (36) |
| 1980 | 1792 (39) | 671 (17) | 2343 (27) |
| 1981 | 1832 (39) | 681 (56) | 2334 (46) |
| 1982 | 2087 (35) | 678 (21) | 2789 (43) |
| 1983 | 1800 (39) | 778 (41) | 2912 (43) |
| Population (millions) | 5.2 | 4.0 | 8.2 |
| No. of physicians (thousands) 1978–1983 | 10–11 | 7–8.5 | 17–20 |

relation to the number of physicians and population size is well above the international average.

From an intensive monitoring project in Copenhagen it was found that in comparison with the annual mean of spontaneous reports during a 4 year period, about 5% of all ADRs were also reported through the national spontaneous monitoring system. In a recent study on drug induced hospital admissions in Oslo it was found that 7% of the patients were admitted to a medical clinic because of ADRs, and it was estimated that only 3–4% of all ADRs that should be reported in Norway were actually sent to the monitoring centre. Similar studies in Sweden have indicated that about 5% of admissions to medical clinics[1,2] and 8% of admissions to departments for infectious diseases are caused by ADRs.[3] From the latter study a total reporting frequency of 13% was found. However, in Sweden some serious ADRs have been reported more frequently, e.g. Stevens–Johnson's syndrome, 20%; blood dyscrasias, 25–40%; osteitis from BCG-vaccination, 77%; and fatal oral contraceptive-associated thromboembolic complications 100%.[4]

## RESULTS OF THE SYSTEMS

Signals in the monitoring systems, indicating a novel ADR or an increase in known reactions, often lead to special investigations to verify the suspicion or estimate the risk. Such investigations may involve patient studies, intensive monitoring or epidemiological methods using, for example, registers of hospital discharge diagnoses. In the Scandinavian countries detailed information on drug sales is available and also published regularly.[5,6,7] Drug sales are expressed as the number of 'defined daily doses' (DDD) per 1000 inhabitants per day, which allows denominator data to be estimated. In Sweden prescription data are also collected[4,7] from which prescribed daily doses and amounts can be calculated according to age and sex of the patients and indication for drug treatment. Some examples of such studies are presented below.

### Thromboembolic disease and oestrogen content of oral contraceptives

Reports on thromboembolic disorders in connection with the use of oral contraceptives have been analysed regarding the type of preparations used by the affected women. In a joint study in the United Kingdom, Sweden and Denmark a positive correlation was found between the oestrogen dose and the risk of deep-vein thrombosis and pulmonary embolism.[8] This type of study shows the need for international co-operation in order to gather sufficient material to permit statistical evaluation. A follow-up study in Sweden during the period 1975–77 gave results in agreement with the initial data.[9] An analysis of the Norwegian data reported during the period 1978–84 shows four cases of fatal pulmonary embolism associated with low dose oestrogen ($<37.5\,\mu g$). The mean age was 21.5 years (18–26).

### Biguanides and lactic acidosis

The Swedish reports on lactic acidosis and other adverse reactions to phenformin and metformin during 1965–77 were analysed in relation to sales and prescription data.[10] The biguanides accounted for 0.6% of all reported ADRs, but for 6% of the fatal cases (all phenformin). A nationwide prescription survey disclosed no differences in age and sex between patients receiving phenformin and metformin. During 1975–77 the two drugs were used in similar amounts in Sweden. The relative incidences of ADRs in relation to sales did not differ. However, significantly more cases of lactic acidosis and deaths were reported for phenformin than for metformin. Since then the reports of lactic acidosis during metformin treatment have been closely monitored. The reported incidence remains low at about 1 per 10 000 patient years, and is strongly related to high age and impaired renal function.

## PATIENT STUDIES

In two Swedish studies the monitoring system has been used as a register to find patients with a special ADR for supplementary investigations. Through the co-operation of the reporting physicians it was possible to arrange acetylator phenotyping of 31 patients with hydralazine-induced lupus. All but one of them were slow acetylators.[11]

Likewise it was possible to phenotype seven patients with phenformin-induced lactic acidosis for hydroxylator status using deprisoauine as a probe drug. Of these only one was a slow hydroxylator – a young woman on a low phenformin dose. The other six patients were rapid hydroxylators, and they all had other contributory reasons for developing lactic acidosis such as cardiac failure, excessive alcohol intake, etc.[12]

### Metoclopramide associated tardive dyskinesia

By relating ADR reports to sales and prescription statistics and information from a continuous patient related prescription data base it was possible to show that longterm use of metoclopramide by elderly people was associated with a substantial risk of developing tardive dyskinesia.[13]

### Drug-induced liver reactions

By analysis of ADR reports collected in Denmark during a 10 year period a thorough description of 1,200 drug-induced liver reactions has given valuable knowledge about the type and severity of liver damage seen with different drugs.[14]

### Piroxicam-associated gastrointestinal bleedings

During the first years of marketing piroxicam in Norway 66 reports of gastrointestinal ulcer or haematemesis were reported, which clearly demonstrated that this new NSAID had the same ulcerogenic potency as its forerunners, especially when used in high doses or in combination with other analgesics.[15]

### Guillain–Barré syndrome following zimeldine treatment

As a final example the detection of a hitherto unknown rare, but serious, ADR to a new antidepressant will be described. Zimeldine was introduced in Sweden in March 1982. The drug differs chemically from other antidepressants, and has unique pharmacological properties as it selectively blocks the reuptake or serotonin in the neurons. Clinically the major advantages seemed to be a reduction of anticholinergic and cardiovascular side-effects, and it was also less toxic when overdosed. However, suspected hypersensitivity reactions resembling acute attacks of influenza had been reported to occur during the clinical trials.

During the first 6 months an increasing number of reports of hypersensitivity reactions were received. These reactions most commonly developed after 7–14 days of treatment, when the patients became acutely ill with high fever and severe myalgia and/or arthralgia. Liver transaminases were often elevated, and the patients often complained of severe headache and nausea. Sometimes the syndrome mimicked meningitis, and two patients who were taken to hospital actually showed signs of aseptic meningitis. In September 1982 there was a report of one patient who had developed signs of polyradiculitis, and in December the Swedish ADR Centre received a report of one patient who developed a complete Guillain–Barré syndrome after a hypersensitivity reaction. The manufacturer then reported that they had seen a similar case in a clinical trial in 1979, but at that time specialists in neurology and infectious diseases had judged this as being unassociated with zimeldine treatment. After these three cases appeared in the Swedish ADR Committee's bulletin in May 1983 another eight reports were received during the summer. All 11 cases were similar in their presentation, the Guillain–Barré syndrome appearing shortly after a hypersensitivity reaction.

In Uppsala a recent survey of 'spontaneous' Guillain–Barré Syndromes (GB) revealed an annual incidence of about 2.5 per 100 000 adults.

Zimeldine sales during the period in question were 4.2 million DDD (DDD = 200 mg) and the average prescribed daily dose was about 170 mg. Zimeldine exposure could thus be calculated to equal about 14 000 patient years during the first 16 months of marketing. The natural occurrence of GB would be 0.35 cases in such a population compared with six probable and three possible cases of GB among the zimedine-treated patients.[16] These data were presented to specialists in neurology and psychiatry and to the manufacturers, and in September 1983 the manufacturers decided to withdraw the drug from the world market.

## FUTURE MONITORING

The monitoring centres in the Scandinavian countries are now recognized institutions having good relations with the medical profession. In spite of under-reporting the potential for identifying new rare ADRs is clearly shown by the zimeldine story. The centres are all acting to improve reporting, and they all have the advantage of having access to drug utilization data. Supplementary methods are also used, for example intensive monitoring in Denmark and case-control studies in Sweden. Thus there is an ambition within the centres to develop and improve all aspects of drug monitoring.

## References


1. Beerman, B., Biörck, G. and Groshinsky-Grind, M. (1978). Admissions to a medical clinic due to drugs and intoxications. *Läkartidningen*, **75**, 959–960 (summary in English)
2. Bergman, U. and Wiholm, B.-E. (1981). Drug related problems causing admission to a medical clinic. *Eur. J. Clin. Pharmacol.*, **20**, 193–200
3. Jorup-Rönnström, C. and Britton, S. (1982). The nosocomial component of medical care. *Scand. J. Infect. Dis.*, (Supp 36), 150–6
4. Wiholm, B.-E. (1984). Spontaneous Reporting of ADR. Cross-fertilization with register data on morbidity and drug utilization in detection and prevention of adverse drug reactions. In Boström, H. and Ljungstedt, N. (eds.) *Skandia International Symposia*, pp. 152–167. (Stockholm: Almqvist & Wiksell International)
5. Nordic Statistics on Medicines. (1982). I, II Nordic Drug Index with Classification and Defined Daily Doses. *NLN Publications Nos 8 & 9*, Nordic Council on Medicines, Box 607, S-75125 Uppsala, Sweden
6. The Drug Consumption in Norway, yearly publication by the *Norwegian Medicinal Depot*, PO Box 100, Veituet 0518 Oslo 5, Norway. CISBN 82-903-1204-0, ISSn 0332-67535
7. Svensk Läkemedelsstatistik, yearly publication by the National Corporation of Swedish Pharmacies (Apoteksbolaget), S-10514 Stockholm, Sweden
8. Inman, W. H. W., Vessey, M. P., Westerholm, B. and Englund, A. (1970). Thromboembolic disease and the steroidal content of oral contraceptives. A report to the Committee on Safety of Medicines. *Br. Med. J.*, **2**, 203
9. Böttiger, L. E. Boman, G., Eklund, G. and Westerholm, B. (1980). Oral contraceptives and thromboembolic disease. Effects of lowering oestrogen content. *Lancet*, 1097–101
10. Bergman, U., Boman, G. and Wiholm, B.-E. (1978). Epidemiology of adverse drug reactions to phenformin and metformin. *Br. Med. J.*, **2**, 464–6
11. Strandberg, I., Boman, G., Hassler, L. and Sjöqvist, F. (1976). Acetylator phenotype in patients with hydralazine-induced lupoid syndrome. *Acta Med. Scand.*, **200**, 367
12. Wiholm, B.-E., Alván, G., Bertilsson, L., Säwe, J. and Sjöqvist, F. (1981). Hydroxylation of debrisoquine in patients with lactic acidosis after phenformin. *Lancet*, **2**, 1098–9
13. Wiholm, B.-E., Mortimer, Ö., Boethius, G. and Häggström, J. E. (1984). Tardive dyskinesia from metoclopramide. *Br. Med. J.*, **288**, 545–7
14. Dossing, M. and Andreasen, P. B. (1982). Danish drug-induced diseases of the liver. A 10-year survey shows halothane contributes a hefty share. *Scand. J. Gastroenterol.*, **17**, 205
15. Laake, K., Kjeldaas, L. and Borchgrevink, C. F. (1984). Side-effects of piroxicam (Feldene). A one-year material of 103 reports from Norway. *Acta Med. Scand.*, **215**, 81–3
16. Fagius, J., Osterman, P. O., Sidén, Å, Wiholm, B.-E. (1985). Guillain–Barré syndrome following zimeldine treatment. *J. Neurol. Beurosurg. Psychiatry*, **48**, 65–9

# 11
# Spain

J.-R. LAPORTE

The purpose of this chapter is not only to give an account of the development of methods for drug monitoring in Spain, but also to explain how drug monitoring activities have been set up and are carried out in a country where the development of a rational drug policy is urgently needed.

## DRUG PRESCRIBING AND MONITORING IN SPAIN

The population of Spain is approximately 37.5 million. The total number of doctors in 1983 was about 83 500. The population covered by the National Health Insurance System (*Seguridad Social*) is 32.6 million (87%). Of these, 5.9 million are pensioners, who obtain their medication free of charge. The remaining 26.7 million pay 40% of the costs of the medicines they are prescribed directly to the pharmacists[1].

The situation in Spain regarding drug prescribing and monitoring is far from ideal. Some of the problems which are currently encountered are listed below.

*Pharmaceutical supply*: 2477 chemical entities, 7256 proprietary brands (trademarks), 18 291 pharmaceutical forms. Fixed-dose combinations account for 55.7% of all proprietary brands. Only 57% of pharmaceutical products on the market can be considered of great value or, at best, of questionable value.[2]

*Drug information*: promotional activities by the pharmaceutical industry, which have very little educational value,[2–6] are the main source of information used by physicians.[3,4]

*Prescription of medicines*: drugs prescribed by doctors in the *Seguridad Social* closely reflect the low quality of the pharmaceutical market.[7] 'Cerebral vasodilators' are the group of drugs most prescribed to elderly people.[8,9] Consumption patterns of antibiotics,[10] psychotropic drugs,[11,12] antidiabetics,[13,14] and anti-hypertensive drugs[15] consistently differ from general recommendations in international literature. Hospital data[8,11,16] and surveys on current knowledge of the pharmacological properties of the most frequently prescribed drugs[10,17] show a worrying degree of 'wrong' therapeutic practice. Sixty per cent of the market would disappear if stricter criteria were applied[4,18] (Therapeutic Formulary for GPs., 1980[19]). Only 41% of the 500 most prescribed drugs in 1980 have a clinical pharmacological rationale for their use in therapy. (i.e. 59% were considered ineffectual or inappropriate in any circumstances).[20]

*Use of drugs by patients*: several surveys suggest that patients have an inadequate knowledge of the medicines they take.[9,21] Thirteen per cent of randomly selected elderly people interviewed at home were taking additive doses of the same drug (the most frequently found being phenylbutazone, barbiturates, corticosteroids, diazepam and codeine) contained in two or more proprietary brands without knowing it.[21]

*Drug monitoring*: no official system of drug monitoring is in operation, although a law which came into force in 1973 established that reporting of ADRs to the '*Centro Nacional de Farmacobiologia*', a national agency for drug control, was compulsory for pharmaceutical firms and for physicians.

The above mentioned law also established that post-marketing surveillance must be carried out by means of compulsory reporting of adverse drug reactions, either by physicians or by pharmaceutical firms.[22] Since then, however, reporting forms have never been circulated among doctors by the 'Centro', and reports on gathered information (if any) have never been released. Furthermore, the former Director General of Pharmacy and Drugs declared to the lay press that 'no adverse reactions have been reported, and those who cite anecdotal reports are seeking self-promotion, publicity, and scandal'[23].

The outlook was somewhat different in Catalonia:

(1) A formal course in clinical pharmacology, officially included in the medical curriculum, has been taught in the Autonomous University of Barcelona to more than 4000 young doctors since 1974. This course includes specific training in drug evaluation and epidemiology, in addition to other aspects of clinical pharmacology and therapeutics.[24]

(2) The Catalan Academy of Medical Sciences, a medical society to which approximately one half of the Catalan physicians are voluntarily affiliated, has been organizing and developing programmes of continuing education, among which the preparation and distribution of more than 20 000 free copies of the therapeutic formulary for GPs has been a useful point of reference for the changing situation.

In this setting a growing number of doctors inside and outside hospitals are following a more critical approach to drug selection and prescription,[25] and this is the most promising trend on which drug surveillance initiatives are based.[26,27] The main objective of all current efforts is to counterbalance the negative tradition which was outlined earlier in this chapter. The techniques, strategies and fields of investigation in drug monitoring are selected taking into account their educational value. At the same time research abilities are built up to confirm and strengthen existing evidence and to produce original data.

Before briefly presenting the specific content of the continuing programmes, it should be emphasized that the common aim of all of them is to establish permanent and reliable networks of drug surveillance.

## THE IMPLEMENTATION OF THE VOLUNTARY REPORTING SYSTEM (VRS)

Until the beginning of 1982, drug monitoring in Spain had been restricted to two programmes which had been set up by the Division of Clinical Pharmacology of the Autonomous University of Barcelona: the first, a scheme of intensive monitoring using the methodology of the Boston Collaborative Drug Surveillance Program (BCDSP), had been in operation for one year in a paediatric hospital in Barcelona,[28] and the second, a cohort of more than 600 ambulatory patients chronically treated with the oral anticoagulant acenocoumarol, had been systematically followed up since 1979.[29]

In May 1982 the '*Fondo de Investigaciones Sanitarias de la Seguridad Social*' funded a research project to implement a voluntary reporting system in Catalonia (5.6 million inhabitants, 17 750 doctors). A drug utilization computerized file was set up using consumption figures as 'denominators'. An advisory board was constituted, with members from all medical specialities together with one epidemiologist and one biostatistician. The Department of Health of the Autonomous Government, the Catalan Academy of Medical Sciences, and the two Faculties of Medicine of both Universities accepted the patronage of the programme. A yellow leaflet explaining the need for drug monitoring, the purposes of the VRS and how it works was mailed to all doctors in October 1982. A reporting form (yellow card) was designed, and Catalan and Spanish versions of it were circulated among doctors in November of the same year. During its first 6 months of operation, the VRS was presented at seven meetings of the staff and residents of the most important hospitals in the area, and at meetings of the Catalan Society of Pharmacology, the Spanish Society of Clinical Pharmacology, and the Association of Medical Staff of the Pharmaceutical Industry. In August 1983 our centre was nominated as the Spanish representative in the WHO International Drug Monitoring Program.

Reporting forms are mailed every 6 months to all doctors. Special yellow letters are also sent out at varying intervals to stimulate reporting. The first issue of a yellow Bulletin devoted to the findings and methodological aspects of the VRS was mailed to all physicians in February 1984, and a more in-depth yellow Annual Report has been published and sent to all reporters and to other health professionals on request. Steps are now being taken to include one form in the official (monthly) medical journal of the 'Academy' and to insert yellow reminders into the prescription pads used by GPs in the National Health Insurance System (*Seguridad Social*). During the first year of operation 541 reports have been received, containing enough information for analysis and processing on 533 ADRs.

Reports are now requested only from members of the medical profession. Regarding the question of what to report, all kinds of reports are obviously welcome, but those concerned with severe and unusual events and those occurring with recently-marketed drugs are particularly solicited. All reporters receive an acknowledgement of their contribution in the form of a (yellow) letter, in which additional information or therapeutic consultation is offered on request.

Reports from other continuing drug monitoring programmes (see above) are also included in the programme. Local literature is systematically screened, and adverse drug reactions reported in the form of 'letters to the editor' or short communications go into the ADR-system. After some months of operation some unsolicited reports of ADRs were received from pharmaceutical companies, and these are also included in the data base. Table 1 shows the distribution of the reports according to the methods used for reporting.

In some cases (approximately 15–20%) attempts are made to obtain additional information, mostly by telephone, in order to validate the reports. Data such as possible underlying disorders, other drugs administered that were not mentioned in the original report, effects of the same or other similar drugs taken before by the patient, or other relevant information not detailed by the reporter, such as dose, route of administration, duration of the treatment, age, etc. are elicited.

**Table 1** Voluntary reporting system: source of the reports received during the first year of operation

| | *No. of reports* | *(%)* |
|---|---|---|
| Yellow card | 372 | (69.8) |
| Yellow cards from hospitals collaborating with the programme | 91 | (17.1) |
| Other specific drug monitoring programmes | 39 | (7.3) |
| Medical journals | 22 | (4.1) |
| Drug companies | 9 | (1.7) |
| *Total* | 533 | |

Reports are presented and evaluated at weekly meetings of the programme secretariat, which includes six clinical pharmacologists who are responsible for different areas of drug monitoring. Advice is sought when judged necessary by members of the Advisory Board. After processing, a copy of the report (in which patient and doctor names have been omitted) is sent to the manufacturer(s) of the suspected drug(s). Reports are then coded for storage and processing. The data stored are those required by the WHO Collaborative Centre plus details concerning items of the Karch and Lasagna algorithm,[30] which is applied with some modifications.

The need for a critical review of this decision table soon became apparent. For example, it was difficult to accept that 'relapse on rechallenge' had to occur if an event was to be classified as 'definite': respiratory distress followed by vascular shock, with pruritus and urticaria, appearing within minutes after the administration of penicillin to a patient without any antecedent of respiratory difficulty, would be an event that could only be assessed as 'probable'. Similarly, no fatal reaction could be classified as 'definite', since 'relapse on rechallenge' is obviously impossible! On the other hand, an assessment which could fit the rules adopted by the WHO International Programme, and could be more easily 'translated', was felt desirable. The alterations introduced in the algorithm are mainly related to the loss of valuable information when answering its questions in terms of a yes–no dichotomy. Let us take the example of the item 'known response pattern to drug'. For some associations only anecdotal cases have been described, while for others well-designed studies and a wide clinical and epidemiological experience strongly support a causal relationship. Hence, the response to this question could tentatively be summarized in four ways: (1) there is an extensive background of knowledge on the association in question (e.g. venous thrombosis in a woman who has been using oral contraceptives with high oestrogen content for some years); (2) either anecdotal cases have been published (e.g. hepatitis associated with ranitidine in 1982–83[31]) or there is conflicting evidence from different epidemiological studies (e.g. infantile pyloric stenosis associated with the use of Bendectin during pregnancy[32,33]); (3) to our knowledge, this association had never been described up to now, and (4) the pharmacological profile of the drug in question is contrary to the observed event (e.g. mydriasis after the administration of an anticholinergic agent). It is clear that categories (1) and (2) are equivalent to the category 'Yes' of the algorithm, and categories (3) and (4) are equivalent to the category 'unknown response-pattern to drug'. This method of assessment is now being tested, and will be evaluated when 1000 ADRs have been processed (by the end of 1984).

The severity of the reported reactions is another issue which has deserved special attention. The efficiency of a drug monitoring system does not depend on the number of adverse events it is able to collect, but rather on the number of *new* events not previously described, and on the severity of these events (i.e. their clinical, epidemiological and

**Table 2** Voluntary Reporting System. Distribution of reports according to their source and degree of severity

| | *Minor* | *Moderate* | *Severe* | *Fatal* |
|---|---|---|---|---|
| Yellow card | 262 | 80 | 25 | 5 |
| Yellow card, hospitals | 31 | 23 | 35 | 2 |
| Other specific drug monitoring programmes | 16 | 3 | 17 | 3 |
| Medical journals | — | 14 | 8 | — |
| Drug companies | 3 | 5 | 1 | — |
| *Total* | 312 | 125 | 86 | 10 |

community health consequences). Hence, ADRs have tentatively been classified into four groups: (1) fatal reactions (in which the drug has or may have contributed to this outcome); (2) severe, directly life-threatening reactions (e.g. pulmonary thromboembolism, agranulocytosis, or hyperkalaemia); (3) moderate, i.e. those which, according to the information given in the report, lead to admission to hospital or absence from work or school, without being life-threatening (e.g. extrapyramidal reaction, hallucination, cholestatic hepatitis, etc.), and (4) minor, a group which includes all other ADRs (obviously this group may include ADRs which in fact had been of moderate severity, but, according to the information contained in the report, may not be considered as such). Table 2 shows the distribution of ADRs according to the method of reporting and their severity.

Strict confidentiality as regards to patients and doctors is maintained. This does not mean that gathered information is not circulated, and that specific information cannot be given to health professionals on request. Accordingly, the annual publication of cumulative summaries of suspected reactions, using the drug trade name when it is a fixed-dose combination, is envisaged in the near future.

A proposal by the Director General of Drugs to extend the VRS to other regions of Spain is now being discussed after training of personnel in the Barcelona centre.

## SETTING UP A SCHEME FOR INTEGRATED DRUG MONITORING

Conceptually, a comprehensive system of drug surveillance requires the following elements:

(1) Spontaneous adverse reaction reporting.

(2) Follow-up studies of large cohorts of persons exposed to specific drugs to detect a range of events that are important, but too

**Table 3** Some integrated activities of drug monitoring (Division of Clinical Pharmacology, Autonomous University of Barcelona)

| *System/Subject* | *Methodology* | *Observations* |
|---|---|---|
| 'Yellow card' | VRS[26,27] | covers in-patient and health care by general practitioners; 541 reports during the first year |
| International study on agranulocytosis and aplastic anaemia | case-control surveillance[36] | the catchment population in the Barcelona area is 4 050 000 inhabitants; a network of 20 Haematology services collaborate in the ascertainment of cases |
| Analgesic nephropathy | case-control study | cases included have been patients in haemodialisis programme in the Great Barcelona Area |
| Congenital malformations | case-control surveillance | cases included have been patients in haemodialysis programme in the Great Barcelona Area |
| ADRs among in-patients | in-hospital intensive monitoring[37] | |
| *Ad hoc* studies aimed at specific problems | descriptions of series | role of marketed drugs in the aetiology of severe self-poisoning[38], previous use of amiodarone among patients with pulmonary fibrosis[39], haemorrhagic risk during chronic treatment with acenocoumarol[40] |

infrequent to be detected in clinical trials. Generally, such studies cannot be expected to identify very rare events, and they can be expensive, since, unless cohort studies are very large – either in terms of numbers or of years of follow-up – they may be unable to detect important but relatively uncommon events.

(3) Case control studies and case control surveillance[34] of diseases generally too uncommon to be detected by follow-up studies. In the case control approach, subjects with selected diseases are identified, and comprehensive histories of prior drug use are obtained. Any association between a drug and a disease is evaluated in detail to determine whether or not a causal hypothesis could be considered. A case control study aimed at verifying a specific hypothesis is more efficient, more rapid, and usually less costly in obtaining the same information that could be obtained by case study. Although it is often claimed that case control studies are more subject to bias than cohort studies, a more accurate claim would be that both methods are subject to various forms of bias; in both, however, problems of bias in selecting subjects and in obtaining information can be minimized in many situations.[35]

(4) Intensive monitoring of hospitalized patients.

(5) *Ad hoc* studies and techniques to test hypotheses generated from any one of the approaches described above, or to intensively monitor recently-marketed drugs.

Some of these methodologies have been developed in our centre (see Table 3) with the aim of complementing the educational as well as the informative and preventive role of the voluntary reporting system.

## References

1. Anonymous. (1982). Apéndice estadistico. Análisis de resultados. *Papeles de Economia Española*, **12/13**, 93–106
2. Erill, S. (1974). Clinical pharmacology in Spain. *Clin. Pharmacol. Ther.*, **16,** 597–604
3. Erill, S. (1981). Información sobre medicamentos y su repercusión en la prescripción farmacológica. In Laporte, J. and Salvá, J. A. (eds.) *Avances en Terapéutica, vol. 11*, pp. 18–28. (Barcelona: Salvat)
4. Arnau, J. M. (1982). *La selecció de medicaments a Catalunya. L'Index Farmacològic i la utilització de les fonts d'informació sobre medicaments pels metges i farmacèutics*. (Doctoral thesis). (Bellaterra: Universitat Autònoma de Barcelona).
5. Erill, S., Du Souich, P. and Garcia Sevilla, J. A. (1975). Chloramphenicol-containing drugs. A report from Spain. *J. Clin. Pharmacol.*, **15,** 401–4
6. Cami, J., Laporte, J., Gutiérrez, R. and Laporte, J. R. (1977). Estudio de los preparados que contienen anfetamina existentes en el mercado farmacéutico nacional. *Med. Clin. (Barc.)*, **68,** 57–62
7. Laporte, J. R., Erill, S. and Garcia Sevilla, J. A. (1974). El médico ante las especialidades farmacéuticas. Análisis de 1356 prescripciones. *Anales Med. (Barc.)*, **60,** 973–9
8. Laporte, J. R., Martin, M., Puig, J., Segura, A. and Blanquer, A. (1979). Consumption

and prescription of 'cerebral vasodilator' drugs in Spain. In Tognoni, G. and Garattini, S. (eds.) *Drug Treatment and Prevention in Cerebrovascular Disorders*. pp. 110–20. (Amsterdam: Elsevier/North-Holland)

9. Mas, X., Laporte, J. R., Frati, M. E., Busquet, L., Arnau, J. M., Ibáñez, L., Séculi, E., Capellà, D. and Arbonés, G. (1983). Drug prescribing and use among elderly people in Spain. *Drug Intell. Clin. Pharm.*, **17**, 378–82
10. Drobnic, L., Beni, C., Canela, J., Ezpeleta, A. and Castell, E. (1984). El uso de los antibióticos en la asistencia primaria de Barcelona. *Med. Clin. (Barc.)*, **82**, 567–71
11. Laporte, J. R., Capellà, D., Gisbert, R., Porta, M., Frati, M. E., Garcia Santesmases, M. P. and Garcia Iñesta, A. (1981). The utilization of sedative–hypnotic drugs in Spain. In Tognoni, G., Bellantuono, C. and Lader, M. (eds.) *Epidemiological Impact of Psychotropic Drugs*. pp. 137–49. (Amsterdam: Elsevier/North-Holland)
12. Laporte, J. R., Capellà, D., Porta, M. and Frati, M. E. (1983). Patterns of use of psychotropic drugs in Spain in an international perspective. In Gram, L. F., Usdin, E., Dahl, S. G., Kragh-Sørensen, P., Sjöqvist, F. and Morselli, P. L. (eds.) *Clinical Pharmacology in Psychiatry. Bridging the Experimental–Therapeutic Gap*. pp. 18–31. (London and Basingstoke: Macmillan)
13. Laporte, J. R., Porta, M., Capellà, D. and Arnau, J. M. (1984). Drugs in the Spanish health system. *Int. J. Health Serv.*, **14**, 635–48
14. Barbeira, J. M., Levy, M. and Garcia Iñesta, A. (1983). Consumo de medicamentos antidiabéticos. Uso relativo de antidiabéticos orales respecto a insulinas. *Inf. Ter. Segur. Soc.*, **7**, 112–8
15. Capellà, D., Porta, M. and Laporte, J. R. (1983). Utilization of antihypertensive drugs in certain European countries. *Eur. J. Clin. Pharmacol.*, **25**, 431–5
16. Gómez, J. and Erill, S. (1979). Image of systemic antimicrobial agents as perceived by physicians in a 900 bed hospital. *Eur. J. Clin. Pharmacol.*, **15**, 127–32
17. Laporte, J., Du Souich, P. and Erill, S. (1976). Conocimiento por parte del médico de la composición y propiedades de las especialidades farmacéuticas más prescritas. *Rev. Clin. Esp.*, **140**, 269–74
18. Laporte, J. R. and Arnau, J. M. (1982). Guias farmacológicas para la asistencia médica primaria. In Laporte, J. and Salvá, J. A. (eds.) *Avances en Terapéutica, Vol. 12*, pp. 135–53 (Barcelona: Salvat)
19. Comissió Redactora. (1980). *Index Farmacològic 1980*. (Barcelona: Acadèmia de Ciències Mèdiques de Catalunya i de Balears)
20. Laporte, J. R., Porta, M. and Capellà, D. (1983). Drug utilization studies: a tool for determining the effectiveness of drug use. *Br. J. Clin. Pharmac.*, **16**, 301–4
21. Mas, X., Laporte, J. R. and Martin, M. (1981). Drugs and the elderly. *Br. Med. J.*, **282**, 824
22. Ministerio de la Gobernación. Orden de 12 de noviembre de 1973 sobre Farmacovigilancia. *Boletin Oficial del Estado*, **287**, 23190–1
23. González Oti, R. Declarations to the Journal *El Pais*, December 13, 1981
24. Divisió de Farmacologia Clinica, U.A.B. (1984). *Farmacologia clinica i Terapèutica. Programa i Guions*. (Bellaterra: Universitat Autònoma de Barcelona)
25. Arnau, J. M. and Laporte, J. R. (1983). Fuentes de información sobre medicamentos utilizadas por médicos y farmacéuticos. *Arch. Farmacol. Toxicol.*, **9**, 109–14
26. Laporte, J. R., Porta, M., Capellà, D. and Frati, M. E. (1982). La notificación voluntaria de reacciones adversas a medicamentos. *Med. Clin. (Barc.)*, **79**, 287–91
27. Capellà, D. and Laporte, J. R. (1984). La notificació voluntària de reaccions adverses a medicaments. La targeta groga. *Ann. Med. (Barc.)*, **70**, 17–21
28. Laporte, J., Laporte, J. R. and Frati, M. E. (1979). Vigilancia farmacológica hospitalaria. In *IV Reunión Nacional de la Asociación Española de Farmacólogos*, pp. 111–31 (Santiago de Compostela: Asociación Española de Farmacólogos).
29. Laporte, J. R., Arboix, M., Arnau, J. M., Busquet, L., Frati, M. E. and Mas, X. (1981). Drug utilization among hospital out-patients treated with acenocoumarol. In Hollmann, M. and Weber, E. (eds.) *Drug Utilization Studies in Hospitals*. pp. 65–9. (Stuttgart: Schattauer)
30. Karch, F. E. and Lasagna, L. (1977). Toward the operational identification of adverse drug reactions. *Clin. Pharmacol. Ther.*, **21**, 247–54

31. Barr, G. D., and Piper, D. W. (1981). Possible ranitidine hepatitis. *Med. J. Austr.*, **2,** 421
32. Eskenazi, B. and Bracken, M. B. (1982). Bendectin (Debendox) as a risk factor for pyloric stenosis. *Am. J. Obst. Gynecol.*, **144,** 919–24
33. Mitchell, A. A., Schwingl, P. J., Rosenberg, L., Louik, C. and Shapiro, S. (1983). Birth defects in relation to Bendectin used in pregnancy. II. Pyloric stenosis. *Am. J. Obst. Gynecol.*, **147,** 737–42
34. Slone, D., Shapiro, S. and Miettinen, O. S. (1977). Case-control surveillance of serious illnesses attributable to ambulatory drug use. In Colombo, F., Shapiro, S., Slone, D. and Tognoni, G. (eds.) *Epidemiological Evaluation of Drugs*. pp. 59–70. (Littleton, Massachusetts: PSG Publishing Company)
35. Sackett, D. L. (1979). Bias in analytic research. *J. Chron. Dis.*, **32,** 51–63
36. International Agranulocytosis and Aplastic Anemia Study. (1983). The design of a study of the drug etiology of agranulocytosis and aplastic anemia. *Eur. J. Clin. Pharmacol.*, **24,** 833–6
37. Arnau, J. M., Camps, A., Curull, V., Muñiz, R. and Laporte, J. R. (1984). Programa de detección de reacciones adversas a medicamentos en pacientes hospitalizados. Métodos y resultados de la fase piloto. *Med. Clin. (Barc.)*, **82,** 433–7
38. Frati, M. E., Marruecos, L., Porta, M., Martin, M. L. and Laporte, J. R. (1983). Acute severe poisoning in Spain: clinical outcome related to the implicated drugs. *Hum. Toxicol.*, **2,** 625–32
39. Morera, J., Vidal, R., Morell, F., Ruiz, J., Bernadó, L. and Laporte, J. R. (1983). Amiodarone and pulmonary fibrosis. *Eur. J. Clin. Pharmacol.*, **24,** 591–3
40. Arboix, M., Laporte, J. R., Frati, M. E. and Rutllan, M. (1984). Effect of age and sex on acenocoumarol requirements. *Br. J. Clin. Pharmac.*, **18,** 475–9

# 12
# The United States of America

J. K. JONES, G. A. FAICH and C. ANELLO

## HISTORICAL PERSPECTIVES

Formal arrangements for drug monitoring in the United States have existed since the early 1950s, when chloramphenicol-associated aplastic anaemia was first described. This first took the form of a registry of adverse reactions to chloramphenicol[1]. Subsequently, the American Medical Association (AMA) formed a general registry for adverse reactions. At the same time, the Food and Drug Administration (FDA) developed a similar registry in the early 1960s. In the late 1960s, the American Medical Association turned over their effort to the FDA which became the primary site where voluntary spontaneous reports were collected[2]. This complemented the reports from pharmaceutical manufacturers who are required by regulation to report all events thought to be associated with an approved new drug[3].

About the same time, other drug monitoring programmes were set up, most notably the Boston Collaborative Drug Surveillance Program (BCDSP) (see also Chapter 17), followed by the Boston Drug Epidemiology Unit (DEU) in the early 1970s. Inspired by the haematological registry, a number of other adverse reaction registries were spawned; these are described later. In the meantime, there was considerable official concern about drug monitoring in the United States. This resulted in an FDA Special Committee on Drug Experience in the early 1970s and calls by the US Congress, notably Senator Edward Kennedy in 1976, for a concerted effort in drug monitoring, in turn resulted in the formation of a Joint Commission on Prescription Drug Use[4]. This Commission, in concert with the FDA and the US Department of Commerce, co-funded a large contract – the Experimental Technology Incentives Program (ETIP) contract, to study the entire subject of drug monitoring. This effort, carried out from 1978 to 1981, provided a useful review of the current state of the art in post-marketing surveillance (PMS)[5–7]. The funding agencies and contractors also developed the concept of a multi-faceted *system* of drug monitoring, as opposed to a single 'turnkey' method for PMS, which might be useful in all cases. In the mid-1970s, the FDA began to fund various drug epidemiology efforts, such as the BCDSP and DEU. They also aggressively pursued the development of new methods and resources for PMS, resulting in the active exploration and use of record-linkage data-bases, such as those provided for health maintenance organizations (HMOs) in Seattle, Puget Sound and by Kaiser in Oakland, and by the Medicaid Management Information System. On February 22 1985, new FDA regulations were published focusing post-marketing reporting of ADRs on the Division of Drug and Biological Product Experience of the Center for Drugs and Biologics of the FDA. A requirement for '15 day Alert" reports has been established. Fifteen day alerts are defined as 'serious and unexpected' events and include estimates of the frequency of ADRs. All other periodical reports are submitted quarterly for the first 3 years and annually thereafter. Internally, the FDA has developed clear guidelines for ADR reporting, and has begun to use and publish ADR and drug use data.

## ESTIMATING DRUG EXPOSURE

In order to put ADRs in perspective, it is necessary to determine the context of each report. To accomplish this, the FDA has had to obtain data from other sources. These data fall into two classes: data used to determine the extent of drug exposure, and those which provide information both about exposure and adverse events and which permit the estimation of risk ratios in defined populations. At the present time, there are over 32 000 named products in the United States. A major problem in estimating drug exposure data is the difficulty inherent in the large number of drug names and the constant changes in the content of products. This complicates attempts to set up a stable monitoring system. There is no universally accepted drug classification scheme, and several trade names can be applied to a similar product.

Much of the data on drug exposure in the United States comes from continuing marketing surveys. In this category, the largest and most comprehensive data base is that supplied by IMS America, Inc. (Ambler, PA.) which collects and sells many types of data, primarily for marketing purposes. IMS collects data from pharmacies, hospitals and practitioners, and extrapolates to provide estimates of national experience. These data provide crude estimates of overall drug use.

The National Prescription Audit (NPA) is an audit at pharmacy level which samples over 600 pharmacies and tabulates data on dispensed prescriptions which are then extrapolated nationally. The National Disease and Therapeutic Index (NDTI) samples the prescribing of 525 physicians representing the major specialties, such as family practice, internal medicine, gynaecology, cardiology and dermatology. The sample is based on every 'patient-encounter' and drug prescription over a sample period of 48 hours within each quarter of the year. This complements the NPA Data Base. The National Drugstore and Hospital Audit provides kilogram estimate of drug sales. All of these data bases have recently been combined into an integrated data base called IMSPACT which allows appropriate searches in response to various types of question.

At the present time, data on hospital drug exposure are very limited. Although the National Hospital Audit provides kilogram estimates of hospital purchases, there are no comprehensive estimates of patient exposure. Recently, the FDA carried out a feasibility study for a national hospital data base and found that this would be difficult to implement.[8,9]

There are several smaller marketing services which carry out other types of sampling of drug exposure or prescribing and various *ad hoc* consumer surveys which the FDA have not yet used. At the present time, for example, there are meagre data on over-the-counter (OTC) drug consumption. In the US, OTC drugs are not only sold in drug stores, but also in groceries, supermarkets, variety stores and by mail order.

One major resource, the Medicaid Management Information System, records all drugs and diagnoses for over 25 million patients who receive medical care from state and federal government funds. So far, only data from certain states such as Michigan, Florida and Tennessee have been used for this purpose. The data include patient demographics, geographic location and details of drugs dispensed by a pharmacy by date of service. Diagnostic data, tabulated by the International Classification of Diseases, 9th edition (ICD-9CM), is also recorded by date of service, and this produces a longitudinal profile of medical or pharmacy encounters over time. The Medicaid system has been described elsewhere,[10] and its epidemiological uses are discussed in Chapter 16. Several investigators have made use of the data from Michigan, Minnesota and Tennessee Medicaid systems to study drug use. There are also data bases developed by the US National Center for Health Statistics which provide patient-based estimates of drug exposure.[11]

## IDENTIFYING DRUG PROBLEMS

### Spontaneous reports

The FDA has been collecting spontaneous reports of ADRs since the early 1960s. In 1969, a formal computer system was developed which has now accumulated over 230 000 individual case reports.

Before 1980, approximately 9–12 000 reports were received each year. In 1981, there was a large surge in their number, possibly resulting from publicity about a possible teratogenic effect of Bendectin (Debendox), the antinausea drug used during pregnancy, and increased interest in the PMS field. Foreign case-reports were included and, from 1983, about 40 000 reports were received annually.

At the present time, the manufacturers responsible for all approved new drug application (NDA) products (which comprise a large proportion of the prescription products in the United States) are required, within 15 days, to report to the FDA, using the FDA's report form 1639, any adverse event, whether or not it is thought to be related to the drug. This requirement includes reports of any new or unusually serious adverse effects or any increase in frequency of a previously recognized serious effect. Other less serious ADRs are to be reported to the FDA at less frequent intervals. These reports comprise over 85% of the FDA data-base. In parallel, the FDA also receives reports from physicians, pharmacists, and other health professionals.

In 1984, a method of direct reporting by computer using the American Medical Association GTE Computer System was initiated and is being evaluated. As before, the Division of Drug Experience collects spontaneous reports derived from letters or telephone calls. The Division also reviews over 180 Medical Journals for new and unexpected adverse effects which are summarized in the Current Drug Evaluation Literature (CDEL), published monthly in the American Society of Hospital Journal.

In the US, all products are comprehensively 'labelled' by means of product package inserts which list the known side-effects. The reports of suspected ADRs are compared with the label in the light of their seriousness and possible causal relationship to the drug. Up to mid-1984, medical or pharmacist reviewers assessed the presence or absence in the label of serious or causally related reactions, and then selected one or more adverse reaction coding (COSTART) term to describe the reaction, which was then entered into the computer.[12] Because this procedure was labour-intensive, from late 1984 the COSTART coding terms have been applied without complete review, and all reports entered into the computer immediately. Individual evaluation by the reviewers is now restricted to reports which describe previously unrecorded or serious ADRs, (typically, those qualifying for 15-day reports).

New, unusual or serious reports are reviewed at a weekly 'Alert' meeting in which the array of serious adverse effects are considered. Any reports meriting follow-up, such as those which might be causally related, those which were new or which resulted in hospitalization or death were assigned to epidemiologists who discussed appropriate follow-up strategies. These would include a thorough search of documented evidence supporting the suspected drug-effect association, including other cases recorded in the FDA's ADR data-base or known to the manufacturer, and those recorded in the literature.

The 'Alerts' are circulated as memoranda to the regulatory staff in the FDA, and are sometimes incorporated in monographs called *ADR Highlights* which are distributed within the FDA to provide some basis for labelling or other regulatory changes. *ADR Highlights* are also distributed to regulatory agencies in other countries and, in some cases, when thought to be particularly important, are published in the *FED Drug Bulletin* or in Journals, usually as 'brief reports' or 'letters to the editor'.

Data from the spontaneous reports are sent on tape on a regular basis to the World Health Organization Centre for Drug Monitoring in Uppsala, Sweden.

The data from spontaneous reports have several uses. First, they signal new problems, particularly with new drugs. Examples of important problems include hepatic toxicity associated with ticrynafen (subsequently withdrawn from the market), hepatotoxicity associated with ketoconazole, and a number of other serious drug effects. Secondly, case-reports provide useful 'profiles' of adverse effects to identify demographic groups which may be at especially high risk. It has previously been shown that in the majority of reported ADRs, the demographic characteristics are similar to those of the population exposed to the drug. Special situations do occur, however, where a particular subgroup is at unique risk.[13,14] The profile can often describe the spectrum of problems specific to one drug group. This has predictive value for those responsible for reviewing new additions to a family of compounds, for example, non-steroidal anti-inflammatory agents.

The FDA's spontaneous reporting system is now undergoing modernization. A 5-year subset of the ADR data base is currently available on-line. This allows for efficient reviewing and generation of reports to various users. On-line reporting not only by the AMA GTE system but also by tape or electronic mail from manufacturers is being contemplated.

## Registries

To complement the spontaneous reporting system, there are several adverse reaction registries currently in operation. These registries stem from the historical development of the original Adverse Reaction Registry of chloramphenicol-induced aplastic anaemia. The FDA has encouraged the development of registries since the early 1960s, most notably the Tissue Reaction to Drugs Registry at the Armed Forces' Institute of Pathology developed by Nelson Irey. This registry includes a large series of cases and pathological material relating to adverse reactions to drugs.[15] In the 1970s, Dr W. H. Shehadi developed the Registry of Radiologic Contrast Media which can produce estimates of the frequencies of various reactions to these agents.[16] More recently, the FDA has funded three further registries: the National Registry of Hepatic Reactions,[13] the Ocular Reactions Registry,[17] and the Dermatology Registry.[18] Consideration has been given to the need to establish other registries. These registries have taken different forms.

In some cases, they have collected data from physicians, such as opthalmologists who might not otherwise report adverse reactions. In other cases, the presence of a person interested in drug associated disease has probably stimulated colleagues to report and develop case series relating to this issue. Overall, registries have provided valuable information, usually to corroborate the data in the FDA's Spontaneous Report Data-Base.

Finally, the FDA supported data-bases described below have also generated hypotheses about possible drug-associated effects. The Medicaid data enables the diagnoses of large cohorts of patients exposed to drugs to be compared with age/sex-matched controls not exposed to drugs. This can generate risk estimates for all diagnoses in the ICD code for use as a crude signalling tool. Similar types of comparisons can be carried out in patients in the record linkage of the Puget sound (HMO), although in this case diagnoses are limited to hospitalizations only. The Boston Drug Epidemiology Unit, in its focus on specific drug-induced diseases such as peptic ulcer, myocardial infarction, birth defects or breast cancer, has developed a number of hypotheses such as the negative association of aspirin and myocardial infarction, or of thiazide diuretics and gallbladder disease, etc.[19,20]

## EPIDEMIOLOGICAL DATA RESOURCES

There are two major approaches to developing epidemiological data on suspected drug-event associations: case-control and cohort studies.[21,22] Case-control studies focus on the disease, and develop estimates of relative risk of a disease in patients who have or have not been exposed to drugs. This methodology has the advantage of being useful in exceedingly rare diseases where the exposure is relatively common, but the disadvantage of being dependent upon retrospective information, often collected by interview with the doctor or patient, with its inherent biases. With increased use of computerized drug histories, this bias can sometimes be avoided. Selection of truly appropriate controls is most difficult, although the methodology for this has advanced considerably in the past 10 years.

Cohort studies, in contrast, identify an entire group of patients exposed to a drug and, ideally, compare them with an age/sex-matched group of patients not exposed to the drug, but resembling the treated group with regard to the majority of major characteristics (especially diagnosis and concurrent therapy). Many studies are carried out without control cohorts, and this limits the ability to interpret the association between effects that have been discovered, and particularly to distinguish those which might be associated with the disease under treatment and those due to the treatment itself. Cohort studies tend to be useful for more commonly occurring adverse reactions. Over the past decade, the FDA has expanded its use of facilities for case-control and cohort studies. Many centres can conduct both types of

**Table 1** Selected US epidemiological resources for post-marketing drug surveillance

| *Resource* | *Characteristics* |
|---|---|
| Boston collaborative drug surveillance program Hospital data base | 40 000 monitored medical hospital patients in 1970 |
| Puget Sound health maintenance organization, Seattle, Washington | 280 000 persons with record linkage of all drugs since 1976 and hospitalizations. Access to original medical chart |
| Drug epidemiology unit | 40 000 hospitalized patients with data on previous drug exposures, focus on patients with drug-induced diseases (cancer, peptic ulcer, myocardial infarction, etc) |
| Medicaid MMIS | record linkage data by date of service on drugs, diagnoses for the 10 + % of each states population covered by Medicaid. Data accessed in over 8 states = population 5 million |
| Kaiser Hospitals Los Angeles* | HMO covering 2 million patients with recent (1984) development of computer pharmacy data with link to medical records |
| Kaiser Oakland* | HMO with record linkage of pharmacy date to medical date including state cancer registries for 140 000 patients 1969–73 |
| Committee on Professional Hospital Activities (CHPA)* | a resource containing roughly 40% of all hospital discharge diagnoses in the US. Not linked to drugs except at special sites (Puget Sound, etc.) |

*These three resources have been used in the past, but are not currently funded by the FDA

study, but most use the case-control approach because cohort studies frequently demand such a large population in order to identify or measure events of interest that very few data-bases of sufficient size exist. A current list of resources is included in Table 1.

One of the most exciting, but also perplexing, resources is the Medicaid Management Information System (MMIS), a record linkage of billing information for drugs and medical providers for 25 million Medicaid patients in individual states. In 1978, the FDA funded development of this resource in two states, Michigan and Minnesota, as a potential resource for PMS. Since that time, it has been used in a number of studies of both drug utilization and quantitation of drug associated disease entities.[10,23] Recently, the FDA has completed a validation study of this data-base. Although the preliminary studies appear promising, the data have many perplexing characteristics. It is apparent that each type of drug-event problem must be approached individually. Each state has different rules for billing, recording, and paying for various medical and pharmacy services, and this makes interstate comparisons difficult. The incentives for including or excluding diagnoses vary from state to state and possibly from practice to practice. Nonetheless, the validation studies suggested that the drug exposure data are quite reliable. The validity of the diagnostic data, on the other hand, was not so well defined in the study, and its use in practice remains to be established.

The Drug Epidemiology Unit, in operation since 1972, has been carrying out an ongoing multiple case-control study design which has been described in detail elsewhere.[24,25] The most compelling aspect of this design is its concentration on the ability to link certain diseases thought to be associated with drugs (e.g. peptic ulcer, myocardial infarction, and aplastic anaemia) with exposures to all drugs. The aplastic anaemia study, for example, will provide a useful data base for determining the relative risk associated with a wide variety of individual drugs in several countries.[26]

The BCDSP, which derives data from hospitalized patients, has continued to be useful, but does not produce information about many new drugs.[27] However, the development by Dr Hershel Jick of the Puget Sound HMO record linkage scheme has shown considerable potential particularly for long-term monitoring.[28] The HMO record links hospital discharge diagnosis and outpatient drug use, and has been used to study birth defects, various diseases associated with phenylpropanolamine, and a variety of other problems.[29–31]

A number of special studies have been developed. For example, there have been several case-control studies of birth defects[32] and there has been a greater focus on geriatric drug problems,[33] including a National Institute on Ageing study of drug exposure in three states.

Finally, drug abuse, although not always included in drug monitoring, is included in the FDA's responsibility. The Drug Abuse Warning Network, a sample data-base of both emergency room visits and coroners' experience, has been highly useful in developing national estimates of problems associated with abuse of such drugs as propoxyphene, butyl nitrite, and phenylpropanolamine.[34] Likewise, poisoning by drugs and other substances has recently been included in the drug monitoring area, and data are collected on a regular basis from a large number of poison control centres. Data collection using optical character reading allowing rapid data entry may be adopted in this and other areas of drug monitoring.[35]

## INDUSTRY PHASE-FOUR STUDIES

Since interest in PMS developed in the mid-1970s, a number of pharmaceutical manufacturers have developed their own approaches to post-marketing surveillance of specific drugs, particularly new molecular entities such as cimetidine. Some of these efforts have been requested or were part of the basis of approval by the FDA; more recently studies have been developed to provide both marketing and medical PMS data. A review of the early results suggests that these PMS studies provided little that a good spontaneous reporting system could not provide.[36] Nonetheless, considerable interest in the entire area of epidemiological surveillance has been shown by the pharmaceutical industry. At least five manufacturers have developed active programmes and are funding efforts to study comparative effects of drugs in the postmarketing period.

## A PERSPECTIVE ON US DRUG MONITORING, 1984

At the present time there is no clear definition of drug safety or drug risk even for those drugs used in particular groups such as rheumatoid arthritics, healthy young women, etc. Only recently has there been an effort to compare drug risk with that of other types of societal risks, such as car accidents, infectious disease and the like. Such an effort is now being made, and this suggests a future with a more rational and balanced approach towards drug surveillance. The other side of this coin is the fact that, given limited resources, there are also limits to the number of interesting and significant drug events that can be measured in an acceptable way, and this calls for acceptance of priority decisions.

There is considerable work still to be done in the US. Most drug monitoring methodologies are well understood. Many resources are available and are being further developed. The task for the future is to develop appropriate ways of making the best use of these tools.

## References

1. Moser, R. H. (1971). The obituary of an idea. *J. Am. Med. Assoc.*, **216,** 2135–6
2. Lee, B. and Turner, W. M. (1978). Food and Drug Administration's Adverse Drug Reaction Monitoring Program. *Am. J. Hosp. Pharm.*, **35,** 929–32
3. United States Code of Federal Regulations. **21,** 310, 300–4
4. Melmon, K. L. (1976). Editorial. The clinical pharmacologist and scientifically unsound regulations for drug development. *Clin. Pharm. Ther.*, **20,** 125–9
5. Melmon, K. L. (1980). An Experiment in Early Post-Marketing Surveillance of Drugs. Task A and Task A Appendix. FDA Contract #223-78-3007. *National Technical Information Service (US)* (PB#288577-AS)
6. Melmon, K. L. (1980). An Experiment in Early Post-Marketing Surveillance of Drugs. Task B FDA Contract #223-78-3007. *National Technical Information Service (US)* (PB#139090)
7. Melmon, K. L. (1981). An Experiment in Early Post-Marketing Surveillance of Drugs. Task C FDA Contract #223-78-3007. *National Technical Information Service (US)* (PB# 1149759)
8. Forbes, M. L., Burke, L. B. and Jones, J. K. (1981). Need for uniform data elements in hospital drug use review. *Am. J. Hosp. Pharm.*, **38,** 711–5.
9. Baum, C., Forbes, M. B., Kennedy, D. L. and Jones, J. K. (1983). Patient drug profiles and medical records as sources of hospital drug use information. *Am. J. Hosp. Pharm.*, **40,** 2191–3

10. Jones, J. K., Van de Carr, S. W., Rosa, F. W., Morse, L. and LeRoy, A. (1984). Medicaid Drug-Event Data: an emerging tool for evaluation of drug risk. *Acta Med. Scand. Suppl.*, **683,** 127–34
11. Koch, H. National Center for Health Statistics, (1982). The collection and processing of drug information: National Ambulatory Medical Care Survey, United States, 1980. *Vital and Health Statistics.* **Series 2**, No. 90. DHHS Pub. No. (PHS) 82-1364. Public Health Service. (Washington DC: U.S. Government Printing Office)
12. Jones, J. K. (1984). Regulatory use of adverse drug reactions. In *Detection and Prevention of Adverse Drug Reactions.* pp. 203–14. (Stockholm: Almquist and Wiksall)
13. Jones, J. K. (1981). Suspected drug-induced hepatic reactions reported to the FDA's Adverse Reaction System: An overview, *Sem. in Liver Dis.*, **1,** 157–67
14. Matta, L. (1984). Approaches to Structure-Related prediction of drug toxicity by analysis of human toxicity data, *PhD Thesis,* American University, Washington D.C. U.S.A.
15. Irey, N. S. (1976). Adverse reactions and death. *J. Am. Med. Assoc.*, **236,** 575–8
16. Shehadi, W. H. (1974). Adverse reactions to intravascularly administered contrast media. *Am. J. Roentgen*, **124,** 145–52
17. Fraunfelder, F. (1976). *Drug Induced Ocular Side Effects and Drug Interactions.* (Philadelphia: Lea and Febiger)
18. Stern, R. S. and Brown, H. L. (1983). Adverse drug reactions. *Arch. Int. Med.*, **143,** 1631
19. Jick, H. (1978). Regular aspirin use and myocardial infarction. In Breddin, K., Dorndorf, W., Loew, D. and Max, R. (eds); *Acetylsalicylic Acid in Cerebral Ischemia and Coronary Heart Disease*, pp. 151–2. (Stuttgart: Schattauer Verlas)
20. Rosenberg, L., Shapiro, S., Slone, D., Kaufman, D. W., Miettinen, O. S. and Stolley, P. D. (1980). Thiazide and acute cholecystitis. *N. Engl. J. Med.*, **303,** 546–8
21. Anello, C. (1977). *Identification of Adverse Reactions to Marketed Drugs in the United States and the United Kingdom.* (DHHS, CDB, OEB)
22. Jick, H. (1977). The discovery of drug-induced illness. *N. Engl. J. Med.*, **296,** 481–5
23. Jones, J. K., Van de Carr, S. (1983). Zimmerman, H. and Leroy, A. Hepatotoxicity associated with phenothiazines. *Psychopharm. Bull.*, **19,** 24–27
24. Slone, D., Shapiro, S., Miettinen, O. S. *et al.* (1971). Drug evaluation after marketing. *Ann. Int. Med.*, **90,** 257–61
25. Slone, D., Shapiro, S., Miettinen, O. S. (1977). Case-control surveillance of serious illnesses attributable to ambulatory drug use. In Colombo, F., Shapiro, S., Slone, D. *et al* (eds.) *Epidemiologic Evaluation of Drugs.* pp. 59–70. (New York: Elsevier/North Holland)
26. International Agranulocytosis and Aplastic Anemia Study. (1983). The design of a study of the drug etiology of agranulocytosis and aplastic anemia. *Eur. J. Clin. Pharmacol.*, **12,** 653–8
27. Miller, R. R. and Greenblatt, D. J. (1976). Drug Effects in Hospitalized Patients. *Experiences of the Boston Collaborative Drug Surveillance Program, 1966–75.* New York: John Wiley)
28. Jick, H., Madsen, S., Nudelman, P. M., Perera, D. R. and Stergachis, A. (1984). Post marketing follow-up at Group Health Cooperative of Puget Sound. *Pharmacology*, **4,** 99–100
29. Aselton, P., Jick, H. and Hunter, J. R. (1985). Phenylpropanolamine exposure and subsequent hospitalization for malignant hypertension, arrhythmia, neuropsychiatric illness, and nonhemorrhagic stroke (letter). *J. Am. Med. Assoc.*, **253,** 977
30. Jick, H., Holmes, L. B., Hunter, J. R., Madsen, S. and Stergachis, A. (1981). First trimester drug use and congenital disorders. *J. Am. Med. Assoc.*, **246,** 343–6.
31. Jick, H. (1984). Adverse drug reactions: The magnitude of the problem. *J. Allergy Clin. Immunol.*, **74,** 555–7
32. Rosa, F. and Jones, J. K. Drugs in pregnancy: 25 years after thalidomide. *Keynote address, WHO conference on Drugs in Pregnancy, October 28, 1984* Schlangenbad, W. Germany (Manuscript in preparation)

33. Moore, S. R. and Teal, T. W. (1985). *Geriatric Drug Use – Clinical and Social Perspectives.* (New York: Pergamon Press)
34. National Institute of Drug Abuse – Annual Data. (1983). *Data from the Drug Abuse Warning Network*, Statistical Series I, No. 3
35. Veltri, J. and Litowitz, T. (1983). 1983 Annual Report of the American Association of Poison Control Centers National Data Collection System. *Am. J. Emerg. Med.*, **2,** 420–43.
36. Rossi, A. L., Knapp, D. E., Anello, C., O'Neill, R., Graham, C., Mendelis, P. and Stanley, G. (1983). Discovery of adverse drug reactions: a comparison of selected Phase IV studies with spontaneous reporting methods. *J. A. Med. Assoc.*, **249,** 2226–8

# 13
# The World Health Organization

J. F. DUNNE

---

## INTRODUCTION

The development of the international research-based pharmaceutical industry has acted as a powerful cohesive force in medicine over the past 40 years; with relatively few exceptions, the same range of basic drugs is now used throughout the world in orthodox medical practice. Nonetheless, the responsibility for drug registration remains firmly entrenched in the national domain. In all major industrialized countries new drugs qualify for registration only if they have emerged satisfactorily from a precisely prescribed toxicological and clinical screening procedure, and the measure of these requirements has become more exacting with the recognition that animal models can be fallible as predictors of long-term safety of new drugs in clinical use.

Internationally applicable guidelines for the evaluation of the safety and efficacy of drugs have been elaborated from time to time under the aegis of the World Health Organization.[1] However, despite the existence of these norms, differences have occurred between national provisions that have given rise to potential commercial barriers, and this has led, in turn, to several moves to redress these differences through harmonization of registration procedures between major trading partners particularly within Europe and more widely among highly developed countries under the aegis of the Organization for Economic Co-operation and Development (OECD).[2]

## THE MONITORING ROLE OF WHO

International co-operation stands on somewhat firmer ground when post-registration surveillance of drug performance is considered. Here it has particular appeal since the likelihood of detecting infrequent unanticipated adverse reactons should bear a direct relationship of the magnitude of the monitored population. Various methods are employed to obtain relevant information on suspected adverse reactions on an international scale. The simplest expedient for the regulatory agencies is to impose, as a condition of registration of a drug, an onus on any manufacturer operating internationally to forward without delay all information on serious incidents possibly attributable to his product, wherever they may occur. In many countries, however, doctors are encouraged to report such events directly to officially designated national monitoring centres that are closely related to or integrated with the regulatory agencies: a system that provides obvious scope for close intergovernmental collaboration. In addition, a number of centres sponsor independent intensive monitoring units that may also serve as integral parts of a wider international network.

A factor of crucial importance to the success of the intergovernmental activity that has developed in this context over the past 15 years has been the co-ordinating role of the World Health Organization.[3–6] In 1962, as a direct consequence of the thalidomide tragedy, it was requested by the Member States that WHO should initiate an international programme for exchange of information on safety and efficacy of drugs. This resolution was supplemented the following year, first by an appeal to all countries to notify the Organization immediately of decisions to prohibit or limit the availability of specific drugs as a result of demonstration of unacceptable toxicity, and secondly by a request to the Organization to arrange for the systematic collection of information on adverse drug reactions (ADRs).

As a result, since 1963, WHO has notified Member States, on a confidential intergovernmental basis, of all restrictive regulatory decisions taken on considerations of safety that have been brought to its attention. However, since assessments of risk and benefit may differ from country to country, national authorities do not necessarily respond in consonant terms to an alert of drug toxicity. The notification system consequently has an inherent bias since only countries taking restrictive action have a commitment to report and, on occasion, other authorities have experienced difficulty in determining the relevance of these warnings to their own circumstances. This has underscored a need for WHO to issue edited commentaries that review and contrast the responses of the various national agencies to major problems of drug-induced toxicity.

## ESTABLISHING THE WHO CENTRE

The active involvement of WHO in drug-monitoring activities started 5 years later in 1968, when a feasibility study into a collaborative international scheme was undertaken. Ten countries from Australasia, Europe and North America agreed to pool all reports notified to their pre-existing national centres with a primary objective of 'identifying at the earliest possible moment the liability of a drug to produce undesirable effects which were not detected during its clinical trials'. An internationally staffed co-ordinating unit was established by WHO in Alexandria, Virginia, on funds provided by the government of the United States of America, and this was charged with the responsibility of devising suitable techniques, acceptable to all the participating centres, for recording, storing and retrieving incoming reports of suspected reactions, and to explore possible methods of analysing the implications of information in the data base.

All the basic elements of the system (which are now available to national centres wishing to develop compatible mechanisms) were fully developed within the initial 3-year feasibility phase before the co-ordinating unit was transferred to WHO Headquarters in Geneva, Switzerland, where it became operational in 1970.

During 1978, as the result of an agreement between WHO and the government of Sweden, the operative elements of the international system were moved to a Collaborating Centre within the Swedish Department of Drugs. WHO retained full responsibility for the co-ordination of the programme and the admission of additional centres. Furthermore, in view of the understandings previously established concerning the confidentiality of the data, the organization remained accountable for publication and dissemination of all information generated within the programme. The centres themselves, however, now exert a direct influence on its management. A rotating advisory group of representatives of national centres has been formally established that re-evaluate the basic functions of the system and consider whether systematic changes are required in the nature of the input or output of the system.

## Coding system

Among the operational elements fundamental to the success of the system was the creation of a standardized, multi-tier classification of ADR terms suitable for use in a computerized file.[7] The International Classification of Diseases (also developed by WHO) is, as yet, unsuited to this purpose, but the possibility of incorporating the existing terms into a future edition of the ICD may now be explored. Similarly a means of cross-referring proprietary drug names – and particularly combination products – was created to enable suspected reactions to identical products or generic equivalents to be grouped together, and to allow participating centres to identify the composition of drugs used under different names in other countries.[7]

Opinions canvassed from the participating centres on the data required for a critical assessment of the case-reports emphasized the importance of the following elements: a country code; a case identification number; an indication of whether the report was an initial notification or a follow-up; the category of informant (general practitioner, specialist, dentist); the sex and age of the patient, the description of the suspected ADR; the identity of each drug administered whether or not a causal relationship was suspected, the indications for which it was administered, and the definitive outcome of the event. A strong case can also be made to include additional information establishing, for example, the time relationships of the various events, and provision for supplementary data of this nature was included in the standardized case-report form. However, the experience which has accumulated in this and many other activities to show that complicated notification forms frustrate collaborative effort suggests the decisions initially taken might usefully be re-examined.

## Validation and retrieval

To devise an efficiently compiled computerized data-base for the storage and retrieval of this information, some of which was submitted on stereotyped report forms and some on magnetic tape, presented a complex programming exercise.[8] A series of internal testing routines became essential to check the compatibility of incoming information and to ensure its correct location within the data-base. Versatile retrieval programmes were required to subserve specific search requests efficiently and to compile summarized data. Moreover, as the data-base expanded, automated signalling devices became indispensable to identify suspected reactions that were new to the system and unanticipated clusters of identical reactions.[9–11]

Without the active commitment of well-established national centres to share their experiences and to revise their own systems in the interest of conformity of approach and compatibility of method, nothing tangible could have been achieved and, in order to protect the coherence of the programme, other centres that have subsequently entered the scheme have been expected to conform to identical terms.[12] Also, with a view to maintaining the quality of the input, admission has been made contingent upon an assurance of reasonable continuity of staffing, the existence of appropriate facilities for collecting and transmitting data, and an evident capacity to validate specific reports and to follow up suspicious leads as necessary.

Considered in terms of the interest and collaboration it has evoked, the programme has flourished. The number of actively participating centres has increased from 10 to 24, and at no stage has any country withdrawn its participation. The data-base now contains more than 250 000 reports which have been added latterly at a rate of approximately 2000 per month. Although these reports derive predominantly from the industrialized world, a number of developing countries, aware of a need to monitor the consequencs of the rapidly increasing use of drugs within their communities, have also demonstrated an active interest in the scheme. In return, they have obtained access to the data-base and to a series of routinely-prepared collated reports. In addition to an annual catalogue of reports each centre is provided with a quarterly print-out citing all reports relating to malignancy and congenital deformity, reactions that are new to the system, those occurring with unexpected frequency, and those ascribed to the most frequently reported drugs. Further investigation of suspicions generated by these reports is now regarded, in general, as a responsibility of the participating centres, although the co-ordinating unit is able to contribute to research objectives by searching the data-base for ancillary information on request, and by circulating commentaries on data relating to specific reactions as occasion demands.

## PROGRESS

On the basis of experience obtained over the past decade the values and the weaknesses of the scheme, as it is now implemented, have gradually emerged.[6] One obvious, although admittedly intangible, benefit is the support offered to national centres servicing relatively small countries, through the provision of a large, internationally-based catalogue of adverse reactions. Criticisms are frequently voiced that the information has limited value since, in general, it is not amenable to formal statistical analysis. Certainly, few would contest that the rate at which serious drug-induced reactions are notified is everywhere disappointingly low, and that the reports received are unlikely to provide an accurate reflection of true patterns of incidence of iatrogenic disease. Nonetheless spontaneous monitoring systems have an inherent flexibility that can be exploited advantageously, particularly since all doctors are notionally involved and all patients under medical supervision are notionally covered. Used responsibly by experienced, medically-qualified personnel there is no cause to assume that inferences cannot, on occasion, be made from the available data with reasonable confidence.

## CONFIRMATION OF 'SIGNALS'

As yet, the potential responsiveness of the system has been decisively demonstrated in only three instances.[13] Within a matter of weeks of the initial published description of a possible connection between practolol and delayed oculocutaneous reactions,[14] substantial numbers of confirmatory reports were sent to several national centres. Coincidentally, this information suggests these lesions, in their florid form, are virtually pathognomic for practolol since scant evidence has subsequently emerged to associate other beta-adrenergic blocking agents with this hazard. Similarly, the rarity with which suspected cases of clioquinol neurotoxicity have been reported outside Japan,[15] and the paucity of suspected cases of bismuth-induced encephalitis identified outside France,[16] suggests the existence of strong geographically linked factors in the aetiology of these conditions.

## Limitation of primary signalling method

Since no alternative practicable method is at hand which could feasibly provide such rapid and decisive confirmation of previously unsuspected serious reactions and at the same time possibly delimit their incidence, the survival of spontaneous monitoring is presumably assured. However, the limitations of the international scheme need to be appreciated and, in particular, its dubious potential in providing early warnings of unanticipated events rather than confirmatory evidence of their existence, needs to be considered dispassionately. A number of shortcomings are inherent:

(1) Virtually by definition, unsuspected reactions tend not to be reported spontaneously by doctors since they are not alert, in these instances, to the possibility of a drug-related aetiology, and may have no grounds for suspicion. Reactions that masquerade as common spontaneously occurring conditions, or which only become evident after a long period of latency, are particularly likely to escape attention: no-one would report a carcinoma of the breast, for example as an ADR unless *a priori* strong evidence existed to support the hypothesis.

(2) Considerable time can elapse before reports are incorporated into – and retrieved from – the international data-base. The average period is of the order of 9 months, and when national centres forward reports relatively infrequently greater delays can occur. The consequences of this are most evident in the case of newly-introduced drugs. Data forwarded to national centres have recently provoked the withdrawal of benoxaprofen[17] and zomepirac[18] before the information entered into the international domain. Intensive promotion of newly-introduced drugs coupled with intensive post-registration monitoring of their performance seems destined to confirm this trend.

(3) A critical analysis and exhaustive investigation of all possible leads contained within the international data-bank would be a gargantuan task. Moreover, a suspicion of a previously unsuspected reaction that is discernible only from evidence gleaned internationally seldom leads to action at national level, if only because there is usually no collateral information available to provide independent confirmation of the provisional hypothesis.

## Need for follow-up

The possibility of promoting direct international collaborative effort in the follow-up of these suspicions remains largely unrealized. On occasion commision of appropriately designed prospective or retrospective studies might be justified; in other situations a general request to doctors for specific information could be more appropriate. There is an ever-present problem, however, that public anxiety may be aroused unnecessarily or prematurely by uninformed speculation on the need for consequential action. In the public domain the ultimate responsibility for the availability of pharmaceutical products rests with the national agency responsible for their registration. An international agency, acting solely as a trustee of information submitted by national centres, has an obligation to refrain from any action or any disclosure of data liable to embarrass or compromise these authorities in their statutory functions.

Nonetheless, closer liaison between countries in the investigation of suspicions raised by reports collected internationally could pay dividends. The prospective assessment of long-term clofibrate therapy under the aegis of WHO[19] was immediately recognized as a classic venture in international collaboration. Its outcome was salutary in that, whereas treatment was associated with significantly increased mortality, the causes were varied and were unlikely to have been detected other than in a controlled study. Its impact was also salutary in that its international provenance lent it an authority that has remained largely unquestioned. International collaboration in the prospective monitoring of drugs, however, remains to a great extent unexploited. Its potential is worthy of closer examination.

## References


1. *WHO Technical Report Series*, No. 563 (1975). Guidelines for Evaluation of Drugs for Use in Man. Report of a WHO Scientific Group. (Geneva: WHO)
2. Organization for Economic and Cultural Development (1981). *Guidelines for Testing of Chemicals.* (Paris: OECD)
3. Royall, B. W. (1971). International aspects of drug monitoring: role of the World Health Organization. *WHO Chronicle*, **25**, 445
4. Royall, B. W. (1971). International aspects of the study of adverse reactions to drugs. *Biometrics*, **27**, 689
5. Royall, B. W. (1973). Monitoring adverse reactions to drugs. *WHO Chronicle*, **27**, 469
6. Dunne, J. F. (1977). Success and shortcomings of WHO international drug monitoring programme. In Gross, F. H. and Inman, W. H. W. (eds.) *Drug Monitoring* (New York: Academic Press)
7. Royall, B. W. and Venulet, J. (1972). Methodology for international drug monitoring. *Methods of Information in Medicine*, **11**, 75
8. The use of computers in international drug monitoring. Edited report of a scientific consultation on computer systems in drug monitoring (1973). *WHO Chronicle*, **27**, 476
9. Finney, D. J. (1974). Systematic signalling of adverse reactions to drugs. *Methods of Information in Medicine*, **13**, 1
10. Mandel, S. P. H., Levine, A. and Belẽno, G. E. (1976). Signalling increases in reporting in international reporting of adverse reactions to therapeutic drugs. *Methods of Information in Medicine*, **15**, 1
11. Levine, A., Mandel, S. P. H. and Santamaria, A. (1977). Pattern signalling in health information montitoring sysems. *Methods of Information in Medicine*, **16**, 138
12. *WHO Technical Report Series, No. 563 (1972). International Drug Monitoring. The Role of National Centres. Report of a WHO Meeting (Geneva: WHO)*

13. Lawson, D. H. (1979). Detection of drug-induced disease. *Br. J. Clin. Pharmacol.*, **7,** 13
14. Wright, P. (1974). Skin reactions to practolol. *Br. Med. J.*, **2,** 1081
15. *WHO Drug Information*, Oct.–Dec. 1977. Clioquinol and SMON, p. 9
16. *WHO Drug Information*, Apr.–June, 1977. Bismuth salts and ecephalopathy, p. 8
17. Anonymous. (1982). Benoxaprofen, *Br. Med. J.*, **2,** 459
18. US Food and Drug Administration. Zomepirac. *FDA Press Release*, 8 March 1983
19. Oliver, M. F., Heady, J. A., Morris, N. and Cooper, J. (1980). Report of the Committee of principal investigators. WHO Co-operative Trial on primary prevention of ischaemic heart disease using clofibrate to lower serum cholesterol: Mortality follow-up. *Lancet*, **2,** 379

# 14
# The pharmaceutical industry – drug monitoring by Ciba – Geigy

I. T. BORDA and G.-C. BERNEKER

## HISTORICAL BACKGROUND, CONCEPTS

During the last three decades, emphasis on drug safety has increased for several reasons: the introduction of many new drugs since the Second World War; the long-term treatment of common chronic diseases exposing a large number of individuals to drugs for long periods; the recognition that no biologically active substance can be completely safe and the degree of 'unsafety' cannot be fully determined; and the growing public interest in drug-related problems coupled with an increasingly critical attitude towards current drug safety control mechanisms.[1] With these facts in mind, it is axiomatic to state the drug monitoring is important in modern medicine.

While both the lack of drug safety standards and the responsibility of the manufacturer were shown as early as 1938 by the fatalities from sulphanilamide in a diethylene-glycol base,[2] it was in the wake of the thalidomide tragedy that drug-induced disorders prompted public demands for a government role in drug safety and more rigorous methods for their control. The occurrence of the practolol syndrome, 13 years after the lessons of thalidomide, demonstrated that the safety procedures by then in force were insufficient to prevent this second major drug calamity.[3] The importance of the practolol episode lay not only in proving that drug safety measures at the time were inadequate, but also in revealing a common interest shared by the pharmaceutical manufacturer, the Regulatory Authorities, the prescribing physician and the patient. This interest was simply to find and implement the most effective and economical methods for early detection of drug-related problems. Contrary to the views of some critics, this is no less the goal of the pharmaceutical manufacturers than it is of Drug Regulatory Authorities. Both sides wish to ensure that acceptable safe and effective drugs are marketed without delay, realizing that tardy approval of useful drugs can cause hardship to the individual patient deprived of medications. But they are also aware that hasty introduction of a dangerous drug can cost the manufacturing company more in loss of money and reputation than earlier drug sales could bring in. The major effort of Drug Regulatory Bodies has been directed towards the protection of public health, requiring manufacturers to prove the safety and efficacy of their drugs. Initially the industry responded with a defensive attitude and policy. Later, however, research-based pharmaceutical companies came to realize that both the clinical and marketing performance of a drug would be fostered by appropriate monitoring of safety and efficacy; they also became increasingly conscious about an ethical and legal duty of care with respect to their products.

The setting up and development of the Drug Monitoring Subdepartment (DM) at Ciba-Geigy reflected and paralleled these changing concepts, the growing importance and gradually accumulating knowledge in this relatively new area of scientific endeavour.

In spite of the demonstration of drug-induced blood dyscrasias and the establishment of a registry to compile them, throughout the 1950s most clinical information on drug effects came from a variety of studies organized by the manufacturer before marketing. This was supplemented by the results of clinical trials conducted before the drug became available for general use and also by published individual case reports. Formal programmes for spontaneous reporting emerged only after thalidomide in the early 1960s. Until the merger of Ciba Ltd. and Geigy Ltd. and the amalgamation of their two respective adverse drug reaction centres into the DM in 1970, the drug monitoring system of each company rested mainly on spontaneous voluntary reports of suspected adverse drug reactions.

The progress made in drug monitoring over the last decade has been due to experience with more and more new drugs. These efforts were undoubtedly stimulated by a few unexpected calamitous events precipitated by drugs. As the medical community as a whole was learning more about adverse drug effects so was Ciba–Geigy; the strongest and most sobering of these lessons for the Company was that of clioquinol and subacute myelo-optic neuropathy (SMON).[4]

This story, which began to unfold in the early 1970s, stimulated intensive activities to determine whether or not there was a link between drug and alleged event, and undoubtedly had a strong impact on the company's philosophy and policies. The need to develop ways of detecting, defining and reacting to all unexpected effects of the company's drugs was recognized, whether these were newly marketed or had been used for decades. Although spontaneous voluntary reporting continued to constitute an important part of the input to DM, its limitations became clear: that it cannot by itself, generate hypotheses on previously unsuspected adverse reactions except by fortuitous observation; cannot confirm or deny the generated hypothesis with complete certainty; and cannot quantify the rate of occurrence of adverse reactions in a given population.[5] Drug monitoring could no longer be regarded merely as a passive process of gathering data, different techniques had to be evolved to include an active and effective follow-up, along with means to gather detailed information about the patients receiving the drugs as well as estimate the numbers exposed to a drug in a given setting.

The surveillance of a drug is a continuous process which begins with the establishment of an overall pharmacological and toxicological profile of the substance in one or more animal species in the early stages of drug development, followed by extrapolation of the profile obtained to man from comparative pharmacodynamic and pharmacokinetic data. The spectrum of clinical evaluation is progressively broadened throughout the lifetime of all products containing the drug. Data on the drug's performance can be gathered under various clinical conditions from several sources, commencing with the efficacy and tolerability data gained during clinical trials; observations from intensive hospital drug monitoring schemes; published or spontaneously reported individual cases and extending to information accumulated in national computer-linked data registers; and into the data banks of drug epidemiology programmes. It became necessary for DM to co-operate more closely with Clinical Research and Drug Registration inside the company as well as with members of academia, regulatory authorities and other pharmaceutical firms. As interest increased dialogues began for the development of computerized data processing comparable with that of the WHO drug monitoring system to allow data exchange between various countries reporting such information on drug reactions to the WHO.

## ORGANIZATION, RESPONSIBILITIES, WORKING PROCEDURES IN CIBA–GEIGY (BASLE) DM

Drug monitoring is one of three subdepartments within the Ciba–Geigy Basel Medical Department (Figure 1). It consists of three sections: Clinical Drug Safety, Information Processing, and Surveillance (Figure 2). The following objectives of the DM are formally laid down to express the company's interest and feeling of responsibility for the patient's welfare:

(1) To act as an early warning system, with its prime aim being the identification of adverse reactions or signals at an early stage which indicate the possibility of an adverse drug reaction and to take action to inform prescribers.

(2) To systematically collect, evaluate and process data on unwanted effects of marketed Ciba–Geigy drugs, and to adopt, improve and

* Some of these concepts and developments are illustrated in the three drug case-histories outlined in the Appendix.

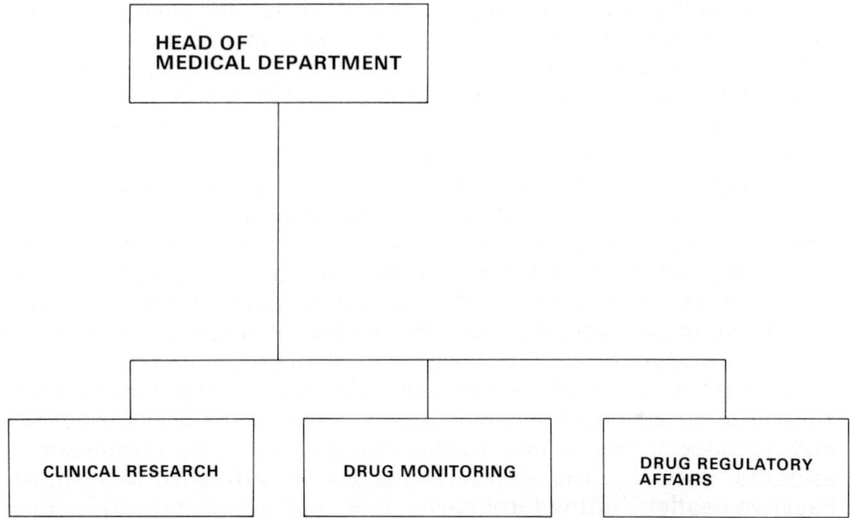


**Figure 1** The place of Drug Monitoring within the medical department

further develop monitoring technologies including epidemiologic methods.

(3) To act as a central office for the collection of ADRs from and for our group companies world-wide, and to foster the continued development of an international Ciba–Geigy Drug Monitoring organization.

(4) to maintain and further develop contacts with Industry and with other organizations such as monitoring centres, academic centres, national and international agencies carrying out work related to drug monitoring.

## The Clinical Drug Safety Section (CDS)

CDS is the core of the DM of Ciba–Geigy Basel. Its basic responsibility is the critical medical evaluation of all incoming data on adverse drug reactions associated with marketed Ciba–Geigy drugs. The activities of CDS include: conducting an ADR reporting system; handling individual enquires received from group companies or other sources; preparing various types of reports for internal and external information; co-operating with all sections and departments within the company, but particularly with Clinical Research, Medical Data Analysis, Research, Drug Regulatory Affairs and CDS-Sections in Group Companies; maintaining permanent contact with outside centres (e.g. the Swiss Adverse Drug Reaction Centre, Swiss Toxicology Centre, Adverse Drug Reaction Centres of the other 'Inter-pharma' Companies); actively participating in the Package Leaflet Editing Group, the Medical Editorial Team and the 'Trade Mark Committee'; maintaining and periodically updating a brochure entitled 'Information on overdosage with Ciba–Geigy Pharmaceuticals'.

All medical specialty areas are represented by specialists called Monitors. These Monitors are physicians with broad experience in drug usage as well as expertise in a particular clinical area such as haematology, cardiology, neurology, gastroenterology, dermatology, endocrinology, etc. Each monitor is also responsible for a certain therapeutic area, for example CVS or CNS. In view of the linguistic problems and the increasing drug monitoring activity in Japan one member of CDS handles matters related to drug monitoring at Ciba–Geigy, Japan.

DM is represented on the Company's 'Pharma Development Board'. Members of the CDS are appointed to many committees and groups to represent their areas of expertise. These appointments may occur on an *ad hoc* basis, e.g. Task Forces (see p. 186), or may be permanent, e.g. Package Leaflet Editing Group.

All incoming reports with adverse reactions are 'screened' by the Head of Clinical Drug Safety who will channel the report to the appropriate Monitor responsible for that particular medical specialty.

The CDS Monitor checks and evaluates all incoming data from the point of view of the medical specialist and in the light of previous experience. If necessary, the monitor also consults the sponsor of Clinical Research or the Medical Services Section of Drug Regulatory Affairs. Before the Monitor forwards the data for information processing, the Intensive Surveillance Group checks the Monitor's evaluation for quality and consistency, particularly regarding causality assessment. The routine method of processing data and the channels of communication therefore ensure that multiple cross-checks are built into the system.

Although basic pharmacologic data may not be sufficient to anticipate all the adverse effects which may occur in large scale use of drugs, it will facilitate evaluation of later reports on drug effects. In accordance with this view much attention is being paid to drug safety data during early clinical pharmacological studies (Phase 1 – conducted by the Biology Subdepartment). This responsibility is taken over by Clinical Research during clinical trials (Phase 2 to Phase 4); DM is represented by the Head of DM in the planning of these trials. When a drug is introduced to the market the Heads of the Biology Subdepartment and Clinical Research Subdepartment ensure that all available information on tolerability is provided to DM which at this point assumes responsibility for surveillance of the drug throughout its lifetime.

Once a drug is on the market it is taken by the patient under conditions possibly very different from those of the pre-marketing stage. Consequently the emphasis of monitoring shifts to a close watch on the pattern and frequency of the reported problems, and to an immediate follow-up by direct personal contact with the reporting physician whenever possible. While a particular watch is kept for the emergence of isolated, unusual reactions, the pattern of reported events (or any systematic change in it) may also signal problems for a specific drug, group of drugs or therapeutic area.

*Sources of information*

Drug adverse reaction reports present a wide spectrum in the nature, quality and quantity of data they contain. Most provide at least a preliminary assessment of the clinical information even if this is only an impression that a clinical event may be related to a drug.[6]

The following types of information are processed:

*Spontaneous Reports:* The oldest source of information on adverse reactions arriving in a largely unsystematic way from physicians, pharmacists or patients is sent either directly, or more often indirectly through the Medical Departments of Ciba–Geigy affiliates or the national monitoring centres of different countries. The reports usually refer to single cases, and although they are very important sources of information on drug-related events they have well known major deficiencies: they are subject to various observer biases; they provide no estimates of the number of patients exposed to the drug in question (denominator); and their numerator estimates are unreliable (mainly due to underreporting). In addition the evaluation of single case spontaneous reports offers particular problems: interactions with pre-existing and intercurrent disease states, concomitant therapy and nutritional–genetic–environmental factors may all be present without being accessible to evaluation because of incompleteness of data. Under certain circumstances, however, adverse drug effects can be identified even from spontaneous reporting alone, particularly if the relative risk of the reaction is high, the drug is widely used, and the effect is immediate and unrelated to the disease under treatment. Any growing number of similar observations derived from spontaneous reports should stimulate further studies with more sophisticated epidemiological methods.

In order to simplify the processing of adverse drug reaction reports, standard forms conforming to WHO requirements have been developed in-house. These range from short forms for routine clinical use (e.g. to record data from telephone calls) to more detailed forms (particularly for serious or interesting cases). These forms are sent by the company to the doctor reporting an ADR requesting him to fill in 'boxes' indicating vital statistics of the patient (initials, sex, age, occupation, height, weight), the name and batch number of the drug; the dosage and duration of treatment; the particular reaction, its management and outcome; the indication for prescribing the drug (including a brief history, relevant clinical and laboratory findings) and details of concomitant drug therapy. Two additional forms are used if teratogenic effects are suspected: the first for drugs ingested during pregnancy and a second for use in cases of possible congenital defects. The questionnaires exist in different languages. After the completed questionnaire has been returned to DM Basel each report is assigned a CDS reference number, and its data checked clerically for completeness and internal consistency. The report then goes to the appropriate CDS Monitor who evaluates the elements of the available information. Naturally the monitoring physician may initiate further direct follow-up of the case with the reporting physician to amplify available details and to clarify apparent discrepancies. These steps are taken most often through the appropriate group company; CDS, however, ensures that the existence of the report and its essential features are made known to all interested parties. A decision is made at this point as to what if any action is needed. In the event of an unusually serious adverse drug reaction the information is brought to the immediate notice of the Head of the Medical Department. If necessary national and international Regulatory Authorities are also notified, so that there is no delay in response to the situation. When it appears unlikely that there is further information to come in about the case, and after quality and consistency checks by the Intensive Surveillance Group have been completed, the report is passed on to the Information Processing Section for recording and storage in the data bank for single cases.

*Medical Literature and Reports from National Regulatory Authorities:* Publications from the medical literature containing information on Ciba–Geigy products are sent to DM by the Ciba–Geigy Documentation Centre. Reports from National Regulatory Authorities may reach DM regularly or intermittently.

Cases from both sources are recorded in a data bank as individual single cases if this is permitted by the structure of the documentation. If the data does not distinguish between individual patients, the information is entered into the separate data bank for multiple cases. The informational content of publications, and reports from authorities, varies from excellent in the case of detailed accurate case records to practically useless. Reports from national authorities may supply highly informative case records or merely list unwanted effects. Publications with the average information level of medical reports are classified as 'normal'. Such a classification based on the information value makes data retrieval on a qualitative basis possible.

There may also be difficulties with case identification, which means that in spite of cross-checks, the risk of reporting the same case more than once can never be completely excluded. For this reason 'suspicious' data are recorded and stored separately in subfiles. Single case reports are often not as stringently scrutinized by editorial reviews as other scientific publications. As a result unjustifiable conclusions based on inadequate clinical investigation may be published, and consequently become available for citation.

Notwithstanding its deficiencies the main value of this type of data lies in the fact that it comes from widely spread, 'real-life' usage of a drug. This implies an increased chance of detecting relatively rare adverse events when compared with drug experience data from clinical trials. An indication of the overall incidence rates of the more common events can also be gained, provided that there is some estimate of the extent of drug usage.

*Comprehensive Hospital-Based Drug Monitoring:* Intensive hospital drug monitoring initiated by the Boston Collaborative Drug Surveillance programme[7] in 1966 is a method of observing several facets of drug exposure in hospitalized patients with and without adverse reactions. In-depth data collection in a standardized format supplies both numerator and denominator data; formal investigations can be initiated based on the observations. The limited number of drugs used, the finite number of patients monitored and a relatively short period of observation, place restrictions on this methodology. There is now a programme of comprehensive hospital monitoring for drug effects in Switzerland[8] which is mainly supported by the three major Swiss pharmaceutical companies (Ciba–Geigy, Roche, Sandoz). This programme, called Comprehensive Hospital Drug Monitoring Bern (CHDMB) was initiated in 1970 by Professor R. Hoigné and Professor P. Stucki, and is conducted in two university-affiliated teaching hospitals in Bern. To date, a data bank on over 20 000 monitored patients is available from this programme with an annual accrual rate of approximately 3000 patients. The programme provides very useful information both on drug-usage and adverse reaction 'profiles'. The system produces alerting signals, and has already led to the detection and description of new ADRs (Dipyrone and hypotension;[9] nomifensine and drug-fever).[10]

*Competitive Product File:* This file contains data regarding possible or proven factors implicated in unwanted drug effects which came to the notice of Drug Monitoring. These mainly concern competitive pharmaceutical preparations, chemical substances, household products, cosmetics, agrochemical preparations, tobacco, alcohol, occupational and environmental factors in a broad sense of the word. The main sources of data for this file are abstracting and telephone services such as Ringdoc, Inpharma, Medical Letter, Reactions, Medline printouts, etc.

*Output Reporting Activities*

(1) *Tolerability Reports*: These reports are produced periodically for any given product or formulation, and deal with specific problems of a particular drug. They contain all the data known to Ciba–Geigy from the time of the first clinical trial with the drug up to the date of the report. Therefore, the Tolerability Reports, unlike *Ad Hoc* and Flash Reports (see below) are usually extensive.

(2) *Ad Hoc* Reports are prepared in reply to a definite question about a preparation, a group of preparations, a symptom or a group of symptoms (for example oral contraceptives and blood pressure, cardiotoxicity of tricyclics). These reports are prepared on request, or whenever the extent, nature or importance of the information justifies providing such a report.

(3) *Flash Reports* are designed to draw attention to a potential danger (e.g. a change in the reporting frequency, or first occurrence of a symptom for a given drug) on the basis of available, often incomplete, possibly not well-founded, information. The Flash Report also proposes measures to clarify a particular situation.

All three types of report are revised from time to time whenever justified by the receipt of new data. Other types of report are produced in printout forms (e.g. Signalling Reports on first-time reported reactions).

The CDS monitoring system aims both at retrieving stored information on known or suspected drug effects, and also at picking up signals that may lead to the detection of previously unknown drug reactions.

Information emanating from the different reports of CDS may initiate changes and recommendations for the usage of a product, or for aproaches to national and international drug regulatory bodies; but first of all for appropriate, accurate, and up-to-date information for the prescriber.

**Information Processing Section (IP)**

This Section is responsible for the recording, storage, retrieval and statistical evaluation of the information received from various sources. The range of the Section's functions includes the development and maintenance of monitoring systems as well as of computer assisted methods of data evaluation. The IP consists of four groups (Figure 2): the 'System Development and Maintenance Group' (concerned with the further development and maintenance of the retrieval and reporting software); the 'Innovation, Data Quality Control and Statistics Group' (ensures that appropriate retrieval procedures and statistical methods are used for selecting and evaluating the data); the 'Data Collecting, Input' and Maintenance Group' (responsible for the processing of all published and unpublished information); and the 'Dictionaries Codes and Nomenclature Group' (maintains control of all standardized terminologies in use in Drug Monitoring).

**Electronic Data Processing System (EDP)**

The data from detailed questionnaires (adapted to WHO requirements) as well as any information obtained from internal and external sources are recorded interactively, (at optical display or typewriter terminals). This allows for the checking and if necessary immediate correction of errors. It is possible to feed a symptom into the system in clear text and have its coding performed automatically. The data or modifications flow first into data buffers; then the new checked/corrected data can be entered from these data buffers into the appropriate bank via a batch job. Entry of this information also activates an 'Early Warning' system which can be programmed to signal a certain set number of occurrences of a new ADR report to any specific drug.

The desired information can be recalled by a simple telegram style enquiry, either directly at the terminal (provided the information flow is not too large) or via a batch job, started through the terminal. The elements of information and the format, decoding and sorting of records can be preselected at will.

With the command for update the computer automatically starts printing an index card; this card is colour-coded manually, and contains all information leading to a microfiche listing all relevant documents. Single case cards are for individual cases reported on questionnaires or for cases described in detail in the literature. Multiple Case Cards are for the recording of global data from publications, reports or listings. These index cards permit rapid retrieval of information. Since the data from the various sources differs in content, significance and relevance each source must be evaluated, processed and stored separately.

Thus there are two systems of information available for data retrieval: computer printouts for data classification and programmed data compilation as required; and the Colour Coded Manual Card Index for quick access to the original reports (microfiches).

The modular structure of the system makes extension possible (such as linking to other systems, statistical evaluations, graphic presentations, etc.) The system is designed to meet increasing information requirements, and to enable us to detect relevant signals.

## Surveillance Section

In the continuous process of monitoring for drug safety three stages can be identified: alerting, verification (positive or negative) and acting upon the findings.[11] The Surveillance Section is involved in all these stages. In close co-operation with the Clinical Drug Safety Section it aims at early detection of signals (Intensive Surveillance); it maintains appropriate and efficient working methodologies in order to follow-up signals requiring further investigation (Active Surveillance) and ensures that appropriate measures are undertaken in accordance with the findings (Task Forces). The three groups have complementary functions and common objectives: namely to identify, assess and react to a specific drug safety problem.

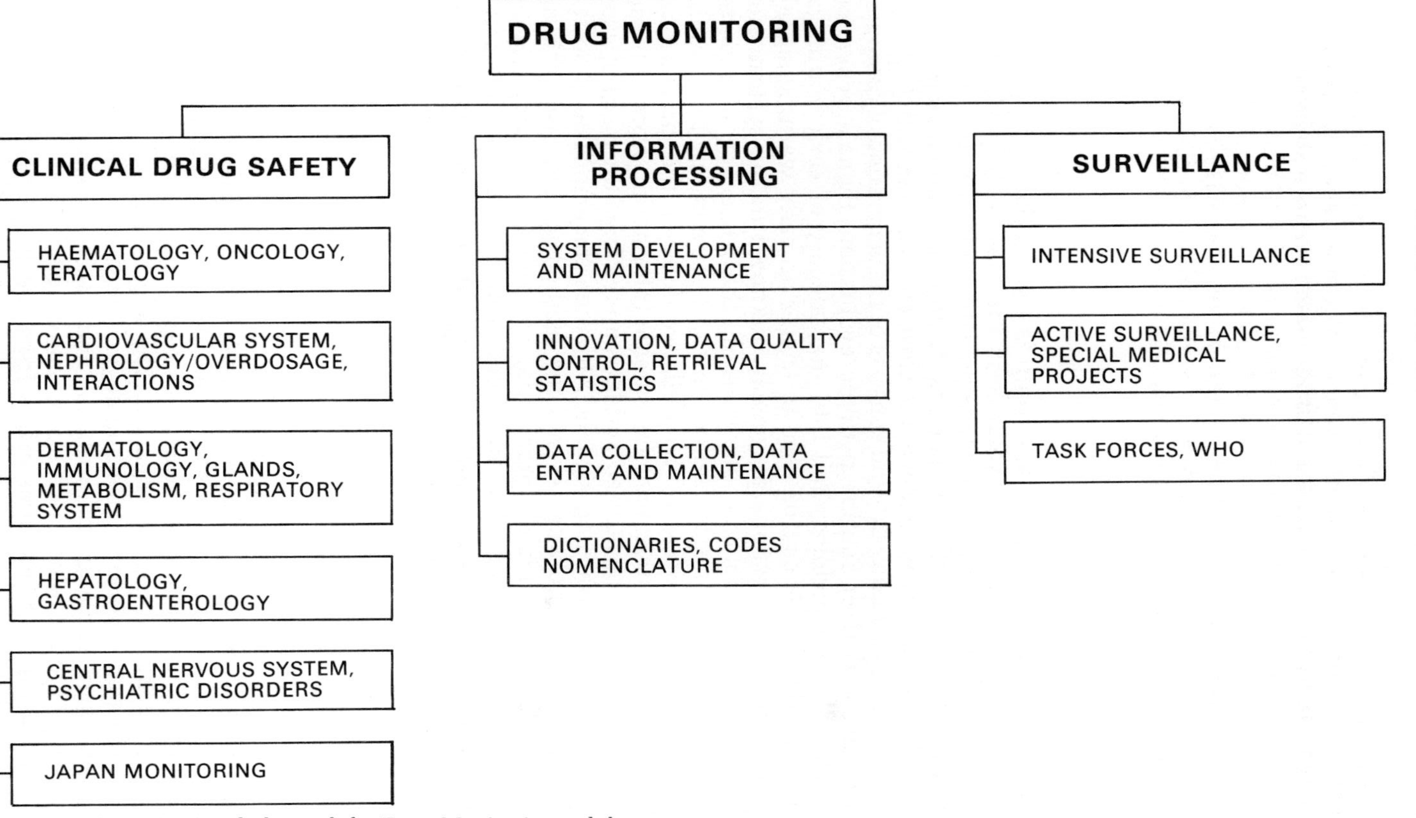


**Figure 2** Organizational chart of the Drug Monitoring subdepartment

The therapeutic benefits of a drug may be so great as to allow some given incidence of reactions even of moderate severity. However, unexpectedly serious or frequent drug-related events may be signalled by animal experiments, studies in humans or patient monitoring. The nature of these data may be such that they cannot be dealt with through the normal routine channels of the CDS section; the Surveillance Section takes over the responsibility to follow-up such problems potentially related to Ciba–Geigy drugs.

### *Intensive Surveillance Group*

The main responsibility of this group is the regular and systematic scrutiny of all information available in the files of Drug Monitoring with the aim of detecting, as early as possible, signals indicative of the occurrence of events that are potentially important and may be drug-related. This activity is conducted in close co-operation with CDS and Information Processing (IP) and consists of the generation of computer printouts and their routine periodic evaluation. Signals generated through this methodology fall into the category of early warnings. Different thresholds can be used to trigger an early warning signal, such as adverse reactions previously unknown to the system; particularly severe reactions; increases in the frequency of reports; changes in morbidity or mortality figures, etc. In addition to scrutinizing all DM files Intensive Surveillance follows the professional literature and any other relevant outside information from different sources. These will be utilized and interpreted from the point of view of potential early warning signals. Although the emphasis is on the identification of untoward events the method should also pick up previously unrecognized therapeutic, diagnostic or prophylactic properties of a drug. An additional routine duty of Intensive Surveillance is to check the quality, plausibility and consistency of the causality assessment made by the CDS Monitors on individual ADR-reports.

### *Active Surveillance Group*

This group (somewhat vaguely and imprecisely, but frequently equated with Post-Marketing Surveillance) plays a three-fold role: (1) it evaluates (in co-operation with CDS and Intensive Surveillance) early warning information from the point of view of identifying signals that require further special investigation; (2) it selects the most appropriate and efficient working methodology, especially in regard to epidemiology for a given problem; and (3) if necessary designs, implements and evaluates special monitoring schemes.

A need for such activities arises from the belief that knowledge about a drug when it is marketed is very rapidly found to be insufficient. The need for Active Surveillance is also explained by the recognition that while spontaneous (voluntary) reporting is an important source of adverse drug reaction signals it has serious limitations, cannot by itself be relied upon for alerting, and much less for verification. In order to find the appropriate study-design, Active Surveillance may use experimental or non-experimental, prospective or retrospective, controlled or uncontrolled methods; cohort, case control or record-linkage approaches. Depending on the problem on hand and the degree of suspicion, the correct sequence of studies for each problem is also important.[12] In order to fulfil these tasks Active Surveillance must keep abreast with the professional literature, and obtain from different sources comparable information related to drug monitoring. It is the logical prerequisite for this group to maintain and further develop working relationships outside the Company both within the industry (including our own Group Companies) and with non-industry, and to have contacts with experts and opinion-makers in national/international organizations including the World Health Organization. As an additional duty the Active Surveillance Group provides, if requested, assistance for the Departments within and outside the Company (e.g. to Group Companies) in the form of expert medical advice on matters related to adverse drug effects.

### *Task Forces Group*

A Task Force (TF) is an *ad hoc* multi-disciplinary group of representatives of various departments of the Pharma Division. It deals with special problems concerning the safety (and at times the efficacy) of a particular Ciba–Geigy pharmaceutical product. A new TF is created whenever proposed by the Head of Drug Monitoring and/or the Head of the Medical Department. The Head of the TF Group acts as Chairman and reports to the Head of DM. He has the authority to approach the TF liaison member of the Pharma Division Management Committee or any other line manager directly. The TF has the authority to allocate work to all Departments represented in it through the respective members, and such assignments take priority over normal day-to-day operations. The main duty of the TF group is to maintain and co-ordinate activities related to a given problem associated with a Ciba–Geigy drug. Its aim is to support and defend the product, observing professional ethics and scientific objectivity. It is the responsibility of the TF to propose effective and appropriate measures to the relevant authorities within and outside the company after clarification of the scientific, medical and technical factors involved in the case under assessment. The TF is also concerned with dissemination of relevant information in and outside Basel and with co-ordinating the implementation of Headquarters policy in respect to pharmaceutical products. A TF is disbanded when its tasks have been completed and/or the particular circumstances that have necessitated its establishment cease to exist.

## POST-MARKETING SURVEILLANCE

Post-Marketing Surveillance (PMS) must be among the most frequently used terms in the medical literature of the last decade. Concluding a conference on this topic Lasagna[13] wrote in 1976: 'The conferees agreed that the question of *whether* or not post-marketing surveillance should be done is idle; . . . post-marketing surveillance is an absolute necessity for assessing the benefit/risk ratio of a new drug . . .' Although all parties may agree on the principle (and the pharmaceutical industry in particular is committed by virtue of its responsibility for the surveillance of its products), a wide variety of opinions is expressed over the definitions, objectives and particularly over the choice of methodologies of drug surveillance after marketing. The fact that 7 years after Lasagna's statement expert committees on both sides of the Atlantic still debate these matters suggests that the term PMS means different things to different people.

It is beyond the scope of this chapter to analyse the philosophical, technical, medical, political and financial aspects of PMS, therefore we will limit ourselves to some general remarks and a few suggestions for the near future regarding PMS at Ciba–Geigy DM.[14]

It has been stated that quantification of adverse drug effects of established drugs can be achieved with routine surveillance systems. These systems, however, appear inadequate for the evaluation of newly marketed drugs, mainly because they cannot accumulate a sufficient number of patients within a reasonable period of time.[12]

Because it may not be possible to conduct formal PMS studies on *every* new drug, a choice has to be made about *what* to follow-up and *how*. The determining factors depend largely on the problem at hand, but also on how rapidly the drug comes into widespread use and on the frequency of the event potentially related to the use of the drug. If the drug is very commonly used (e.g. conjugated oestrogens) and the question is whether it may cause some type of cancer (e.g. endometrial carcinoma), case control surveillance should be able to detect the relationship, even if there is a time lag of several years between administration of the drug and the appearance of the event. If the drug in question is used moderately often (e.g. practolol) and the event (e.g. eye symptoms) is also fairly common, a record-linkage system may reveal the relationship even if the disease condition is not severe enough to result in hospitalization. However, in such a case the record-linkage system would have to include out-patient clinics, and specialty organizations. If it is anticipated that certain drugs will be used relatively rarely a decision has to be made as to which drug should be followed, since costs are likely to be very high for such a methodology. Selection criteria may be based either on pre-marketing suspicions: (e.g. a potential for damage by extension of the known pharmacological effect;) or on the fact that the drug is for long-term use; or on its known metabolic, neurological, or cardiovascular effects. Although a recent retrospective analysis[15] of the most important drug-related calamities concluded that retrospective cohort studies would *not* have detected such adverse events it is generally believed that the establishment and follow-up of a prospective cohort population is important for PMS. For a seldom-used drug the search for relatively rare events (e.g. 1 per 1000 individuals exposed) the problem of detection is difficult and expensive; with existing surveillance systems the discovery of such adverse effects cannot be presumed. For a drug of great public health importance the adverse effects can be studied sequentially with several methods; if one methodology (e.g. spontaneous reports) signals adverse effects, further clinical studies and/or clinical trials targeted at the specific problem offer a chance for verification. For the determination of long-term drug effects (e.g. carcinogenicity of drugs) the combination of case-control studies and record-linkage looks the most promising.[16]

For Ciba–Geigy DM the primary objective of PMS is to minimize the potential harmful consequences, and maximize the optimal use of all the Company's drugs at the earliest possible time. Since DM assumes responsibility for drug safety at the time when the drug is introduced on the market, all its activities are considered to be related to PMS, although more specific tasks in this area are carried out by the Active Surveillance Section.

The continued importance of single descriptive non-experimental methods is recognized by DM, and combined with mechanisms for generating and testing hypotheses. As no single experimental design can accomplish all the goals of post-marketing surveillance, PMS is conceived as a flexible network where different elements of several methodologies can be and should be combined. This will allow the adoption of the best approach to any of a variety of events arising in connection with the large number of the company's drug products, as well as adaptation of PMS plans to particular countries' drug policies and drug safety standards. At the end of this Chapter three examples of potential drug-event relationships are described. They are presented to underline the great diversity of problems demanding different approaches and methodologies, as well as the varying depth and extent of investigations. These 'drug case-histories' also illustrate the company's reactions to urgent drug-related problems and the increasing experience of DM in dealing with them. Many other recent examples have also been investigated: e.g. beta-blockers and intestinal fibrotic reactions; interaction between beta-blockers and monoamine oxidase inhibitors; antidepressants and convulsions; pyrazolon-derivatives and agranulocytosis; anticonvulsants and endocrine disorders, etc.

Co-operation and consultation with expert individuals and groups outside Ciba–Geigy is considered indispensable. This can be arranged either on an *ad hoc* basis to study a specific problem or by plugging into the programme of one or more of the major academic centres engaged in PMS. Permanent associations have distinct advantages: access to a large body of data collected by good methodology and handled with proven expertise, availability of advisors in different disciplines (clinicians, epidemiologists, biostatisticians) and the possibility of obtaining advice and data on urgent problems. The selection of centres may be directed by the need for different methodologies (e.g. case-control method in one place, record-linkage in another), as well as by the need to cover different geographical areas. Ciba–Geigy currently maintains close contact with the Southampton Drug Surveillance Research Unit in the UK, and collaborates with the Boston University Drug Epidemiology Unit (USA). There are hopes of establishing similar working relationships with the Department of Epidemiology at the School of Publich Health, University of Texas, Houston. Good progress has been made towards co-operation with the World Health Organization in matters of drug safety.

## THE NEAR FUTURE

Having discussed Ciba–Geigy DM's present structure, operation, and its PMS concepts, it is in order to present a few thoughts for the near future.

### *Spontaneous reporting*

This system will probably remain the most important source of our early ADR signals. Although spontaneous reporting will never provide fully comprehensive information, these reports originate from using the drug in practice, where clinical observation cannot be replaced, but only complemented by other methodologies. Under-reporting is considered the Achilles heel of spontaneous reporting. The two main reasons for this are: failing to recognize the event–drug connection, and a failure to report the ADR (perhaps owing to lack of time required to complete the form).

There are a variety of ways to improve the doctors' 'compliance':

(1) *The use of visual reminders* (e.g. check boxes on hospital discharge summaries, desk set calendars, flags, etc.).

(2) *Automated verbal reporting* by reducing or eliminating writing. The doctor's interest in reporting, and the demand to complete a form are two opposing forces. Verbal reporting is easier and more attractive, and it can also be instantaneous and complete. A charge-free telephone reporting centre with around-the-clock service could receive ADR reports, manned by trained clerical personnel and using automatic recording devices after hours. The reports would be scrutinized daily by ADR-specialists. Follow-up in writing or by personal visit to the reporting physician could complete the documentation. Such systems are operational and successful (e.g. the American Academy of Dermatology Adverse Drug Reaction Reporting System). Alternatively, small tape-recor-

ders could be distributed to medical practitioners, the tapes collected at regular intervals and follow-up procedures initiated.

(3) *Personal contacts* with physicians stimulate ADR reporting and follow-up. While company representatives carry out this role well, the multifaceted work related to adverse reaction reporting and follow-up could be separated from marketing functions and raised to a higher scientific level. Retired physicians and pharmacists as well as medical and pharmacy students (part-time employed) could form a cadre of professionals to generate more interest and involvement in ADR reporting. These ADR specialists could obtain detailed data on the cases, discuss causality assessment, provide relevant literature, advise on management of ADRs, supply feed-back information quickly and authentically, and establish a constant liaison with the reporting doctor.

(4) *Feed-back information* is very important. It has often been said that adverse drug reaction reporting cannot be a one-way street if interest in reporting is to be maintained. The feed-back should be prompt (i.e. arrive within a reasonable period of time before the case is forgotten), practical (i.e. come up with an answer after evaluating the case) and personalized (whether endorsing the reporting physician's assessment or explaining a different view).

(5) *Causality assessment* is likely to improve the overall quality of information derived from spontaneous reporting and work on further refinement of this technique is continuing.

### *Clinical trial reports*

In looking at PMS as a continuous spectrum of data bearing on drug safety the results of clinical trials are valuable sources of information. Clinical trial documents are usually fully analysed only at the termination of the trial. There can thus be a delay in detecting tolerability problems, and the opportunity for prevention and quick intervention may be lost. Early involvement of DM in both the organization of clinical trials and in a periodic review of the record forms during the trial is assured and will be reinforced.

### *Comprehensive hospital monitoring*

It is important to note that in the Boston Collaborative Drug Surveillance Program the monitors are nurses, but in the Bern Programme medical doctors perform the monitoring. Their present tasks are: to promote observation and reporting of any possible ADRs by the house-staff and the nursing team; to record the data; to participate in data processing and at meetings; to present cases with adverse drug reaction along with the reviewed pertinent literature; and to assist in preparing publications. This valuable programme can be expanded by increasing the number of monitors, so they could play a more active role in detecting and following-up ADRs, and undertake *ad hoc* investigations of specific problems.

*Reports from national ADR centres*

The full data stored by these agencies or by the World Health Organization is seldom received by pharmaceutical companies. The watch-dog role of these centres, and their sensitive relationship towards industry in the past have limited the two-way flow of information. This situation is now changing favourably. Information on adverse drug reactions is provided by the Regulatory Authorities in Canada and in the United Kingdom, and similar arrangements can be anticipated in other countries.

Continuing discussions between representatives of the industry and WHO have resulted in valuable exchanges of information on some drug-related problems. Ciba–Geigy recently formulated, and is now implementing, a new policy on acute infectious diarrhoeal diseases.[17] This policy was constructed in close consultation with WHO; one of the elements of this programme is the gradual phasing-out of clioquinol, thus solving a long-debated problem.

**Expansion of PMS**

*Primary and secondary prevention studies* These studies conducted with beta-blockers and sulphinpyrazone are carefully designed and controlled and provide a large and valuable body of data. These drugs are important and widely-prescribed, and an increased use of tolerability data gained from these programmes will be most informative.

*Input from Group Companies* In assessing the role of Group Companies in PMS the importance of the following inter-country variables should be weighed: (1) the level of awareness of ADRs and interest in reporting; (2) the presence and strength of an ADR-unit; (3) the methodology used and the extent of co-ordination with DM Basle. National drug policies and regulations as well as medical practices show enormous differences in drug safety standards, which must be taken into account in planning for and in expectations from drug monitoring activities. Japanese PMS appears promising, and a study to compare this system with others is planned. Closer co-operation between Ciba–Geigy Basle and Group Companies (France, Germany, Italy, UK, USA) in PMS-activities will be achieved. The current state of ADR reporting in a country does not necessarily truly reflect the interest in drug safety of the respective medical communities and health authorities. While developing their national drug policies many countries, that until now engaged little in drug surveillance (e.g. Italy, Indonesia, Brazil), are becoming increasingly active in this area. In Italy the Ciba–Geigy group Company is planning a drug monitoring centre in co-operation with the University Hospital of Milan.

In countries where drug-surveillance does not exist or is minimal, a logical start would be to stimulate interest in, and wherever possible create a nucleus for ADR-reporting. Support of drug surveillance activities by Ciba–Geigy could focus particularly on those regions in which the company is strongly involved. Group Companies in countries where Drug Surveillance and reporting is at a higher level represent the most important current input-sources and in these (USA, Canada, UK, France, Japan, Germany) efforts will be directed towards optimizing the procedures. (For example by increasing the completeness of ADR information, introducing standardized evaluation procedures, scrutinizing clinical trial reports prospectively, rapidly reporting significant and urgent data, and an increasing use of telex and international data-transfer networks including the Ciba–Geigy 'Informatrics' System.[18]

*Corporate monitoring* Such a programme could be initiated by Ciba–Geigy alone or in co-operation with other companies in selected countries. Regional Surveillance Centres located in multi-practice areas and/or based in University Centres/Clinical Pharmacology Departments could be established to monitor the drugs of the sponsoring companies. The Ciba–Geigy Medicines Safety Centre[19] at the University of Cape Town, South Africa is already operational, and is the only collection agency for adverse drug reaction reports in that country. Such Centres could conduct hospital-based monitoring programmes; implement regional intensified ADR Reporting Systems (e.g. similar to the New Zealand programme),[20] support drug-related aspects of local health registries and actively engage in teaching drug safety and drug monitoring.

## THREE EXAMPLES OF POTENTIAL DRUG-EVENT RELATIONSHIPS

### Rauwolfia and breast cancer

The hypothesis of an association between the ingestion of rauwolfia alkaloids and an increased risk of breast cancer was first suggested in a paper[21] published in the *Lancet* in September, 1974, from the Boston Collaborative Drug Surveillance Program (BCDSP, 1974). This was based on routine analysis of discharge diagnoses and pre-admission drug histories of 5000 patients hospitalized in Massachusetts. Two other reports on this topic had been orchestrated to appear in the same issue of the *Lancet*, one from Oxford,[22] the other from Helsinki;[23] the authors of both reports had had advance information about the Boston Study (Armstrong *et al.*, 1974;[22] Heinonen *et al.*, 1974).[23] The BCDSP paper claimed that there was a more than three-fold increase in the risk of breast cancer for women exposed to reserpine compared with women not so exposed, and suggested a causal association. The British and Finnish studies both confirmed the Boston hypothesis although their estimates of the statistical strength of the finding were less strong.

The three papers immediately stimulated many letters and editorials in medical journals. These, as well as even more numerous comments and references in the lay news media, gave rise to concern among doctors who had prescribed rauwolfia as well as among patients who had taken it. The belief that rauwolfia had a carcinogenic potential rapidly led to a marked decline in use of this effective and heretofore popular antihypertensive. From 1975 onwards, further epidemiological studies began to be reported.

These were the subject of three major reviews. One, the Report of the *Ad-Hoc* Committees on Reserpine and Breast Cancer, published in May, 1978,[24] came to no clear conclusion about the first seven papers (DHEW, 1978). The Chairman of this Committee had previously prepared her own systematic review,[25] concluding that the association between rauwolfia and breast cancer might be valid but very weak, and not likely to be causal (Henderson, 1977). Labarthe's review of 1979 covered nine publications and supported Henderson's views; both pointed out potential methodological difficulties in the case-control studies (Labarthe, 1979).[26] However, none of these three reviews rejected either the original hypothesis of an association between rauwolfia and breast cancer, or the alternative possibility of a chance association.

At least seventeen studies were published on this subject between 1975 and 1980. Ten did not support the hypothesis that rauwolfia derivatives initiate or promote breast cancer; four suggested a 'possible small relationship', or 'low-level', 'not statistically significant' or 'weak' association; the authors of three papers could not come to a conclusive answer.

In 1980 the situation appeared to be as follows:

> the chances of having previously been exposed to rauwolfia were slightly higher in patients with breast cancer than in patients with a variety of other conditions, but although the raised risk-ratio was unlikely to be due to chance, it was not possible to decide that the association is causal. However, even if the association were thought to be causal, the small increased risk to public health presented by the continuing availability of rauwolfia would probably be out-weighed by the risks attendant upon its withdrawal.

Since 1980, there have been further reviews and comments, but two recent studies,[27,28] which have both failed to confirm a causal hypothesis (Friedmann, 1983; Shapiro, 1983), are significant. The latter[28] is particularly interesting because Shapiro was one of the authors of the original *Lancet* paper in 1974. After the subsequent establishment of the Drug Epidemiology Unit at Boston University

Medical School, his group carried out a second, similar study on breast cancer and previous medication history with improved methodology. Their conclusion is that rauwolfia does not increase the risk of breast cancer; Shapiro considers that the original association found in 1974, based on small numbers, was probably due to chance. In a recent lecture, indeed, he considered that the 1974 paper should probably not have been published.

During this time, 82 meetings of the Ciba–Geigy Basle 'Task Force Reserpine' were held, the first on June 26, 1974 (i.e. some 3 months before the date of the initial publications: initial notice of the finding had very constructively been provided to the Company by a senior author, on the understanding that no unauthorized use would be made of the information). The last – so far – occurred on November 20, 1979. At first the meetings were weekly; around the time of the publication they occurred daily and sometimes even lasted all day. Their purpose was to ensure that available information was correctly evaluated by internal and external consultants, in animal toxicology as well as epidemiology; to identify gaps in knowledge of the group of alkaloids involved and to arrange for these to be filled as quickly and accurately as possible; to notify Group Companies and, through them, Health Authorities, of developments; and, naturally, to defend one of the Company's most important products from unjustified charges by answering questions from physicians, to media and others as well. Despite the fact that not only reserpine was implicated, the initial publication referred to this alkaloid only, (the authors and the editor of the *Lancet* declined to change the title). Ciba–Geigy, as the discoverer of the anti-hypertensive action of the pure alkaloids of *R. serpentina*, and subsequently the foremost market leader of the product, took the initiative in informing other leading manufacturers and arranged three Task Force meetings with representatives of its major competitors. From the end of 1974, the frequency of meetings dropped again to weekly, fortnightly and, by the middle of 1975, to monthly. No meetings were held between February 1976 and January 1979, when the results of a new animal study were reviewed.

Many points could be made about this activity. In retrospect, it may seem to have been due to lack of experience with what was at that time a new kind of adverse reaction: a frequent, severe and life-threatening illness, a very small proportion of which was alleged to be due to the ingestion of a widely used and highly effective medication, prescribed up to 10 or 15 years earlier.

Finally, the problem turned out to be a non-problem. This is not necessarily to agree with Shapiro that the original study should not have been published; but to suggest that as much care should be taken in interpreting observations about alleged causal relations between drugs and untoward events if they are derived from epidemiological studies as if they come from observations upon single cases. Methodology for determining the weight that should be attached to scientific reports so that information from different sources can be combined, exists (Hammond and Joyce, 1976).[29]

## Hydralazine and cancer

Hydralazine hydrochloride is an antihypertensive agent, which has been widely used all over the world since 1952 in the treatment of essential hypertension, and since 1975 in treating hypertension due to toxaemia of pregnancy. The efficacy of hydralazine as well as the spectrum of its adverse effects have been well established. During an estimated 28 million patient-years of treatment no clinical evidence has emerged regarding an association between hydralazine and human cancer.

In 1978 Toth[30] reported a significantly increased incidence of lung tumours (adenomas and adenocarcinomas) in Swiss albino mice given hydrazinophthalazine hydrochloride in drinking water during their lifespan. The results were not analysed appropriately, due to the unusual design of the experiment whereby a control mouse was killed each time a treated mouse died. The purity of the compound (93%) was also lower than USP standards (98%). Although interpretation of this paper was difficult, in view of the therapeutic importance of hydralazine a Task Force was formed in Basle. Ciba–Geigy alerted all its Group Companies to the report, and a review with all available data on hydralazine was sent to the Group Companies with a request to transmit the information to their respective Health Authorities.

Two human studies relevant to the potential carcinogenicity of hydralazine were available. The first (Perry, 1963)[31] compared patients suffering from malignant hypertension who developed hydralazine toxicity with other recipients of the drug who did not. He found a higher incidence of cancer in the first group. Because of the small number of patients and confounding variables (more females in the group with toxicity, no data on smoking) no conclusions could be drawn from this paper.

A second paper by Williams[32] (1978) compared cases and controls in a large National Breast Cancer Screening Project and reported an elevated relative risk estimate for breast cancer in hydralazine users. The results of this study were not statistically significant, concomitant use of other drugs was not sufficiently considered, and there was also a question regarding selection bias in the patient population under study.

In order to clarify the relevance of Toth's results Ciba–Geigy decided to review the literature on mutagenicity and initiate new studies, and conduct long-term rodent experiments.

No clear-cut answer emerged from the literature (Tosk, 1979; Shaw, 1979; and Williams, 1980)[33–35] concerning the mutagenicity of hydralazine. Between 1979 and 1981 Ciba–Geigy conducted eleven mutagenicity tests with nine different systems; the findings were positive in three and negative in eight tests.

A study on carcinogenicity of hydralazine in C57/Bl mice, initiated by Ciba–Geigy in Japan, was concluded in 1981. The investigator reported that the results had not provided evidence of a carcinogenic effect of hydralazine, but a careful evaluation of the data by Ciba–Geigy Basle found that markedly reduced survival rate in the high dose group and a spilling accident in the low dose group invalidated the study.

Another Ciba–Geigy study using Fischer 344 rats treated with hydralazine showed evidence of a carcinogenic effect with respect to the overall number of tumour-bearing rats. No carcinogenic effect could be recognized for individual tumours or groups of neoplasms. This study was also considered inconclusive for two reasons; excessive mortality in all groups (the study had to be terminated prematurely after 22 months); and of the 400 rats used in this study 95 were not available for data analysis.

In September, 1980, the International Agency for Research on Cancer[36] (World Health Organization) summarized the evaluation on hydralazine as follows:

> 'The experimental data, while providing limited evidence for the carcinogenicity of hydralazine hydrochloride were difficult to interpret due to certain aspects of experimental design and analysis. The epidemiological data were insufficient. In view of the extensive use of this drug further studies should be undertaken.'

In the light of equivocal, even contradictory results from both mutagenicity and rodent studies and with hardly any information on humans it seemed very important to clarify this issue. Most views within the Company were in favour of carrying out human epidemiological studies. Outside experts were consulted, who expressed the opinion that while further careful mutagenicity and animal studies might tip the inconclusive balance of similar previous studies one way or the other, the relevance of such data to humans would still remain limited at best.

Once it was agreed that human epidemiological studies were necessary, the questions of feasibility, location and duration of such a study remained. Several months of exploratory discussions with clinical and epidemiological centres in Europe and in the USA followed. The news was discouraging. No centre with a sufficiently large number of hypertensive patients treated with hydralazine and analysed with appropriate methodology could be found in Europe. In the United States the Mayo Clinic in the period between 1960–1970 had treated 70 000 hypertensive patients, only 129 with hydralazine, most having received other antihypertensive agents (among them rauwolfia).

A case control surveillance programme,[37] conducted by the Drug Epidemiology Unit, Boston University Medical School to study correlations between cancer and previous life-time drug use appeared promising. When discussions with this group began (1981), they had approximately 1500 cases of newly diagnosed breast cancer on their files with additional cases accruing at the rate of about 750 per year. 5000 patients with various types of cancer and about 45 000 patients with non-cancerous conditions were available in their data bank. About 1% of the breast-cancer cases had been exposed to hydralazine; and this prevalence appeared high enough to render a case control study feasible (but only with a very large number of subjects, estimated at approximately 5000 at the time). It was proposed to investigate the relation of hydralazine to newly diagnosed breast cancer in women between the ages of 40–69. Such questions as controls, method of analysis, selection bias, information bias, confounding bias (in the latter particularly the concomitant use of other anti-hypertensive drugs) were considered. The duration of the study was estimated at 4 years. It was finally agreed that from the point of view of public health only the relation of hydralazine use to the risk of common cancers should be studied, since even an increased risk of a rare cancer is relatively unimportant.

Therefore, the study was designed to explore the relationship of cancer of the breast, large bowel and lung to hydralazine use. A preliminary analysis on hydralazine and breast cancer based on 1236 newly diagnosed cases and 5774 controls found 17 hydralazine users among the cases and 48 among the controls, giving an age-adjusted relative risk estimate of 1.0 with an upper 95% confidence limit of 1.8. Reserpine use was not associated with breast cancer in this group of patients; indeed the relative risk estimate for hydralazine among patients who had also used reserpine was 0.8, among those who had not used reserpine the estimate was 1.1. These initial results suggested that hydralazine does not increase the risk of breast cancer, but the results are only tentative because of the small numbers.

This study has been in progress since 1982. Approximately 3000 cases of breast cancer have so far been enrolled. Completion of the study is expected by the end of 1984 or early 1985.

## Potassium chloride – preparations and gastrointestinal lesions

Reports of ulceration of the upper gastrointestinal tract associated with solid potassium chloride preparations appeared soon after these products were introduced internationally in 1965. Two recent studies[38,39] (McMahon, 1982, Barkin *et al.*, 1983) compared the effects of a new micro-encapsulated potassium chloride preparation (Micro-K produced by Robbins – USA) with that of a wax-matrix KCl formulation (Slow-K – produced by Ciba-Geigy). The first study conducted by McMahon, and sponsored by Robbins, was originally presented by the author at the Tulane University Medical School Clinical Therapeutic Symposium in June, 1982. In both studies high doses (96 mEq, per day) of solid KCl had been given to normal male volunteers for one week with concomitant administration of an anticholinergic agent. Endoscopic examination of the upper gastrointestinal tract was performed at the conclusion of therapy. Both studies showed a higher incidence of asymptomatic erosive lesions from wax-matrix KCl than from the micro-encapsulated form. It was postulated by the authors of these papers that micro-encapsulated KCl is less injurious because of its wide dispersion in the stomach.

Following the publication of McMahon's paper the FDA requested all manufacturers of solid potassium chloride products to perform similar studies, and later suggested that labelling for solid potassium chloride products other than Micro-K should be modified to reflect the available new information.

A Ciba-Geigy Task Force was formed to co-ordinate action between Basle and the group company in Summit (USA). A circular letter and a statement was dispatched to all Ciba-Geigy Group Companies. This included an outline of the developments concerning Slow-K, comments and criticisms about the clinical relevance of the study, and information that the company was sponsoring further relevant investigations initiated in the United States. The Group Companies were requested to pass on all information to their respective Health Authorities.

The clinical relevance of the studies reporting a surprisingly high incidence of upper gastrointestinal lesions from wax-matrix KCl was questioned on the following grounds: (1) almost five times the normal daily dose (96 mEq) of potassium supplements was used; (2) it is not known to what extent the concomitant administration of anticholinergic agents simulates decreased gastric emptying, a clinical condition in which the possible occurrence of occasional serious gastrointestinal side-effects from Slow-K is known; (3) the high (33%) incidence rate of mild ('Grade 1') lesions in the subjects receiving placebo was not distinguishable from the rates seen in those receiving solid potassium preparations.

The reported high incidence of erosive lesions with wax-matrix KCl seemed inconsistent with the fact that there are only sporadic reports of such complications in patients receiving these products. The re-analysis of adverse drug reaction experience with Slow-K performed jointly by Ciba-Geigy in Basle and in Summit showed that Slow-K has been used since 1965 in 60 countries by over 14 million patients. A total of 239 cases of gastrointestinal side-effects of all types have been reported in association with Slow-K. 118 of these were classified as minor, of the remaining 121 cases 26 were instances of lesions/ bleeding in the stomach and duodenum, irrespective of causality. It could thus be estimated that the approximate incidence of gastrointestinal lesions was less than 1 per 100 000 patient years.

In view of the difficulties in interpreting the studies, and also because of the inconsistencies between their conclusions and the Company's adverse drug reaction experience with this product,[40] Ciba-Geigy initiated a series of endoscopic investigations to clarify the safety issue. Four studies[41,42] were conducted in the United States (at the Hershey Medical Center, Pennsylvania and the University of Arizona).

The first of these studies[42] simulated normal clinical conditions by treating the subjects with 48 mEq of KCl (2.5 times the normal daily dose) given after meals. Other compartments of this study as well as three others were conducted under more extreme conditions. Subjects were exposed to 91–96 mEq of potassium supplements administered on an empty stomach, and also received high doses of a potent anticholinergic. These four studies came to the following main conclusions;

(1) All solid KCl preparations may cause mucosal lesions of the upper gastrointestinal tract, but the incidence is low;
(2) Erosions and ulcers in subjects given wax-matrix KCl were not significantly more frequent in those given micro-encapsulated KCl.

These conclusions were complemented and supported by an epidemiologic study,[43] in which no evidence was found for a positive association between wax-matrix KCl use and upper gastrointestinal bleeding in over 15 000 intensively monitored hospitalized patients, 1050 of whom had received solid KCl by mouth.

In March 1983 an FDA Advisory Committee concluded that: 'From several studies the lesions caused by Micro-K or other wax-matrix products seem to be generally mild, clinically insignificant and not differing in incidence by orders of magnitude'.

A 'Medical Summary' including the overall results of the newest data was submitted by Ciba-Geigy to the FDA in June 1983, with a request that the proposed labelling for Micro-K and Slow-K be reconsidered.

## ACKNOWLEDGEMENTS

This chapter is based in part upon one appearing in the first edition of this book entitled 'The pharmaceutical industry – Philosophy and practice of drug surveillance within Ciba–Geigy' by Drs M. Crawford, G.-C. Berneker and O. de S. Pinto. The authors also wish to acknowledge discussions with Dr M. Crawford during preparation of an early draft of the present manuscript, and express their thanks, to Professor C. R. B. Joyce for his helpful comments.

### References

1. Gross, F. H. and Inman, W. H. W. (eds.) (1977). *Drug Monitoring*. pp. ix–x (London/New York: Academic Press)
2. Geiling, E. M. K. and Cannon, P. R. (1938). Pathogenic effects of elixir of sulfonilamide (diethyleneglycol) poisoning. *J. Am. Med. Assoc.*, **111,** 919
3. Editorial. (1977). After practolol. *Br. Med. J.*, pp. 1561–2
4. Gent, M. and Shigematsu, I. (1968). *Epidemiological issues in reported drug-induced illnesses – S.M.O.N. and other examples*. pp. 119–267. (Hamilton, Ontario: McMaster University Library Press)
5. Drury, V. W. M. (1977). Monitoring ADRs in general practice. In Gross, F. H. and Inman, W. H. W. (eds.) *Drug Monitoring*, pp. 117–22. (London/New York: Academic Press)
6. Doll, Sir Richard. (1969). Recognition of unwanted drug effects. *Br. Med. J*, **2,** 69

7. Slone, D. *et al.* (1966). Drug Surveillance Utilising Nurse Monitors, An Epidemiological Approach. *The Lancet*, **2,** pp. 901–3
8. Hoigné, R., Streit, C., Stocker, F. *et al.* (1981). Drug Monitoring and Epidemiologie von Arzneimittel-Nebenwirkungen. In Borelli, S., Düngemann, H. (eds.) *Fortschritte der Allergologie und Dermatologie. Klinik für Dermatologie und Allergie*, pp. 169–74 (Basel Neu Isenburg Wien: Davos and IMP. Verlagsgesellschaft)
9. Zoppi, M., Hoigné, R., Keller, M. F., Streit, F. and Hess, T. (1983). Blutdruckfall under Dipyron (Novaminsulfon-Natrium). *Schweiz.* Med. *Wschr.*, **113,** 1768–70
10. Hunziker, T., Fehlmann, U., Kummer, H., Spengler, H. and Hoigné, R. (1980). Arzneifieber auf das Antidepressivum Nomifensin (Alival). *Schweiz. Med. Wschr.*, **110,** 1295–300
11. Venning, G. R. (1983). Identification of adverse reactions to new drugs. II. How were 18 important adverse reactions discovered and with what delays? *Br. Med. J.*, **286,** 365–8
12. IMS America, Ltd. (October 24th, 1978). Final Report – Task A. An Experiment in Early Post-Marketing Surveillance of Drugs. Joint Commission on Prescription Drug Use, Inc. Rockville, Maryland 20852
13. Lasagna, L. (1976). Post-marketing surveillance of drugs. p. 6. (Washington, DC: Medicine in the Public Interest, Inc.
14. Borda, I. (1981). Drug surveillance and postmarketing surveillance *Ciba-Geigy-Basle-Document*, 36–52
15. Venning, G. R. (1983). Identification of adverse reactions to new drugs. I. What have been the important adverse reactions since thalidomide? *Br. Med. J.*, **286,** 199–202
16. Slone, D., Shapiro, S., *et al.* (1979) Drug Evaluation After Marketing. *Ann. Int. Med.*, **90,** 257–61
17. Ciba-Geigy policy on control of diarrheal diseases – CIBA–GEIGY – BASLE-DOCUMENT – October 1982
18. Bieri, R., Palmer, N., Penin, L. and Turri, M. (1982). 'Informatrics': the clinical trial system of CIBA-Geigy. *Proc. Med. Informatics Eur.*, **16,** 596–601
19. Biersteker, E. and Folb, P. I. (1982). A simple and effective drug information system. *The Practitioner*, **226,** 605
20. McQueen, E. G. (1980). New methods in PMS (New Zealand). In Inman, W. H. W. (ed.) Monitoring for Drug Safety. 1st Edn.pp. 201–6 (Lancaster: MTP PRess)
21. Boston Collaborative Drug Surveillance Program (1974). Reserpine and breast cancer. *Lancet*, **2,** 669–71
22. Armstrong, B., Stevens, N. and Doll, R. (1974). Retrospective study of the association between use of rauwolfia derivatives and breast cancer in English women. *Lancet*, **2,** 672–5
23. Heinonen, O. P., Shapiro, S., Tuominen, L. and Turunen, M. I. (1974). Reserpine use in relation to breast cancer. *Lancet*, **2,** 675–7
24. Department of Health, Education and Welfare (1978). *Reports of the* Ad Hoc *Committee on Reserpine and Breast Cancer*. DHEW, Washington DC
25. Henderson, M. (1977). Reserpine and breast cancer – a review: In Colombo, F., Shapiro, S., Slone, D. and Tognoni, G. (eds.). Elsevier.
26. Labarthe, D. R. (1979). Methodologic variation in case-control studies of reserpine and breast cancer. *J. Chron. Dis.*, **32,** 95–104
27. Friedman, G. D. (1983). Rauwolfia and breast cancer. No relation found in long term users age 50 and over. *J. Chron. Dis.*, **36,** 367–70
28. Shapiro, S., Persells, J. L., Rosenberg, L., Kaufman, D. W., Stolles, P. D. and Schottenfeld, D. (1984). Risk of breast cancer in relation to use of rauwolfia alkaloids. *Eur. J. Clin. Pharm.*, **26,** 143–6
29. Hammond, K. R. and Joyce, C. R. B. (1977). Psychological influences on human judgment, especially of adverse reactions. In Gross, F. H. and Inman, W. H. W. (eds.) *Drug Monitoring*. pp. 269–87 (London: Academic Press)
30. Toth, B., Tumorigenic effect of 1-hydrazinophthalazine hydrochloride in mice. *J. Natl. Cancer Inst.*, **61,** 1363–5
31. Perry, Jr. H. M. (1963). Carcinoma and hydralazine toxicity in patients with malignant hypertension. *J. Am. Med. Assoc.*, **186,** 1020–2

32. Williams, R. R., Feinleib, M. Connor, R. J. and Stegens, N. L. (1978). Abstract: Case-control study of antihypertensive and diuretic use by women with malignant and benign breast lesions detected in a mammography screening program, *J. Natl. Cancer Inst.*, **61,** 327–35
33. Tosk, J., Schmeltz, I. and Hoffman, D. (1979). Hydrazines as mutagens in a histidine-requiring auxotroph of *Salmonella typhimurium. Mutat. Res.*, **66,** 247–52
34. Shaw, C. R., Butler, M. A. Thenot, J.-P. Haegle, K. D. and Matney, T. S. (1979). Genetic effects of hydralazine. *Mutat. Res.*, **68,** 79–84
35. McMahon, F. G., Akdamar, K., Ryan, J. R. and Ertan, A. (1982). Upper gastrointestinal lesions after potassium chloride supplements: A controlled clinical trial. *The Lancet*, **2,** 1059–61
36. IARC Working Group. (1980). Hydralazine and hydralazine hydrochloride summary of data reported and evaluation. In *IARC Monographs on the Evaluation of the Carcinogenic Risk of Chemicals to Humans.* Vol. 24, pp. 85–100. (Geneva: WHO)
37. Slone, D., Shapiro, S., Miettinen, O. S. (1977). Case-control surveillance of serious illnesses attributable to ambulatory drug use. In Colombo, F., Shapiro, S., Slone, D. *et al.* (eds.). *Epidemiologic Evaluation of Drugs.* pp. 59–70 (NewYork: Elsevier/ North Holland Biomedical Press)
38. Williams, G. M., Masué, G., McQueen, C. and Shimada, T. (1980). Genotoxicity of the antihypertensive drug hydralazine. Science **210,** No4467, 329–30
39. Barkin, J. S., Harary, A. M., Shamblem, C. E. and Lasseter, K. C. (1983). Potassium chloride and gastrointestinal injury. *Ann. Intern. Med.*, 262
40. Data on file; Ciba Pharmaceutical Co.
41. Patterson, D. J., Weinstein, G. S. and Jeffries, G. H. (1983). Endoscopic comparison of the effects of solid and liquid potassium chloride supplements on the upper gastrointestinal tract. *Lancet*, **2,** 1077–8
42. Patterson, D. J. and Jeffries, G. H. (1983). Spectrum of mucosal injury from oral potassium chloride supplemes in normal volunteers (abstr.) *Gastroenterology*, **84,** 1271
43. Aselton, P. J. and Jick, H. (1983). Short-term follow-up study of wax-matrix potassium chloride in relation to gastrointestinal bleeding. *Lancet*, **1,** 184

# Section 2: SPECIALIZED MONITORING

# Editor's Introduction and Commentary

The first section of this book has been mainly concerned with the generation of 'signals' or hypotheses that something adverse may be happening as a result of the administration of a drug. This second section describes various systems which have been developed to measure the strength of these signals, and to balance the *risk* or probability that something bad will happen with the *benefit* or probability that something good will happen as a result of treatment. We are concerned with the problems of determining *relative risk* and *absolute risk*, in other words, of distinguishing events which may be related to drug use from those which occur spontaneously. We are also concerned with the measurement of the *incidence* of new events occurring within a given time period and the *prevalence* or background frequency of similar events.

To clarify these terms, let us imagine, for example, that we have examined a representative sample of 10 000 people and have found that 200 patients are diabetic. The prevalence of diabetes is 2%. Suppose we re-examine the same 10 000 patients one year later and find that 10 patients who were previously normal have now developed diabetes. This represents an annual incidence of 0.1%. If all 10 000 patients survived, the prevalence at the end of one year would be 2.1%. Some diabetics, however, would have been expected to die and be replaced by newly diagnosed diabetics so the prevalence would tend to remain more or less the same from year to year.

Some drugs prevent or cure diseases, so that over a period of time the prevalence as well as the incidence of a disease may decrease. Others preserve the lives of people who would otherwise die from a disease, so the prevalence may actually increase while the incidence remains static. If an important cause of death such as tuberculosis or malaria is eliminated by treatment, more people will survive to eventually die of something other than tuberculosis or malaria. Indirectly, the successful treatment of one disease may be linked with an increase in some other disease. When we compare seemingly identical populations, matched for age, sex, race, health and so on, who differ only with regard to the treatment they are using, we may see differences in the frequency with which certain illnesses are recorded. We may, for example, find that diabetes is more prevalent or has a higher incidence in hypertensive patients treated with diuretics. Since most patients with significant disease or symptoms received some kind of treatment, nearly all judgements of risk and benefit are made on the basis of *relative* risks and *relative* benefits of various treatments. Absolute risks can hardly ever be measured because untreated controls, certainly those with serious diseases, cannot be studied. In the Commentary to Section 5 we will consider a third type of risk – perceived risk – which is not measurable in epidemiological terms of absolute or relative risk, but depends on how people interpret these risks.

Drug risks on the whole are miniscule in relation to familiar risks such as those involved in travelling, sport, smoking or certain occupations. They are also very small in relation to the risk of most of the diseases for which they are used. These risks are important when the consequences of treatment turn out to be worse than the disease being treated, or when an equally effective alternative treatment is available which avoids these risks. If a drug was effective for the treatment of a life-threatening disease but was shown to cause cancer in 1% of patients who used it, there would be massive adverse publicity, and the drug would almost certainly be banned. Assuming that there were no alternative treatments, it would be of little consequence, however, if one in every hundred patients died from cancer attributable to the drug, when one in five or one in six of the population die anyway from cancer unrelated to treatment.

Various attempts have been made to develop risk scales which would help us to compare the risks of treatment with other more familiar risks.[1,2] The risks of dying from cancer, coronary disease or stroke during any one year are all within the same order of magnitude (between 1 in 100 and 1 in 999). The risk of dying from arthritis, asthma, cirrhosis, diabetes, road accidents, burns, falls or suicide are all two orders of magnitude less (1 in 10 000 – 1 in 99 999). In the United Kingdom, thanks to the almost indiscriminate use of antibiotics in the treatment of sore throats and febrile illnesses in children, acute rheumatic fever now kills less than 1 in 10 000 000 of the population each year, a risk which is in the same order as that of being fatally struck by lightning or bitten by a snake. National vital statistics of this nature, however, are of little interest to a patient suffering from a disease. What he wants to know is the risk of death or permanent injury caused by that disease and the risks of treating that disease.

Set against a scale of risks of diseases, the risks of drugs used to treat them are very small. The risk of jaundice from benoxaprofen poisoning, for example, was small even for elderly people who took too much. The risk of aplastic anaemia induced by phenylbutazone was two to three orders of magnitude smaller than the risk of dying from the complications of arthritis. Zomepirac, with a world reported incidence of fatal anaphylaxis of less than one in 2 000 000 may have been 10 000 times less dangerous than the complications of arthritis, indeed, most of the anti-inflammatory drugs which were removed from the market between 1982 and 1984 were at least a hundred times safer than some of the diseases they were used for.

It is worth remembering that thalidomide affected a very high proportion, possibly more than 90%, of fetuses that were exposed to it during the vulnerable period of organogenesis. Practolol may have caused serious damage in more than 1% of those who used it for more than a year. Almost all the other serious drug reaction problems which have been identified during the past quarter of a century, have occurred at a frequency which is two or more orders of magnitude less than that induced by practolol.

The main objective of most of the schemes which are described in the second section of this book is to assess the safety of drugs and measure their risks before very large numbers of patients have been affected. These schemes are not designed to replace voluntary anecdotal reporting nor are they designed to identify very rare ADRs. None of them will prevent accidents from happening. Whatever the public expectation may be, all applications of technology are associated with some risk that the unforeseen will occur. Many people have suggested that slowing the rate of introduction of new drugs, for example, by curbing advertising, will increase safety. It is more likely, however, that this could merely delay the detection of the more serious ADRs which are quite rare and likely to come to light only when large numbers of patients have been treated. Alertness to unexpected side-effects depends on novelty, and the best way to establish safety is to ensure that the largest possible number of patients are monitored as soon as a drug is marketed.

The three most important developments in post-marketing surveillance during the past 20 years have been the scheme for hospital based monitoring, originally developed by Jick and his colleagues in Boston (see Chapter 17) which produce high quality data on rather limited numbers of patients, the use of outpatient data assembled in the Medicaid programme (Chapter 16) and the nation-wide Prescription-Event Monitoring (PEM) scheme developed in England by the Drug Surveillance Research Unit (DSRU) which is described in Chapter 15. PEM is the only new scheme to be developed since the first edition of this book appeared 5 years ago, and is the first large scale development of the principle of event monitoring described by Finney (Chapter 31) which was first tested in a modified form by Skegg (Chapter 19). We are uniquely fortunate in England that the National Health Service is served by a special health authority known as the Prescription Pricing Authority (PPA) which processes prescriptions written by general practitioners so that pharmacists may be remunerated for the drugs that are dispensed. Each prescription provides a unique opportunity to identify a doctor, a patient and a drug exposure. The main limitation of the system is the number of questionnaires that doctors are prepared to complete. PEM has been developed to the point where it should be possible to include all new chemical entities marketed for use in general practice in such a way that at least the first 10 000 or more patients are monitored. It is very unfortunate, for patients as well as from the point of view of development of measures to improve drug safety, that almost from the moment that this stage was reached in June 1984, the number of innovative products reaching the market has dwindled almost to vanishing point. This is probably due to loss of confidence by the pharmaceutical industry after the sudden spate of drug withdrawals during the period 1982–1984, to generic substitution, and to a hardening attitude by the Licensing Authority to the introduction of new drugs; hopefully, the late 1980s will see a resumption of innovation.

Doctors are enthusiastic supporters of PEM, they use it as a more rational approach to decision-making than systems depending on spontaneous reporting, and they co-operate because the scheme does not involve very much work, because it does not require them to make judgements about the relationship between drug treatment and adverse events and because it does not carry any medico-legal risk. General practitioners appear to have had no difficulty understanding the difference between event monitoring and ADR monitoring and the level of co-operation has consistently been excellent.

Non-steroidal anti-inflammatory drugs (NSAIDs) are used to illustrate how PEM works, and already some important results have been obtained. It is not possible to extrapolate to all NSAIDs, but a study of five of them calls into question the traditional view that gastrointestinal bleeding or perforation may be a very great risk when these drugs are used. With all five the case rate for the complications of peptic ulcer was approximately equivalent to one in 200 patient-years of exposure, and this was probably very little different from the rate in patients who had ceased to use NSAIDs or who had switched to alternative treatment. It should not be forgotton that a very high proportion of arthritic patients use other analgesics in addition to NSAIDs, and that there is little or no information about the incidence of ulceration or haemorrhage in untreated arthritic patients.

Another interesting finding was the fact that the drug least expected to cause dyspepsia was in fact associated with the largest number of events of this type. The reason for this paradox is almost certainly that whenever a drug is claimed to cause fewer side-effects than its competitors, it is likely to be used in patients who are particularly prone to these effects which are then recorded more frequently as adverse events. This may also be an important source of bias in voluntary reporting systems. Particular attention should be drawn to Table 6 in which the authors compare and contrast the strengths and weaknesses of the yellow card system and Prescription Event Monitoring. Ten strengths or weaknesses are identified, and in every case the strength of one system is a weakness in the other. The two schemes are thus entirely complementary and not competitive. In this second edition, we welcome a new feature, the contribution by Morse and Le Roy of Health Information Designs Inc. (HID) and Strom of the University of Pennsylvania School of Medicine. Just as PEM in England makes use of the largest available source of patients who have been treated with drugs, in other words doctors' prescriptions, the 'COMPASS' scheme utilizes the facility for identifying patients provided by the vast state-sponsored Medicaid programme established 20 years ago in the United States. Unlike PEM where cohorts have to be built up prospectively once a decision to study a particular drug has been made, the 'COMPASS' scheme utilizes an existing data base which provides information both about drugs and diagnoses. It would be possible, for example, to select a cohort of patients suffering specifically from rheumatoid arthritis who had been treated with phenylbutazone. In PEM it would only be possible to identify rheumatoid sufferers after the doctor had supplied the follow-up information in response to a general enquiry about all patients who had been treated with phenylbutazone.

'COMPASS' currently embraces ten state Medicaid data bases covering a population of 5.3 million patients. Medicaid patients are probably not truly representative of all US citizens with respect to certain factors, especially poverty which may be related to health problems. There is, for example, a relative deficit of employed males and a large relative excess of young children. Nevertheless, the 'COMPASS' data has wide applications in the study of drug safety in general.

In both PEM and 'COMPASS' access to primary medical records is possible with the collaboration of the prescribing physician. Clearly the use that is made of them is limited both by the time available for follow-up work and by the need to avoid overburdening doctors with requests for detailed information. Both are event reporting systems which do not depend on the extent to which individual doctors perceive the possibility that events may be ADRs. Both groups have studied non-steroidal anti-inflammatory drugs extensively and some interesting differences and similarities are apparent. For example, 'COMPASS' data showed that upper gastrointestinal bleeding was relatively more common among males, while in the PEM data the incidence was no different in males or females receiving NSAIDs. Both groups on the other hand have recorded a high use of indomethacin for gout. Medicaid is less likely to suffer from the biases which afflict case control studies, especially recall bias, and the problems that are associated with the selection of controls. PEM has similar advantages in this respect but only in situations in which related drugs are compared. It is also worth noting that both schemes are considerably less expensive on a cost-per-patient basis than nearly all other methods of PMS.

The highly successful Boston Collaborative Drug Surveillance Program (BCDSP) is described in Chapter 17 by Professor David Lawson who has been responsible for one of its international satellites in Glasgow. One outstanding observation among the wealth of data he presents is the rarity of fatal ADRs in hospital. There were only 20 deaths in 26 462 consecutive admissions, and most of those who died were seriously ill before the ADR. This reinforces the general conclusion that serious ADRs are most uncommon and refutes speculations which were frequently made, particularly in the early 1960s, that ADRs were a major cause of hospital admission.

Several examples are quoted of the ability of hospital-based monitoring to link toxicity with dosage, with the patient's age or diagnoses, or with concurrent drug treatment. Hospital based schemes also provide evidence of drug interactions which are unlikely to be evaluated by spontaneous monitoring or by schemes such as PEM. As Lawson points out however, major interaction problems are very rare. Although books have been written about them, the majority may be anticipated on the basis of pharmacological knowledge obtained prior to marketing, and serious problems are rare in routine clinical practice.

Special attention is drawn to the rarity of drug-induced gastrointestinal haemorrhage as a reason for hospital admission. This tends to confirm the results of PEM already referred to, and runs contrary to long held and perhaps wrongly held views of the risks of treating patients with NSAIDs. The results of work by the BCDSP, HID and the DSRU may well lead quite soon to a radical rethinking of attitudes about the safety of medicines.

The BCDSP and the DSRU have shown negative associations between aspirin and at least two of the five NSAIDs that have been studied and myocardial infarction. This finding makes biological sense, and suggests that anti-inflammatory drugs may well be candidates for both primary and secondary prevention studies in coronary disease. Indeed, Lawson suggests that the very low risk of haemorrhage with aspirin may make it an acceptable candidate for prophylactic cardioprotection.

Obviously the main limitation of the BCDSP is the relatively small number of patients treated with any one newly introduced drug. The BCDSP is not, for example, an appropriate arrangement for detecting ADRs which have a true frequency of 1 in 10 000. Professor Lawson's chapter contains a great amount of thought-provoking data. Those who are not familiar with the methodology should make use of the very extensive bibliography he provides.

Complementary to the BCDSP is the 'Aberdeen–Dundee System' described in Chapter 18. This owes much to the inspiration of the late James Crooks who with Roy Weir and Dorothy Moir (*née* Coull) established a patient-drug file in Aberdeen in 1968 which was linked with hospitals in Dundee in 1972. The system is concerned mainly with hypothesis testing, and is likely only to measure comparatively frequent events occurring with commonly used drugs. As with the BCDSP and the DSRU, the value of patient-drug files increases as the files become larger.

Professor Skegg (Chapter 19) describes an early experiment in medical record linkage conducted in general practice in the Oxford area, and reviews other linkage systems in various countries. Medical record linkage (MRL) must be regarded as the 'Philosophers Stone' of drug surveillance. Modern computer technology has advanced enormously since post-marketing surveillance commenced after the thalidomide tragedy and, if doctors could be persuaded to throw away their pens and their manual records, MRL could become a reality. One cannot help feeling, however, that the technology has advanced far more rapidly than attitudes to medical practice, and that the benefits of MRL may not be realized until the twenty-first century. Skegg's study commenced in 1974 and anticipated PEM by 8 years in the sense that it was the first attempt to develop the principle of event monitoring as opposed to mere ADR reporting. Admittedly, the scale was small, only six practices involving 20 general practitioners and a population of about 42 000 patients. Even on this scale, however, it was shown that the study would probably have identified the practolol problem had it been in operation in the 1970s. Skegg points out that positive evidence of safety can only be obtained from studies (like PEM) that do not depend on doctors' suspicions. He anticipated that confidentiality should not be a problem, and this has been confirmed in PEM as far as co-operation by general practitioners is concerned. However, Skegg's hope that computerization of the Prescription Pricing Authority should facilitate more widespread MRL, is unlikely to be realized, because patient's identities are not to be included in the computer records of prescriptions processed by the Authority.

Margaretha Helling-Borda, has provided a comprehensive review of computer development in the context of drug monitoring (Chapter 20). This requires little editorial comment except to acknowledge this important initiative by WHO. In the editorial to Section 1 of this book, attention was drawn to the achievements of WHO in bringing people together, and we should also recognize the pioneer work by WHO in bringing together international post-marketing data.

With Professor Dundee's chapter on monitoring of anaesthetics (Chapter 21), we move to a number of specialized areas of drug safety not covered by general practice schemes or by most of the hospital schemes so far developed. Anaesthetics are *distributed* rather than *prescribed* in the usual sense and, in most hospitals it is necessary to monitor case records in order to identify patients who had been anaesthetized with certain agents, since there is no direct link between the pharmacy who supply anaesthetics to the operating theatres in bulk, and individual patients who receive them.

Dundee suggests that a 'yellow card' issued by the CSM is unsatisfactory for use by the anaesthetist. It should not, however, be forgotten that yellow cards were almost the only source of information available to Inman and Mushin[3] who were able to reach a conclusion, unpopular at the time but now generally accepted by anaesthetists, that there was a relationship between the number of rechallenges with halothane and the time of onset of jaundice in the small number of patients who are sensitive to this agent. Quite rightly, of course, Dundee points out that most of the reactions to anaesthetics are observed by the anaesthetist while the patient is in the theatre. Each procedure could be likened to a pharmacological experiment. In other fields it is very rare for the physician to be in attendance throughout the period in which the intended pharmacological effects of his treatment are manifest, and during which most of the more dangerous ADRs will occur.

As with anaesthetics, radio-contrast media (Chapter 22) are not 'prescribed' in the usual way out but, like anaesthetics, their acute effects will become apparent while the patient is still in the X-ray department. Various studies of intravenous urography are quoted in which the mortality ranged from 1 in 14 000 to 1 in 117 000, and the risk of one procedure is thus similar to the risk of one year's treatment with phenylbutazone. The design and conduct of a massive investigation involving 247 hospitals, possibly the largest monitoring scheme ever mounted in a hospital environment, is described in considerable detail. The mortality recorded in this study, four deaths in 173 000 patients, was similar to that encountered in earlier surveys.

The special problem of radio pharmaceuticals (Chapter 23) are not associated with the 'active' chemical substances involved since the concentrations of radioactive material are measured in millionths of the concentration of impurities normally present in the analytical grade chemicals. Many products cannot be subjected to the usual controls because they often have to be 'manufactured' and used on the same day. The problems that do arise are usually related to the excipients or carriers used to formulate the radioactive material. These have led, for example, to fairly large numbers of anaphylactic reactions, and also to neurological disasters when injected intrathecally.

While many surveillance schemes have been drug-orientated, Dr Bruinsma's File of Adverse Reactions to the Skin (Chapter 24) is one of the few schemes which is event-orientated. He is the first person to use 'FDR' (favourable drug reaction) in sharp distinction to 'ADR', and he points out that FDRs may become as important as ADRs in the future. Skin reactions are more numerous than any other class of ADR and, though rarely fatal, are the cause of considerable morbidity.

Professor Fraunfelder's National Registry of Drug-induced ocular Side-effects (Chapter 25) was inspired by his visit to Moorfields Hospital in 1975 where much of the work needed to identify the problem of ocular toxicity with practolol was conducted. Drug-induced blindness is certainly the most feared event next to death. Fortunately it is extremely rare and because of this, individual doctors may never encounter a case during the course of their professional lifetime. For this reason a reference centre for ocular effects is especially important.

Professor Scott (Chapter 26) reminds us that although the thalidomide tragedy was immediately and visibly horrific, the induction of vaginal cancer by diethylstilboestrol in the female offspring of treated women, was perhaps more sinister. Surprisingly this latter incident in the United States did not attract much attention from the press in spite of the knowledge that pregnancies are frequently accidentally exposed to contraceptive or other sex hormones. Fortunately no other examples of carcinogenesis, passed from mother to fetus have so far come to light. Other special problems which Professor Scott calls to our attention are those associated with the use of hormonal replacement therapy in post menopausal women, and of the need to find alternatives to sex hormones for the present generation of women of child-bearing age whose mothers used oral contraceptives, revealing risks such as those of thromboembolism and others such as uterine or breast cancer which are still greatly feared.

The natural companion to Scott's chapter is that of Professor Smithells on teratology (Chapter 27). Paradoxically perhaps, although drug monitoring during the last quarter of a century started with thalidomide, the arrangements for monitoring for congenital defects are the least well developed of all forms of post-marketing surveillance. No area of PMS is as rife with stories of alleged drug-induced injury. Unproven and perhaps unprovable arguments about anti-emetics such as 'Debendox' ('Bendectin'), hormone pregnancy tests, oral contraceptives and anticonvulsants and their possible relation to congenital abnormalities have raged for 20 years. These arguments often cause immense suffering to parents who have been encouraged to believe that their child's deformity may have been drug-induced, even though the balance of scientific evidence points to the fact that the abnormalities are probably spontaneous. Repeatedly, the CSM has reviewed the evidence against 'Debendox' and denied that it is a teratogen. Nowhere has the problem of bias in case-control studies been so evident. Worst of all have been the attempts to use maternal recall of drug exposure in many of the studies. Once publicity has been given to the possibility of a link between a drug and an abnormality there is no way in which the recall of a mother of an abnormal baby can be regarded as unbiased.

Dr Chambers (Chapter 28) can view the forensic scene as a doctor and as a lawyer, since he is doubly qualified and became a coroner after experience in the pharmaceutical industry. He gives us a fascinating insight into the possible role of drugs in the cases he has heard. In one example he quotes the possibility that high doses of chlorpromazine may have interfered with its own metabolism. The conflicting discussions surrounding this proposition lead him to question the ability of juries to settle scientific problems of this nature.

Dr Chambers touches on the subject of death certification. Death certificates are a potentially useful source of information, but their accuracy leaves very much to be desired. This is particularly true of elderly patients in whom ADRs are most frequent and who are less likely to come to autopsy.

Coroner's inquests are usually covered by the press, and Chambers quotes 'the opinion of Gavin Thurston, (who was once a part-time field worker with the Committee on Safety of Medicines), that reporting a death to the CSM may be a more appropriate procedure than an inquest'. He suggested that an inquest into a death following the use of the pill by a young woman may do more harm than good.

In Chapter 29, Dr Haler provides technical advice for the pathologist who should be constantly mindful of the possibility that a death may have been drug-induced, and he deals exclusively with the steps which must be taken to ensure proper reservation of fluids and tissues for subsequent investigation.

Finally in Chapter 30, Dr Volans describes the contribution to drug safety made by the Poisons Information Services. It is significant that his predecessor, Dr Roy Goulding was involved at the very start of the yellow card scheme by the Committee on Safety of Drugs, immediately before the editor of this volume became responsible for its management. There are no sharp distinctions between drugs and poisons, and many of the more serious ADR problems could be avoided by closer attention to dose and indication. In contrast to the CSM, the Poisons Information Centre is linked to laboratory services and also functions as an information centre. It can supply information required by the clinician for the management of acute poisoning over the telephone, and much of its success must be attributed to the almost instant availability of its various services. This contrasts strongly with the Committee on Safety of Medicines whose permanent officers are deterred by bureaucracy, by fear of medico-legal involvement and by the Official Secrets Act from providing a similar service for ADRs. The quality of service provided by Dr Volans' unit in the United Kingdom provides the strongest argument for separation of ADR monitoring from regulatory activity. There might even be advantages in combining poisons and ADR units established on a regional basis to assemble toxicity and ADR data and provide information.

## References

1. Urquhart, J. and Heilmann, K. (1984). *Risk Watch. The Odds of Life*. Facts on File. New York
2. Inman, W. H. W. (1985). Risks in Medical Intervention. In Cooper, M. G. (ed.) *Risk: Man-made Hazards to Man*. pp. 35–53 (Oxford: Oxford University Press)
3. Inman, W. H. W. and Mushin, W. W. (1978). Jaundice after repeated exposure to halothane. *Br. Med. J.*, **2**, 1455–6

# 15
# Prescription – Event Monitoring

W. H. W. INMAN, N. S. B. RAWSON and L. V. WILTON

## INTRODUCTION

About 10 years after the thalidomide disaster many hundreds of patients treated with practolol suffered severe complications associated with the oculomucocutaneous syndrome. A small number of deaths were attributed to sclerosing peritonitis, and several patients were blinded after developing corneal ulceration. Many more suffered less severe ocular, auditory or skin reactions. Probably because the early manifestations of the syndrome took the form of skin lesions resembling psoriasis or conjunctivitis and 'dry eye', conditions which are commonly encountered in general practice, the majority of doctors failed to appreciate their significance and there was no Yellow Card 'signal'. By the time the problem was recognized about 100 000 patients had been treated with practolol, some of them for as long as 2 years, and it emerged, retrospectively, that many hundreds had been affected.

The practolol incident led to the recognition of the severe limitations of voluntary reporting as the sole method for detecting adverse drug reactions (ADRs), and to several proposals for schemes based on the identification of patients by means of prescriptions. These were intended to provide populations of known size, in which the incidence of ADRs could be measured. The first proposal for a scheme, known as 'Recorded Release', was presented at a conference in Honolulu in January 1976.[1] Special personalized prescription pads would be issued for individual patients treated with new drugs, which would be known as 'Recorded Drugs'. The pads would incorporate three-part (no carbon) stationery to produce two copies of the prescription. The patient would take his prescription to the chemist in the usual way. Simultaneously, the first copy would be posted to the monitoring agency so that the patient would be 'recorded'. The second copy would be part of a larger document incorporating a questionnaire, retained in the patient's notes for a pre-arranged period and then sent to the monitoring agency together with a record of any events that had occurred since treatment was commenced. The prescription pad would also include 'repeat' prescriptions, and each item would be marked with a unique identification number. Once a patient had been recorded, the monitoring centre could circulate reminders to doctors at the appropriate time requesting that the second copy should be returned. Doctors would be discouraged from prescribing the drug if they were not prepared to collaborate.

A number of minor variations on the Recorded Release theme, such as 'Registered Release',[2] were subsequently proposed, but none was adopted by the Department of Health and Social Security. In 1979, another prescription-based scheme known as 'Retrospective Assessment of Drug Safety' was proposed by the Committee on Safety of Medicines (CSM), but was also turned down. Since it was clear that any further attempt to set up a research scheme of this kind within a government department was unrealistic, the former Medical Assessor of Adverse Reactions to the CSM established an independent Drug Surveillance Research Unit (DSRU) at the University of Southampton. From this base, a scheme known as Prescription-Event Monitoring (PEM) has been developed. This has proved to be highly successful, attracting the active participation of perhaps as many as 75% of general practitioners in England.[3,4]

The DSRU is supported by unconditional ('no strings') grants from about 30 manufacturers in addition to the Department of Health and Social Security. At the present time, the Unit does not enter into contractual relationships with individual companies. The choice of drugs for inclusion in PEM is made by the Director on the basis of scientific interest and clinical importance and not in response to pressure from sponsors. In practice, nearly half the drugs that have been studied are manufactured by non-sponsoring companies. Funds have been raised by the Director on the basis of an enlightened attitude on the part of an industry which generally recognizes the significance of post-marketing surveillance by a non-industrial, non-regulatory and non-contracting institution. The industry recognizes that, while most drugs will turn out to be safe, (a result which will encourage their successful promotion), there will be rare occasions when harm to patients will be minimized by early detection of a serious hazard. Either way, the manufacturer, the medical profession and above all the patient, stand to benefit from support given to the Unit.

## EPIDEMIOLOGICAL BACKGROUND

In an affluent society, almost all patients with any significant disease or symptom receive some form of treatment. It is almost impossible to establish baselines for the incidence of the events occurring in untreated 'control' populations because there are no controls. Even if patients with untreated disease could be found, they would be atypical for several reasons. For example, they would be likely to have less severe disease. Almost all decisions, therefore, have to be based on comparisons of the *relative* incidence of events in groups of patients who receive different medicines for the same disease.

Before attempting to design any scheme for post-marketing surveillance, it is important to understand what can and cannot be done with study groups of various sizes. The greater the true incidence of an event, the smaller is the number of patients required to measure it. The acceptable level of toxicity of a drug is related to the severity of the disease being treated, and the amount of risk a patient is prepared to take. If the disease is very serious, it may be reasonable to use a drug which produces a relatively high incidence of serious or even fatal reactions. If, on the other hand, the drug is used to treat symptoms of non-lethal illness, the acceptable level of risk is much smaller. Large risks in the order of 1% may be identified in a few hundred patients, while a very small risk in the order of 0.001% might require a study involving a million patients.

Since the cost of a survey is related to the number of patients involved, it is unlikely that any scheme will ever enable very low levels of risk to be measured. There is no way, at a price any nation could afford, that all the minor remedies on the market could be successfully tested by any known method of post-marketing surveillance.

The main objective of PEM is to detect and quantify comparatively large risks which are, nevertheless, too small to be detected in clinical trials. Initially, it was decided that the minimum cohort of patients should be 10 000. If only one-third of doctors responded to requests for information, this would allow events with a true frequency of one in 1000 to be identified with a high degree of certainty. PEM would improve the chance that accidents such as the practolol incident would be minimized. It was not intended to replace the CSM's Yellow Card system which is capable of identifying very rare events even though it cannot measure their incidence.

## THE ROLE OF THE PRESCRIPTION PRICING AUTHORITY

PEM depends on the identification of patients and their doctors as the prescriptions pass through the Prescription Pricing Authority (PPA). This is a special health authority set up by the Secretary of State (but independent from the Department of Health) to provide him and local Family Practitioner Committees (FPCs) with information about the quantity and cost of drugs provided through the health service, and for the purposes of remunerating pharmacists for the medicines they dispense. The PPA currently consists of 16 members, comprising the Chairman, four pharmacists, three doctors, four representatives of FPCs, three members representing the officers employed by the Authority, the Community Health Councils, and the Department of Health and Social Security, respectively, and one academician familiar with the work of the Authority who is currently a Professor of General Practice (and author of Chapter 42 of this book).

There are 90 FPC areas in England, and the prescriptions are processed by the 11 processing divisions of the PPA. Between April 1st 1983 and March 31st 1984, a total of 341 million prescriptions were processed. The input from individual FPCs ranged from less than one million to more than 11 million. The total number of chemist's accounts was 9322. On average, each doctor issues about 15 000 prescriptions per year or about 60 in each working day. The total cost of the drugs dispensed in England each year is approximately two billion pounds.

The fact that the PPA is divided into 11 divisions and the country into 90 FPC areas allows the DSRU to collect prescriptions for different drugs in different areas. At present, the limit to the number of drugs that can be studied by any division of the PPA at any one time is four, the largest number that can be readily memorized by the pricing clerks who have to pick out individual prescriptions as they work at high speed to price each item. According to skill and experience, each pricing clerk processes up to 7000 prescriptions per day. In 1982/83, the authority supplied the DSRU with photocopies of 362 000 prescriptions, roughly one in every thousand prescriptions written in England as a whole during that year.

The DSRU conducts PEM in England only. It was anticipated that there would be enormous problems with the identification of patients in Scotland, Wales and Northern Ireland because of the high frequency of patients sharing the same surname. A doctor in Cardiff, for example, could easily have several patients named 'Jones' receiving prescriptions for the same drug at more or less the same time.

The prescriptions are usually priced between six and eight weeks after being written by the general practitioner. In order to collect prescriptions for the whole country it is necessary to brief up to 2000 staff at the processing divisions. As each prescription required for PEM is encountered, it is photocopied and then returned to the pricing stream. Monthly batches of photocopies are sent to the DSRU where they are sorted and processed on an ICL System 25 mini-computer using Apex 25 software provided by Maclaren Computer Systems Ltd. Because more than one doctor in a practice may have prescribed for the same patient, or may have used his partner's prescription pad, the process of sorting can be difficult. The legibility of patients' names or addresses is often poor and details such as the initials or title of a patient (e.g. Mr or Mrs) may be incomplete. The proportion of prescriptions which can be deciphered is usually about 70%, but experienced clerks can often improve on this considerably. Before a questionnaire is printed, the doctor's address on the prescription is checked against the DSRU's dictionary of doctors' addresses, and the computer also checks the entry against a 'list' of addresses of a small number of doctors who have indicated they would prefer not to be involved in PEM. After 3 years, the total number of names on this list is currently less than 100. A machine check also limits the number of questionnaires, usually to a maximum of four per doctor, in order to avoid overloading.

## COLLECTION OF EVENT-DATA

The design of the questionnaire, which is usually referred to as the 'green form', has been kept simple in order to encourage compliance. Each questionnaire includes the following explanatory note and simple example of an event:

> *Definition of an EVENT*
> An EVENT is any new diagnosis, any reason for referral to a consultant or admission to hospital (e.g. operation, accident or pregnancy), any unexpected deterioration (or improvement) in a concurrent illness, any suspected drug reaction, or any other complaint which was considered of sufficient importance to enter in the patient's notes.
>
> *Example*
> A broken leg is an EVENT. If more fractures were associated with this drug they could have been due to hypotension, CNS effects or metabolic bone changes.

The patient's name and address, the name of the drug, the date of the prescription and the doctor's name and address are printed on the green form by the computer. The doctor is asked to supply the date of birth or age and details of events that have occurred during treatment and after stopping treatment where appropriate. It also requests the indication for treatment, whether or not the treatment had been effective and whether or not it was being continued at the time the green form was completed by the doctor.

In most of the studies, the bulk of the response occurred during the first 6 weeks after posting the green forms. A residue of perhaps 10–20% may take several months to reach the DSRU, and occasionally, forms have been returned as long as 3 years after a survey had commenced. The response by doctors has ranged from about 55% to 75% and this is considered to be remarkably satisfactory.

## DATA PROCESSING

The procedure for processing and assessing the data is still being developed, but is essentially simple. Wherever possible, the words used by a doctor to describe an event are matched with an entry in the 'event dictionary', which is divided into 'event groups', such as skin, gastrointestinal, renal, etc. Within each group, the individual terms are arranged alphabetically using a system of high level terms such as 'rash' and low level terms such as 'erythematous' to define diagnostic sub-divisions of the higher level terms. The same dictionary is used for the indication for treatment. It should be remembered that many events entered after treatment has been started actually relate to the reason for the treatment and not to its possible effects. At present it is not possible to code all the information about drugs administered concurrently or subsequently. About 60% of prescriptions for non-steroidal anti-inflammatory agents (NSAIDs), for example, included other drugs. In other studies, such as those of antibiotics, this proportion is lower. Information about concurrent drugs can be retrieved because prescriptions and green forms are permanently stored on microfilm.

## GENERATING AND TESTING HYPOTHESES

PEM can be used both to generate and test hypotheses. We will illustrate both these functions by describing in some detail our study of five NSAIDs, which shows how similar drugs may be compared. We will also describe a large uncontrolled study of ranitidine which illustrates how PEM can be rapidly mobilized to provide a safety profile for a drug. We also investigated the possibility that erythromycin estolate might be a more frequent cause of jaundice than other formulations and that emepronium bromide might be associated with an unacceptable risk of oesophageal ulceration.

### Non-steroidal anti-inflammatory drugs (NSAIDs)

Few drug groups have been associated with as much controversy and concern as the NSAIDs. Benoxaprofen was withdrawn from the market in August 1982 because of reports of jaundice in elderly people. Zomepirac was withdrawn in March 1983 after reports of fatal anaphylactic shock in the United States. We decided to attempt to assess this hazard by identifying patients whose prescriptions were still in the PPA's 'pipeline' immediately after the drug was withdrawn. In September of the same year, a new and sophisticated indomethacin preparation known as 'Osmosin' was withdrawn after reports of small bowel perforation and, once again, we tapped the PPA's pipeline in order to determine if this risk was unacceptable.

Many patients using NSAIDs are elderly and the mortality from degenerative diseases and senility is very high. During the few weeks or months prior to their death, many are admitted to geriatric wards or to old people's homes. In 1984, we commenced a routine enquiry into the cause of all deaths. The main sources of information were copies of the death certificates, supplied by the Office of Population Censuses and Surveys, and the patients' notes loaned by the FPCs with the permission of the patients' general practitioners. In many cases, even after making these enquiries it was not possible to establish whether or not a patient was taking the drug at the time of death or in the period immediately preceding it.

Approximately 104 000 green forms relating to patients who had been prescribed NSAIDs were posted to general practitioners and 60% were returned. Many forms provided no useful information. Some doctors had moved, retired or died during the interval between writing the prescription and receiving the green forms. Many patients changed practices and others could not be traced. In some cases the doctor had no record that the drug was ever prescribed, although we know, of course, that a prescription had been issued.

Zomepirac had been promoted as a general purpose analgesic as well as an NSAID and doctors recorded 110 different indications, including terminal cancer in which the drug had been exceptionally useful for treating the pain of bone metastases. The four other drugs were used mainly for musculoskeletal disease of which osteoarthritis accounted for about half. Rheumatoid arthritis accounted for about 20% of the indications for benoxaprofen and about 10% of those for fenbufen, piroxicam and indomethacin.

If drugs produce no side-effects, we would expect the pattern of events to be independent of whichever drug is employed. If treatment was generally beneficial, we would expect indication-related events such as joint pain to be less frequent while a patient was receiving treatment. ADRs, on the other hand, would show up as a *relative excess* of events during treatment in comparison with the post-treatment period, while unexpected benefits should show as a *relative deficit*. Because patients attend the surgery less frequently after treatment has been stopped, the overall rate of recording of events tends to be lower than during the treatment period. Some patients, however, change to another NSAID after a period of treatment with the drug under surveillance and this may affect the subsequent pattern of events.

Even a summary of the data on the five NSAIDs in the form of a simple listing of events is a formidable 100-page computer print-out. Many different presentations and analyses have been considered, but the two methods that seem most appropriate are, first of all, to express the events occurring during treatment as the *rate per 1000 patient-years of exposure*, thus allowing various drugs to be compared and, secondly, to prepare profiles of events occurring during and after stopping treatment, expressing the events as the *number per 1000 events* or as a percentage. This form of profile analysis closely resembles the 'adverse reactions profile' described in Chapter 1. It allows comparisons to be made between the profile or pattern of events associated with the various drugs, and between the treatment and post-treatment period with individual drugs. A relative excess or deficit of events during treatment may reflect a risk or benefit of treatment.

In practice, even though the five NSAIDs were studied at different

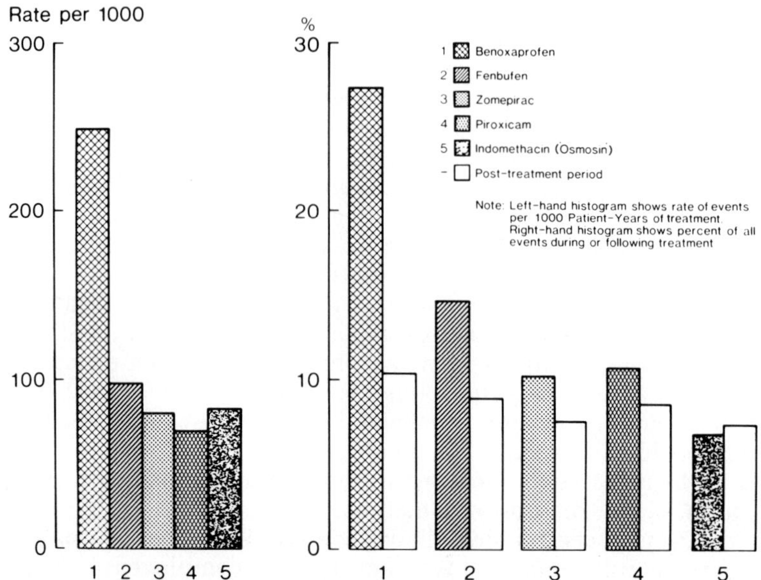


**Figure 1** Skin Events

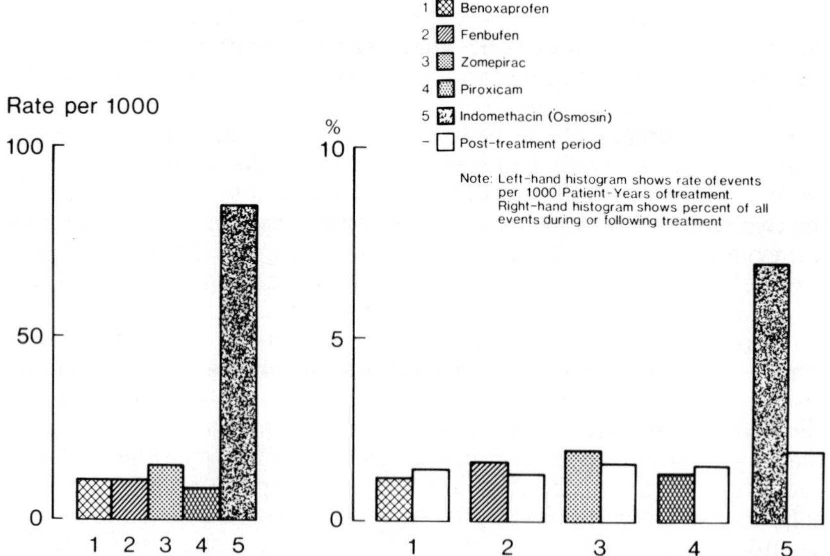


**Figure 2** Headache

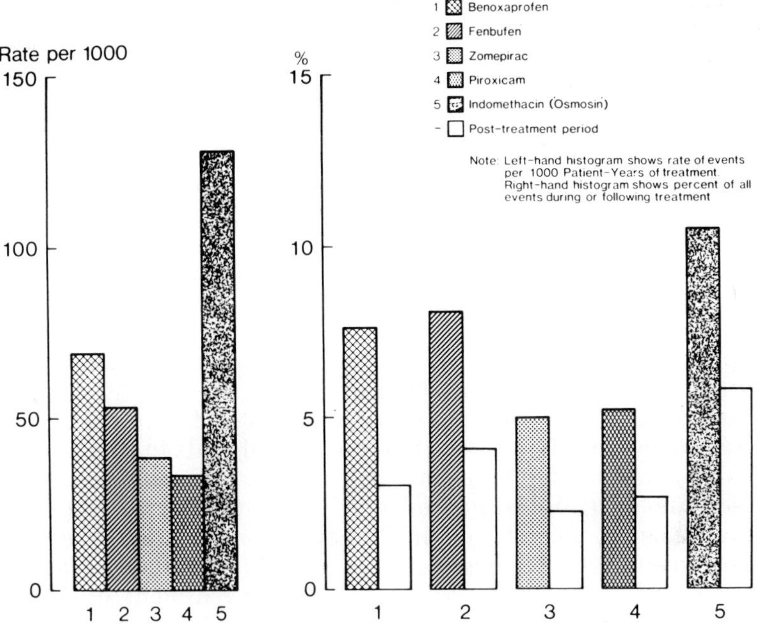


**Figure 3** Gastrointestinal events

times for different periods of observation and against a background of increasingly adverse publicity, the data have been remarkably consistent. Previously recognized ADRs have shown up clearly as an excess of events during treatment and, as we shall see, one potentially important benefit has been strongly signalled.

For purposes of illustration, selected data are presented here in a series of figures. Each is composed of two sets of histograms. On the left of each figure, the absolute rates occurring during treatment are shown for the five drugs, and on the right, five pairs of bars show the relative percentage of each event during and after stopping the drug or changing to another NSAID. The data obtained after stopping each drug are shown as the unshaded bar on the right of each pair.

The pattern of skin events is shown in Figure 1. It can be seen that the rate of skin events with benoxaprofen was two to three times greater than with the other drugs, and that they accounted for more than a quarter of all events recorded during treatment. This was because of the very high incidence of photosensitivity and onycholysis which were the principal ADRs to this drug.

In Figure 2, headache associated with indomethacin was reported about eight times more frequently than with the other four drugs. This is probably a genuine side-effect of indomethacin. In Figure 3, cases of dyspepsia and gastritis appear at first sight to be more common with indomethacin in the form of 'Osmosin', a drug that was specifically promoted because the active ingredient was released slowly as the capsule passed down the alimentary canal thus, it was hoped, causing less irritation. It can be seen that dyspepsia and gastritis still account for a greater proportion of events after 'Osmosin' had been removed than during the corresponding post-treatment period with the other four drugs. The reason for this is quite simply that 'Osmosin' was deliberately selected for use in patients who were particularly prone to gastrointestinal disturbances. This illustrates a very important general principle. Whenever a new drug is promoted as a product which causes few side-effects, it is likely to be used in patients in whom such effects are more common. This may well be an important source of bias in reports to spontaneous ADR monitoring systems of the kind described in Section 1 of this book.

Figure 4 illustrates perhaps the most important finding in our study of NSAIDs. It should be noted that the vertical scale in this figure has had to be increased ten times in order to show the comparatively rare but serious gastrointestinal effects, including haematemesis and perforated peptic ulcer. No significant or important differences can be seen between these five drugs, nor is any difference apparent in the proportion of these events reported during treatment or after the patients have stopped or switched NSAIDs. These serious events occurred about once in every 200 patient-years of observation.

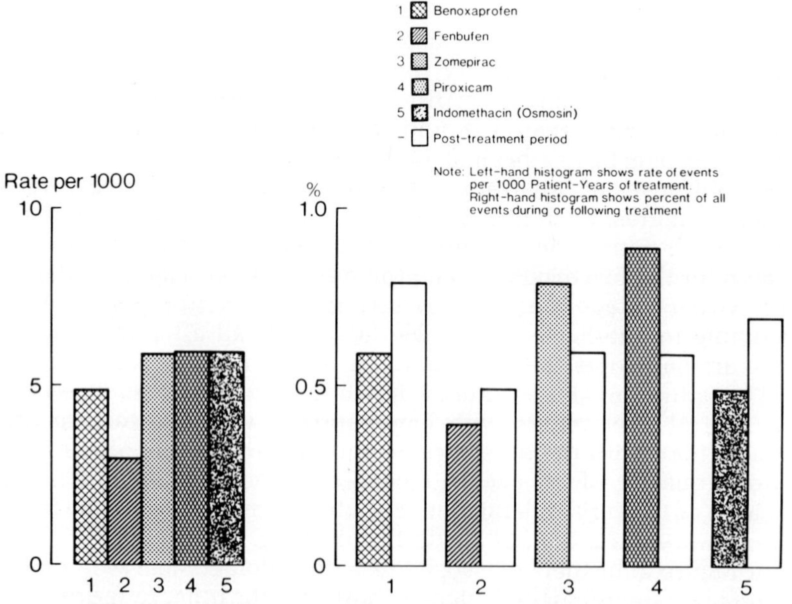


**Figure 4** Upper gastrointestinal haemorrhage and perforated peptic ulcer. (vertical scale × 10 compared with Figures 1–3.)

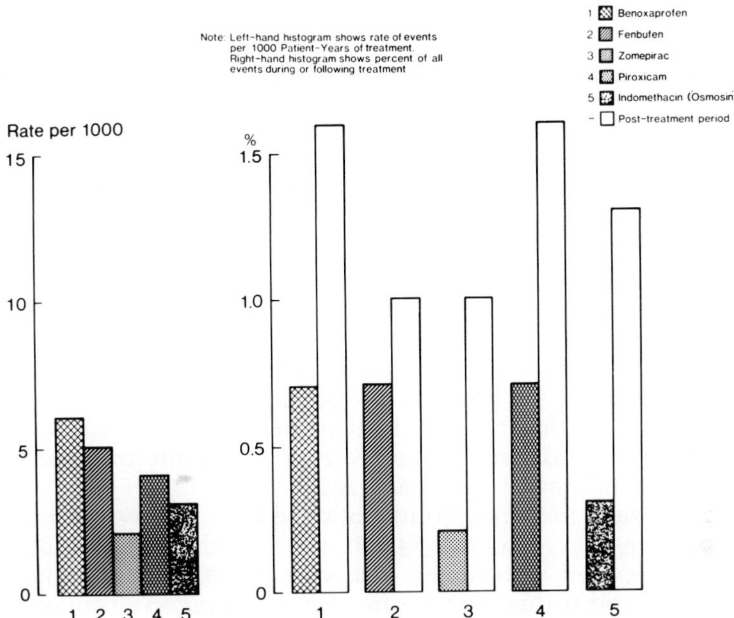


**Figure 5** Myocardial infarction. (vertical scale × 10 compared with Figures 1–3.)

Figure 5 shows a most interesting example of how PEM may uncover potentially beneficial events. This was first noticed when analysing the data for zomepirac. It seemed that there were remarkably few cases of myocardial infarction while patients were using the drug in relation to the number recorded after the drug had been withdrawn from the market. Subsequently, inspection of the data obtained for the other drugs showed a similar marked deficit with 'Osmosin', a less marked one with piroxicam and benoxaprofen but virtually no effect for fenbufen. A number of factors have been identified which could have accounted in part for the deficit of deaths during treatment, but the trend was apparent for non-fatal cases. Moreover, a similar trend was suggested in the data for thrombotic stroke and pulmonary embolism even though the number of cases was very small. It is not possible to say with anything approaching certainty whether or not these results prove a cardioprotective effect of NSAIDs. Nevertheless, it is quite likely in view of the effects of this group of drugs on the prostaglandin system. It is to be hoped that this hypothesis will be tested in other studies.

Three of the five NSAIDs were withdrawn from the market after reports of serious adverse reactions, all of which were encountered as very rare events in our studies.

*Jaundice and benoxaprofen*

Our study of benoxaprofen commenced before attention had been drawn to the problem of hepatorenal damage and was unfairly criticized for not, apparently, identifying this problem. As can be seen in Table 1, a number of cases of jaundice and renal failure were recorded and efforts were made over a period of many months to obtain more information about them. Not unexpectedly, most of the cases were found to be due to cancer, gallstones, cirrhosis, or pre-existing renal damage. There remained one probable case and 11 possible cases, six of which had been placed in this category by default because no further details were obtained. Some of these cases were identified during the course of a subsidiary study in which, in addition to sending green forms requesting a detailed account of events, doctors were sent lists of other patients in their practices for whom benoxaprofen had been prescribed and were asked simply to record any serious ADRs that might have occurred.

The total size of the study group obtained both by green forms and by the supplementary lists was 24 000, and even this large population of patients exposed to benoxaprofen was insufficient to allow any estimate of mortality due to benoxaprofen poisoning to be obtained. It seems likely that the incidence of deaths from this cause is in the region of one in 25 000, a figure which would not be incompatible with the reports of the CSM derived from the whole population of more than half a million patients who were using the drug.[5] It is important to realize from these results that, while all adverse reactions are events, by no means all events are adverse reactions which is why it is so important to follow up individual reports of suspected adverse reactions in order to exclude alternative explanations for the events that are reported.

Practitioners have been most helpful, supplying additional information and putting us in touch with hospitals in which patients with

**Table 1** Follow-up of cases of hepatic or renal failure occurring during or after treatment with Benoxaprofen

| *Relationship of jaundice and/or renal failure* | *Cases identified in approximately 24 000 patients treated with Benoxaprofen (deaths in parentheses)* | |
|---|---|---|
| Probably related to benoxaprofen | 1 | |
| Possibly related to benoxaprofen | 11* | (5) |
| Association unlikely | 15 | (6) |
| Unrelated | 27 | (11) |
| Total | 54 | (22) |

*Includes 6 cases rated 'possible' by default, where no detailed information has been obtained

serious events were admitted. The greatest difficulty we have encountered is in determining whether or not patients were continuing to take the NSAID at the time of hospital admission or death.

Because of the publicity associated with the benoxaprofen affair and the removal of zomepirac and 'Osmosin', we believe it is unlikely that many cases of jaundice or renal failure, anaphylactic shock or intestinal perforation with the three drugs respectively will have been missed, although we cannot be completely certain about events which might have occurred after patients had left the care of the general practitioner who prescribed a drug for them, e.g. possibly developing a serious side-effect or dying.

*Anaphylaxis with zomepirac*

There were 94 records of acute skin reactions and 26 of asthma in patients who took 'Zomax'. Of four reports of anaphylaxis, none of which was fatal, two were regarded as probably related to zomepirac, one possibly related and one unrelated (see Table 2). No patient went into shock. In one case the patient had had one or more previous courses of zomepirac and developed itching, headache and rigors lasting for several hours after taking a single tablet. A second patient had used the drug for 5 months and had developed angioedema half an hour after taking a tablet. The third patient developed headaches, diarrhoea and vomiting after the first tablet, whether this was an anaphylactic reaction is doubtful. The fourth patient had a past history of angioedema and developed a recurrence 2 months after stopping zomepirac.

Seventeen acute skin reactions were considered to be probably related to zomepirac and 22, including six cases of urticaria, were thought to be possibly related to it. The remaining 46 acute reactions were either unlikely to be related to the drug or occurred after treatment had been stopped. Seven cases were attributed to other NSAIDs, two to penicillin and two to the use of a beta-blocking agent.

Three asthmatics seem to have been worse while taking the drug, but there was no relationship with treatment in 23 other asthmatic patients. One asthmatic died in his sleep but was not taking zomepirac.

There were thus no deaths and no cases of anaphylactic shock

**Table 2** Possible allergic reactions to zomepirac

| | *Relation to zomepirac* | | | | |
|---|---|---|---|---|---|
| | *Probable* | *Possible* | *Unlikely* | *Unrelated* | *Total* |
| Anaphylaxis | 2 | 1 | — | 1 | 4 |
| Urticaria | — | 6 | 2 | 8 | 16 |
| Other rashes | 17 | 16 | 16 | 25 | 74 |
| Asthma | — | 3 | 6 | 17 | 26 |
| Total | 19 | 26 | 24 | 51 | 120 |

which was the original reason why the drug had been withdrawn in the United States. The incidence of skin reactions was about one in 500 and of non-fatal anaphylaxis, about one in 5000. The world reported incidence of fatal anaphylaxis due to zomepirac is thought to be in the order of one in two million.

*Intestinal perforation with 'Osmosin' (indomethacin)*

'Osmosin' had been removed from the market because of reports of intestinal perforation. In our series of nearly 13 000 patients, there was one report of a patient who died from perforation of the small bowel which occurred 1 month after he had been taken off the drug and put on the standard preparation of indomethacin known as 'Indocid'. We regard this case as a 'possible' because he might have kept some 'Osmosin' tablets and taken one or more of them several weeks after being advised to stop.

We have also included a study of 'Indocid', the original intention being to explore the possibility that 'Osmosin' and 'Indocid' might show different rates of gastrointestinal disorder. The results of this experiment were very instructive from the methodological point of view. Many patients in the 'Indocid' group had been using the drug for very long periods, sometimes as long as 20 years. The number of events recorded was much lower than with the other five preparations and the data are considered not to be comparable. Many doctors complained that it took too much of their time to record events in patients who had used 'Indocid' often for many years and asked us not to embark on other studies of well-established drugs.

*Co-prescribed drugs*

We have studied samples of some 500 prescriptions issued to patients treated with benoxaprofen, piroxicam and 'Osmosin' and have established the pattern of drugs prescribed at the same time as the NSAID which was similar for all three drugs. It is, of course, possible that other drugs are prescribed on different prescriptions during other visits to the surgery, and it is certain that some patients will purchase drugs over the counter without a prescription.

In Table 3 it can be seen that about 40% of NSAID prescriptions do not include an additional item, about 30% include an additional item and a further 30% include between two and eight items.

Table 4 shows that patients using an anti-inflammatory drug frequently require additional analgesics to carry them through periods when the pain is worse than usual. Very often these are the so-called compound analgesics of which the combination of dextropropoxyphene and paracetomol ('Distalgesic') was the most frequent. It was noteworthy that 2–3% of patients also received a second NSAID on the same prescription, but less than 1% received one of the 'disease-modifying' drugs, gold or penicillamine.

About 90% of the 'sedatives' were benzodiazepines used as minor

**Table 3** Percentage of prescription forms including additional treatment

| *Number of additional items* | *Benoxaprofen (*n = 597)* | *Piroxicam (n = 696)* | *'Osmosin' (n = 651)* |
|---|---|---|---|
| None | 42 | 40 | 43 |
| 1 | 32 | 30 | 33 |
| 2 | 17 | 19 | 16 |
| 3 | 5 | 7 | 5 |
| 4 | 3 | 3 | 2 |
| 5–8 | 1 | 1 | 1 |

*n = Number of Prescription Forms

tranquillizers or sleeping tablets. Between a quarter and one third of the co-prescribed drug were those used to treat hypertension or heart failure, and about half of these were diuretics, an important consideration in the light of the fairly slow metabolism and excretion of drugs such as benoxaprofen.

**Table 4** Percentage distribution of co-prescribed drugs

| *Co-prescribed drug* | *Benoxaprofen (*n = 575)* | *Piroxicam (n = 748)* | *'Osmosin' (n = 604)* |
|---|---|---|---|
| Compound analgesic | 12 | 11 | 11 |
| NSAID | 3 | 2 | 3 |
| Other analgesic | 7 | 6 | 9 |
| Sedative, Hypnotic | 16 | 14 | 14 |
| Antidepressant | 3 | 4 | 4 |
| Diuretic (+/− potassium supplement) | 13 | 17 | 11 |
| Hypotensives and β-blocker | 7 | 8 | 9 |
| Gastrointestinal | 9 | 7 | 8 |
| Iron and vitamins | 3 | 4 | 3 |
| Systemic corticosteroid | 2 | 3 | 2 |
| Topical corticosteroid | 3 | 2 | 2 |
| Other drugs | 22 | 22 | 24 |

*n = Number of co-prescribed drugs

## Ranitidine

For our second example of the use of PEM as a method for raising hypotheses we have chosen ranitidine.

The $H_2$-receptor antagonists are probably one of the most significant advances in therapeutics in recent years. There was a long interval between the introduction of cimetidine, the first in the series, and the second, ranitidine. Originally we planned to study both drugs and we collected prescriptions for ranitidine from the moment it was first marketed together with a large sample of prescriptions for cimetidine.

In February 1983, we decided to conduct a pilot experiment in order to learn more about the population of patients receiving ranitidine so that we could plan a larger study of both drugs. The pilot study was based on patients who had commenced treatment during the period October 1981–June 1982. Approximately 18 000 green forms were dispatched to doctors and more than 10 500 (58%) were returned. In 9% of the cases, the forms could not be completed, most frequently because the patient had moved, and this left a total of approximately 9600 forms for assessment. It was in fact possible to complete a preliminary analysis of these forms only 11 weeks after the decision to initiate the study. These 11 weeks included the time required to print the green forms, to transfer the patients' and doctors' details to them, to post them and to analyse those forms that were returned.

The average period of observation, during or after stopping the drug was 12.5 months. Thirty per cent were still receiving ranitidine when the period of observation was terminated, and 70% had discontinued treatment after an average of only 3.5 months. In the latter, it was therefore possible to study the pattern of events which occur 'off treatment'. Obviously, the patients who discontinued treatment after a short period are not strictly comparable to those who continued with treatment, at least with regard to the pattern of gastrointestinal symptoms. Nevertheless, some general impressions about the events that occur in patients treated with the drug can be obtained by comparing the event pattern recorded during approximately 50 000 patient-months of treatment with another similar period in the group of patients who had stopped treatment.

Ranitidine had been prescribed for peptic ulceration or haemorrhage in 52% of the patients, for hiatus hernia, oesophagitis, reflux or stricture of the oesophagus in 22%, for dyspepsia, gastritis or duodenitis in 21% and for gastric cancer in 0.5%. In a further 2% of the patients, ranitidine had been prescribed to treat disorders caused by steroids or NSAIDs, and a wide variety of conditions were listed as indications in the remaining 2.5%.

Where it had been possible to assess efficacy, 83% of doctors reported that ranitidine had been effective. In these patients, 66% had stopped treatment, whilst in those in whom it had not been effective, 94% had stopped treatment.

Three hundred and eighty-eight patients (4.0%) had died. In 101 cases, the doctors were not able to report the cause of death because the patient's notes had been returned to the FPCs. Ninety-four patients died from cardiovascular disease and 137 patients died from cancer, including 66 who had cancer of the oesophagus, stomach or duodenum. Remarkably, in view of the fact that more than 5000 patients had a history of peptic ulcer, only three deaths were attributed to gastrointestinal haemorrhage during treatment and two more in patients who had ceased treatment. These results are remarkably similar to those which have recently been reported by Colin-Jones *et al.* in a prospective study of cimetidine.[6]

Skin events were reported in 274 patients while taking ranitidine and in 218 after treatment had been stopped. Rashes were attributed to other drugs in seven and nine patients, respectively. Herpes was reported in 28 patients on treatment compared with only 13 off treatment. The manufacturers very kindly re-examined their clinical trial results in the light of this observation and found that there had been five reports of herpes in 1108 patients treated with ranitidine, and no cases in 1094 patients treated with placebo. Although the meaning of this 'signal' is not yet clear, it is an excellent example of the power of PEM to raise hypotheses and also of the value of close collaboration with the manufacturers.

A difference which at first sight seemed odd was the 25 patients who underwent orthopaedic surgery whilst on treatment compared with only eight who had stopped treatment. These events are linked with the use of ranitidine to control the complications of NSAIDs.

No cases of liver disorder were attributed to ranitidine, but it was interesting to note that 26 cases of gallbladder disease were diagnosed during the treatment period compared with only 11 after treatment. In contrast, cholecystectomy was performed in 53 patients who had stopped treatment compared with only 10 who had taken it up to the time of operation. It seems likely that the underlying cause of the symptoms for which ranitidine had been prescribed (gallstones) was only revealed for the first time after the drug had been started.

For a number of reasons, we did not initiate a green form exercise for cimetidine. The drug had been marketed several years earlier, and although many ranitidine-treated patients had been using cimetidine (some were cimetidine failures), the reverse could not be true. It was clear that the two groups would not be comparable in other respects. Our subsequent experience with 'Indocid', already referred to, suggests that our decision not to attempt a study of cimetidine was probably correct. The main value of the ranitidine data will be for comparison with any new $H_2$-receptor antagonist which may be marketed in the future.

## USE OF PEM TO TEST HYPOTHESES

Although, as we discovered in our study of 'Indocid', PEM is probably not an appropriate method for generating hypotheses for older established products, it has been used to test specific hypotheses in these products. General practitioners are not prepared to copy out all the events that may have been recorded in the patient's notes over many years, but they are prepared to answer specific questions such as 'did the patient develop jaundice?' This is illustrated here with our studies of erythromycin and of emepronium bromide.

### Jaundice and erythromycin

In 1982, some 5300 general practitioners were invited to participate in a study designed to test the hypothesis that erythromycin estolate might be more commonly associated with jaundice than other preparations of this antibiotic. Reports to the CSM suggested that the relative risk might be as much as 20 times greater with the estolate. However, the hypothesis had never been tested and the true incidence of jaundice caused by the drug is unknown. In 1973, when the CSM first became concerned, erythromycin estolate accounted for only half the market for all forms of erythromycin but for 95% of all reports of jaundice.

We collected prescriptions for 'Ilosone' (erythromycin estolate) during January and February 1982, together with a one month sample of prescriptions for 'Erythrocin' (erythromycin stearate) collected in February, from 19 of the 90 FPC areas in England. Forms relating to 12 000 patients were dispatched and 76% were returned. Sixteen green forms recorded jaundice as an 'event'. All 16 patients with jaundice were followed up and in every case the doctor was able to provide additional information regarding its probable cause. Four of the cases were attributable to gallstones, three to cancer, six to infective hepatitis (hepatitis A virus was identified in three), and there were three cases in which the antibiotic could be considered to have been a possible cause of jaundice.

Jaundice attributable to erythromycin characteristically occurs within 2 weeks of commencing treatment, or sometimes earlier, if a patient has previously been exposed to the drug. It is invariably transient, and to our knowledge, no patient has ever died. It is of great interest that the only three cases which would fit this pattern occurred with erythromycin stearate, rather than the estolate. Although these results do not rule out the estolate as a cause of jaundice, and we did not prove that it is a less common cause than the stearate, we can be reasonably confident that the incidence with the estolate is less than one in 1000 and probably considerably less.[7]

The manufacturers of 'Ilosone' have always included warnings about jaundice in their sales literature, and it is probable that the relatively large numbers of cases of suspected estolate jaundice referred to the CSM have been reported selectively. These results emphasize the need for caution in assessing the results of voluntary reporting. The Yellow Card system certainly suggested the relatively large excess of reports linking the estolate with jaundice was probably evidence of a greater risk.

## 'Cetiprin' (empronium bromide) and oesophageal symptoms

In April 1983, we asked doctors to complete modified green forms which had been designed to record oesophageal symptoms in patients using 'Cetiprin' for enuresis. 7150 doctors returned forms relating to 15 920 patients. Rather surprisingly, a total of 447 of these patients (2.8%) were reported to have had swallowing difficulty or upper gastrointestinal symptoms of varying severity. We, therefore, designed a second questionnaire and distributed this in July 1983. Unfortunately, 169 of the cases could not be traced because the photocopies of the prescriptions which were the only means of identifying them, and which had been sent to the general practitioner with the green forms, had not been retained. It is believed that any serious cases of oesophageal damage which might have been included in this group of 169 would have been remembered if their symptoms were sufficiently severe, for example, to require admission to hospital. Seventy-eight per cent of the patients were female and 59% were aged over 70 years. About 12% had neurological disease, such as multiple sclerosis, which might interfere with swallowing, and the majority of patients were taking other drugs which are frequently associated with upper gastrointestinal symptoms. Eleven per cent, for example, had received potassium supplements and 37% were taking NSAIDs. The drug was reported to have been effective in 80% of patients. Fourteen per cent of patients had a past history of hiatus hernia, 7% a past history of oesophagitis, 2.5% had a previous oesophageal stricture and 31% had a history of dysphagia or dyspepsia. In only six cases was dysphagia noted immediately after an attempt was made to start treatment.

The results of the assessments are shown in Table 5. In 19 cases (7%), the symptoms were considered to be serious and 170 (61%) were rated mild to moderate in severity. In 23 cases (8%), it was considered that the symptoms were probably due to 'Cetiprin', but in only one patient were they serious. This patient had severe oesophagitis which was attributed to 'Cetiprin' by her doctor, but he had reservations about the true cause because the patient was emotionally labile and frequently presented with similar symptoms after domestic upsets.

No patient in the series died as a result of taking 'Cetiprin' and there were no cases of oesophageal perforation. We could find no relationship between oesophageal symptoms and the number of tablets taken.

One reason for studying 'Cetiprin' was the knowledge that an improved formulation, 'Cetiprin Novum', had been developed which should overcome some of the oesophageal problems experienced with the existing formulation. Since the incidence of serious problems with the latter is so low, however, it is difficult to see how PEM could be used to demonstrate that the new tablets are superior in this respect.

**Table 5** Assessment of role of 'Cetiprin' (emepronium bromide) in oesophageal symptoms

| *Severity* | *Serious* | *Mild to moderate* | *Trivial* | *Total* |
|---|---|---|---|---|
| Relation to 'Cetiprin': | | | | |
| Probable | 1 | 14 | 8 | 23 |
| Possible | 6 | 91 | 41 | 138 |
| Unlikely | 2 | 35 | 31 | 68 |
| Unrelated | 10 | 30 | 9 | 49 |
| Total | 19 | 170 | 89 | 278 |

## ADVANTAGES AND LIMITATIONS OF PEM

Undoubtedly, the most encouraging feature of PEM is the high degree of compliance by doctors who have been requested to complete the green forms. The scheme has been running for 3 years without any noticeable fall-off in the response. Only a tiny minority of doctors have asked to be excluded from the scheme. Nevertheless, there must be a limit to the number of forms that 23 000 general practitioners are prepared to fill in each year, and we believe that a realistic target is 120 000 per year, or roughly one per doctor per 2 months on average. Such a throughput should be more than adequate to provide cohorts of around 10 000 or more patients who receive each new chemical substance as it is marketed.

The reasons for the excellent response by general practitioners are not hard to find. Of paramount importance is the independence of the DSRU from both government and industrial influences. Next is the feedback in the form of PEM NEWS. Although only three editions have been produced, practitioners have indicated their appreciation of the Unit's attempts to inform without overloading, and to remind them periodically that the results of their efforts to fill in green forms are worthwhile. It is clear that doctors appreciate the fact that each green form focuses their attention on one patient who has received one drug and that they are not required to decide whether or not events are drug related. They also seem to appreciate that PEM is capable of producing a more balanced appraisal of the risks and benefits of treatment than could ever be possible through any form of reporting scheme which does not measure numerators (events) and denominators (drug exposures). They see PEM as a system which should lead to more appropriate regulatory decisions, rather than the all-or-nothing drug withdrawals which have dominated the scene during the past 3 years. They are constantly reminded that PEM is not a substitute for the Yellow Card scheme.[8,9]

Table 6 lists ten strengths or weaknesses of the Yellow Card and Green Form systems. It can be seen that the two schemes differ in every respect, the strength of one being a weakness of the other, thus demonstrating how the two schemes complement each other. The Yellow Card scheme is limited to opinions that an event might be drug related. It is complied with by only a minority of doctors, and is only moderately effective in hypothesis generation because of the difficulty of distinguishing drug-related from spontaneous effects. It cannot measure incidence, allows only limited scope for hypothesis testing and does not provide information about events which occur when patients are not taking the drug (non-drug reactions).

On the other hand, its great strengths are that it can be applied to all drugs all the time and can function immediately a new drug is marketed provided doctors are on the alert. It can identify ADRs occurring at any level of frequency, including those which are extremely rare, and any doctor or dentist can participate. PEM, in

**Table 6** Some strengths and weaknesses of the CSM and DSRU systems

| *Strength or weakness* | *Yellow card (CSM)* | *Green form (DSRU)* |
|---|---|---|
| 1. Criteria for reporting | Only suspected ADRs | Any adverse events |
| 2. Availability | All drugs, all the time | Selected new drugs only |
| 3. Potential speed of problem detection | Fast if doctors on the alert | Minimum of 3–12 months delay |
| 4. Compliance by doctors | Poor | Excellent |
| 5. Hypothesis generation | Fair | Good |
| 6. Dectection of rare events (< 1 in 1000) | Good | Poor |
| 7. Measurement of incidence | None | Good |
| 8. Hypothesis testing | Poor | Good |
| 9. Control data | None | Some |
| 10. Participants | All doctors and dentists | General practitioners only |

complete contrast, can only be applied effectively to recently marketed drugs, and is subject to a minimum delay of 3 months from the time a prescription is written to the time of follow-up (and usually at least 12 months until sales are adequate to provide a worthwhile cohort). It cannot detect rare events and is available only to general practitioners. Its strengths are considerable. It will detect events which are in fact ADRs but which would not be reported to the CSM as such and it is very well supported by doctors. It is good at hypothesis generation and testing, can measure incidence and provides data on events which occur after treatment has been stopped for purposes of comparison.

Clearly, there are many other limitations to PEM. Compliance is not 100% and perhaps 10% of returned green forms are void because the patient has moved to another practice or is otherwise lost to the study. It is never completely certain if a patient is taking the drug at the time an event occurs. Many possibly important events are not reported to the doctor or recorded by him in the notes or not transferred to the green form. It may be difficult to distinguish disease-related from drug-related events. Comparable drug event-profiles may not be available. This will almost always be true when the first of a new series of 'breakthrough' drugs is marketed. Historically, there would have been no close comparison for propranolol or cimetidine, though it would of course have been possible to compare PEM data with other drugs used for the same indication.

## THE FUTURE

Looking to the future of PEM, assuming as is likely that the current 'recession' in drug innovation will last only a few years at worst, we intend to make use of our more sophisticated computer system to expand the number of analyses which can be performed routinely. We hope, for example, to be able to separate the event-profiles of patients with different diagnoses, for example rheumatoid and osteo-arthritis, and to be able to search for differences in the frequency of events in relation to the timing of treatment. It is important to identify events which may be concentrated during the early months of treatment which are more likely to be ADRs. We also plan to individualize the follow-up so that, for example, it is possible to post a green form on the precise anniversary of the first prescription. We have already commenced an exercise which will link the use of a drug with the procedure for cancer and death certification.

Much remains to be done to develop PEM. As a data-base, its value will increase as more drugs are investigated. Already it has shown that the actual levels of risk, even with some drugs that have been removed from the market, are quite low. Erythromycin estolate was under threat of removal from the market when it was shown that the seemingly large incidence of hepatotoxicity, which had been significant, was probably an artefact due to selective reporting. Three NSAIDs were removed from the market because of risks which probably lie within the two orders of magnitude – 1 in 20 000 to 1 in 2 000 000 – levels which would, if generally applied lead to the removal of many drugs used to treat serious conditions. PEM has been hailed by many as the most significant development in drug monitoring since the thalidomide disaster, and certainly it has advanced our ability to study the pattern of events that occur in the 'real life' situation of everyday medical practice rather than under the artificial conditions of clinical trials.

## Acknowledgements

We wish to record our appreciation of the help of Mr Eric Stabler, formerly the Secretary of the Prescription Pricing Authority, for the vital part he played in setting up PEM and, more recently, the help of Dr Gordon Geddes and his successor Mr Richard Bray who, together with the staff of the PPA, almost all of whom have been involved in various capacities, have made this important system a reality. We also wish to thank the Office of the Chief Scientist of the DHSS and nearly 30 pharmaceutical manufacturers for essential financial support, and some 18 000 general practitioners who have collaborated in the scheme.

## References

1. Inman, W. H. W. (1978). Detection and investigation of drug safety problems. In Gent, M. and Shigematsu, I. (eds.) *Epidemiological Issues in Reported Drug-Induced*

*Illnesses*. Honolulu, 1976. (Hamilton, Ontario: McMaster University Library Press)
2. Dollery, C. T. and Rawlins, M. D. (1977). Monitoring adverse reactions to drugs. *Br. Med. J.*, **1,** 96
3. Inman, W. H. W. (1981). Postmarketing surveillance of adverse drug reactions in general practice **I**: Search for new methods. *Br. Med. J.*, **282,** 1131–2. **II:** Prescription-event monitoring at the University of Southampton. **282,** 1216–7
4. Inman, W. H. W. (1984). Prescription-event monitoring in benefit-risk evaluation. Detection and prevention of adverse drug reactions. *Skandia International Symposium*, October 18–20 1983, Stockholm. pp. 133–141. (Stockholm: Almqvist and Wihsell International)
5. Inman, W. H. W. (1985). Let's get our act together. Annual Essay 1985. Side-effects of Drugs Annual 9. Dukes, M. N. G. (ed) xv–xxiii. (Amsterdam: Elsevier).
6. Colin-Jones, D. G. Langman, M. J. S., Lawson, D. H. and Vessey, M. P. (1983). Post-marketing surveillance of the safety of cimetidine: 12 month mortality report. *Br. Med. J.*, **286,** 1713–16
7. Inman, W. H. W., and Rawson, N. S. B. (1983). Erythromycin estolate and jaundice. *Br. Med. J.*, **286,** 1954–5
8. Inman, W. H. W. (1983). Yellow cards and green forms. *Practitioner*, **227,** 1443–9
9. Inman, W. H. W. (1985). Risks in medical intervention. In Cooper, M. (ed.) *Risk: Man-Made Hazards to Man.* (Oxford: Oxford University Press)

# 16
# COMPASS: a population based postmarketing drug surveillance system

**M. L. MORSE, A. A. LE ROY and B. L. STROM**

## INTRODUCTION

Post-marketing drug surveillance (PMS) programmes collect information about the effects of drugs after marketing and when in customary use. While valuable surveillance systems have existed for decades, many have been voluntary efforts which yield data limited by under-reporting, under and over-ascertainment, and a lack of information on the number of exposed patients needed in order to determine rates of disease. The type of PMS programme needed to complement existing programmes is a *system* of post-marketing drug surveillance which quickly, systematically and comprehensively links drug use information to diagnostic information in a defined population. Unfortunately, the magnitude of the study populations needed for PMS and the sophistication of the automated data processing system necessary to monitor these populations have, until now, presented logistical and economic barriers to their utility.

The limitations inherent in existing post-marketing surveillance systems in the United States prompted the US Food and Drug Administration (FDA) in 1978 to examine new and innovative approaches to meeting its responsibilities of ensuring the safety and efficacy of drugs available to the American public. One such approach, which has been under investigation since 1978, is the use of Medicaid data through a system known as the Computerized On-Line Medicaid Pharmaceutical Analysis and Surveillance System (COMPASS$^{TM}$). This chapter describes the conceptual basis of COMPASS, and the epidemiological routines available with this large data base for performing PMS.

## MEDICAID: THE HEALTH CARE PROGRAMME

Title XIX of the US Social Security Act established a programme of medical assistance for certain low-income individuals and families. The programme, known as Medicaid, became federal law in 1965. It is administered by each state within certain broad federal requirements and guidelines, and is the primary source of health care coverage for the economically disadvantaged. In addition, states may provide medical assistance to the 'medically needy'. This usually means people who fit into one of the categories covered by the cash welfare programmes (aged, blind, or disabled individuals, or members of families with dependent children when one parent is absent, incapacitated, or unemployed), who have enough income to pay for their basic living expenses (and so are not recipients of welfare), but not enough to pay for their medical care. It is important to note that Medicaid does not provide medical assistance to all of the poor. Low income is only one test of eligibility; resources are also tested. Most important, to be covered one must belong to one of the groups designated for welfare eligibility. Medicaid accounted for some $35 billion in federal and state expenditures in the financial years 1984–85. Medicaid is financed jointly with state and federal funds, with the current federal contributions to the programme ranging from 50 to 77.55%.

Title XIX of the Social Security Act requires that certain essential services *must* be offered in any state Medicaid programme: in-patient hospital services; out-patient hospital services; laboratory and X-ray services; skilled nursing facility services for individuals aged 21 years and older; home health care services for individuals eligible for skilled nursing services; physicians' services; family planning services; rural health clinic services; and, early and periodic screening, diagnosis, and treatment services for those under the age of 21. In addition, states may provide a number of optional services, such as drugs, spectacles, private-duty nursing, intermediate care facility services, in-patient psychiatric care for the aged and persons under 21, physical therapy and dental care. With respect to the use of Medicaid data for PMS, variation between states with respect to these 'optional' services – particularly drugs – poses some problems regarding the comprehensiveness of the data, as well as the compatability of a multi-state data base for purposes of data collection.

Individual states determine the scope of services offered; for example, they may limit the type or quantity (days of hospitalization) of service covered. Also, since states determine the eligibility level for the welfare programmes, they exercise a great deal of control over the income eligibility levels for Medicaid. All of these variations – in benefits offered, in groups covered, in income standards and in levels of reimbursement for providers – result in a wide variation in Medicaid programmes from state to state.

Medicaid operates as a vendor payment or 'third-party' programme. Payments are made to medical service providers, not to the patient.

Claims have to be made, and providers are then paid. The necessity of paying providers, and the maintenance of orderly medical services reimbursement records, generates computerized billing data. These data, which are in effect a by-product of an already developed billing system, can be used for clinical and epidemiologic research. Health care researchers can, theoretically, use these data, turning data collected for administrative reasons into useful medical information.

One of the first research related applications of Medicaid data to investigate drug use was the introduction of drug utilization review (DUR) programmes in the late 1960s. These early DUR programmes were conducted in the states of Florida, California, North Carolina, Massachusetts, Maine, Arkansas and Pennsylvania. The discovery of irrational drug use patterns through the review of Medicaid patient drug history profiles established the potential of the Medicaid billing data as a resource for studying out-patient drug use. For example, in Florida the drug use characteristics of approximately half a million Medicaid beneficiaries were routinely monitored by eight regional DUR committees. From January to December 1975, over 20 000 potential drug therapy problems were identified resulting in more than 4700 physician inquiries. Over 3100 (68%) of the physicians contacted expressed a willingness to reconsider and alter the drug therapies in question.

The early DUR programmes were handicapped by the absence of diagnosis data to complement drug use patterns presented on the drug history profile. The Medicaid drug benefit programmes of the late 1960s and early 1970s were often administered under contract to drug claims processing firms and thus physician and hospital information was not part of the DUR data base. However, as more and more states adopted a federally certified uniform Medicaid Management Information System (MMIS), the ability to tap one single data base for both drug and diagnosis data became a reality. By the mid-1970s, approximately 15 states were able to link, through MMIS, out-patient drug use to out-patient and in-patient physician/hospital diagnoses. Today, 49 state Medicaid programmes operate under a certified MMIS, with the potential of linking diagnoses to drug use in tens of millions of people.

## THE MEDICAID MANAGEMENT INFORMATION SYSTEM: THE DATA SOURCE

COMPASS exclusively utilizes data processed by and contained within the Medicaid Management Information System (MMIS). Therefore, the capabilities and limitations of COMPASS should be viewed relative to the parent system – MMIS.

The Medicaid Management Information System is divided into six functional areas or subsystems:

(1) Recipient subsystem
(2) Provider subsystem

(3) Claims processing subsystem
(4) Reference file subsystem
(5) Surveillance and utilization review subsystem
(6) Management and administrative reporting subsystem

The initial input of data varies between states, but is generally performed by either a manual (key punch) or automated process, which includes optical character recognition or tape-to-tape transfers. The Recipient, Provider, Reference file, and Claims processing systems, in a sense function together to process and pay each provider for all valid claims. The Surveillance and Utilization review subsystem and the Management and administrative reporting subsystem are basically involved in data consolidation, organization and presentation in a manner that will enable managerial control over the Title XIX Programme. Once claims are paid, the Surveillance and Utilization review subsystem analyses the payment characteristics of the provider and beneficiary population and identifies any patterns that may represent fraud or abuse. This is a major intended use of the MMIS data base – detection of fraud and abuse.

From January 1980, the US Health Care Financing Administration requires that all State Medicaid programmes report disease/disorders using the International Classification of Diseases-9th Revision Clinical Modification (ICD-9-CM). Thus, compatibility of diagnosis data between states is generally obtainable with little or no modification. On the other hand, drug data are reported by a variety of coding mechanisms, thereby presenting significant compatibility problems.

Although a necessary and essential responsibility for the management of such a large fiscal programme, the accounting system of MMIS has tended to inhibit the active consideration of MMIS data for medical research purposes. However, MMIS data have been found to be useful to many researchers in a variety of health care research areas. Federspiel *et al.* used the Tennessee Medicaid data base to analyse physician practice and drug prescribing habits, and to review the effects of physician education programmes.[1] Buck and White used the California Medi-Cal data to study the impact of Professional Standards Review Organizations on physicians' practice patterns.[2] Eisenberg and Nicklin used Pennsylvania Medicaid data to evaluate the utilization of diagnostic services by physicians in the community.[3] Morse, LeRoy *et al.* continue to use multi-state Medicaid data to assess the impact of inappropriate drug therapy on hospitalizations.[4] More recently, Avorn and Sumerai have used Medicaid data to assess the effect of information aimed at physicians on their prescribing patterns.[5]

## COMPASS – A POPULATION-BASED PMS SYSTEM

The Computerized On-Line Medicaid Pharmaceutical Analysis and Surveillance System (COMPASS) is a very large computerized data base of MMIS Medicaid billing data. It is designed to permit a researcher to enrol and analyse cohorts of patients exposed to a drug (or drugs), or patients with specific diseases, and compare them with matched or unmatched control groups of patients.

COMPASS was originally conceived by Health Information Designs, Inc. (HID), and has been under development by HID since 1978, and is funded by FDA. Initially, an extensive on-site evaluation of MMIS systems in six states was undertaken, and it was decided, based on this evaluation, to obtain MMIS data from Michigan and Minnesota (initial Medicaid population of 1.2 million) because of the high quality of their MMIS data files. Since 1981, the addition of the Florida, Missouri, Nebraska, Arkansas, Mississippi, Ohio, Virginia and Colorado Medicaid data sets brings the total COMPASS population to approximately 6.0 million patients. Discussions are underway to add other states and to add non-Medicaid sources of data, e.g. private insurance programmes.

The Claims processing subsystem of MMIS serves as the resource for all the data used by COMPASS. Although dozens of data elements are contained on claim forms, COMPASS uses only a small set of discrete data elements with which to link out-patient drug exposures to patient disease/disorders.

The essential data elements include:

Confidentialized patient identification code,
State and county,
Age, sex and race,
Out-patient drugs prescribed (national drug code specific),
In-patient or out-patient diseases/disorders treated (coded by the International Classification of Diseases 9th Edition, Clinical Modification),
Dates of services for both drugs and physician services,
Quantity of drug prescribed,
Days supply of drug prescribed,
Procedures (laboratory, radiological, etc.) provided,
Provider type (hospital, physician or pharmacy), and
Provider identification.

In addition, death data from a number of state's vital statistics files have also been merged into the COMPASS file.

A key data element in the COMPASS data base is date of service, for it shows the temporal relationship between various medical/pharmacy events. These temporal relationships, observed in tens of thousands of patients, provide a basis for assessing causality between drug exposure and clinical outcome. Additional drug data – quantity dispensed and days supply (an estimate submitted by the dispensing pharmacist on the pharmacy claim form – permit insight into the patient's exposure to the drug, particularly when dosages are being prescribed that exceed approved levels.

COMPASS is composed exclusively of 'paid claims' information.

Claims which are rejected due to input discrepancies, omission of required information, ineligibility of beneficiary/provider/service, or erroneous billing amounts are by definition excluded from the COMPASS data base. With respect to the accuracy of the data submitted by Medicaid providers for payment, the Surveillance and utilization review subsystems in each state maintain active, and often aggressive, field audit programmes, which permit state medical audit teams to verify the validity of claims submitted for payment against the patients' medical records in the physician's office or in hospitals. In general, these ongoing audits help to ensure the reliability of reimbursement data.

The COMPASS software is currently installed on a minicomputer manufactured by WANG Laboratories. Drug and diagnosis data processed by each state's MMIS are extracted and forwarded to HID's offices. The extract tape is sorted by patient identification number, service type/code, and date of service, and then edited for incomplete or erroneous data elements.

During the edit stage, specifically developed binary codes are assigned to each National Drug Code (NDC) and International Classification of Diseases (ICD-9-CM) code. This maximizes the on-line storage capacity of the patient history files. Data are organized by patient history profiles, and can be accessed interactively or by batch processing. Tables 1 and 2 list some of the most frequently used drugs and the most frequent diagnoses, respectively, listed in the 1984 COMPASS data base.

Information on drugs and diagnoses can be accessed using a variety of coding methods. For drug information, data can be accessed using NDC codes, generic codes, specific therapeutic class codes or user-defined code groupings. Similarly, it is possible to access diagnosis information using ICD-9-CM codes, disease category class codes or user-defined code groupings.

COMPASS diagnosis profiling and patient history profiling capabilities also provide the basis for developing and conducting case control studies. Patients with a history of, or currently presenting with, specific diseases or conditions are gleaned from the data base using standard sort procedures. Often, however, specific morbidities are listed under different descriptions within ICD-9-CM, thus necessitating the construction of morbidity groupings containing all ICD-9-CM codes associated with a particular condition or disorder. The use of multiple ICD-9-CM codes in morbidity files accommodates the inherent redundancy within the ICD-9-CM coding convention, and permits a high degree of refinement in the subject selection process.

Conditions such as vertigo and flushing provide good examples of the use of singular and multiple ICD-9-CM morbidity sort file designs. The condition of dizziness can be expressed by three unique ICD-9-CM coded terms: lightheadedness (code 770.5), dizziness (code 385.0), and vertigo (code 770.4). Physicians may use any one of these three codes to relate dizziness as the description of the condition for which a

**Table 1** Selected frequently used drugs – 1984 COMPASS system

| *Generic drug name* | *Estimated number of patients** |
|---|---|
| Codeine phosphate | 1 684 128 |
| Amoxicillin | 1 412 674 |
| Penicillin | 1 373 569 |
| Sulphamethoxazole | 772 632 |
| Hydrocortisone | 742 819 |
| Cephalexin | 740 296 |
| Trimethoprim | 730 468 |
| Ergocalciferol | 731 244 |
| Promethazine HCl | 655 708 |
| Hydrochlorothiazide | 544 399 |
| Ibuprofen | 489 755 |
| Ethinyloestradiol | 471 221 |
| Norethindrone | 414 445 |
| Miconazole Nitrate | 396 890 |
| Furosemide | 361 123 |
| Clotrimazole | 346 562 |
| Mestranol | 293 704 |
| Cefaclor | 290 505 |
| Metronidazole | 282 708 |
| Cimetidine | 280 477 |
| Digoxin | 276 105 |
| Propoxyphene HCl | 270 995 |
| Doxycycline (Hyclate) | 270 995 |
| Hydroxyzine HCl | 265 216 |
| Chlordiazepoxide HCl | 261 340 |
| Potassium chloride | 255 209 |
| Betamethasone (Valerate) | 244 783 |
| Norgestrel | 226 037 |
| Flurazepam HCl | 225 345 |
| Thiamine Mononitrate | 222 916 |
| Diazepam | 215 914 |
| Amitriptyline HCl | 215 112 |
| Propoxyphene napsylate | 196 527 |
| Hydrocortisone acetate | 179 626 |
| Gentamicin (Sulphate) | 179 111 |
| Naproxen | 178 114 |
| Propranolol HCl | 176 086 |
| Nitroglycerin | 176 055 |
| Methyldopa | 169 558 |
| Prednisone | 169 140 |
| Sulindac | 154 554 |
| Diphenoxylate HCl | 152 331 |

* Estimates based on COMPASS Generic Drug Ranking Reports. System population 6.0 million

professional service claim was submitted for payment. Therefore, to ensure that all dizziness cases are captured from the COMPASS data base, the dizziness sort file will contain all three ICD-9-CM codes, and

**Table 2** Selected frequently reported diagnoses – 1984 COMPASS system

| *ICD-9-CM diagnosis* | *Estimated number of patients** |
|---|---|
| Acute upper respiratory infection | 1 622 036 |
| Acute pharyngitis | 1 241 285 |
| Otitis media (NOS) | 933 083 |
| Bronchitis (NOS) | 874 728 |
| Abdominal pain | 868 071 |
| Urinary tract infection (NOS) | 804 341 |
| Chest pain (NOS) | 654 366 |
| Non-infectious gastroenteritis (NEC) | 640 251 |
| Pneumonia, (organism NOS) | 620 463 |
| Anaemia (NOS) | 578 829 |
| Vaginitis (NOS) | 577 876 |
| Acute tonsillitis | 568 835 |
| Dermatitis (NOS) | 529 048 |
| Acute bronchitis | 488 955 |
| Headache | 425 899 |
| Hypertension (NOS) | 417 060 |
| Chronic sinusitis (NOS) | 389 400 |
| Influenza with respiratory manifestations (NEC) | 345 366 |
| Normal delivery | 324 562 |
| Pregnancy state, incidental | 318 101 |
| Cystitis (NOS) | 306 727 |
| Diabetes uncomplicated adult | 304 957 |
| Absence of menstruation | 303 284 |
| Respiratory abnormality (NEC) | 296 715 |
| Streptococcal sore throat | 278 962 |
| Myalgia and myositis (NOS) | 261 282 |
| Supervized other normal pregnancy | 253 775 |
| Gastritis/duodenitis (NOS) | 244 068 |
| Single liveborn – in hospital | 225 996 |
| Coronary atherosclerosis | 225 365 |
| Non-specific skin eruption (NEC) | 220 043 |
| Cervicitis | 216 773 |
| Allergic rhinitis (NOS) | 214 531 |
| Hypothyroidism (NOS) | 207 601 |
| Viral infection (NOS) | 207 490 |
| Anxiety state (NOS) | 202 823 |
| Female pelvic inflammatory disease (NOS) | 202 812 |
| Pregnancy exam – pregnancy unconfirmed | 202 014 |
| Diabetes mellitus uncomplicated | 200 968 |
| Backache (NOS) | 199 456 |
| Asthma (NOS) | 193 745 |
| Benign hypertension | 160 116 |
| Cardiac dysrhythmia (NOS) | 157 845 |
| Asthma without status asthmatica | 156 288 |
| Congestive heart failure | 154 806 |
| Death | 134 495 |
| Acne (NEC) | 133 769 |

*Estimates based on COMPASS Diagnosis Banking Reports. System population 6.0 million

a match with any one of these codes will trigger a case-select program. 'Flushing', however, has no other coding synonym in the ICD-9-CM thesaurus file; therefore, sorting on code 775.3 will yield discrete cases of flushing within the data base.

Interaction with the system is menu driven. The user may choose between a number of epidemiological routines displayed on the terminal screen. A selected list of these is presented in Table 3. For example, the relative risk signal generator takes a user-defined cohort of drug exposed patients and a user-defined control group and automatically calculates relative risks and 95% confidence intervals for all ICD-9-CM diagnosis codes, all NDC or generic codes, and all procedure codes, or any defined subset of these. Analogously, the odds

**Table 3** Selected epidemiologic procedures available on-line in COMPASS

| *Procedure* | *Description* |
|---|---|
| Cohort enrolment | Enrolment of all patients exposed to a certain drug or with a certain disease |
| Challenge/rechallenge analysis | After finding an apparent drug–disease association, this routine searches for those patients who have a second appearance of the disease subsequent to a second drug exposure |
| Diagnosis rankings | A count of the number of people suffering from each diagnosis in any specified group of patients, ranked by disease incidence, code number, etc. |
| Drug/disease admissibility screens | A requirement that patients must have had a medical service of some type in the beginning of and end of a specified time period, to assure they were eligible for reimbursement in the interim period |
| Drug exposure rankings | A count of the number of people exposed to each drug in any specified group of patients, ranked by utilization, code number, etc. |
| Odds ratio signal generation | see text |
| Period of exposure analyses | Analysis of exposures in a specified time interval relative to an illness or another exposure, e.g. in the first trimester of pregnancy |
| Random age/sex/morbidity matched control patient selection | Development of control groups for any specified cohort, matched for age, sex, diagnosis, and/or drug |
| Relative risk signal generation | see text |
| Temporal analysis | Examination of the temporal relationship between a drug and a subsequent diagnosis |

ratio signal generator takes a user-defined case group of patients suffering from a particular disease and a user-defined control group and calculates odds ratios and 95% confidence intervals.

Primary medical records can also be obtained from physicians, hospitals, etc., as long as the number of requests is relatively limited.

COMPASS provides a resource for constructing large and diversified cohorts of patients. These cohorts can be constructed to include groups of drug-exposed and non-exposed populations either matched or unmatched for age, sex, existing morbidities, etc. Both retrospective cohorts and prospective cohorts can be developed within this system, including either patients from the system's current data base or patients recruited prospectively, as new patients enter the COMPASS data base over time.

The performance of case control studies in COMPASS is similar in both concept and design to the recruitment of cohorts. In the case-control model, patient selection is based upon the presence or absence of specific disease/condition encounters, rather than selection by the presence or absence of drug exposure.

The COMPASS data base is unique in providing opportunities to observe drug use experiences in large and diversified patient populations. By virtue of Medicaid eligibility requirements, this data base is rich in young children, women of childbearing age and the elderly, but this skewed population limits the inferences that can be drawn from the data base to the population as a whole. However, valuable insight into the drug use experiences of several patient populations, previously only studied to a limited extent, but prevalent within the Medicaid system, can be discerned from the data base.

For example, COMPASS maintains a paediatric cohort (PEDIATRIC base) within which paediatric drug use is studied. Young children are rarely included in most pre-clinical trials and pre-marketing studies, because of ethical restrictions. Thus, paediatric drug usage has received relatively limited study, most of which has been in the hospital environment. Large scale out-patient studies of paediatric drug usage are uncommon in the literature. Currently, the COMPASS data base contains the drug use and disease histories of over approximately 2 million children under 12 years of age. Nearly 400 000 of these children are under 2 years of age, thus providing a unique opportunity to study drug use in the infant. Given the longterm potential complications of many of today's drugs, this cohort could provide an insight into the long range effects of drug exposure at early ages.

As another example, drug effects on the fetus have been widely publicized. Although pregnant women are cautioned against the use of medicines during pregnancy, many continue to use a variety of prescription and non-prescription products. The effects of these drug exposures on the fetus are difficult to examine, principally due to the absence of complete data on drug use during pregnancies. Data obtained by history are subject to possible recall bias. Due to the large number of women of childbearing age in the COMPASS data base, large cohorts of pregnant women can be enrolled early in their pregnancy and monitored for drug exposures until term. To date, birth outcome data and trimester specific drug use experience is available for over 150 000 deliveries in COMPASS. Children born with birth defects can be linked to their mothers' drug/disease history profiles, and possible associations between the drug exposures and the birth anomalies can be examined. Additionally, the pregnant mothers' drug usage patterns may reveal interesting relationships with the illness patterns of their offspring during childhood.

COMPASS employs a number of routines to permit system-wide signalling for adverse drugs reactions (ADRs). The process of signalling involves the automatic scanning of large numbers of patient medical history files relating drug therapies to suspected adverse reactions. Interrogation of patient files can be conducted on a routine basis, either monthly or quarterly, and measurements of discrepancies and disproportions are made on selected drugs and reactions. Measurements exceeding selected thresholds generate

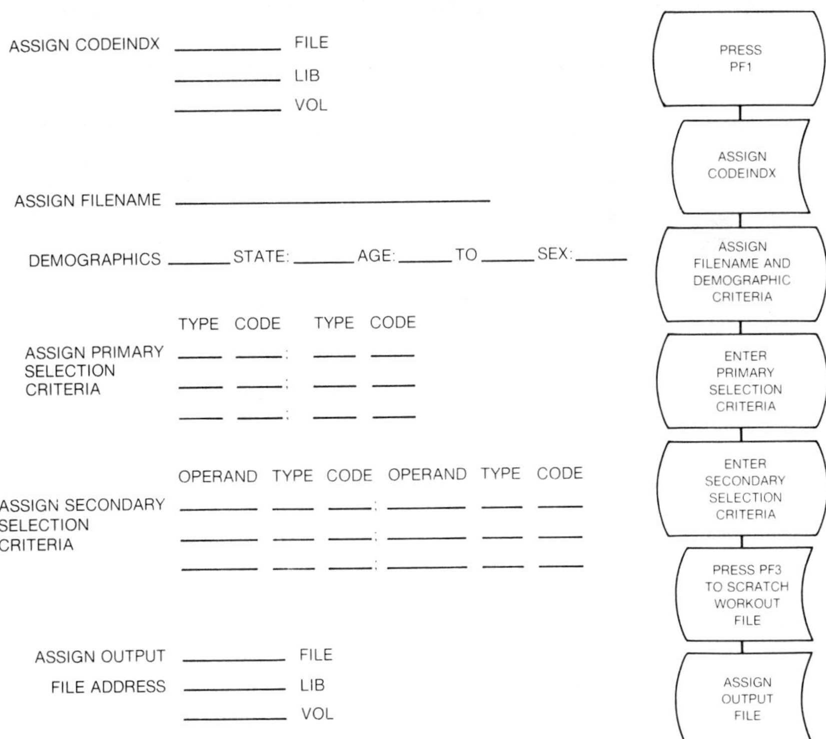


**Figure 1** Cohort/case control enrollment module

signals, which serve to indicate suspicious associations between drugs and reactions.

The COMPASS data base provides a framework around which a number of signalling protocols can be programmed and implemented. Because COMPASS is an event reporting system, physicians in the Medicaid program do not initiate drug-specific ADR incidence reports, but rather report the condition or diagnosis for which a medical service was provided. In contrast, ADR reporting to national or international drug surveillance centres is always based on perceived drug specific post-exposure reactions. Despite the limitations inherent to the COMPASS data base, the data do provide a basis for intense clinical and epidemiological examination using COMPASS or other more clinically oriented surveillance systems.

## Experience with COMPASS

As one of a number of examples of the use of COMPASS to explore drug–disease associations, a study is underway investigating gastro-intestinal bleeding associated with use of non-steroidal anti-inflammatory drugs (NSAIDs). Funded by FDA, the study utilized 1980 Medicaid billing data from Michigan and Minnesota, and yielded over 100 000 users of NSAIDs.[6] Based on these data, gastrointestinal bleeding was confirmed as an event associated with the use of NSAIDs. In addition, significant differences in the incidence of gastrointestinal bleeding associated with the use of different NSAIDs were noted. Both dose–response and duration–response relationships were documented. This study reproduced many known facts, including: the incidence of upper gastrointestinal (UGI) bleeding increases with age; there is a higher frequency of UGI bleeding among males than among females; and patients with alcohol-related diagnoses taking NSAIDs may bleed up to ten times more frequently than those without an alcohol-related diagnosis. Drug utilization patterns were also as expected: ibuprofen was used more frequently for dysmenorrhea, indomethacin and phenylbutazone were used more frequently for crystal arthropathy. Also, patients with pre-existing abdominal conditions prior to dispensing of a NSAID bled more frequently than those without these factors.

As another example of uses of COMPASS, a study performed to explore the relative incidence of allergy and/or anaphylaxis among different non-steroidal anti-inflammatory drugs was commissioned by McNeil Pharmaceuticals.[7] A case-control study was first used as a validation study, documenting the system's ability to reproduce known drug causes of allergy and/or anaphylaxis. This was then followed by a series of retrospective cohort studies. Many known associations with anaphylaxis have been reproduced, for example a higher rate in females than in males. The results of this study were a key factor in the recommendation by the FDA's Arthritis Advisory

Committee to allow the remarketing of zomepirac.

In another study using COMPASS, funded by the FDA, the association between oral contraceptives and gallbladder disease, including a dose–response relationship, was reproduced.[8] Also reproduced were associations between gallbladder disease and obesity, thiazides, diabetes mellitus, pancreatitis, pregnancy, etc.

Examples of other studies which have been performed on COMPASS include investigations of the associations between oral contraceptives and thromboembolism, ticrynafen and liver disease, ampicillin and skin rash, phenothiazines and liver disease, and sulpha drugs and thrombocytopenia. All these studies confirmed known associations. Other studies now underway include prospective cohort studies of newly marketed drugs, inexpensively meeting the manufacturers' regulatory requirements for PMS studies; retrospective (historical) cohort studies of suspected drug effects, e.g. the relative incidence of gastrointestinal bleeding following the use of different potassium chloride preparations, and the relative incidence of blood dyscrasias following the use of different procainamide preparations; and retrospective cohort studies screening drugs for unsuspected drug effects, e.g. isotretinoin.

## Advantages of COMPASS

The principal advantage of COMPASS is the very large population it includes – currently over 6 million, also, it is important to note that it is population-based, allowing the calculation of incidence rates.

Both prospective and retrospective cohort enrollment protocols can be incorporated into longitudinal studies, with relatively low rates of attrition associated with patient relocation or changes in physician. Traditional cohort attrition factors, such as patient relocation or election to obtain medical services from non-study participating health care providers, are not relevant within the COMPASS population, in that all health care services, regardless of provider, are paid for by the same state agency. Neither relocation (as long as it is within the same state) nor the use of multiple health care providers interferes with the continuity of patient medical history development within the COMPASS data base.

Unlike most other PMS systems, COMPASS includes both in-patient and out-patient diagnoses. The data it includes are not dependent on recall or subject to interviewer bias. For example, since the system does not use interviewers and questionnaires as a source of data, asymmetrical influences attributable to variations in the interview techniques or the use of non-standardized questionnaires are absent. Furthermore, both pre- and post-study drug exposure data are collected systematically without consideration of any drug effect, thereby minimizing physician reporting bias.

Finally, as a system which uses data collected in an ongoing way as a byproduct of an administrative process, it is relatively inexpensive, and can be used to quickly address questions of regulatory or clinical importance.

COMPASS also has some advantages specific to conducting either cohort or case-control studies. Cohort studies of drug effects compare treated with untreated patients, looking for differences in clinical outcome. This approach has several advantages: direct calculation of relative risks and incidence rates; the ability to observe multiple outcomes; and lack of subject recall bias, since individuals are enrolled prior to the onset of disease. The major disadvantage of this approach is that it often requires a large number of subjects to be followed over a long period of time. This is not a problem, however, when using an existing data base like COMPASS to perform retrospective cohort studies.

Case-control studies compare diseased patients with non-diseased patients, and look for differences in antecedent drug exposures. Proper control groups selection is a critical aspect of case-control study design; unless cases and controls are at equal risk of exposure to the factors being investigated, study results may be biased. Selection bias will exist when either the cases or controls are differentially selected in a way that may effect the probability of exposure to a study drug. Given COMPASS' ability to survey the *census* of either drug exposed patients or patients exhibiting a suspected adverse effect, the impact of selection bias can be minimized. In COMPASS, controls may be randomly selected from the entire non-diseased population, with or without matching for age, sex, race, drug(s), and/or other disease(s). These 'cohort-based case-control studies' allow researchers to take advantage of the strengths of case-control studies, for example the ability to study many different possible causes of a single disease, while avoiding their main potential problems, i.e. selection of a biased control group and recall bias.

## DISADVANTAGES OF COMPASS

Certain limitations of the COMPASS system are also known. Currently, despite its size, COMPASS cannot be used to study *very* rarely prescribed drugs or extremely rare adverse reactions. There is also a 2 month lag period between the time a drug is dispensed and the time it appears on the monitoring system. COMPASS is limited to billing data, making it impossible to control for some potentially important confounding variables, e.g. smoking, diet and occupation. To date, it contains only Medicaid patients and, so, its results may not be applicable to other populations. However, this is more likely to be a problem for descriptive studies than for analytical studies – if a drug causes an adverse effect, it is likely to do so whether one is rich or poor. It does not include any data on in-patient drug usage. Additionally, patients drop out from the COMPASS data base, most often because of termination, suspension of their eligibility or death. The extent to which this affects the continuity of the data base must be controlled using specific admissibility and history screening techniques.

The most important potential limitation in a system using billing data is the inevitable question raised about the validity of its data. An FDA-funded validation study of COMPASS was recently completed, comparing COMPASS data to its primary sources, i.e. data from hospitals, physicians, pharmacies, etc. The results of this study indicate that the demographic and drug data appear to be of extremely high quality. Within pre-established limits, year of birth agreed in 94% of sampled patients, and could not be determined from the medical records in another 2.5%; sex agreed in 95% of patients, and could not be determined from the medical records in another 4%; and the date of a pharmacy's dispensing of each drug agreed in 97% of sampled prescriptions. Regarding medical services, of the records that could be evaluated, 93% of the services in COMPASS could be found in the provider records searching within 1 week of the COMPASS data; in 17% of those, the provider record included a previous or subsequent visit that was not in COMPASS. Diagnostic agreement to at least three digits of the ICD-9-CM code occurred in 41%, agreement within a broad diagnostic category in another 16% (i.e. same body system and/or type of illness), no diagnosis was present on the provider record in 12%, a single diagnosis in 3% and there was no agreement in 28%.

Clearly, this study raises important concerns about the validity of the diagnosis data in COMPASS. However, this validation study has serious methodological problems itself. Physicians were sampled from two urban areas, which may not reflect the accuracy of the diagnostic information in the entire system. Only 55% of physicians participated. Of the remainder, 9% could not be located, 5% had no records available and the remainder refused to participate. Although at one extreme one could interpret the results as showing 60% disagreement, one has to realize that included in that 60% were 12% in which the provider record had no diagnosis, 3% in which the provider record probably was missing diagnoses, and 16% in which there was agreement on at least the same body system and/or type of illness. Even the remaining 28% await additional analyses regarding the seriousness of the discrepancy. Thus, included as 'disagreement' would be situations such as a diagnosis of myocardial infarction in one of the data sources and a diagnosis of chest pain in the other. Moreover, the study only checked records from the physicians' primary practice site and never attempted to get information from sites such as other offices or an Emergency Room. In Michigan and Minnesota, 50% of physicians have such other practice sites. Probably most importantly, however, was that this was not a study of validity, but a study of disagreement. This is especially important in view of a previous study of billing data which suggested that, when there was disagreement, the claims diagnoses were more useful than the chart diagnoses.[9] Certainly, the FDA-funded study provides further evidence of the limitations of physicians' medical records.

The findings of the FDA funded validation study must also be interpreted in the context of the ongoing drug monitoring experiences of COMPASS' sister system DURbase. Each month thousands of patient-specific drug risk alerts, based on DURbase software designed to identify irrational drug use patterns observed in the COMPASS data base, are sent to the physicians and pharmacists involved in the patients' management. These alerts request that the practitioner verify the accuracy of the billing data, and if they agree with the basis of the alert, modify their patient's drug therapy regimen to minimize the risks for a possible drug therapy-induced illness. Over 70% of the cases identified are responded to by the practitioners involved, and less than 1% of their responses indicate that the medical event data, upon which the risk was generated, were erroneous.

There is other significant evidence to suggest that the data from the system is valid, including: the existence of federal MMIS certification requirements; the identities of drugs and procedures which determine the level of reimbursement for them and, therefore, they are closely audited; and the data have face validity (i.e. the right drugs appear with the right diagnoses and in the right sequence). Most important, however, are the number of studies which have been performed using COMPASS, by both the Food and Drug Administration and the Clinical Epidemiology Unit of the University of Pennsylvania School of Medicine. In all cases, COMPASS confirmed known associations, including, in many of them, a dose–response relationship. Thus, if there is a signficant error in the diagnosis data, it is likely to be random, and overpowered by the available sample size.

Thus, although the findings of the validation study remain to be fully clarified, the data in COMPASS appear to be sufficiently valid to be useful. Nevertheless, in using COMPASS, one must always remain aware of the potential for invalidity, building into each study tests for validation. For example:

(1) The preliminary case-control study we included in the NSAID-anaphylaxis study;
(2) Using the more certainly valid drugs and procedures in combination with diagnoses to define illnesses;
(3) Stratifying cases by the certainty of their diagnosis (e.g. using the presence or absence of hospitalization, drug treatment, multiple appearances of the same or related diagnoses, etc.);
(4) Where necessary, getting primary records on patients of particular interest and importance.

## FUTURE PERSPECTIVES

The importance of developing and improving mechanisms for studying the effects of drug use in a post-marketing environment is recognized throughout the world. Use of medical event data from private and national health systems, however feasible in concept, is constrained by enormous political and economic barriers. Among these barriers are patient confidentiality and cost of data generation.

The substantial growth of COMPASS over the past 4 years is due in part to consideration of two critical barriers. Firstly, demonstrating that significant improvements in patient care can be realized by confidentially sharing with the practitioners involved in the patient's management the medical history profiles of those patients exhibiting irrational drug use patterns. This provides a more palatable basis for the establishment and use of a patient-specific medical event data base.

Secondly, monitoring drug use relative to patient compliance, contraindicated conditions, and iatrogenic complications yields significant reductions in drug therapy-induced hospitalizations and outpatient remedial care services.[4] The economies realized through monitoring risks for drug-induced illness provide a strong financial incentive for health care programmes to dedicate manpower, computer time, and other resources to developing and maintaining the medical/pharmacy event data base. Facing increasing costs and diminishing revenues, private health care programmes as well as national health care systems are increasingly employing cost-containment mechanisms for improving care and reducing costs. COMPASS can justify itself on cost through its DURbase monitoring component, providing, as a by-product, a rich resource for post-marketing drug surveillance and adverse drug reaction monitoring.

In summary, COMPASS now provides a large, growing, and important source of drug use/diagnosis experience data for the FDA, the pharmaceutical industry and academic institutions. With a population of over 6 million patients, it can quickly, comprehensively and relatively inexpensively enroll large numbers of patients exposed to a drug or patients with a specific diagnosis and investigate drug–disease associations. It is unlikely that any single data source will ever fulfil all of the diverse data needs of PMS, certainly, none now does. However, inasmuch as it complements the characteristics of the existing data sources, COMPASS represents a major new resource for PMS.

## References


1. Federspiel, C. F., Wayne, R. A. and Schaffner, W. (1976). Medicaid records as a valid data source: The Tennessee Experience. *Med. Care*, **14,** 166–72
2. Buck, C. R. and White, K. C. (1974). Peer Review: impact of a system based on billing claims. *N. Engl. J. Med.*, **291,** 877–83
3. Eisenberg, J. M. and Nicklin, D. (1981). Use of diagnostic services by physicians in community practice. *Med. Care*, **19,** 297–309
4. Morse, M. L., Le Roy, A. A., Gaylord, T. A. and Kellenberger, T. (1982). Reducing drug therapy-induced hospitalizations: impact of drug utilization review. *Drug Inform., J.*, **16,** 199–202

5. Avorn, J. and Sumerai, S. (1983). Improving drug-therapy decisions through educational outreach. *N. Engl. J. Med.*, **308,** 1457–63
6. Carson, J. L., Strom, B. L., Morse, M. L., Stolley, P. D., Soper, K. A. and Jones, J. K. (1983). The relative gastrointestinal toxicity of the non-steroidal anti-inflammatory drugs. *Clin. Res.*, **31,** 230A
7. Strom, B. L., Carson, J. L., Morse, M. L. and West, S. L. (1984). Anaphylactoid reactions to zomepirac and other non-steroidal anti-inflammatory drugs. *Clin. Res.*, 229A
8. Strom, B. L., Tamragouri, R. N., Morse, M. L. *et al.* (1984). Oral contraceptives and gallbladder disease: validation of a computerized data base. *Clin. Pharmacol. Ther.*, **35,** 278
9. Studney, D. R. and Hakstian, A. R. (1981). A comparison of medical record with billing diagnostic information associated with ambulatory medical care. *Am. J. Pub. Health*, **71,** 145–9

# 17
# Intensive monitoring studies in hospitals: – I The Boston Collaborative Drug Surveillance Program

D. H. LAWSON

## INTRODUCTION

In 1966 Slone *et al*[1] commenced a small pilot scheme for monitoring medical in-patients for acute undesired drug effects occurring during hospitalization. The system they adopted proved so successful that it has since been expanded to include a wide variety of medical wards in several different countries. By 1976 information had been collected from over 35 000 consecutive medical in-patients providing a data resource of great scope. In 1977 further accrual of information from medical wards was greatly reduced, and in several of the participating hospitals data collection was switched to surgical in-patients. By 1982 the first report from this surgical programme involving a review of over 5000 patients was in press.[2] Running in parallel with the medical in-patient study and using similar methodology, the group also reviewed a small number of patients in paediatric wards[3] and some in psychiatric wards.[4] These studies constitute the main body of information now commonly referred to as the Boston Collaborative Drug Surveillance Program. As a result of findings from this programme a second type of study was undertaken in 1972. This involved collecting hospital discharge diagnoses and details of medication histories from 25 000 consecutive patients in hospitals throughout the Greater Boston area in Massachusetts.[5] The resulting information permitted the investigators to mount a large series of case-control investigations to test for associations between commonly used drugs and common disorders. Finally, since 1978 members of the group have collaborated with investigators in a pre-paid health care plan in Seattle – Group Health Co-operative – in analysing information from their computerized pharmacy and record systems relevant to possible drug toxicity.[6]

## INTENSIVE IN-PATIENT MONITORING FOR ADVERSE DRUG REACTIONS

The aims of this study are to provide information on drug use in hospitals; to give details of acute adverse effects attributed to drugs used in hospital, and to seek to determine whether particular subgroups of the hospitalized population are at greater than average risk of experiencing these effects; to give information on the frequency of certain events occurring during hospitalization, whether these effects be drug-related or not; and to identify associations between diseases and the use of medications on an out-patient basis. The methodology employed in this study has been described in detail elsewhere.[7]

During the course of analysing the medical data, it has emerged that there are wide differences in drug utilization between participating centres. When drug use was compared in a matched group of Scottish and American medical in-patients it was found that the latter received twice as many drugs for most indications as did the former.[8] Adverse drug reactions likewise appeared more prevalent in the American patients, although for each administered drug similar rates of reactions were reported from the two countries.

### Adverse drug reactions (ADRs)

Drug-related deaths have proved rare amongst medical in-patients; only 24 instances have been uncovered among 26 462 consecutive admissions.[9] Most of these patients were seriously ill prior to the drug-related event which, in the opinion of the investigators, contributed to their death. In only six patients (approximately 1 per 4500 admissions) did it seem possible that the death may have been preventable.

Analysis of information on life-threatening adverse reactions attributed to drugs in one of the participating centres revealed that these were significantly more common in patients with malignancy[10] – providing further evidence that severe ADRs are, on the whole, uncommon in medical in-patients suffering from otherwise benign conditions.

One of the benefits of the uniformity of data collection and the large number of patients studied is that rare effects of drugs which occur acutely after taking the drugs can be studied. In a recent publication, Porter and Jick[11] gave details of 119 episodes of drug-attributed anaphylaxis, convulsions, deafness or extrapyramidal symptoms occurring in 38 812 patients who had received over one-quarter of a million courses of drug treatment. In a similar study, Miller and Jick[12] emphasized that severe colitis, associated with antibiotic use, was a rare event especially in the American hospitals participating in the Program.

A detailed analysis of the characteristics of the group of patients receiving each drug in the study is undertaken at regular intervals. Regular searches of the data are undertaken to highlight possible subgroups of the recipient population who are at greater than average risk of developing adverse effects of drug treatment.

### *Heparin*

A review of 2656 recipients of sodium heparin showed that bleeding was a dose-related phenomenon which occurred most commonly in women, severely ill patients and those who received aspirin during therapy. In addition, heavy alcohol drinkers were at substantial risk of major bleeding during heparinization. During a 7-day course of therapy the cumulative risk of bleeding was over 9%, with the third day being the time of greatest risk.[13]

### *Flurazepam*

Greenblatt and his colleagues[14] have recently analysed the accumulated information on flurazepam – a widely used hypnotic both in the USA and Europe. This drug, while overall showing a commendably low adverse reaction rate of 3.1% (reaction usually being excessive drowsiness), appears to have a great propensity for over-sedating the elderly, particularly if given in high dosage (Table 1). This type of analysis is likely to prove of value to practising clinicians since it emphasizes not only the great safety of the drug in the majority of patients, but also the substantial risks of overdosage in a minority.

**Table 1** Frequency of adverse effects of flurazepam (percentages in parentheses)

| | *Adverse Effects* | |
|---|---|---|
| *Age (years)* | *Daily dose* ($<$ *30 mg*) | *Daily dose* ($>$ 30 mg) |
| $<$ 49 | 10/795 (1.2) | 5/140 (3.6) |
| 50–69 | 16/952 (1.7) | 13/96 (13.5) |
| $>$ 70 | 17/517 (3.3) | 16/41 (39.0) |

### *Methyldopa*

A study of 1067 patients receiving the anti-hypertensive agent methyldopa highlights one important aspect of the continuing monitoring project – the constraints on interpretation of the data.[15]

Methyldopa is used for the long-term management of hypertension. Only those undesired effects which occur within a short period of commencing the drug are seen in measurable amounts in this programme. Thus the commonest undesired acute effect noted was hypotension, which apart from being dose-related was also commoner in younger patients, in low-weight subjects and in those with renal impairment. All these factors were acting independently, and so differences in the frequency of hypotension as great as eight-fold were detected in different subgroups of the recipient population. The information derived from this study should allow safer prescribing of this drug in future, by encouraging low starting doses especially in non-obese, young patients particularly if they manifest any degree of renal impairment.

The group have analysed information from a large number of other drugs some of which are shown in Table 2.

**Table 2** Drugs described in detailed reports from Boston Collaborative Drug Surveillance Program*

| | | |
|---|---|---|
| Digoxin | Ampicillin | Prednisolone |
| Frusemide | Amoxycillin | Allopurinol |
| Ethacrynic acid | Tetracycline | Phenytoin |
| Spironolactone | Cotrimoxazole | Aspirin |
| Potassium Chloride | Isoniazid | Tricyclic antidepressants |
| Theophylline | Pethidine | Nitrazepam |
| Lignocaine | Propoxyphene | Flurazepam |
| Procainamide | Oral Contraceptives | Chlordiazepoxide |
| Propranolol | Dipyrone | Diazepam |
| Practolol | Oestrogens | Chlorpromazine |
| Reserpine | | Chloral Hydrate |

*For references apply to Dr H. Jick, Boston Collaborative Drug Surveillance Program, 400 Totten Pond Road, Waltham, Massachusetts, USA

In reviewing the information on adverse reactions to particular drugs it is occasionally observed that these occur with greater than expected frequency in patients who exhibit some abnormality in routine blood tests performed on admission to hospital.

### *Diphenylhydantoin*

One such association was seen amongst recipients of diphenylhydantoin – a commonly-used anticonvulsant drug. Reactions attributed to this drug were reported in 11.4% of 88 patients with an admission serum albumin concentration lower than 3.0 g/100 ml and in 3.8% of 234 patients with concentrations above this level. This association between toxicity and low levels of serum albumin concentration was independent of age, dose of phenytoin, renal function, type of reported reaction or primary diagnosis of the recipient, and was sufficiently strong to suggest a causal link between these two factors. A likely explanation of this association is the fact that phenytoin is strongly bound to serum albumin, and has a low therapeutic index. Thus even small increases in free phenytoin levels are likely to have disproportionate effects on the recipients. This is confirmed by the well-known dose-response relationship with this drug, however from the data presented by the Boston Program[16] it would appear that it can also arise at constant dose-levels by alterations in the albumin concentration – a fact predicted by kinetic studies, but not previously demonstrated in the clinical setting.

*Tetracyclines*

Another clinically relevant interaction between a drug and a biochemical parameter seen in the data is the association between the use of the tetracycline group of drugs and drug-attributed rises in blood urea nitrogen concentrations.[17] In this study, which was confined to a set of diuretic users, tetracycline recipients experienced clinically significant rises in blood urea nitrogen approximately three times as often as expected. Moreover, the magnitude of the differences between the tetracycline recipients and the controls was greater in those with pre-existing normal renal function than in those with renal impairment, suggesting that these differences were indeed causally related to the antibiotic use. This particular study is of special interest since the link between drug and event was not made by the attending physicians, but rather was discovered from within the data-base. This discovery depended upon the patients coincidentally receiving a drug(s) which is suspected of having an undesired effect upon blood urea nitrogen concentration, and which, therefore, led the prescribing physicians to monitor these concentrations. Thus this analysis had to be confined to diuretic recipients, since it was only in this cohort that blood urea nitrogen levels were monitored frequently enough and any subsequent abnormality reported. Invariably the reported abnormalities were attributed to the diuretic, not to the tetracycline.[17]

*Chloral hydrate – warfarin*

Drug interactions are rarely recognized as a major problem in this series of patients. One such interaction illustrates a major strength of the study. In 1970 Sellers and Koch-Weser[18] reported that, contrary to the commonly held view at the time, the hypnotic chloral hydrate, which is metabolized to trichloracetic acid, enhances the anticoagulant activity of warfarin. The suggested mechanism for this enhancement was the displacement of warfarin from binding sites on plasma albumin by the metabolite trichloracetic acid. Were this hypothesis true it might be expected to be seen in the data of the Boston study – data which had been collected prior to the publication of the Sellers and Koch-Weser article and hence would be free of bias due to prior knowledge of the interaction on the part of the prescribing physicians. Moreover, in view of the nature of the proposed interaction, its duration would be expected to be brief since any displaced warfarin would rapidly be excreted by the kidney and the previous *status quo* resumed. To test this hypothesis, patients anticoagulated during hospitalization were divided into three groups receiving continuous, intermittent or no chloral hydrate during the first 10 days of warfarin therapy. Those receiving continuous chloral hydrate treatment required significantly less warfarin during the induction phase than those receiving no chloral hydrate, with the occasional chloral recipients requiring an intermediate dose.[19] This convincingly demonstrated both that the interaction was a clinically relevant one, and that prescribers could compensate for it by measuring prothrombin times, and adjusting warfarin doses even though they were unaware of the chloral effect.

### *Smoking and drug effects*

Although drug interactions are not a major recognized cause of drug toxicity, a significant number of drug effects are modified by the smoking status of the recipients.[20] The results are compatible with the hypothesis that substances in cigarette smoke induce hepatic microsomal enzyme activity, thereby increasing the rate of drug metabolism. The analgesic propoxyphene appears to be significantly less effective in heavy smokers (20%) than in light smokers (15%) or non-smokers (10%), and this is true independently of the underlying condition being treated. With the benzodiazepines, diazepam and chlordiazepoxide there was a strong dose-related positive association between smoking and drug-attributed drowsiness, although (perhaps surprisingly) no such association was found between daily alcohol intake prior to admission and drowsiness. Nor was there any association between smoking and phenobarbitone-attributed drowsiness; the absence of this is presumably due to the fact that phenobarbitone recipients already have maximally-induced enzymes. An alternative explanation of the diazepam information is to suggest that there are more central receptors for benzodiazepines in the smoking population than amongst non-smokers.

With the phenothiazine, chlorpromazine, which was studied primarily in information from psychiatric hospitals, again a strong negative association was seen between drug-attributed drowsiness and smoking; some 3% of heavy smokers being particularly drowsy after treatment as compared with 11% of light smokers and 16% of non-smokers.

Clearly, therefore, smoking status should be taken into account in everyday prescribing habits, and also in clinical trials of new drugs which are significantly metabolized by the hepatic drug-metabolizing enzyme system.

### *Heparin and Ethacrynic acid*

Early in the course of the study, when information from only 4000 patients had been collected, a review of the prevalence of gastrointestinal bleeding during hospitalization showed this to be greater than expected amongst patients who received intravenous ethacrynic acid. This association was true whether or not the patients had also received heparin.[21] Further analysis of data as they accumulate continue to demonstrate this propensity of intravenous ethacrynic acid to cause gastrointestinal haemorrhage – a feature shared with no other commonly used diuretic (Table 3).

**Table 3** Gastrointestinal bleeding in ethacrynic acid recipients and controls according to heparin administration (percentages in parentheses)*

| | *Frequency of gastrointestinal haemorrhage* | |
|---|---|---|
| | *Ethacrynic acid* | *Controls* |
| Heparin recipients | 16/40 (40) | 14/83 (17) |
| No heparin | 16/117 (14) | 50/1298 (4) |

*For details see Slone *et al.*[21]

### *Drug induced rashes*

By 1973, after the American hospitals had been joined by two Israeli ones, it became apparent that there was a greater than expected frequency of drug-attributed rashes amongst the Israeli patients, and further that this excess was confined to the 42% of Israeli patients who received the analgesic dipyrone: a drug rarely used in USA because of the risk of agranulocytosis. After exclusion of patients who were transfused, the standardized rates for drug rashes (irrespective of the drug incriminated) were 2.3% for American patients, 2.6% for Israeli patients not receiving dipyrone and 6.6% for Israeli dipyrone recipients.[22] A detailed examination of the dipyrone recipients showed that in few was the observed rash actually attributed to this drug, despite the close temporal relationship between drug exposure and onset of rash. It was concluded that dipyrone is a drug which regularly causes rashes in Israeli patients.

Skin rashes occur with a frequency of 2–3% in patients in medical wards. Moreover, since most patients receive drug therapy in hospitals and most rashes seen in hospitalized patients are thought to be drug-induced, this reaction is an ideal one to review independently of the attending physician's or clinical pharmacologist's views on the aetiology of the rash. At a time when there were 22 227 patients in the study there were 507 allergic drug-induced skin reactions reported in some 491 patients. Data analysis was undertaken using a sequential procedure whereby patients exposed to known allergens were sequentially removed from the series. Since penicillins and blood products are known to be major rash-producers (on *a priori* grounds), all patients receiving these preparations were initially excluded from the study. This involved 38% of the patients and 70% of the patients with a rash. For the remaining patients recognition of drugs causing skin reactions depended on the frequency of rashes in treated patients being at least twice that of the untreated ones, and on the fact that there was a clustering of rashes in the days following first exposure to the drugs.[23] Using this procedure some 57 drugs were identified as rash-producers and, perhaps as importantly, many commonly-used drugs were shown not to be associated with allergic reactions.

*Drug induced gastrointestinal haemorrhage*

Using similar techniques, Jick and Porter[24] recently described an analysis of drug-induced gastrointestinal haemorrhage in a series of 16 646 medical patients who had no known medical illness which predisposes to such haemorrhage. This study indicated that major gastrointestinal haemorrhage was rare, occurring in only 57 medical patients (0.3%). Drugs which predispose to this condition were mainly anticoagulants, corticosteroids, ethacrynic acid and aspirin-containing compounds.

## Pre-hospital drug use and reason for hospitalization

Part of the data collected by the monitors when a patient is hospitalized includes a history of previous drug consumption. The format of this question involves a detailed record of drug consumption in the 3 months prior to admission and for those drugs which were taken during this time, a record of the amount consumed (total daily dosage) and the duration of its consumption (length of treatment period). Thus if a patient regularly took drugs for a period which ended 4 months prior to hospitalization this would go unrecorded by the group. While this is regrettable, it was felt that because of selectivity of recall, histories preceding the 3-month period would be so inaccurate as to require more formal confirmation than was possible for economic reasons. Interpretation of the various findings of the programme must be done with this limitation in mind.

An early analysis of the medication history information was published in 1973 by Lawson[25] who sought, unsuccessfully, for an association between regular use of aspirin or aspirin-containing compounds and hospitalization, either for renal disease or with evidence of significant renal disease in the form of elevated levels of blood urea on admission or urinary abnormalities on routine testing. This study proved negative, indicating that substantial numbers of patients may consume analgesics, both containing salicylates alone and in mixtures with other compounds for long periods without evidence of major renal disease. Although essentially a negative study, interpretation of this report should be undertaken with the realization that it contains within it a strong negative confounder in the nature of the initial questionnaire which limits the drug consumption history to the preceding 3 months. Thus if a patient consulted his doctor about symptoms relevant to renal impairment and was found to be a heavy analgesic consumer, that individual may be advised to discontinue analgesics. Were he subsequently to be admitted, say 6 months later, the history of analgesic abuse would go unrecorded. This bias in the data is unlikely to have led to a major distortion in the study referred to above, since analgesic consumers are well known to be unable to discontinue the habit.[26] Nevertheless, the realization of this potential problem led the group to collect an additional piece of information on all new patients interviewed after 1975 – whether the primary discharge diagnosis (and, therefore, presumably the reason for hospitalization) had been made *for the first time* on that occasion. Clearly if that were so, knowledge of the existence of the condition was not present before admission and so could not lead to distortion of the patient's drug-taking habits.

Review of this new study material revealed a strong negative association between regular aspirin intake and non-fatal myocardial infarction.[5] Several reasons for this negative association must be considered, since it is at least biologically a credible one. Aspirin is known to have substantial effects on platelet aggregation and on prostaglandins, both of which may, at least theoretically, be important factors in the genesis of myocardial infarction. The statistical significance of the observed relationship was strong, and has been repeated in two independent studies. Confounding by age, sex, hospital and indication for aspirin can be ruled out on the basis of the data available. Moreover, the association was present among diabetics, hypertensives, those with previous infarctions and those with a secondary diagnosis of arthritis. Information on factors such as personality, diet and exercise were not available, and could, therefore, be potential confounding factors. Likewise since all patients were hospitalized, a similar result could appear were aspirin consumers to suffer a selectively early mortality upon sustaining an acute myocardial infarction, although this is highly unlikely.

Finally, the quality of history-taking was not biased with regard to the hypothesis at issue, since there was no such hypothesis at the time of the first report. Moreover the quality of the history-taking in other respects between patients with myocardial infarction and those with other diagnoses gives good cause to believe that there were no problems with this aspect of the data.

Thus the results of the first study, repeated in two other independent ones, are consistent with the hypothesis that there is a protective effect of aspirin against non-fatal acute myocardial infarction, while by no means establishing the association is definitely a causal one. Final interpretation of these data will await results of several prospective trials currently under way; however, it should be emphasized that these trials will all look for an effect of *aspirin in the secondary prevention of acute myocardial infarction in otherwise healthy people*. As well as giving new impetus to these prospective trials the Boston studies will indicate that if these trials produce a positive result, the aspirin effect reported by the BCDSP applies also to primary prevention and to patients with other predisposing factors such as hypertension, diabetes, etc.

In addition to details of medication history the group collect information on smoking, hot beverage and alcohol consumption. Review of this information by routine scanning of data by the computer revealed a substantial positive association between coffee-drinking and non-fatal myocardial infarction. This association was not due to confounding by age, sex, previous myocardial infarctions, hypertension, congestive heart failure, obesity, diabetes, smoking or occupation, nor was it explained by the use of sugar with the coffee. The study suggests that individuals drinking more than five cups of coffee daily have about twice as great a risk of having an acute myocardial infarction as people drinking none at all.[27] However, like all case-control studies various explanations for this relationship other than a causal one must be considered. In particular an unknown proportion of the patients had had a previous myocardial infarction, and may therefore have increased their coffee consumption in consequence of this. Potential importance of the association between drugs and myocardial infarction was sought from the separate cross-sectional study mounted in 1972 (see below).

Using a case-control approach Stason and colleagues[28] sought for an association between alcohol consumption and non-fatal myocardial infarction. In this study there were 399 cases and 2486 control subjects. No overall association, either positive or negative, between alcohol use and acute myocardial infarction was detected, although there was some evidence of a lower rate in patients consuming six or more drinks daily.

## CROSS-SECTIONAL STUDY OF DRUG USE IN HOSPITALIZED PATIENTS

The aim of this study was to collect a large body of information on pre-hospital drug use from patients admitted to both medical and surgical wards in a circumscribed area of the world. The methods employed in its conduct have been fully described elsewhere.[5] Briefly, patients hospitalized in general medical and surgical wards of 24 hospitals in the greater Boston area were studied. These 24 hospitals contained

6571 beds representing about 45% of the total number of general hospital beds available in the greater metropolitan Boston area which has a population of about 2 800 000.

A review of the information obtained from the 25 000 participants in this study indicates that if the drug-taking habits of this community are representative of Americans in general then at least 75 million adults in the USA take one or more drugs regularly, i.e. at least once per week and usually daily. Over 15 million take aspirin regularly, over 10 million take hypotensive drug therapy and over 5 million take oral contraceptives, with similar numbers taking benzodiazepines and antacids. Approximately 20% of the population consume psychotropic drugs during a 3-month period. Use of such drugs is commoner in females (25%) than males (15%). There is a gradual trend towards increased use in the sixth decade.[29]

## Adverse drug reactions

The information in this study can be used to generate and/or test hypotheses, and to quantitate hazards of drug treatment in the out-patient setting.

An early observation concerned the frequency of fatal drug reactions in patients admitted to surgical services in the participating hospitals.[30] As has been mentioned previously we have good information on the frequency of fatal drug reactions in medical patients.[9] However, it is important not to assume that such events occur with equal frequency in other services. Indeed it can be assumed that their frequency is greatest among medical in-patients who are most likely to be suffering from generalized diseases affecting multiple-organ systems. This assumption is borne out in the information available from this second study. Out of 10 281 surgical patients only 29 died in hospital. Of these, nine died from disseminated cancer, and had not been operated upon during their admission. Of the remaining 20 deaths, nine died as a consequence of complications of operation (six had an infection and three had a haemorrhage); the remainder died of other events post-operatively. Records of all 11 patients whose death was not attributable to operative complications were reviewed in detail. In only two instances was death in part related to adverse effects of drug therapy – a rate of 0.19 drug related deaths per 1000 surgical in-patients (95% confidence limits 0.02–0.71 per 1000). Both deaths occurred in women over the age of 60 years and were associated with bleeding during heparin therapy, i.e. they fall within the high-risk category already defined for heparin recipients in the continuing intensive hospital surveillance programme.[13].

The observed death rate of 0.19 per 1000 surgical in-patients should be compared with that of 0.9 per 1000 medical in-patients.[9]

The data accumulated in this study have been subjected to several routine screening analyses to look for associations between drugs and disease. In such routine analyses many associations are detected, some of which are by their very nature predictable; others are obviously spurious, and yet others require detailed follow-up and careful evaluation.

*Aspirin use and myocardial infarction*

As already indicated, this study was initially undertaken to evaluate independently the negative association between regular aspirin use and acute myocardial infarction seen in the in-patient medical monitoring survey. This it did, showing a similar trend to the previous results, thereby increasing confidence that the reported association was a real one.

*Aspirin use and gastrointestinal haemorrhage*

In a further analysis the relationship between regular use of aspirin-containing compounds and hospital admissions, first for newly-diagnosed peptic ulcers and secondly for major upper gastrointestinal bleeding in the absence of known predisposing conditions, was reviewed.[31] For patients admitted with newly-diagnosed, uncomplicated benign gastric ulcer there was an association with aspirin use on a regular basis for 4 or more days weekly. A similar association existed for those admitted with major gastrointestinal haemorrhage. By contrast aspirin taken regularly for 4 or more days per week was not significantly associated either with bleeding or uncomplicated duodenal ulceration. Nor was there evidence of significant associations between less heavy use of aspirin and these conditions. Assuming that the patients reviewed in this study are drawn from a population of approximately 1.3 million, it is estimated that there were 780 000 people between the ages of 20 and 75 at risk from being included in the study. Thus the data can be used to estimate the incidence rates for hospital admissions for these conditions which are attributable to aspirin use. Overall 10 per 100 000 users per annum appear to be admitted for uncomplicated gastric ulcer, and 15 per 100 000 users per annum for major gastrointestinal haemorrhage. This study, therefore, provides further evidence in favour of an extremely low risk of major gastrointestinal pathology from the consumption of aspirin – a risk which might well be acceptable were this drug to protect against the onset of acute myocardial infarction.

*Oestrogens and gall bladder disease*

Compared with non-users the risks of surgically confirmed gallbladder disease amongst oral contraceptive-taking women between the ages of 20 and 44 years was increased twofold (95% confidence limits for relative risk 1.4 and 2.9). Using the population figures already referred to above, the estimated annual attack rate attributable to oral contraceptives was 79 per 100 000 users. This strong association is unlikely to be due to confounding, and may well be related to changes in bile constituents.[32] A similar association was also seen for post-menopausal oestrogen therapy. Compared with non-users the risks of surgically confirmed gallbladder diseases amongst post-menopausal women aged 45–69 taking oestrogens was increased 2.5 times (95% confidence limits 1.5 and 4.2). The estimated incidence rate attributable to oestrogens was 131 per 100 000 women at risk per annum.[33]

*Oestrogens and venous thromboembolism*

Using techniques similar to those in the above studies, it can be shown that there is a strong relationship between idiopathic venous thromboembolic disease and oral contraceptive use: the risks being increased 11-fold for users as compared with non-users (95% confidence limits 5.2 and 25). In this situation, however, the disease itself is rare amongst non-pregnant women aged 20–44 years. The attack rate is 6 per 100 000 non-users and 66 per 100 000 oral contraceptive users.[34]

There was no significant association between venous thromboembolism and post-menopausal oestrogen therapy, perhaps because the dose of oestrogen given to post-menopausal women is less than that used for oral contraceptive purposes. The overall prevalence of idiopathic venous thromboembolism in this study of women aged 45–69 was estimated at 11 per 100 000 population at risk per annum.

In 1976 Meade *et al.*[35] reported that increased concentrations of coagulation factors in oral contraceptive users was associated with a compensatory increase in fibrinolytic activity in non-smokers but not in smokers. This raised the possibility that smoking may predispose to thromboembolism in oral contraceptive users. In order to test this hypothesis pooled data from both the intensive monitoring programme and the cross-sectional study were reviewed. There were 63 patients admitted primarily because of uncomplicated venous thromboembolism, and for each such patient three controls were sought: matching cases and controls by age, study source and hospital of admission. Both patients and controls were current oral contraceptive users. The prevalence of smoking was equal amongst cases and controls, and there was no association between duration of contraceptive use and thromboembolism within the smoking population. This study, therefore, provides strong evidence against a major effect of smoking on the risk of thromboembolism in a group of otherwise healthy contraceptive users.[36]

*Regular drug use and cancer*

In view of the prevalent concern that drug-use could induce cancer, the accumulated information was reviewed to determine whether any associations could be detected between regular drug usage and the newly diagnosed tumours in 800 patients aged 20–75 years in this cross-sectional study. Drug-use in these patients was compared with that in 3443 patients admitted because of acute illnesses which were not related to cancer or to any need for regular drug-use. Some 56% of the cancer patients and 50% of the controls had used one or more drugs on a regular basis prior to hospitalization. However, since drug-use increases with age, and patients with cancers are on average older than those hospitalized with acute illnesses, when the data were examined by age strata the proportion of regular users of drugs was equal amongst cancer patients and controls. Detailed analysis of these patients indicated that the point estimate of risk ratio for any regular drug-use amongst the group of cancer patients was 0.88 when compared to controls (the 90% upper confidence limit was 1.02). Thus the available information indicates with 90% confidence that less than 1% of cancers identified in this study were likely to have been caused by recent regular drug-use.[37] One caveat to this study is that the numbers of patients with cancer of any one site was small, with the exception of breast and lung where there were 159 and 110 subjects, respectively. In particular there were only 15 patients with gastric cancer, 20 with renal tumours, 21 with pancreatic tumours and 22 with uterine cancer. Thus a drug which infrequently induces any of these relatively rare tumours would not appear with sufficient frequency to be detected by this approach. Moreover, any regular drug which was discontinued up to 3 months before hospitalization would not be recorded in this study, and hence any excess cancer risk due to discontinued regular drug-use will not be accounted for in these analyses. The method is, however, sensitive enough to detect an association between cigarette smoking and cancer in males. Thus for males contrasting the smoking histories of cancer patients and controls, there was an estimated risk of being a current smoker of 1.92 relative to non-smokers in this series (90% confidence limits 1.53–2.42). Further analysis of the data indicated that about 48% of the tumours seen in male smokers could be attributable to smoking, and that amongst the male population in general some 25% of cancers could be due to smoking. Comparable figures for females were 21% and 8%, respectively. Thus although most of the carcinogenic effects of smoking are seen in the lung, they are sufficiently strong to be detected even when all tumours are considered together.

*Reserpine and breast cancer*

Perhaps the report from this study which generated the greatest controversy was that indicating a positive association between reserpine use and breast carcinoma.[38] In brief, a case-control study was undertaken comparing the use of anti-hypertensive drugs in 150 women with newly diagnosed breast tumours and 1200 controls, 600 from medical in-patients and 600 from surgical in-patients. Of the women with breast tumours 11 (7.3%) gave a history of using reserpine-containing drugs as compared with 13 of the medical and 13 of the surgical controls (2.2% each). By contrast use of other anti-hypertensive agents was similar in the three groups (4.7%, 4.3% and

4.8%, respectively). Thus the risk ratio point estimate for breast cancer among reserpine users relative to non-users was 3.5 (95% confidence limits 1.6–8.0). The association was not due to confounding by age, nor was it due to interview bias since it was entirely unsuspected. It appeared to be unrelated to hypertension since other anti-hypertensive drugs were not also associated with the tumour. Nor was it due to selection bias for cases or controls.

Since the association appeared a strong one and has obvious major public health importance, two other studies were commissioned before the results were published. Both showed similar trends, although with neither was the association so strong as in the original study.[39,40] When published, these three studies aroused considerable concern, particularly in countries where reserpine remained a commonly used anti-hypertensive agent whose use might well increase in view of the intensive campaign under way to bring hypertension under control.

The original three studies have since been followed by many others (for review see Henderson).[41] At the time of writing it appears that, on balance, there is an association between reserpine and breast cancer, but that the relative risk lies somewhere between 1.5 and 2.0, i.e. at the lower end of the 95% confidence limits of the first report. Risk ratios of this magnitude are clearly important for such a common disease, but equally clearly the risk of associations of this magnitude arising as a result of confounding are not insignificant. At the present time the demonstrated association appears to be real, but it remains to be proven that it is a causal relationship.

*Hormone replacement therapy and uterine cancer*

It is worth mentioning that the association between hormone replacement therapy (HRT) and uterine cancer[42] was not detected by this second study. There were 22 patients with newly diagnosed uterine cancers in the study and only one was taking hormone replacement therapy, this type of therapy being uncommon on the eastern seaboard of the USA in 1972 when the study was undertaken. The association between HRT and uterine cancer was not detected because it had not occurred in the Boston area at that time. In women with intact uteri in Boston in 1972 less than 0.5% aged 50–75 years had been taking this treatment for more than 5 years. Thus at most 400 women with intact uteri taking HRT for more than 5 years were living in the catchment area of the hospitals surveyed. With a risk ratio of 7–8 times (expected use of HRT in uterine cancer patients), the association could have been detected amongst 22 patients had HRT been more prevalent in the area of the study.

*Smoking and the menopause*

The relationship between cigarette smoking and a natural menopause was evaluated in both sets of data – the intensive monitoring study and the cross-sectional study. In both studies, for each year between ages 44 and 53, more current smokers were post-menopausal than non-smokers.[43] This association seems likely to be a causal one, and has important effects on the interpretation of several investigations of illnesses which are thought to be related to the menopause. In particular Kannell *et al.*[44] reported a higher rate of coronary heart disease in menopausal women when compared to pre-menopausal ones of the same age. Since smoking is strongly correlated with coronary heart disease and was not controlled in the above analyses, apparent association between menopause and coronary heart disease may be confounded by smoking.

## POPULATION-BASED STUDIES

Group Health Co-operative (GHC) is a pre-paid consumer-owned health care plan with approximately 280 000 members primarily resident in the Seattle area. Members in this plan are provided with free drugs, out-patient care and hospital services. Since 1976 all prescriptions written for members receiving out-patient medical attention have been computerized. Likewise diagnostic information obtained during hospitalizations can be obtained from computerized sources in such a manner that out-patient drug usage patterns can be related to events such as hospitalization. A detailed description of the methods used in this programme have been given previously.[6] To date several analyses of this large body of information have been published. The programme is particularly suited to providing information on reasonably common events which arise in patients, either at specific times in their lives (e.g. during pregnancy) or during long-term use of medicines which are in frequent use in the community.

### *Hormones and cancer*

In 1980 Dr Jick and his colleagues reported that although the incidence of breast cancer was similar in women aged 45 years or under, whether or not they were oral contraceptive users, in pre-menopausal women over 45 years of age there was a positive association between *current* oral contraceptive use and breast cancer. Moreover, this association was stronger in women aged 51–55 years than in those aged 46–50 years.[45] These results are the first to demonstrate a significant relationship between oral contraceptives and breast cancer in women over 45 years, although a similar relationship is discernible in data published in 1975 by Fasah and Paffenberger[46] and in 1979 by Vessey *et al.*[47] In view of the these findings the group then went on to review the relationship between replacement oestrogens and breast cancer in menopausal women aged between 45 and 64 years.[48] No relationship was found between replacement oestrogens and breast cancer in women who had had a hysterectomy, whereas there was a positive association between current oestrogen use and breast cancer in naturally menopausal women aged 45–54 years. This relationship was much weaker in older women (aged 55–64 years). Further studies of these associations were undertaken in 1979 when a greater number of subjects were available for review. In this later study,[49] it was reported that rates of breast cancer in this population remained stable in women aged 30–44 and aged 55–64 during the period 1972–79 despite considerable variations in the frequency of use of oestrogen-containing drugs during this period. By contrast, rates of breast cancer in women aged 45–54 appeared to have fallen since 1977 in association with a substantial fall in oestrogen use in women of this age group. In view of the relatively small numbers of subjects involved these results should be regarded as tentative, and the findings need to be repeated in other centres. Nevertheless, they are consistent with a role for current exogenous oestrogen usage in breast cancer in middle-aged women with intact uteri.

Using the same population, Dr Jick and his group showed a sharp downward trend in the incidence of endometrial cancer which paralleled the reduction of prescriptions for replacement oestrogens in Seattle from July 1975 after the studies of Ziel and Finkle.[42]

### *Drugs and congenital disorders*

This system is an ideal one to review possible teratogenic effects of drugs, since virtually all deliveries in Seattle take place in hospital and in all instances, prescriptions filed by members during the preceding 9 months and the dates when they were filed are known. During the period 1977–79 there were 6837 live births, and of those 80 (1.2%) had a congenital disorder. No drugs were taken in greater than expected amounts by the mothers of these abnormal infants. Of particular interest in view of the publicity surrounding these drugs is the fact that the mixture of doxylamine succinate and pyridoxine hydrochloride ('Bendectin' – UK, 'Debendox') was not associated with any disorder.[50] By contrast there was evidence of an association between certain congenital disorders and the use of vaginal spermicides in the time intervals before conception.[51] Although there was no well-defined syndrome seen in these offspring, this may in part be due to variations in timing of use of these compounds in early pregnancy. As the programme at GHC is a continuous one this source will be of increasing value as the experience with pregnancies both normal and abnormal continues to grow.

## *AD-HOC,* CASE-CONTROL STUDIES

As indicated above, the continuing intensive monitoring programme gives reasonably accurate estimates of the acute hazards of drugs used in hospitalized patients. The cross-sectional study undertaken in 1972 gave reasonably accurate information on the drug-consuming habits of a wide variety of patients hospitalized with the most common diseases, and permitted discovery of drug–disease relationships by utilizing case-control analyses. However, the latter study provided little information on conditions which rarely occur in the community under review, and could not uncover associations between infrequently used drugs and conditions which are only moderately prevalent in the community (e.g. uterine cancer). For this reason the group have undertaken a series of *ad hoc* studies into specific problem areas.

*Oestrogens and vascular disease*

In 1975 Mann and his colleagues[52] published information which suggested that there was a considerably increased risk of developing acute myocardial infarction in young women taking oral contraceptives. Because of the widespread publicity surrounding this publication and three other reports, subsequent case-control studies of this problem were likely to face insuperable problems of bias, since the drug at issue was likely to be contraindicated in patients with known risk-factors for the disease in question. For this reason the Boston group decided to utilize data collected in the first 6 months of 1975 (i.e. prior to the Mann report). The source of this information was the Commission on Professional and Hospital Activities (CPHA) – a group collecting demographic and discharge diagnoses from 40% of all hospitals in the USA. Patients under 46 years of age were identified, all of whom survived hospitalization due to acute myocardial infarction. After receiving permission from the patient's hospital and practitioner, all were interviewed by telephone using a standardized questionnaire, and details of their prior drug and disease history was obtained. Using this technique, 26 otherwise healthy pre-menopausal women who had survived an acute myocardial infarction were interviewed. Of these, 20 (77%) were oral contraceptive users compared with only 14 of the 59 women (24%) in the control group: the relative risk estimate being 14, with 90% confidence limits of 5.5 and 37. Moreover, all but two of the 26 women with myocardial infarction were cigarette smokers. Thus this study demonstrated that while myocardial infarction is rare in otherwise healthy young women, the risk in women over 37 years who both smoke and take oral contraceptives is substantial.[53] The risk in non-smoking patients taking oral contraceptives appears much lower.

In addition, this study showed a strong relationship between non-contraceptive oestrogen use and non-fatal acute myocardial infarction; in this case the relative risk estimate was 7.5 (90% confidence limits 2.4 and 24). Again the risk appeared to be localized, or at least predominant amongst cigarette smokers.[54]

Following the success of the above studies, Jick and his colleagues conducted a further study directed towards elucidating the relationship (if any) between oral contraceptives and stroke. The data came from the combined in-patient and cross-sectional studies. They reported that amongst 14 healthy pre-menopausal women who survived hospitalization with a stroke, 11 (79%) were taking oral contraceptives as compared with seven of 56 otherwise healthy control women (13%). The relative risk estimate for stroke amongst users as compared to non-users was 26 (lower confidence limit = 7). In this study, cigarette smoking was only weakly linked to stroke.[55]

## DRUG TOXICITY IN PERSPECTIVE

In a detailed review of the information accumulated by the BCDSP to 1974, Jick concluded that the evidence pointed to the fact that although ADRs annually affect millions of people in the USA and cause hundreds of thousands of hospitalizations, the rates and severity of reactions to individual drugs are remarkably low when consideration is given to their pharmacological potency. The high prevalence of drug-related morbidity and mortality is a reflection of widespread drug-use rather than intrinsic toxicity of particular drugs. Unnecessary drug toxicity was present in only one area of therapy – that of fluid and electrolyte treatment. In this area apparently avoidable drug deaths do occur.[9,56]

Using the techniques described above it is the view of the Boston group,[57] that most common, serious diseases acquired as a result of drug-use can be detected and quantitated. Particular gaps in our knowledge arise, for example, in the case of newly-marketed drugs, where information of the type referred to above is inadequate, and separate studies will be required to evaluate their toxicity in the early post-marketing phases.[58–61] The use of large data-collecting systems such as the Commission on Professional and Hospital Activities adds a new dimension to the type of information available, since this approach permits for the first time the identification of significant numbers of patients suffering from rare diseases who can then be the subjects of case-control investigations for the search for possible drug-related aetiologies.

It should be appreciated that one limitation which is of particular concern in the data collected both by this group and others is the duration of drug history. In particular we have no information on possible drug–disease relationships arising where the causative drug has been given for a period of time (long or short) and then discontinued for several months before the onset of the disease. Nevertheless, providing the limitations of the case-control method are appreciated fully [62] it is our view that this approach can be a powerful tool for elucidating drug–disease relationships.

### Acknowledgement

The author wishes to thank Dr Hershel Jick for his assistance in preparing this chapter.

## References


1. Slone, D., Jick, H., Borda, I., Chalmers, T. C., Feinlieb, M., Muench, H., Lipworth, L. and Bellotti, C. (1966). Drug surveillance utilising nurse monitors. *Lancet*, **2,** 901
2. Danielson, D. A., Porter, J. B., Dinan, B. J., O'Connor, P. C., Lawson, D. H., Kellaway, G. S. M. and Jick, H. (1982). Drug monitoring of surgical patients. *J. Am. Med. Assoc.*, **12,** 1482
3. Lawson, D. H., Shapiro, S., Slone, D. and Jick, H. (1972). Drug surveillance: problems and challenges. *Ped. Clin. N. Am.*, **19,** 117
4. Swett, C. (1974). Adverse reactions to chlorpromazine in psychiatric patients. *Dis. Nerv. Syst.*, **35,** 509
5. Boston Collaborative Drug Surveillance Program. (1974). Regular aspirin intake and acute myocardial infarction. *Br. Med. J.*, **1,** 440
6. Jick, H., Watkins, R. N., Hunter, J. R., Dinan, B, J., Madsen, S., Rothman, K. J. and Walker, A. M. (1979). Replacement Estrogens and Endometrial cancer. *N. Engl. J. Med.*, **300,** 218
7. Jick, H., Miettinen, O. S., Shapiro, S., Lewis, G. P., Siskind, V. and Slone, D. (1970). Comprehensive drug surveillance. *J. Am. Med. Assoc.*, **213,** 1455
8. Lawson, D. H. and Jick, H. (1977). Drug prescribing in hospitals: an international comparison. *Am. J. Pub. Health*, **66,** 644
9. Porter, J. and Jick, H. (1977). Drug related deaths among medical inpatients. *J. Am. Med. Assoc.*, **237,** 289
10. Lawson, D. H., Hutcheon, A. W. and Jick, H. (1978). Life threatening drug reactions amongst medical inpatients. *Scot. Med. J.*, **24,** 127
11. Porter, J. and Jick, H. (1977). Drug induced anaphylaxis, convulsions, deafness and extrapyramidal symptoms. *Lancet*, **1,** 587
12. Miller, R. R. and Jick, H. (1977). Antibiotic-associated colitis. *Clin. Pharmacol. Ther.*, **22,** 1
13. Walker, A. M. and Jick, H. (1980). Predictors of bleeding during heparin therapy. *J. Am. Med. Assoc.*, **244,** 1209
14. Greenblatt, D. J., Allan, M. D. and Shader, R. I. (1977). Toxicity of high dose flurazepam in the elderly. *Clin. Pharmacol. Ther.*, **21,** 355
15. Lawson, D. H., Gloss, D. and Jick, H. (1978). Adverse reactions to methyldopa with special reference to hypotension. *Am. Heart J.*, **96,** 572
16. Boston Collaborative Drug Surveillance Program. (1973). Diphenylhydantoin side effects and serum albumin levels. *Clin. Pharmacol. Ther.*, **14,** 529
17. Boston Collaborative Drug Surveillance Program. (1972). Tetracycline and drug attributed rises in blood urea nitrogen. *J. Am. Med. Assoc.*, **220,** 377.
18. Sellers, E. M. and Koch-Weser, J. (1970). Potentiation of warfarin-induced hypoprothrombinemia by chloral hydrate. *N. Engl. J. Med.*, **283,** 827
19. Boston Collaborative Drug Surveillance Program. (1972). Interaction between chloral hydrate and warfarin. *N. Engl. J. Med.*, **286,** 53
20. Miller, R. R. (1977). Effects of smoking on drug action. *Clin. Pharmacol. Ther.*, **22,** 749
21. Slone, D., Jick, H., Lewis, G. P., Shapiro, S. and Miettinen, O. S. (1969). Intravenously given ethacrynic acid and gastrointestinal bleeding. *J. Am. Med. Assoc.*, **209,** 1668
22. Levy, M. (1973). Dipyrone as a cause of drug rashes: an epidemiologic study. *Int. J. Epidemiol.*, **2,** 167
23. Arndt, K. A. and Jick, H. (1976). Rate of cutaneous reactions to drugs. *J. Am. Med. Assoc.*, **258,** 918
24. Jick, H. and Porter, J. (1978). Drug-induced gastrointestinal bleeding. *Lancet*, **2,** 87
25. Lawson, D. H. (1973). Analgesic consumption and impaired renal function. *J. Chron. Dis.*, **26,** 39
26. Murray, R. M., Lawson, D. H. and Linton, A. L. (1971). Analgesic nephropathy: clinical syndrome and prognosis. *Br. Med. J.*, **1,** 479
27. Boston Collabororative Drug Surveillance Program. (1972). Coffee drinking and acute myocardial infarction. *Lancet*, **2,** 1278

28. Stason, W. B., Neff, R. K., Miettinen, O. S. and Jick, H. (1976). Alcohol consumption and non-fatal myocardial infarction. *Am. J. Epidemiol.*, **104,** 603
29. Greenblatt, D. J., Shader, R. I. and Koch-Weser, J. (1975). Psychotropic drug use in the Boston area. *Arch. Gen. Psychiat.*, **32,** 518
30. Armstrong, B., Dinan, B. and Jick, H. (1976). Fatal drug reactions in patients admitted to surgical services. *Am. J. Surg.*, **132,** 643
31. Levy, M. (1974). Aspirin use in patients with major upper gastrointestinal bleeding and peptic ulcer disease. *N. Engl. J. Med.*, **290,** 1158
32. Boston Collaborative Drug Surveillance Program. (1973). Oral contraceptives and venous thromboembolic disease, surgically confirmed gallbladder disease and breast tumours. *Lancet*, **1,** 1399
33. Boston Collaborative Drug Surveillance Program. (1974). Surgically confirmed gallbladder disease, venous thromboembolism and breast tumours in relation to post-menopausal oestrogen therapy. *N. Engl. J. Med.*, **290,** 15
34. Boston Collaborative Drug Surveillance Program. (1973). Oral contraceptives and venous thromboembolic disease, surgically confirmed gallbladder disease and breast tumours. *Lancet*, **1,** 1399
35. Meade, T. W., Brozovic, M., Chakrabarti, R., Howarth, D. J., North, W. R. S. and Stirling, Y. (1976). An epidemiological study of the haemostatic and other effects of oral contraceptives. *Br. J. Haematol.*, **34,** 353
36. Lawson, D. H., Davidson, J. F. and Jick, H. (1977). Oral contraceptive use and venous thromboembolism: absence of an effect of smoking. *Br. Med. J.*, **2,** 729
37. Smith, P. G. and Jick, H. (1977). Regular drug use and cancer. *J. Natl. Cancer Inst.*, **59,** 1387
38. Boston Collaborative Drug Surveillance Program. (1974). Reserpine and breast cancer. *Lancet*, **2,** 669
39. Armstrong, B., Stevens, N. and Doll, R. (1974). Retrospective study of the association between use of rauwolfia derivatives and breast cancer in English women. *Lancet*, **2,** 672
40. Heinonen, O. P., Shapiro, S., Tuominen, L. and Turumen, M. I. (1974). Reserpine use in relation to breast cancer. *Lancet*, **2,** 675
41. Henderson, M. (1977). Reserpine and breast cancer: a review. In Colombo, F., Shapiro, S., Slone, D. and Tognoni, G. (eds.) *Epidemiological Evaluation of Drugs.* p. 211 (North Holland: Elsevier)
42. Ziel, H. K. and Finkle, W. D. (1975). Increased risk of endometrial carcinoma among users of conjugated oestrogens. *N. Engl. J. Med.*, **293,** 1167
43. Jick, H., Porter, J. and Morrison, A. S. (1977). Relation between smoking and age of natural menopause. *Lancet*, **1,** 1354
44. Kannell, W. B., Hjortland, M. C., McNamara, P. M. and Gordon, T. (1976). Menopause and risk of cardiovascular disease. *Ann. Intern. Med.*, **85,** 447
45. Jick, H., Walker, A. M., Watkins, R. N., d'Ewart, D. C., Hunter, J. R., Danford, A., Madsen, S., Dinan, B. J. and Rothman, K. J. (1980). Oral contraceptives and breast disease. *Am. J. Epidemiol.*, **112,** 577
46. Fasah, E. and Paffenberger, R. S. (1975). Oral contraceptives as related to cancer and benign lesions of the breast. *J. Natl. Cancer Inst.*, **55,** 767
47. Vessey, M. P., Doll, R., Jones, K., MacPherson, K. and Yeates, D. (1979). An epidemiologic study of oral contraceptives and breast cancer. *Br. Med. J.*, **1,** 1757
48. Jick, H., Walker, A. M., Watkins, R. N., d'Ewart, D. C., Hunter, J. R., Danford, A., Madsen, S., Dinan, B. J. and Rothman, K. J. (1980). Replacement estrogens and breast cancer. *Am. J. Epidemiol.*, **112,** 586
49. Lawson, D. H., Jick, H., Hunter, J. R., Madsen, S. (1981). Exogenous estrogens and breast cancer. *Am. J. Epidemiol.*, **114,** 710
50. Jick, H., Holmes, L. B., Hunter, J. R., Madsen, S., Stergacluis, A. (1981). First-trimester drug use in congenital disorders. *J. Am. Med. Assoc.*, **246,** 343
51. Jick, H., Walker, A. M., Rothman, K. J., Hunter, J. R., Holmes, L. B., Watkins, R. N., d'Ewart, D. C., Danford, A. and Madsen, S. (1981). Vaginal spermicides and congenital disorders. *J. Am. Med. Assoc.*, **245,** 1329
52. Mann, J. I., Vessey, M. P., Thorogood, M. and Doll, R. (1975). Myocardial infarction

in young women with special reference to oral contraceptive practice. *Br. Med. J.*, **2,** 241
53. Jick, H., Dinan, B. and Rothman, K. J. (1978). Oral contraceptives and non-fatal myocardial infarction. *J. Am. Med. Assoc.*, **239,** 1403
54. Jick, H., Dinan, B. and Rothman, K .J. (1978). Non-contraceptive estrogens and non-fatal myocardial infarction. *J. Am. Med. Assoc.*, **239,** 1407
55. Jick, H., Porter, J. and Rothman, K. J. (1978). Oral contraceptives and non-fatal stroke in healthy women. *Ann. Intern. Med.*, **88,** 58
56. Lawson, D.H. (1974). Adverse reactions to potassium chloride. *Q. J. Med.*, **43,** 433
57. Jick, H. (1974). Drugs – remarkably non-toxic. *N. Engl. J. Med.*, **291,** 824
58: Inman, W. H. W., (1977). Recorded release. In Gross, F. H. and Inman, W. H. W. (eds.) *Drug Monitoring*. pp. 65–78. (London: Academic Press)
59. Dollery, C. T. and Rawlins, M. D. (1977). Monitoring adverse reactions to drugs. *Br. Med. J.*, **1,** 96
60. Lawson, D. H. and Henry, D. A. (1977). Monitoring adverse reactions to new drugs: restricted release or monitored release? *Br. Med. J.*, **1,** 691
61. Jick, H., Walker, A. M., Spriet-Pourra, C. (1979). Postmarketing follow-up. *J. Am. Med. Assoc.*, **242,** 2310
62. Jick, H. and Vessey, M. P. (1978). Case-control studies in the evaluation of drug induced illness. *Am. J. Epidemiol.*, **107,** 1

# 18
# Intensive monitoring in hospitals II: The Aberdeen–Dundee System

D. C. MOIR

## INTRODUCTION

Concern about side-effects of drugs, and the best ways of recognizing them, has repeatedly been expressed in recent years and it would appear that this is justified for two reasons. First, clinical trials of new drugs may not be sufficiently sensitive to detect the occurrence of side-effects unsuspected on the basis of preliminary toxicological investigation in animals; and secondly, since serious adverse effects tend to be infrequent, and may occur only after prolonged administration, all adverse effects may not be revealed until a drug has been in general clinical use for some time. Thus, the primary aim in drug monitoring is to diminish the time between the marketing of a drug and the full recognition of its capacity to produce undesirable effects. This aim can only be achieved if the following facilities are available:

(1) A means of identifying previously unsuspected adverse effects.

(2) A mechanism whereby suspected adverse reactions can be confirmed or refuted, and if confirmed the frequency with which they occur in the population determined.

Two main methods of drug monitoring have been developed in the last 15 years: comprehensive surveillance and voluntary reporting to national early warning systems. The most successful and practical example of comprehensive surveillance in hospitals is The Boston Collaborative Drug Surveillance Program,[1] and while such a system can reliably detect adverse reactions which are of a high frequency, it is not so suitable for low-frequency effects where very large numbers are required to obtain significant results. Indeed the cost involved in setting up such an organization limits its wider application in the routine detection of adverse drug reactions (ADRs). The results achieved by voluntary reporting schemes have also met with limited success, largely because of the low response from doctors. Nevertheless this technique has at the present time an important role to play in the detection of previously unsuspected adverse effects. However, even when a drug is suspected of causing a particular side-effect it is difficult to identify a population which has been exposed to the drug and is, therefore, at risk; thus the advantages of the individual contributions to the centralized early warning system may be lost.

## MEDICINES EVALUATION AND MONITORING GROUP: DEVELOPMENT OF A PATIENT-DRUG FILE

The Medicines Evaluation and Monitoring Group (MEMO) have directed their activities to this later stage in the investigation of adverse effects by developing a patient–drug file which facilitates the identification of:

(1) All patients receiving a particular drug; and subsequently

(2) The number of patients exhibiting a specific adverse effect associated with the administration of that drug.

Thus it becomes possible to investigate reported ADRs including suspicions raised by early warning systems and also to ascertain the clinical importance of recognized effects. Major ADRs are, despite the use of many potent pharmacological agents, a relatively rare occurrence, and the patient–drug file can only be of value if it contains information about the drugs taken by a large number of patients, and if this information is held in such a way as to allow rapid and meaningful analysis.

Accurate medication records are the first requirement for the development of such a file, and the standardized prescription records introduced to the Aberdeen Hospitals in the mid-1960s permitted this.[2] The prescribing records written by doctors, and subsequently used by the nurses when administering the individual doses and by the pharmacists when replenishing ward supplies, were shown to be sufficiently complete to make the routine production of a file worthwhile, and in particular it appeared that the data available in the file would be likely to reflect the true situation in the ward. However, even with access to the data from an entire teaching hospital, it appeared that only frequently prescribed drugs could be evaluated in an acceptable period of time; therefore the introduction of similar records to other centres and the development of compatible files would facilitate national collaboration in the study of low-frequency ADRs. Indeed, similar records were introduced to the Dundee Hospitals in 1972 and these two centres now have compatible files.

Data on each patient discharged are collected from two sources: (1) the inpatient Scottish Morbidity Return and (2) the prescribing records. Patient identification and diagnoses are abstracted from the Scottish Morbidity Return and linked with the drugs from the prescription sheets to form a patient–drug file.[3] Processing of this file, which originated in Aberdeen in 1968, progressed through manual to mechanical methods, ultimately using computer facilities to handle the vast amounts of data generated by the teaching hospital group each year. The Dundee hospitals started contributing data to the file in 1972 and all major hospitals in Aberdeen and Dundee are included, covering some 4300 beds, the discharge rate being approximately 70 000 each year. Each patient receives on average 4.3 drugs per admission; the total number of prescriptions added to the file annually is in the region of 300 000. At the present time the total file comprises data on approximately 525 000 patient discharges and in excess of 2 million prescriptions. The drugs recommended on discharge from hospital are also incorporated in the file whether or not they were prescribed during the relevant hospital admission.

In 1968 the coding of the drugs abstracted by MEMO posed a problem, since at that time existing drug codes were not comprehensive, and included only those drugs for which ADRs had been reported, whereas MEMO wished to enter on the file all drugs prescribed in the hospitals which were contributing to the file. In addition, drug codes were not unique for multiple-ingredient drugs, and it was therefore impossible to obtain rapid retrieval of information about a specific preparation. MEMO therefore developed its own drug index which contained the names of all drugs (including synonyms) used by hospitals feeding data to MEMO, and the names and the corresponding five-digit code number[4] are held in a computer dictionary. The drugs are processed by name only, with automatic coding by the computer. The five-digit code is meaningful and incorporates a therapeutic classification; two additional digits may be added to indicate the pharmacological group of the drug. A facility is included which allows processing by route and frequency of drug administration. The diagnoses are coded using the International Classification of Disease four-digit code.[5]

The data abstraction for such large numbers also produces a problem since records become available spasmodically, making the work load uneven; therefore a method of abstracting the data in the central medical records department without patients' case-notes being out of file for an unacceptable period of time had to be devised. A duplicate prescription sheet was introduced to the wards, and on return of the case-notes to the central department it was possible to remove the copy for data-processing while the original was filed in the case-notes; this method alleviated the problem produced by uneven work load.

The patient identification and diagnoses are abstracted by the medical records department staff and the prescribing data on the duplicate prescription sheet are handled by MEMO staff. The data abstracted are subsequently transferred to punch-cards, and the verified cards are processed using a Honeywell computer installation; a suite of programs allows linkage of the data and information retrieval depending on the drug problem being tackled.

The value of any such file depends on the quality of the data fed in, and it is only possible to draw valid conclusions if the data are complete and accurate. Since the data in the patient–drug file are concerned with the diagnosis and treatment of disease it is of paramount importance that a high standard is maintained in respect of:

(i) The completeness of records; and
(ii) The accuracy with which the original transcription and coding documents are completed.

Although initial studies had shown that a sufficient number of prescribing records were available to make routine production of the file worthwhile, it cannot be assumed that this will remain so; checks were therefore incorporated into the routine data collection. While it is not possible to check that a prescription is correct at the time it is written, the quality of the prescription sheets routinely available for data abstraction are assessed periodically and confirm that a high standard of prescribing has been maintained. In addition there is no routine check on the accuracy of the data transcribed or coded since the error rates were low and acceptable compared with the cost of routinely checking the data. All punched cards are, however, verified and on transference to computer storage are subjected to a data-vet which rejects all cards with obviously incompatible information. Thus the computer would, for example, query data which suggested that a male patient had been discharged with a gynaecological diagnosis. Retrieval of data from the file itself in answer to *ad hoc* queries has also lent support to the good overall quality of the data in the file, for in such circumstances after the initial retrieval from the file has been made, in-depth searches of patients' notes are usually necessary; these have confirmed the accuracy of data in the file.

## USES OF THE PATIENT-DRUG FILE

### Investigation of suspected adverse reactions

In the main, the file has been used to aid *ad hoc* investigations such as suspicions raised by the Committee on Safety of Medicines. The file permits rapid identification of the total population who have received a suspect drug or combination of drugs in hospital and it is, therefore, possible to follow-up such patients by examining their case-records, by interview or by carrying out appropriate investigations to determine whether the patients exhibit the suspected effect. Before any conclusions can be drawn it is usually necessary to determine the frequency with which similar effects occur in a suitably matched population not receiving the drug in question. Controlled studies are necessary to confirm or refute suspicions, and since the file includes parameters such as age, sex, diagnoses and length of hospital stay, it is possible to obtain matched populations according to any of these parameters but differing in respect of the drugs they have taken. Numerous studies have been carried out using the file in this way to investigate suspicions raised by the Committee on Safety of Medicines.

One such study was the investigation of a possible association between the administration of spironolactone and the subsequent development of breast cancer in 1975. The file was searched and 1200 patients identified who had received spironolactone during a hospital admission between 1969 and 1974. Of these, 13 had been hospitalized at some time with a diagnosis of breast cancer but in only two instances was the spironolactone prescribed prior to the diagnosis of breast cancer.

Since it seemed likely that a drug suspected of a carcinogenic effect might have been administered over a long period of time, patients with breast cancer between 1969 and 1974 were also identified and their hospital records searched for any evidence of previous spironolactone administration. The records of two matched control groups were also searched. One control group comprised patients with a cancer other than breast cancer, while the second group comprised patients with non-malignant disorders. Controls were matched by age, sex, year of hospital admission, general practitioner and marital state. Thereafter their general practitioner records were also searched and the records of patients who had died and which were held centrally were scrutinized also. It was ultimately possible to compare the prescribing of spironolactone in 646 matched sets and it was found to be low in all groups; two in the breast cancer group, two in the cancer control and five in the non-malignant control group. The result did not, therefore, support an association between breast cancer and the prior administration of spironolactone.

While the basic principles of numerator/denominator monitoring are followed in each case, each investigation will have certain unique features and it should be possible to manipulate the data in the file to facilitate the investigation, as in the investigation of a suspected association between the administration of methaqualone and peripheral neuritis. In this study the likelihood of peripheral neuritis occurring in patients on long-term therapy was increased, and so patients who had received methaqualone on two consecutive hospital admissions were identified in the file.

The case notes of 50 such patients were studied, but there was no evidence to suggest that any had a peripheral neuropathy. It was also possible to identify all patients who had received methaqualone in hospital and had a diagnosis of neuritis recorded on discharge. The case-notes of 49 such patients were reviewed, but in none of these was methaqualone thought to be the causative agent. A further 17 patients who had received methaqualone and had an adverse reaction to a hypnotic or sedative reported in the discharge diagnosis were also studied; there was no evidence of peripheral neuropathy. Since there was no evidence to support the association, the investigation was discontinued until further suspicions are raised. However, had there been evidence of peripheral neuropathy in some of these patients it would have been necessary to obtain closely matched control patients, except that the controls would not be receiving the suspect medicine.

Other studies involving small numbers of patients, and yet again others involving hundreds of patients and controls, have been carried out and have been reported elsewhere, such as:

The cardiotoxicity of amitriptyline[6]
Rauwolfia derivatives and breast cancer[7]
Psychomimetic effects of pentazocine and dihydrocodeine tartrate[8]
L-dopa and direct antiglobulin tests[9]

Each study is carried out in two stages; the file is searched to ascertain some basic items of information such as the prescribing rate of the drug concerned. Thereafter a few sets of case-notes are searched to identify potential problems. The protocol drafted for the study can subsequently be amended in the light of the information available in the patients' case-records, and this type of preliminary investigation has proved particularly useful. If it appears that the desired information is not available, the study will not proceed to the second stage. On the other hand, if sufficient patients can be identified in the file, and it seems likely that the suspected effect could be recognized, then care must be taken to ensure that bias is not introduced by the observer actively looking for the effect and so disturbing the findings. This can be avoided if the controls are selected appropriately, and in view of the size of the file with the wide range of diagnoses from which controls can be drawn it is usually easy to obtain very closely matched control populations and hence reduce any such bias. Furthermore, during the course of a study, the researchers are not necessarily aware of whether they are studying a case or control, and in this way any bias is reduced still further.

A diagnosis may also be used as the starting point for the investigation of a possible association with a particular drug, as was the case in a preliminary study of gastric carcinoma and cimetidine.[10] All patients discharged from the Aberdeen Hospitals between 1977 and October 1979 with a diagnosis of gastric carcinoma were identified. Thus, the case notes of 304 patients were scrutinized to ascertain whether any of these patients had received cimetidine. Nineteen records were discarded since some had been diagnosed prior to 1977, and others had a cancer other than gastric carcinoma. Eighteen case notes were not available for study, but the remaining 277 were examined. There was no mention of cimetidine in 262 case notes. Cimetidine had been given to the remaining 15 patients as follows: in three, cimetidine was first given after the diagnosis of cancer had been made, and in five cimetidine was given in hospital, before the diagnosis was made, but after the onset of symtoms. In seven patients, cimetidine was given prior to the diagnosis of cancer. These patients had had symptoms for 20 years, 10 year, 5 years, 4 years, 15 months, 6 months and 'after a long time unspecified', and they received cimetidine for 2 months, 3 months, 1 month, 6 months, 3 months, 3 months and less than 3 months, respectively. Two of these patients had radiographically and endoscopically proven gastric ulcers, 4 had duodenal ulcers, while the other had a long standing dyspeptic history with a negative radiograph.

The value of collaborating with other centres with similar data, has already been described, and in this particular instance, 95 patients, who had gastric cancer, were selected at random from those patients discharged between March 1976 and December 1979, from Ninewells Hospital, Dundee. Four of these patients were found to have received cimetidine, but one was discarded because the final diagnosis was lymphosarcoma. Of the remaining three, cimetidine was given to these patients prior to the diagnosis of cancer being made. All had long histories of dyspepsia in excess of 10 years, two patients had received cimetidine for up to 2 months, while the length of treatment in the third patient could not be determined. Two patients had a benign ulcer demonstrated radiographically on the lesser curvature, and the third case had achlorhydria and was found to have an anaplastic carcinoma at the site of an entero-anastamosis.

In the course of this study patients who had received cimetidine were also identified, and of a hundred patients in Aberdeen, and 140 in Dundee, who had received cimetidine during the course of a hospital admission, no cases of gastric cancer were found.

In an attempt to determine the importance of these findings, a study was undertaken to ascertain the frequency with which apparently benign gastric ulcers became malignant. All patients discharged from the Aberdeen Hospitals between 1968 and 1979, with a diagnosis of gastric ulcer, who subsequently had a diagnosis of gastric carcinoma recorded, were identified. 1520 patients had a diagnosis of gastric ulcer and 46 of these subsequently had gastric carcinoma recorded. Nine patients had both diagnoses recorded for the same admission and a further 23 were diagnosed as having gastric carcinoma on a second admission within 4 months; it seems likely that these were missed cases. Fourteen cases of cancer were diagnosed between 4 months and 5 years after the initial diagnosis of gastric ulcer, suggesting that one would expect a gastric carcinoma to occur in less than 1% of the population with diagnosed gastric ulcer, as compared with 4 of the 10 cases of gastric cancer who had had a gastric ulcer previously and had received cimetidine out of 371 cases studied in Aberdeen and Dundee.

The consensus of all these findings was equivocal, and it was not possible to either confirm or refute the possible association between gastric cancer and cimetidine. Scrutiny of case records did however highlight the difficulties experienced in diagnosing gastric carcinoma, and drew attention to the need for vigilance in prescribing cimetidine which could mask undiagnosed cancer.

## Drug–drug and drug–disease interactions

The file also facilitates the identification of patients receiving two or more drugs during the same hospital admission making the investigation of drug–drug interactions possible. Many such drug–drug interactions have now been recognized. On occasions these interactions may be beneficial, but as they can also be undesirable it is necessary to know the clinical importance of these interactions. The file makes it possible to trace people who have or are continuing to receive specified combinations of drugs and who can be examined for the occurrence of the suspected and unwanted effect.

Since the file also includes diagnoses it is possible to study drug–disease interactions which may be of particular value, as in liver and kidney disease where drug metabolism may be altered, often leading to an increase in pharmacological and toxic effects. Thus drug effects can be studied in populations receiving specific drug combinations in association with specified diseases, and drug exclusions can be made if appropriate. Similarly, control populations can be identified from the file, controls receiving only one of the two suspect drugs.

## Hazards of long-term therapy

Patients continuing on specific forms of therapy on a recurrent or long-term basis may have a greater chance of developing ADRs which may not have become apparent in the initial clinical trials or in the early years after the drug has first been marketed. The facility to identify patients on the file for whom long-term treatment has been prescribed in hospital and recommended on discharge is therefore of particular value, and may be used in the investigation of possible carcinogenic, mutagenic or teratogenic effects as in the study of rauwolfia derivatives and breast cancer. As the years go by, the file becomes increasingly useful in this respect, and the data in the file can be retrieved so as to indicate first of all patients who have been hospitalized recently and are continuing with the long-term therapy, or alternatively those who have been given the drug on a previous, but not necessarily the most recent, admission; this latter facility has proved to be of value in the follow-up of patients on beta-blockers. Patients can also be retrieved by other factors such as the distance they live from the hospital, so that in monitoring situations where it is desirable to see the patients and there are large numbers available for study, patients living near the monitoring centre may be studied first, provided this does not introduce bias.

### New drugs

Monitoring of newly marketed drugs also becomes possible. Patients who have received new drugs can be identified on the file and their records searched, and/or the patients investigated to ascertain whether they have experienced any untoward effects. Alternatively, the file can be used to indicate those units within our hospital group which are using a specific new medication, and prospective investigation of patients in these units can be carried out in an attempt to detect adverse reactions to the new drug.

### Drug efficacy

There are of course also problems in determining the effectiveness of a drug, and the facility to identify large numbers of patients receiving specific drugs can also be used to investigate drug efficacy and is likely to be of particular value in patients on long-term therapy. Study of a drug as it is used in everyday clinical practice may produce different results from those obtained during the course of rigorously controlled clinical trials, because of the heterogeneity of factors in the real life situation, variation in types of prescriber and indications for use, the existence of multiple pathology and differences in patients' behaviour, in particular their compliance. In addition to information about the adverse and beneficial effects of drugs, information is also required about the benefits in relation to their cost and methods of carrying out cost–benefit analyses of drugs with similar intent need to be developed.

## IMPROVEMENTS AND DEVELOPMENTS

The main benefit of the type of monitoring approach described above is its simplicity and ability to identify populations at risk. Indeed, the data collection is very limited and rarely can suspicions be confirmed or refuted by using the file alone. In practice, it was of course our intention to return to the original case-record to obtain the necessary information, and upgrading the system to include this would involve a very substantial increase in costs. The data, although limited, are gathered from a complete section of the population likely to have a high exposure to new and potent drugs. Thus it would appear that monitoring of new drugs can most readily be undertaken in the hospital, whereas it may not be the most appropriate place for monitoring drugs given over an extended period of time.

Although relatively few items of information are collected about the drugs prescribed in hospital, MEMO felt it necessary, since the file stood in excess of $1\frac{1}{2}$ million prescriptions, to review the data currently collected and the uses to which they had been put. Interestingly, the studies undertaken in the last 10 years had almost exclusively related to drugs given over long periods of time. Drugs prescribed regularly in hospital were considered to be essential for such activities, and an attempt was subsequently made to estimate the value of storing prescriptions in the file which had been given on one occasion only. Analysis showed that 20% of prescriptions in the file had been given on one occasion only, and these have recently been excluded from the data collection system since it was felt that their continued collection could not be justified. The resources so freed were, therefore, devoted to developing a system for recording drugs given on repeat prescription in general practice. The records of repeat prescription subsequently proved to be sufficiently accurate to make abstraction of data worthwhile, and a repeat prescription file is now maintained for seven practices, staffed by 29 principals in general practice, and comprising information on repeat prescribing for some 75 000 patients. This file facilitates still further the identification of patients on long-term drug therapy and both files can now be used in the follow-up of suspected adverse reactions.

Some drugs given in hospital continue to be prescribed after discharge and may be given over long periods of time, while certain medications are used almost exclusively in the community and monitoring techniques need to be developed for that situation also. For example, the oral contraceptive which has been at the centre of many ADR enquiries appears relatively infrequently in the MEMO file since its use originates in the community. Similarly, files based in hospital tend to have few prescriptions for common-cold remedies and appetite-suppressants although such preparations may be repeated frequently in general practice. The resources freed by discontinuing the collection of once-only prescriptions in hospital are now being devoted to developing the records and systems which will facilitate the retrieval of such drugs taken by patients attending hospital outpatient departments or drugs given repeatedly in general practice. Furthermore the majority of pregnant women are not hospitalized in early pregnancy and so the MEMO file does not contain information about the drugs given at a time when they are most likely to be associated with the occurrence of congenital abnormalities. Since, however, the majority of pregnant women in our area visit the hospital ante-natal clinic at the end of the first trimester, a pilot study is currently in progress to establish the best method of ascertaining information about the drugs taken in the first 3 months of pregnancy. The need to develop systems of monitoring drugs taken in the community is urgent. The hospital files have, therefore, been suspended in Dundee, and the resources are currently being used to develop systems of monitoring the drugs prescribed in general practice.

## GENERAL DISCUSSION

The Aberdeen–Dundee system is primarily a hypothesis-testing base and was not intended as a means of detecting previously unsuspected adverse effects. The patient–drug file has, however, now become a huge data-bank which can be exploited for this purpose. The frequency of ADRs has been shown to increase in proportion to the number of drugs prescribed[11] and as patients receiving large numbers of different drugs during one hospital admission can readily be identified on the file, investigation of such patients may reveal both recognized and unrecognized toxicity. Length of stay has also been shown to correlate with the frequency of ADRs, and investigation of long-stay patients identified in the patient–drug file may also prove an equally valuable starting point in monitoring for previously unsuspected ADRs.

The possibility of exploiting the diagnostic information has also been investigated, for as the data accumulate it is possible to detect changes in the frequency or pattern of known and potential ADRs, e.g. blood dyscrasias. Patients' case-records can be studied in the first instance to ascertain the aetiology of the blood dyscrasia. For example, preliminary studies have shown that while the occurrence of two-thirds of such dyscrasias are readily explicable, including those ascribed to previously recognized ADRs, the remainder are unexplained and may be potentially unsuspected ADRs. Detailed ascertainment of the drugs taken concurrently by such patients may show clustering of a potential reaction around one drug or a group of chemically related drugs, and thus previously unsuspected reactions may be identified. As already described, the file can be used to facilitate the study of long-term hazards, where diagnoses such as blood dyscrasias may be the subject for investigation; so the ability to link diagnoses made on one or subsequent admissions with treatment given in the past is of great value.

Although populations are readily identified on the file there may, on occasion, when an infrequently prescribed drug is suspected of causing an ADR, be an inadequate number of patients to provide a meaningful result in an acceptable period of time. Alternatively, the suspected hazard may be of such severity that protracted enquiries are unacceptable, and hence an experiment using the multi-centre approach was undertaken in the investigation of the possible breast cancer-rauwolfia association.[7] While the participation of more than one centre was certainly advantageous in that situation, the investigators found that some difficulties in communication were inevitable. These were most noticeable during the design of the protocols despite the considerable amount of time spent discussing practical issues as they arose. Interestingly, problems encountered in one centre were subsequently mirrored in another, since it was inevitable that the different centres worked at different speeds. This was the first occasion we had had to work together in this way and we did not achieve absolute standardization between the centres; nevertheless, with hindsight this should not have been impossible. The final analyses and validation of results consequently required a considerable expenditure of resources but it was, nevertheless, reassuring to find the results, considered independently or in combination, consistent. Indeed, the problems due to lack of absolute standardization were compensated for by the larger numbers which allowed more adequate consideration of possibly associated factors.

Even with large numbers and statistically significant associations drug monitoring can never establish with certainty the cause and effect relationship between a drug and an adverse effect, and pharmacological investigation is necessary to elucidate the mechanism of the adverse effect. This information is frequently difficult to come by, and so in the real-life situation decisions whether or not to prescribe a drug have to be made after giving due consideration to the therapeutic benefit achieved by the drug compared with likely adverse effects.

In addition to facilitating studies of drug efficacy and toxicity, information can also be retrieved from the file to demonstrate how adequately agreed procedures are being carried out. This may be of value to medical, nursing and secretarial staff in their practical management of various aspects of the drug-handling systems used in our hospitals. Information about the therapeutic practices of the various clinical teams has also been retrieved and circulated, and the prescribing pattern of new medicines is of particular interest. Subsequent retrieval of identical information will demonstrate whether practice has changed or stayed the same, and while it is important not to overplay this technique it is possible that it may have a role in continuing education and may go some way towards encouraging more rational and economic prescribing.

The time expended on the various studies is closely related to the nature of the enquiry. It is, however, fortunate that the enquiries made of the file are sporadic since investigations such as that of the supected breast cancer–rauwolfia derivative association, involving the follow-up of some 4500 patients, took MEMO staff over 9 months to complete, at an estimated cost in 1974 of £15 000. Thus, even with two centres concentrating virtually all their resources on one problem there was still a 9-month delay from the inception of the study to the availability of a statistically acceptable result. If all the information required to answer this query had been held on a computer file then the result would have been available very much more quickly; the cost of such a system would, however, be prohibitive.

Through the years MEMO has been variously financed by University and Health Boards funds, the World Health Organization and presently by the Department of Health and Social Security and the Scottish Home and Health Department. The policies are formulated by a steering group, two members of which provide the day-to-day supervision in each of the two centres. Only one of these is supported by MEMO, although all other professional staff, e.g. part-time medical staff, research nurses and pharmacists and secretarial and clerical staff are supported by MEMO funds which amount at present to £40 000 per annum. The various activities undertaken by MEMO have been costed, and in 1984 processing prescriptions cost £6 per 100 prescriptions processed. Follow-up of patients cost £4.50 per follow-up attempted and £8 per follow-up completed, since in any study a certain number of patients are not successfully followed up owing to, for example, emigration, failure to meet with certain criteria on follow-up, being temporary residents or being untraceable. Small studies are relatively inexpensive whereas larger controlled studies require considerable resources as already described, for not only must the file be maintained; it is also essential to have staff with the necessary expertise to carry out such monitoring studies when the opportunity arises. While resources are undoubtedly important, this method of investigating drug-induced disease involves many disciplines, and collaboration is also of vital importance. Good communications between patient and nurse, pharmacist and doctor to mention but a few are all essential to the efficient maintenance of the hospital drug-handling system and to the planning and implementation of monitoring projects. Furthermore, when low-frequency reactions are being investigated, collaboration at a national, or even international, level may be necessary in order to confirm or refute the suspected reaction within an acceptable period of time. The aim of the Medicines Evaluation and Monitoring Group was to devise a comprehensive but flexible system which could be used to study various drug problems; while it may not be justified for any single purpose, the wide range of problems concerned with drug usage which it has been possible to investigate makes it viable.

## References

1. Jick, H., Miettinen, O. S., Shapiro, S., Lewis, G. P., Siskind, V. and Slone, D. (1970). Comprehensive drug surveillance. *J. Am. Med. Assoc.*, **213**, 1455
2. Crooks, J., Clark, C. G., Caie, H. B. and Mawson, W. B. (1965). Prescribing and administration of drugs in hospital. *Lancet*, **1**, 373
3. Coull, D. C. (1970). 'Drug monitoring in hospital'. The Development of a Hospital Based Information System for Drug Monitoring. *MD Thesis*
4. Barnett, J. W., Dewell, J. V., Moir, D. C. and Alexander, E. (1973). Drug and medicine coding for computer application to pharmacy. *Pharm. J.*, **210**, 204
5. World Health Organization. (1967). *Manual of the International Statistical Classification of Diseases, Injuries and Causes of Death.* (Geneva: World Health Organization)
6. Moir, D. C., Crooks, J., Cornwall, W. B., O'Malley, K., Dingwall-Fordyce, I., Turnbull, M. J. and Weir, R. D. (1972). Cardiotoxicity of amitriptyline. *Lancet*, **2**, 561
7. Christopher, L. J., Crooks, J., Davidson, J. F., Erskine, Z. G., Gallon, S. C., Moir, D. C., Weir, R. D. and Hunter, K. R. (1977). A multicentre study of rauwolfia derivatives and breast cancer. *Eur. J. Clin. Pharmacol.*, **ii**, 409
8. Taylor, M., Galloway, D. B., Petrie, J. C., Davidson, J. F., Gallon, S. C. and Moir, D. C. (1978). Psychomimetic effects of pentazocine and dihydrocodeine tartrate. *Br. Med. J.*, (In press)
9. Moir, D. C., Wood, A. J. J., Davidson, J. F. and Gallon, S. C. (1975). Levodopa and positive direct antiglobulin tests. *Br. J. Clin. Pharmacol.*, **2**, 173
10. Elder, J. B. *et al.* (1979). Cimetidine and gastric cancer. *Lancet*, 1005–6
11. Hurwitz, N. (1969). Predisposing factors in adverse reactions to drugs. *Br. Med. J.*, **1**, 536
12. Ogilvie, R. I. and Ruedy, J. (1967). Adverse reactions during hospitalization. *Can. Med. Assoc. J.*, **97**, 1447

# 19
# Medical record linkage

D. C. G. SKEGG

## INTRODUCTION

The established methods of drug monitoring described in this book have all proved their usefulness, but experience with drugs such as practolol and benoxaprofen has underlined the urgent need for additional techniques capable of detecting unforeseen hazards. There is a particular need for methods of studying delayed effects, such as the induction of cancer, nephropathies, and congenital malformations.

From an epidemiological point of view, an ideal approach would be to record the drugs received by individuals in a large population, and then to study their morbidity and mortality over a long period. A group of experts convened by the World Health Organization[1] called this approach *population monitoring*, and commented:

> 'Insufficient attention has so far been paid to the organization of these systems, and high priority should be given to research into the most practicable methods of developing them.'

More than a decade later, such prospective surveillance has been attempted on only a limited scale. It is a daunting task unless it can be achieved by *linking* records that are collected routinely for other purposes. In a recent review of the most important adverse reactions since thalidomide, Venning[2] concluded that record linkage offered the best opportunity for early discovery of drug hazards. The purpose of this chapter is to explain the concept of medical record linkage, and to discuss how it can be used in monitoring for drug safety.

## THE CONCEPT OF RECORD LINKAGE

Each of us, during a lifetime, generates a large number of records of vital events (such as birth, marriage, and death) and of medical events (such as prescriptions for drugs, vaccinations and admissions to hospital). These records are stored in many different places. The term *record linkage*, which was coined by Dunn[3] in 1946, refers to the bringing together of different records about a single person.

Linkage of records about specified individuals (or families) is a familiar technique in medical practice. In hospitals, for example, it is now customary for all the clinical records about one patient (at a single hospital) to be bound together in a unit medical record. The term record linkage, however, is more often used to describe the systematic linkage of records about every individual in a large population. This type of linkage of medical records has only recently been made feasible by rapid advances in computer technology. With adequate safeguards for personal privacy, such a system can be an invaluable aid to medical research, patient care and health-service management.[4,5]

A pioneer project of this type, known as the Oxford Record Linkage Study, was begun by Acheson in 1962.[6] Initially, records of births, deaths, hospital admissions and obstetric deliveries were linked for a population of about 350 000 people. Certain other types of record were included later, and the population covered was increased to more than 2 million. The linked records have been used to measure the incidence and recurrence of various conditions; to study the outcome of illnesses and surgical operations; and to search for associations between different diseases.[5,7]

In Scotland, which has a population of 5 million, linkage is possible between records of spells of hospital treatment (in general, maternity and psychiatric hospitals), cancer registrations, school medical examinations, deaths, and stillbirths[8]. Record linkage schemes have also been established in some other countries.

## THE FEASIBILITY OF USING RECORD LINKAGE FOR DRUG MONITORING

If drug prescriptions could be linked with records of events such as hospital admissions, deaths and obstetric deliveries, there would be an excellent opportunity to detect major adverse effects of drugs. Linkage of existing records would not require special facilities for data collection, so it should be possible to monitor a large population, and to continue for an indefinite period. Such an approach would be especially valuable for detection of delayed effects (such as the induction of cancer), sudden deaths outside hospital, and effects on the fetus – all of which are difficult to study by other means.

The possibility of using record linkage for drug surveillance was recognized during the 1960s. Acheson[6] suggested a scheme for monitoring the effects of selected new drugs by means of record linkage, although he considered that the standard of identifying data on prescriptions would have to be improved for this to be possible. Doll[9] and Wade[10] both emphasized the potential of record linkage for detecting delayed effects of medicines. Despite such early suggestions, there have been few attempts to develop methods of drug monitoring using record linkage. Nevertheless, preliminary studies have been carried out in the United States of America, Scandinavia and Britain.

**United States of America**

Opportunities for record linkage are generally best in countries with highly organized health services, such as the Scandinavian countries and the United Kingdom. In the United States of America, however, rather similar opportunities are provided by organizations which offer comprehensive medical care to subscribers who pay in advance. The first significant attempt to detect drug effects by linking records about individuals was carried out by one of these organizations, the Kaiser-Permanente group in California.[11,12]

The study was begun in 1969 at the Kaiser-Permanente Medical Center in San Francisco, where out-patient clinics were providing primary medical care for a population of about 120 000 people. Details of drugs dispensed at the out-patient pharmacy (which dispensed about 80% of the prescriptions issued) and diagnoses recorded in the out-patient clinics were linked together in computer-stored medical records. Preliminary analyses showed that the system was capable of detecting known adverse reactions: for example, yeast infections of the vagina were found to be about twice as common among users of oral contraceptives as among other women of the same age.[11] It was hoped that records of hospital admissions and deaths could also be included in the system, but unfortunately this was not achieved before the funding of the project was stopped.

There appear to have been two main reasons for the initial failure of this project: first, it involved highly complex computer record systems, which proved to be extremely expensive; and secondly, it depended upon special recording of data by doctors.[13] Recently, however, Friedman and Ury[14,15] have demonstrated the potential of record linkage by reporting the incidence of cancer among patients whose prescriptions for various drugs had been recorded between 1969 and 1973.

Jick and his colleagues are making use of computerized data from the Group Health Co-operative of Puget Sound, in Seattle. Again, the population included is rather small (about a quarter of a million) and the period of follow-up is still short. Nevertheless, data have been published on several important drug safety issues – including the risk of breast cancer in women receiving oral contraceptives,[16] replacement oestrogens,[17] and other drugs.[18]

The Food and Drug Administration have been investigating the feasibility of using linked data about drugs and events from the Medicaid system for post-marketing surveillance. Promising results were obtained in a pilot study of 1.4 million patients in Michigan and Minnesota.[19]

## North-Eastern Europe*

The Finnish health service maintains a register of people entitled to free drugs, as well as registers for hospital discharges, cancers, and congenital malformations; all of these can be linked by means of a personal social security number.[20] For an *ad hoc* study to test the hypothesis that treatment with rauwolfia increased the risk of breast cancer, linkage between two of the registers was used to identify patients with and without breast cancer who had received drugs for hypertension.[21] There has been no attempt in Finland, however, to use record linkage for detecting unsuspected effects of medicines.

In Sweden, the computerization of prescriptions dispensed offers great opportunities for drug monitoring, but record linkage systems have not yet been developed.

## United Kingdom

For several reasons, the United Kingdom appears to have an excellent opportunity to use record linkage for drug surveillance. Under the National Health Service, nearly everyone is registered with a general practitioner. The great majority of prescriptions are written in general practice, and they are collected centrally for pricing. Furthermore, records of morbidity and mortality are already being collected routinely in a form suitable for record linkage.

In 1974, a study was begun in Oxford to assess the feasibility of using record linkage for monitoring major adverse effects of drugs. The aim was to develop methods that could be used in the future on a larger scale. The population included in this pilot study comprised about 42 000 people registered with 20 general practitioners (in six practices). An important advantage of defining a population according to general practices is that it simplifies the problem of identifying patients from the information given on prescriptions: prescriptions written by general practitioners always have a doctor's name and address stamped on them, and identification of the recipient becomes much easier if the data on the prescription can be compared with a list of the names, addresses and ages of patients in the practice concerned.

For a period of 2 years, three types of record were obtained for every person in the population:[22,23]

(1) Basic information, such as sex and date of birth. This was obtained from the computer records of an organization called the Oxford Community Health Project, but the same data are held for every general practice in the country by the Family Practitioner Committees of the National Health Service.

(2) Details of prescriptions dispensed. The Prescription Pricing Authority provided photocopies of all prescriptions bearing the stamps of the 20 general practitioners. This method of data collection

*See also Chapters 5 and 10 (Ed.)

involved no work for the doctors, and ensured that only prescriptions actually dispensed were recorded. Prescriptions written by medical assistants and locums were obtained, because such doctors have to use the prescription forms of the principals; however, prescriptions issued by hospital doctors were not available. The method of obtaining prescriptions from the Pricing Authority was validated by collecting carbon copies of prescriptions within the practices periodically.

(3) Records of morbidity and mortality. The information about adverse events was obtained by two approaches, which were compared. For 33 000 people (in five practices), details of all hospital admissions, obstetric deliveries and deaths (in or out of hospital) were obtained from the Oxford Record Linkage Study. For the other 9000 people (in the sixth practice), records of illnesses seen by the general practitioners were obtained.

The records about each person were linked on a computer, with particular care to safeguard confidentiality. The data were then analysed for associations between drugs and events. Taking each drug in turn, the frequency of each diagnosis among users of the drug was compared with the frequency among non-users, controlling for other factors such as sex and age.

An example of a known adverse effect revealed by the preliminary screening analysis is shown in Table 1. Among 220 patients treated with liquid paraffin, four were admitted to hospital or died with a diagnosis of bronchopneumonia, whereas the number expected from the experience of 42 897 other people (adjusted for sex and age) was 1.1. This difference was statistically significant. The association was stronger when the analysis was confined to diagnoses made in hospital (relative risk: 9.6; $\chi_1^2 = 9.9$, $p < 0.01$). The four patients were over 80 years of age, and all had received liquid paraffin (or liquid paraffin emulsion) before developing pneumonia.

In the screening analysis, it was assumed that people who received supplies of a drug were 'users' of that drug, while people who did not

**Table 1** Frequency of admission to hospital or death with a diagnosis of bronchopneumonia, according to use of liquid paraffin

| *Use of liquid paraffin* | *Number with bronchopneumonia* | *Total No. in study* | *Relative risk** |
|---|---|---|---|
| Users | 4 | 220 | 3.7 |
| Non-users | 56 | 42 897 | |

$\chi_1^2 = 4.0$ ($P < 0.05$)*

* Adjusted for sex and age, according to the method of Mantel and Haenszel[24]

receive prescriptions were 'non-users'. Of course neither of these assumptions would always be correct: some 'users' would not have taken the medicines they received, while some 'non-users' could have received prescriptions from other doctors or (in the case of drugs such as paraffin) could have purchased medicines without prescription. Such misclassification does not lead to declaration of false associations: it merely reduces the power of the study to detect real associations. The power could be enhanced much more easily by increasing the size of the study, than by attempting to determine patients' compliance with therapy, which is notoriously difficult.[25]

There was also a statistically significant association between liquid paraffin and 'other diseases of the respiratory system' (*International Classification of Diseases*, Eighth Revision, rubric 519). One of the patients involved was a 3-year-old boy. His case-notes showed that he was mentally retarded (with associated hypotonia), and had been admitted to hospital with a 'chest infection' after suffering a convulsion. It was recorded that he was prone to develop coughs, and was requiring antibiotics for chest infections about once a month. For 2 years, he had received regular prescriptions for Mil-Par (magnesium hydroxide and liquid paraffin).

The increased risk of pneumonia among users of liquid paraffin was not surprising in view of the known tendency of mineral oil to enter the lungs and cause lipoid pneumonia.[26] Inhalation of paraffin is particularly liable to occur in elderly debilitated patients,[27] and it might also be expected in a retarded, hypotonic child. Nevertheless, paraffin had not been suspected as a cause of any of these patients' symptoms.

A full account of the Oxford study has been given elsewhere.[22] The findings suggested that prospective drug surveillance using record linkage would be feasible and effective. It was concluded that the method of choice would be to link prescription data with records of hospital admissions, obstetric deliveries and deaths; that a full-scale project should cover a population of at least half a million people (and preferably ten times that number); and that it should continue for an indefinite period.

## POTENTIAL APPLICATIONS

A drug monitoring scheme based on record linkage could be used for a number of different purposes.

### Generating hypotheses about adverse drug reactions (ADRs)

The most important function of a record linkage scheme would be to detect unsuspected effects of medicines. By systematically searching for associations between drugs and events, hypotheses about adverse drug reactions would be generated.

The hypotheses would need to be tested in *ad hoc* studies. In the Oxford study, many unexpected drug–event associations were found, but these could not be assumed to be due to adverse effects of the drugs, because thousands of drug–event combinations had been tested and some statistically significant associations were bound to emerge by chance. Even if an association were not due to chance, it could have been due to the influence of some confounding variable that was not controlled in the study. The most convenient way of testing hypotheses would usually be to employ the case-control method, which has been described elsewhere in this book.

Unfortunately, the number of drug–event associations signalled by a record linkage scheme would probably be larger than the number that could be investigated in special studies. Friedman[28] has discussed the criteria that should be considered in selecting associations for further study.

## Testing hypotheses about adverse reactions

As well as drawing attention to unforeseen hazards, a record linkage scheme would facilitate studies to test hypotheses arising from other sources. These *ad hoc* studies could involve the use of data already collected, review of case-notes or examination of patients. Two examples from the Oxford study will be mentioned.

After description of the serious effects of practolol on the eye,[29,30] an investigation was carried out to see whether minor eye complaints were also commoner during treatment with practolol. Patients in the study population who had received practolol were identified, and their general practice case-notes were examined to determine the frequency of eye complaints and rashes before and during treatment with the drug. As shown in Table 2, 20% of the 71 patients had eye complaints recorded in their case-notes during treatment with practolol, compared with 6% during an equal period immediately before treatment. There was also an excess of rashes during treatment, and half the patients with eye complaints also developed a rash while receiving practolol. The observations before and during treatment were regarded as 'matched pairs', and analysis of discordant pairs showed that the excess of eye complaints during treatment with practolol was statistically significant (one-tailed $p < 0.01$).

Further examination of the data showed that the excess of eye complaints was not due to greater numbers of attendances during treatment, nor to awareness of the hazards of the drug.[31] The results of this study suggested that practolol affected the eye much more commonly than had been appreciated. The same methods were used to study the 246 patients on propranolol, and here the results were more reassuring.[31]

Another study was carried out to determine whether treatment with psychotropic drugs is associated with an increased risk of road

**Table 2** Frequency of eye complaints and rashes in equal periods before and during treatment with practolol (71 patients)

| *Complaint* | *No. of patients* | | *No. of discordant pairs* | | *One-tailed p-value** |
|---|---|---|---|---|---|
| | *before treatment* | *during treatment* | *positive before treatment* | *positive during treatment* | |
| Eye complaint | 4 (6%) | 14 (20%) | 2 | 12 | 0.006 |
| Skin rash | 8 (11%) | 16 (23%) | 5 | 13 | 0.048 |
| Eye compalint + rash | 1 (1%) | 7 (10%) | 1 | 7 | 0.035 |
| Mean period of observation (months) | 19.1 | 19.1 | — | — | — |
| Mean number of attendances | 14.6 | 17.7 | — | — | — |

Data from Skegg and Doll[31]
* *p*-values derived from analysis of discordant pairs

accidents. Patients who had been admitted to hospital (or had died) as a result of injury were identified, and details of their accidents were obtained from hospital case-notes, general practice case-notes, and coroners' reports. Analysis of the drugs that had been received by patients who were driving vehicles at the time of their accidents (and the drugs received by matched controls) showed that patients given minor tranquillizers have an increased risk of involvement in road accidents.[32]

## Demonstrating the safety of drugs

Although the routine analyses reveal statistically significant drug–event associations requiring further investigation, the majority of diagnoses are not more frequent among users of a particular drug. A record linkage scheme would, therefore, provide evidence for drug safety. This information would be particularly useful when alarms are raised about the safety of a drug. *Positive* evidence for safety can be provided only by a monitoring system that does not rely on doctors' suspicions, but rather involves routine screening of the frequencies of all diseases among users of each drug.

## Studying the prescribing of medicines

Surveys of patients admitted to hospital with drug-induced disease suggest that most serious adverse reactions are due to well-known risks of familiar drugs.[33,34] Attempts to control drug-induced disease must, therefore, be based on knowledge about how medicines are used, as well as about their potential hazards. A record linkage scheme would provide valuable information about the use of medicines.

In the first year of the Oxford study, 60% of the population received drugs from their general practitioners, and 24% received five or more items.[35] Because accurate information was available on the distribution of medicines to individuals in a defined population, it was possible to analyse the distribution according to sex and age. It was also found that whereas psychotropic drugs were prescribed more often than any other class, antimicrobials were given to more people. Nevertheless, 10% of all males in the population and 21% of the females received at least one psychotropic drug during the year.

The general practitioners were provided with feedback about their prescribing during the second year of the study. This was followed by a modest reduction in prescribing; it was not possible, however, to determine whether such a change would be likely to persist. More research is needed into the effects of giving doctors information (in various forms) about their own prescribing habits. It is possible that, in addition to yielding information about the effects of drugs, a record linkage scheme would lead to more rational prescribing.[36]

### Other applications

It has been suggested that studies of this kind would be useful for evaluating the efficacy of drugs, as well as their safety.[37] Their usefulness in this respect would be limited, however, because the outcome of treatment with different drugs (say, two anti-hypertensives) is bound to be affected not only by the relative efficacy of the drugs, but also by the various factors that lead doctors to choose a particular drug for a particular patient. It is for this reason that the randomized controlled trial is the most reliable tool for evaluating efficacy. Nevertheless, medicines sometimes have beneficial effects unrelated to their indications: oral contraceptives, for instance, protect against benign breast disease.[38] A system of record linkage might well reveal unexpected beneficial effects.

## POSSIBLE CONSTRAINTS

Clearly a record linkage scheme would have many important applications. We must now consider whether there are any constraints which could limit the feasibility of a full-scale project in the United Kingdom.

### Co-operation of doctors

Any drug monitoring scheme depends upon the co-operation of the medical profession. Apart from its scientific merits, the chief factor influencing the acceptability of a particular scheme is probably the amount of extra work involved for doctors.

The methods proposed following the feasibility study in Oxford would involve general practitioners in virtually no extra work.[22] Administrative staff at the practices would occasionally be asked to assist in identifying prescriptions and other records that could not be identified at the monitoring centre, and the practices might have to be reimbursed for this small amount of work. But the fact that a record linkage system would not depend on special provision of data by doctors, would make it more likely to succeed than many other schemes for post-marketing surveillance.

### Confidentiality

Many doctors and lay people are fearful that the storage of medical records on computers would threaten the privacy of individuals. This may be partly due to lack of awareness that computer-based records can be protected more securely than conventional medical records, but there is also concern that a breach of computer security could enable access to large quantities of information.

Concern about confidentiality should not be a special impediment to a drug monitoring project of the type proposed for the United Kingdom, because all the records that would be included are already being collected for other purposes. Nevertheless, any drug monitoring scheme should be designed carefully to ensure the confidentiality of the data entrusted. Moreover, it should be made clear that under no circumstances would the information be used for any purpose other than medical research.

### Cost

Perhaps the most likely constraint on a system of drug monitoring by means of record linkage would be its cost. Estimates based on the feasibility study in Oxford, however, suggest that – using existing sources of data – the overall cost would be moderate.[22] Furthermore, the cost could be greatly reduced as computer-based methods are adopted at the Prescription Pricing Authority; approximately half of the cost of the pilot study arose from coding and input to the computer of prescription data.

A record linkage scheme would not be cheap but, in comparison with the resources spent on prescription drugs, the amount required would seem to be a justifiable investment in drug safety.

## CONCLUSIONS

No single method of drug monitoring could detect all types of adverse effect, but a system of record linkage would remedy several of the deficiencies of current methods. It would be especially useful for the detection of delayed effects, sudden deaths outside hospital and effects on the fetus. The feasibility study in Oxford confirmed that Britain has an excellent opportunity to use record linkage for drug monitoring. The circumstances seem particularly favourable in Scotland, where a pilot study in Tayside[39] has provided further evidence that record linkage would make a valuable contribution to drug safety.

### References

1. World Health Organization (1972). International drug monitoring. The role of national centres. *WHO Tech. Rep. Ser.*, No. 498
2. Venning, G. R. (1983). Identification of adverse reactions to new drugs. *Br. Med. J.*, **286,** 199–202, 289–92, 365–8, 458–60 and 544–7
3. Dunn, H. L. (1946). Record linkage. *Am. J. Publ. Health*, **36,** 1412
4. Acheson, E. D. (1968). Linkage of medical records. *Br. Med. Bull.*, **24,** 206
5. Baldwin, J. A. and Acheson, E. D. (eds.) *A Textbook of Medical Record Linkage* (Oxford: Oxford University Press) (In press)

6. Acheson, E. D. (1967). *Medical Record Linkage.* (London: Oxford University Press)
7. Baldwin, J. A. (1973). Linked record medical information systems. *Proc. R. Soc. Lond. B.*, **184,** 403
8. Heasman, M. A. and Clarke, J. A. (1979). Medical record linkage in Scotland. *Health Bull.*, **37,** 97
9. Doll, R. (1969). Recognition of unwanted drug effects. *Br. Med. J.*, **2,** 69
10. Wade, O. L. (1970). Pattern of drug-induced disease in the community. *Br. Med. Bull.*, **26,** 240
11. Friedman, G. D., Collen, M. F., Harris, L. E., van Brunt, E. E. and Davis, L. S. (1971). Experience in monitoring drug reactions in outpatients. *J. Am. Med. Assoc.*, **217,** 567
12. Friedman, G. D. and Collen, M. F. (1972). A method for monitoring adverse drug reactions. In Le Cam, L. M., Neyman, J. and Scott, E. L. (eds.) *Proceedings of the Sixth Berkeley Symposium on Mathematical Statistics and Probability.* Vol. VI, pp. 367–80. (Berkeley: University of California Press)
13. Anello, C. (1977). *Identification of Adverse Reactions to Marketed Drugs in the United States and the United Kingdom.* (Rockville: FDA)
14. Friedman, G. D. and Ury, H. K. (1980). Initial screening for carcinogenicity of commonly used drugs. *J. Natl. Cancer Inst.*, **65,** 723
15. Friedman, G. D. and Ury, H. K. (1983). Screening for possible drug carcinogenicity: second report of findings. *J. Natl. Cancer Inst.*, **71,** 1165
16. Jick, H., Walker, A. M., Watkins, R. N. *et al.* (1980). Oral contraceptives and breast cancer. *Am. J. Epidemiol.*, **112,** 577
17. Jick, H., Walker, A. M., Watkins, R. N. *et al.* (1980). Replacement estrogens and breast cancer. *Am. J. Epidemiol.*, **112,** 586
18. Danielson, D. A., Jick, H., Hunter, J .R., Stergachis, A. and Madsen, S. (1982). Nonestrogenic drugs and breast cancer. *Am. J. Epidemiol.*, **116,** 329
19. Jones, J .K., Van de Carr, S. W., Rosa, F., Morse, L. and LeRoy, A. (1984). Medicaid drug–event data: an emerging tool for evaluation of drug risk. *Acta Med. Scand.*, (Suppl.) **683,** 127
20. Idänpään-Heikkilä, J. (1977). Population monitoring: medical record linkage for drug safety surveillance. In Gross, F. H. and Inman, W. H. W. (eds.) *Drug Monitoring.* pp. 17–26. (London: Academic Press)
21. Aromaa, A., Hakama, M. Hakulinen, T., Saxén, E., Teppo, L. and Idänpään-Heikkilä, J. (1976). Breast cancer and use of rauwolfia and other antihypertensive agents in hypertensive patients: a nationwide case-control study in Finland. *Int. J. Cancer*, **18,** 727
22. Skegg, D. C. G. and Doll, R. (1981). Record linkage for drug monitoring. *J. Epidemiol. Commun. Health*, **35,** 25
23. Skegg, D. C. G., Richards, S. M. and Doll, R. (1981). Assessment of the 'E' book as a tool for drug monitoring. *J. Epidemiol. Commun. Health*, **35,** 32
24. Mantel, N. and Haenszel, W. (1959). Statistical aspects of the analysis of data from retrospective studies of disease. *J. Natl. Cancer Inst.*, **22,** 719
25. Sackett, D. L. and Haynes, R. B. (1976). *Compliance with Therapeutic Regimens.* (Baltimore: Johns Hopkins University Press)
26. Crofton, J. and Douglas, A. (1975). *Respiratory Diseases*, 2nd Ed., p. 159. (Oxford: Blackwell Scientific)
27. Volk, B. W., Nathanson, L., Losner, S., Slade, W. R. and Jacobi, M. (1951). Incidence of lipoid pneumonia in a survey of 389 chronically ill patients. *Am. J. Med.*, **10,** 316
28. Friedman, G. D. (1972). Screening criteria for drug monitoring. *J. Chron. Dis.*, **25,** 11
29. Committee on Safety of Medicines (1975). Practolol and ocular damage. *Adverse Reactions Series*, No. 11.
30. Wright, P. (1975). Untoward effects associated with practolol administration: oculomucocutaneous syndrome. *Br. Med. J.*, **1,** 595
31. Skegg, D. C. G. and Doll, R. (1977). Frequency of eye complaints and rashes among patients receiving practolol and propranolol. *Lancet*, **2,** 475
32. Skegg, D. C. G., Richards, S. M. and Doll, R. (1979). Minor tranquillizers and road accidents. *Br. Med. J.*, **1,** 917

33. Hurwitz, N. (1969). Admissions to hospital due to drugs. *Br. Med. J.*, **1,** 539
34. Miller, R. R. (1974). Hospital admissions due to adverse drug reactions. *Arch. Intern. Med.*, **134,** 219
35. Skegg, D. C. G., Doll, R. and Perry, J. (1977). Use of medicines in general practice. *Br. Med. J.*, **1,** 1561
36. Crooks, J. (1984). The concept of medical auditing. *Acta Med. Scand.*, (Suppl.) 683, 47
37. Remington, R. D. (1978). Post-marketing surveillance: a comparison of methods. *University of Rochester Medical Center, Center for the Study of Drug Development, Publication Series*, No. 7, 811 (January 1978)
38. British Medical Journal (1976). Oral contraceptives and breast neoplasia (Leading article). *Br. Med. J.*, **1,** 545
39. Crombie, I. K., Brown, S. V. and Hamley, J .G. (1984). Postmarketing drug surveillance by record linkage in Tayside. *J. Epidemiol. Community Health*, **38,** 226

# 20
# Use of computers in drug monitoring

M. HELLING-BORDA, P. MANELL and H. MANDAHL

## INTRODUCTION

The last two decades have seen an extraordinary explosion of information on drugs and their use. New potent drugs have been discovered, knowledge of disease processes and drug action, both desirable and undesirable, has expanded, making it necessary for industrial, professional and regulatory groups to keep abreast of developments. These technological and scientific advances referred to by Lasagna[1] as 'the Pharmaceutical Revolution' are documented in protocols, files, journals, textbooks, etc and stored in libraries and offices all over the world. The necessity for more rational and timesaving approaches for collecting, classifying and retrieving all this information was recognized early, and with the aid of electronic data-processing (EDP) this has been made possible. The 1960s saw the birth of Medlars, the computerized data-base of the United States National Library of Medicines of published medical literature which, in the 1970s, was developed into an on-line interrogatory system (Medline) with centres in several countries in the world. The 1980s will see the revolution of the use of computers as a common aid to rational prescribing and use of drugs, their safety, efficacy and toxicity. It is no longer a gigantic step from a large computerized file such as Medlars, used primarily for reference purposes, to an on-line file of computer-based correlations of patient characteristics and drug-response, available in all hospital and service departments in pharmacies and doctors' offices, a file which will assist in tailoring drug treatment to the needs of the individual patient. With computers becoming commonplace in all facets of our lives and computer-technology developing so rapidly, such a file requires concerted efforts by physicians, pharmacists, administrators and data processing personnel.[2,3] The distributed computer-technology will support the development within the drug area.

Feinstein[4] in his article on 'Computer malpractice', warns against the situation where 'we may begin to regard the computer as the main focus of operation, supplanting the human activities'. He rightly states that 'the most effective usages of both medical and computer technology may come only if we develop the machines as a collaborating adjunct to the human brain, not as a replacement for it'. The data should, therefore, be presented in such a way that they will assist the user in making decisions. Many will recall the awe in which computers were regarded when they were first introduced into medicine. 'Push button' displays are still staged to impress decision-makers in order to get political and financial support. The attitude towards computers in medicine has varied from unreserved acclaim to disenchantment, but will hopefully become balanced with more familiarity. Specific targets and goals should be properly defined when computer systems are being designed. The machine should not be blamed for lack of planning, co-ordination and communication among clinical, statistical and data-processing groups.

## EXAMPLES OF COMPUTER APPLICATION AS AN AID TO DRUG SAFETY

At a conference on Computer Aid to Drug Therapy and Drug Monitoring[5] 1978 the following areas of computer applicability in the drug field were discussed:

— Hospital monitoring of drug effects
— Monitoring of drug effects in out-patients
— Spontaneous monitoring and reporting of adverse reactions
— Drug data-banks in hospitals and regulatory agencies
— Drug distribution in hospitals
— Prescription monitoring and assistance
— Drug utilization – consumption.

A working conference on The Impact of Computer Technology on Drug Information 1981[6] included the following main sessions:

— Computer Technology Relevant for Drug Information
— Drug Information Systems
— Usage and Results

*Mini-workshops at the above conference discussed*:

— Pharmacological classification of drugs
— Requirements of a data-base management system
— Adverse drug reaction reporting
— Drug consumption and utilization
— Impact of computer technology on drug information

Before a drug is marketed the manufacturer, with the aid of computers, also assembles and analyses data on animal toxicity and results from the different phases of clinical trials to submit to the regulatory agencies. In many pharmaceutical companies the computerized processing of clinical data continues to assist in monitoring the safety of drugs after marketing and alerts the company to deviations from what is known or expected.

### Hospital monitoring

As an example of hospital monitoring of drug effects, the Boston Collaborative Drug Surveillance Program[7] (see Chapter 17) has over the past 15 years monitored patients in over 40 hospitals in seven countries to quantitate the acute toxicity of drugs, and has evaluated factors which influence toxicity. The Boston studies have suggested that serious drug problems, such as those experienced with thalidomide, conjugated oestrogens and practolol are exceptional.[8]

### Monitoring in out-patients

At the Los Angeles County-University of Southern California Medical Center, an electronic data-processing system is used to process and analyse drug utilization data from a large out-patient population, and is a practical and integral part of the prescribing and dispensing system.[9,10] Prescription labels are checked against original prescriptions, patient drug files are reviewed before the drug is dispensed, and warnings to alert the pharmacist of excessive quantities or potential interactions are displayed. This has resulted in improved patient care, cost savings and efficiency.[11]

### Spontaneous monitoring and reporting of adverse reactions to drugs (ADRs)

International collaboration in spontaneous drug monitoring was started by the World Health Organization in 1968.[12] Initially 10 countries participated; the number has now increased to 24. The main objective is to identify, from the pooled computerized data-bank, possible drug safety problems which may require further attention and investigation. The input, storage, retrieval and output of the WHO international file (INTDIS) and different national files will be described in detail in this chapter.

### Drug data-banks in institutions and regulatory agencies

As the need for information on drugs transcends national boundaries, the European Community is investigating methods of co-ordinating a system of drug information through the European On-line Information Network or EURONET, which will provide users with direct access to scientific, technical and socio-economic data.[13] Some large drug data banks are connected to EURONET, e.g. INDIS (International Drug Information System) and SWEDIS (Swedish Drug Information System). Other examples of network applications in the drug area are Telenet, Tymnet and Scannet. In government departments in Sweden, Denmark, France, the United Kingdom and Belgium, in institutions in the Federal Republic of Germany, in a pharmacist association in the Netherlands and in a hospital in France, computerized inventories of marketed drugs, their trade and generic names, therapeutic categories, dosage forms, routes of administration, specific indications, warning, contraindications, etc., have been created.[5] These files are, in a few cases, linked with other national subfiles such as those on ADRs, and the data could with proper safeguads be made accessible internationally.

## Drug distribution in hospitals

In Dundee, the late James Crooks[14] and his collaborators have made use of the computer in a hospital drug distribution system, described in Chapter 18.

## Prescription assistance and monitoring

At the conference on computer aid to drug therapy and drug monitoring in Bern, two studies[15,16] described computerized on-line assistance to hospital physicians when selecting and prescribing a drug. One of these projects[16] was terminated, due to lack of acceptance by the physicians, for complex and ill-understood reasons; the other project[15] has been operating for a number of years. It was developed in conjunction with doctors and pharmacists with the purpose of improving the quality of prescribing. This system ensures that the physician has, at the time of prescribing, as much information as possible about the patient and the proposed drug treatment. To achieve safe and effective therapy and ensure rational prescribing for the individual patient, the physician is guided through a number of procedures. Contraindications, cautions, important and common side-effects, drug interactions and dosage regimens for patients with, for example, impaired renal function are displayed, as well as information on particular characteristics of the patient (pregnancy, allergy, etc.) Alternative drugs can be displayed on a screen if the first drug selected is not considered suitable.

For these efforts to succeed, however, it is necessary for the busy physician to have easy access to the terminals, and to follow established formulary criteria. The educational value of a hospital-based computerized drug interaction monitoring and reporting system has been stressed by Morrell *et al.*[17] who have reported on its benefits particularly for junior hospital doctors and medical students.

A first step in this direction was taken in Sweden.[18] At the Department of Medicine at one county hospital a computerized drug prescription system has recently been installed. The system uses a new type of computer terminal, where the Visual Display Unit (VDU) acts as a touch-control panel. The physician can select from a list of alternatives by touching the VDU with his finger or a pencil. The keyboard is normally not used. The system, built on the registering of a diagnosis, is connected to the regular pharmacy computer system at the hospital pharmacy. This prescription system will in the near future also be used for submitting adverse drug reactions via a computer network to the Swedish Department of Drugs, National Board of Health and Welfare.

In primary health care and general practice computers will not only help in planning and monitoring patient prescriptions and recall visits, but can also allow the physician to assess clinical effects and the behaviour of the patient under medication.[19] A report from the Royal College of General Practitioners in the United Kingdom[20] projected in 1980 that 'A compatible computer system could (and should) be in widespread use in general practice in five years' time and be adopted by virtually all practices in ten years'. Morbidity statistics and operational data are other important pieces of information which can serve as links between different health services and authorities.

## Drug utilization statistics

Studies of drug utilization, consumption and prescribing habits, both in hospital and ambulatory practice, are being carried out in the United States[21] and in several other countries.[22] The data are analysed to obtain information on the extent of drug usage, where drugs are used, local differences, the choice of drugs, the amount of drugs prescribed, use in various age-groups and occasionally the diagnosis for which drugs are prescribed. Most countries do not, however, have the infrastructure for collecting these data seen for example in Norway and Sweden, where the national distribution system is centralized, making drug-utilization studies easy to carry out. Drug-utilization figures are also needed for international comparison and research, where ADR reports should be correlated with the utilization statistics. An international research group sponsored by the World Health Organization is currently collaborating in this field, and uses as a unit for statistical comparison the defined daily dosage (DDD) or the mean dose for the main indication of a drug.[22]

Drug sales statistics can further be linked to vital statistics and disease registries to provide the 'intelligence system' needed to help detect unwanted and unanticipated drug reactions.[23] The application of computer technology to the organization, management and control of pharmacy stock and drug usage in hospitals and elsewhere lead to more efficient pharmacy management and the development of more rational prescribing.[24]

## MONITORING FOR DRUG SAFETY

### General

All the above examples are included to illustrate different applications of computers. Since the thalidomide disaster great emphasis has been placed, understandably, on the dangers of drugs. Methods for monitoring ADRs[25] have been developed, and approaches for post-marketing surveillance continue to be discussed.[26] This continuous surveillance is necessary, not only for old and established drugs, but particularly for newly-introduced ones, as we have seen again recently in the case of benoxaprofen.[27] Lately, however, a shift in thinking has taken place, and it is felt that perhaps too much emphasis has been placed on the dangers of drugs and too little on demonstrating their therapeutic importance and effectiveness as well as their relative safety.

## WHO SYSTEM FOR MONITORING ADRs

### Source of data

Physicians and other health personnel submit, on special national forms, reports of suspected ADRs to a designated national centre, which is usually a government agency. The national centre screens, reviews and evaluates the reports, sometimes with the assistance of an advisory committee. The data are then translated and either manually transcribed onto the WHO reporting form in an English or a French version, or transmitted on magnetic tape.

### WHO reporting form

The WHO reporting form originally contained 47 items, 10 of which were essential basic data. Although requested, the basic data were not always reported. Therefore, it was decided, to simplify the reporting system by reducing the number of items to 27. At the same time it was requested that as many as possible of the items in the form should be covered when reporting. This was done in July 1981 when the new reporting form was introduced.

## WHO ADR terminology

Although space is provided on the reporting form for a description in free text of the ADRs that occurred, national centres are urged to select WHO preferred terms and to enter these in the appropriate space for adverse reaction preferred term. The WHO ADR terminology was initially created in 1967 from an amalgamation of terms existing in some early established national centres. It has since been further developed, expanded and structured and now comprises:

approximately 1400 included terms
approximately 1100 preferred terms
514 high-level terms and
30 system organ classes.

## Definitions and uses

*Included terms*

These represent all ADR terms provided by reporting sources when describing reactions in free text. Included terms are used to assist in finding the corresponding preferred term for proper coding on the WHO reporting form. However, these terms may be used on the input side at the national level where need for more detailed recording is required. At the international level the preferred term is considered adequate for the input side.

*Preferred terms*

These terms are used to describe ADRs reported to the WHO system at a level of detail considered sufficient for international monitoring. They are the terms usually used at the input side, but may also be used in some output documents. Each preferred term may be allocated to a maximum of three system organ classes.

*High-level terms*

These are group preferred terms for qualitatively similar, but quantitatively different, conditions; these terms are used to facilitate reading of output documents.

*System organ classes*

These are used for group terms pertaining to the same body organ (e.g. liver and biliary system disorders) or otherwise related terms (e.g. fetal disorders). System organ classes are used in order to find the appropriate ADR term and for grouping reactions in output documents, e.g. for producing an adverse reaction profile. Examples of the ADR terminology and its structure are shown in figure 1.

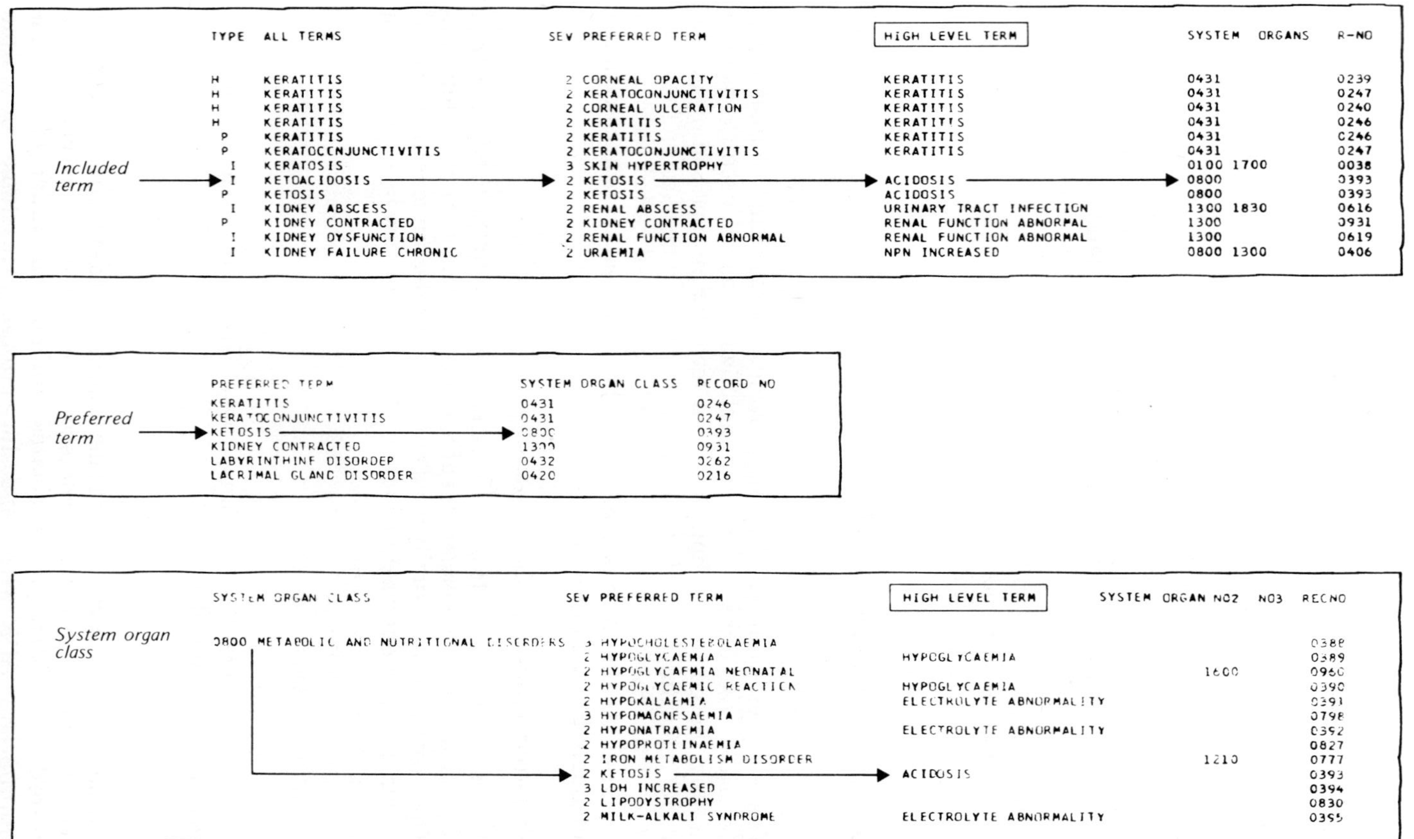



| TYPE | ALL TERMS | SEV | PREFERRED TERM | HIGH LEVEL TERM | SYSTEM | ORGANS | R-NO |
|---|---|---|---|---|---|---|---|
| H | KERATITIS | 2 | CORNEAL OPACITY | KERATITIS | 0431 | | 0239 |
| H | KERATITIS | 2 | KERATOCONJUNCTIVITIS | KERATITIS | 0431 | | 0247 |
| H | KERATITIS | 2 | CORNEAL ULCERATION | KERATITIS | 0431 | | 0240 |
| H | KERATITIS | 2 | KERATITIS | KERATITIS | 0431 | | 0246 |
| P | KERATITIS | 2 | KERATITIS | KERATITIS | 0431 | | 0246 |
| P | KERATOCONJUNCTIVITIS | 2 | KERATOCONJUNCTIVITIS | KERATITIS | 0431 | | 0247 |
| I | KERATOSIS | 3 | SKIN HYPERTROPHY | | 0100 | 1700 | 0038 |
| I | KETOACIDOSIS | 2 | KETOSIS | ACIDOSIS | 0800 | | 0393 |
| P | KETOSIS | 2 | KETOSIS | ACIDOSIS | 0800 | | 0393 |
| I | KIDNEY ABSCESS | 2 | RENAL ABSCESS | URINARY TRACT INFECTION | 1300 | 1830 | 0616 |
| P | KIDNEY CONTRACTED | 2 | KIDNEY CONTRACTED | RENAL FUNCTION ABNORMAL | 1300 | | 0931 |
| I | KIDNEY DYSFUNCTION | 2 | RENAL FUNCTION ABNORMAL | RENAL FUNCTION ABNORMAL | 1300 | | 0619 |
| I | KIDNEY FAILURE CHRONIC | 2 | URAEMIA | NPN INCREASED | 0800 | 1300 | 0406 |

| PREFERRED TERM | SYSTEM ORGAN CLASS | RECORD NO |
|---|---|---|
| KERATITIS | 0431 | 0246 |
| KERATOCONJUNCTIVITIS | 0431 | 0247 |
| KETOSIS | 0800 | 0393 |
| KIDNEY CONTRACTED | 1300 | 0931 |
| LABYRINTHINE DISORDER | 0432 | 0262 |
| LACRIMAL GLAND DISORDER | 0420 | 0216 |

| SYSTEM ORGAN CLASS | SEV | PREFERRED TERM | HIGH LEVEL TERM | SYSTEM ORGAN NO2 | NO3 | RECNO |
|---|---|---|---|---|---|---|
| 0800 METABOLIC AND NUTRITIONAL DISORDERS | 3 | HYPOCHOLESTEROLAEMIA | | | | 0388 |
| | 2 | HYPOGLYCAEMIA | HYPOGLYCAEMIA | | | 0389 |
| | 2 | HYPOGLYCAEMIA NEONATAL | | 1600 | | 0960 |
| | 2 | HYPOGLYCAEMIC REACTION | HYPOGLYCAEMIA | | | 0390 |
| | 2 | HYPOKALAEMIA | ELECTROLYTE ABNORMALITY | | | 0391 |
| | 3 | HYPOMAGNESAEMIA | | | | 0798 |
| | 2 | HYPONATRAEMIA | ELECTROLYTE ABNORMALITY | | | 0392 |
| | 2 | HYPOPROTEINAEMIA | | | | 0827 |
| | 2 | IRON METABOLISM DISORDER | | 1210 | | 0777 |
| | 2 | KETOSIS | ACIDOSIS | | | 0393 |
| | 3 | LDH INCREASED | | | | 0394 |
| | 2 | LIPODYSTROPHY | | | | 0830 |
| | 2 | MILK-ALKALI SYNDROME | ELECTROLYTE ABNORMALITY | | | 0395 |

**Figure 1** Examples from WHO adverse reaction terminology structuring and different output presentations

## WHO drug dictionary and drug reference list

The drugs on the WHO recording form are usually reported as trade names. The reporting physician will make a distinction between the suspected drug (S) and other drugs (O), i.e. those given concurrently with the suspected drug.

In early 1968 when the WHO monitoring activities started, national standardized and computerized drug data files had not been developed, and it was necessary for the WHO to create and build up its own file.[28,29] A separate drug dictionary file was developed to include the active ingredients, classified pharmacologically and therapeutically. The purpose of the drug dictionary, through its linkage to the ADR master-file of ADR reports, is to identify, classify and group drugs reported to the international centre. The Drug Dictionary is continuously updated and annually reprinted as the Drug Reference list – an alphabetical listing on paper and on microfiche, as well as on magnetic tape. It is available to users outside the national centres in the WHO adverse reaction monitoring programme.

## Information transmitted to the WHO centre

The information transmitted to the WHO centre on an individual case can be divided into four categories:

(1) Case identification and patient data
(2) Description of the adverse reaction
(3) Information about administered drugs
(4) Background data and comments by national centre

Each report is identified by a country code and a national identification number. Information is given on the source of the report (e.g. hospital or general practitioner) and on the age, sex and ethnic origin of the patient.

The adverse reaction is described by the preferred terms of the WHO Adverse Reaction Terminology.

In the description of the medication the patient has been taking before the onset of the reaction, the trade name of the drug is preferred. If the trade name is not available, however, the international non-proprietary name (INN) may be given. Space is provided on the form to code dosage regimen, route of administration, duration and indication of treatment for six individual drugs. If more drugs have been used, the total number must be stated. Each report should also contain a notification on which drug(s) is suspected of causing the reaction.

If the suspected drug has been withdrawn (dechallenge) and reinstated (rechallenge), information may be transmitted about possible improvement and/or recurrence of symptoms. Predisposing or contributing conditions, like kidney failure or alcohol abuse, may be stated as well as the outcome of the case (recovery, sequelae or death).

Finally, provision is given for the national centre's assessment of the drug-reaction relationship.

## Handling of reports at the WHO centre. The database INTDIS (International Drug Information System)

The great amount of information gathered in the international system, on adverse reactions and in related registers makes advanced computer techniques necessary for its handling. At the transfer of the Adverse Reaction Monitoring Programme from WHO, Geneva to Uppsala in 1978, the need to modernize the computer facilities was recognized. The main structure and content of the registers have been retained, but a new data base system has been developed based entirely on disc memories which make the data accessible via a computer terminal and considerably accelerate processing.

INTDIS (International Drug Information System)[31] is a relational data base built upon the general data base management system MIMER. Data are organized in tables which are linked together through certain common rows (Figure 2). Any type of information in the data base may be linked to any other item.

This data base solution implies the following characteristics:

— Flexible software, allowing for future expansion
— Interactive and batch updating and search routines
— Searches performed without any programming by means of a query language, MIMAN

## Content of INTDIS

The main section of INTDIS is the case report register which is divided into four parts, corresponding to the structure of an adverse reaction case report (Figure 2).

(1) **Reports; Administrative**, containing case identification and patient data;
(2) **Reports; Adverse reactions**, containing a code description of the reactions;
(3) **Reports; Drugs** with information about the administered medicines;
(4) **Reports, Medical**, containing background information and comment by national centres.

The case report register has several complementary registers.

In the drug registers, divided into seven tables, information is stored on approximately 11 000 proprietary and 4000 non-proprietary names of drugs and substances. The drug information includes the name of the manufacturer, chemical-, pharmacological- and therapeutic clas-

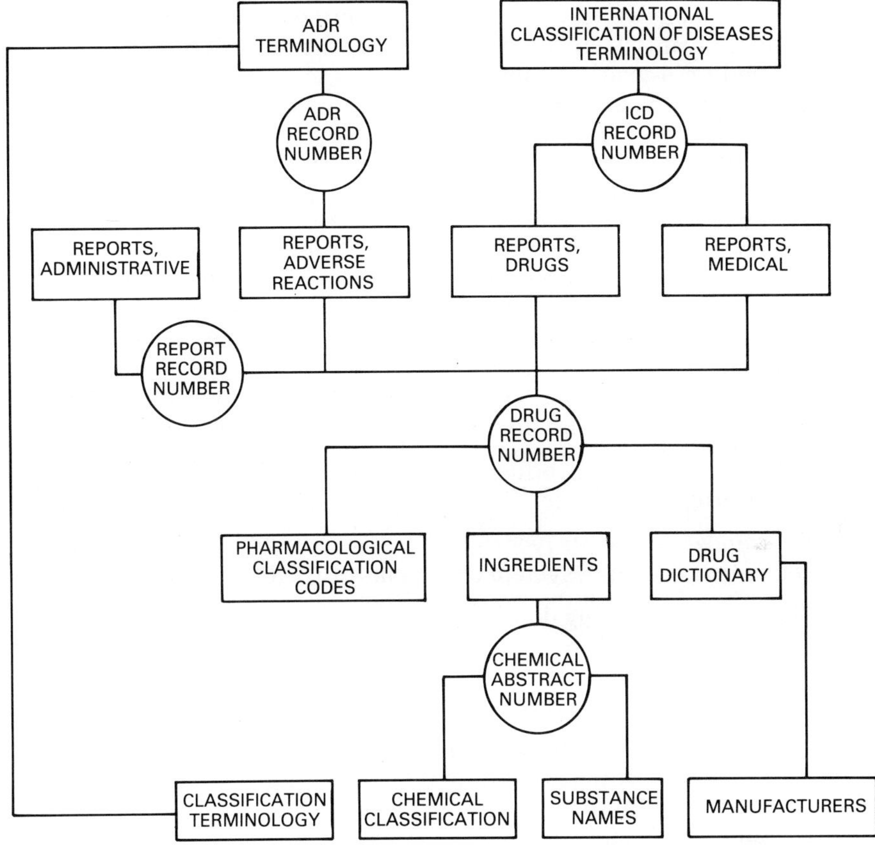


**Figure 2** General outline of the International Drug Information System

sification of each substance, as well as the Chemical Abstract Service number. Around 1000 new names are added to the drug register each year.

## Output from the system

Signalling lists aimed at drawing attention to new, serious or unexpected adverse reactions are produced on a 3-monthly basis. The 'New to the System' list tables all ADR combinations not previously reported. There are four lists which focus on different categories of adverse reactions that need special attention; death, fetal disorders, neoplasms and drug dependence. Reporting frequencies of selected drug–adverse reaction combinations are also presented in a special listing.

A comprehensive review of all incoming reports is produced annually. A printout of the drug register, the Drug Reference list, is also issued on a yearly basis.

Routine listings are produced on paper print, on microfiche or on magnetic tape. In addition to the regular listings a great number of special searches are performed using the query language MIMAN. Every item in INTDIS is searchable.

The participating national centres can also perform searches from remote terminals connected on-line to INTDIS. A number of routine search programs are at the disposal of the participating centres.

Results from special retrievals may be presented in the form of individual case reports, tabulations, graphs or as statistical parameters.

*Document production and information retrieval*

*The output documents produced yearly and quarterly by the WHO computer program include:*

(1) *Reference documents (yearly)*
*Document A:* Drug–system organ class–ADR

(2) Signalling or alerting documents (quarterly)
*Document K:* ADRs new to the system (i.e. reported for the first time)
*Document L:* ADRs of possible interest

(3) Retrieved case-reports: summaries (quarterly)
*Document N:* Deaths (including fetal, neonatal)
*Document P:* Malformations
*Document T:* Neoplasms
*Document D:* Drug dependence

(4) Terminologies, drug classifications and basic reference material
ADR terminology
Drug Reference list (yearly, with quarterly supplements)

## Dissemination of signals

In order to avoid breach of confidentiality and misinterpretation of the data, extreme caution has had to be exercised in the collaborating centre in the dissemination of information to national centres. In the early operation of the program this sometimes exaggerated caution may have caused some delay in the dissemination of information for fear of causing unnecessary alarm. However, if the methods of collection of data and their national characteristics are properly explained, it should be clear that a signal is only the first step towards the early identification of a possible drug safety problem, which may have to be followed up in more detail. Today, caution in the dissemination of data is particularly observed when related to other than national centres.

## Outline specification for a National File

Australia, which has participated in the International Monitoring Scheme since its initiation, first sent its ADR reports to the WHO on manually recorded forms. The increasing rate of reports led to the establishment in 1970 of the Adverse Drug Reactions Advisory Committee, ADRAC, which evaluates the suspected ADRs and distributes relevant information to the medical and allied professions. To assist ADRAC in its work, and to increase the capacity for analysis and dissemination, automatic data-processing was introduced in Australia in 1973.[32]

The computer programs and systems developed in the WHO International Monitoring Centre were made available to the Australian Department of Health, who carried out additions and extensions to the WHO programs to meet the special requirements of ADRAC.[33]

The ADRAC procedure includes:

- Coding of reports
- Computer validation of original reports
- Monthly update of master-file and production of output documents
- Review by the Committee
- Correction and computerized revalidation of reports
- Update of master-file and production of data-tape for despatch to WHO

When received at the international centre, the Australian tape is copied and returned, together with the WHO updated *Drug and Adverse Reaction Dictionaries.*

## PRESENTATIONS OF OUTPUT FROM NATIONAL SYSTEMS

Depending on for what purpose and for whom the output is intended, the output documents vary from one country to another. In Canada and Sweden drug manufacturers receive certain detailed printouts. Usually, however, fairly standardized summary reports are sent to the members of the Adverse Reactions Committees before a Committee meeting. In Australia, for example, ADRAC members receive a number of different printouts before a Committee meeting, and others are used for review and reference purposes at the meeting. Examples of some of these output documents include:

(1) Monthly and total counts of ADRs by broad therapeutic groups;

(2) Expansion of the above with monthly and total counts of reported reactions under each generic name, listed under its therapeutic group;

(3) Monthly summaries of reports where drug/reaction incidence for the reporting month is compared with previous 3- and 12-month periods.

This report is presented alphabetically under generic name with additional information as follows:

| **Generic name** | | | |
|---|---|---|---|
| | **Trade name** | **Report number** | **WHO preferred reaction term** |

An asterisk (*) is placed against any report number or reaction for which death was the outcome and the drug was suspected.

(4) Detailed information, in free text, of each report received under the review period.

Besides other internal documents ADRAC publishes, for registered medical and dental practitioners, a compendium which is a cumulative list of suspected reactions reported to the Australian centre. The compendium is not intended as a comprehensive documentation of ADRs. It is, however, a very useful reference document, in which drugs are presented in alphabetical order under the generic name, followed by the reported trade name and the reaction description (WHO preferred terms) in alphabetical order under each trade name. The total number of reports received and a probability rating (certain, probable, possible and unclassified) for the causal relationship of drug/reaction is also printed, as well as the total number of reactions for each combination.

In the preface the methods of collecting the data are explained and cautions in their interpretation are emphasized, since several sources of bias exist in the way the data are collected. The extent of drug-use, for example, is not known. There is also a tendency to report more frequently on new rather than established drugs, and on serious or fatal reactions rather than trivial reactions such as skin rash.

## USE OF ON-LINE TERMINALS

In the previous sections discussion has centred around transferring and entering information to intermediate coding sheets for input to the computer and batch production of reports and documents on the output side. For certain purposes these procedures will continue to be used. When rapid communication with the computer and the stored data is required, an on-line system with terminals, comprising visual display units, keyboards and printers, is preferable. Data can be entered and retrieved on a much more flexible basis.

A comprehensive integrated computerized on-line drug information system described by Manell[34] and Dagerus *et al*[35] is SWEDIS (Swedish Drug Information System) located at the Department of Drugs. The system has been developed in collaboration with Uppsala University Data Centre, and comprises information on pharmaceutical specialties, reported ADRs, manufacturers/agents, sales statistics, constituents, literature references, diagnoses and therapy survey data, drug effects in clinical chemistry and tablet identification. SWEDIS is the only national system at present where it is possible to correlate adverse reaction report frequencies with drug sale statistics. SWEDIS is used from terminals in drug companies, pharmacies, hospitals and doctors' offices.

The computer technology developed for SWEDIS is used within INTDIS. The SWEDIS-technology is now used as a basis for the computerized adverse drug reaction information system in Norway. Implementation of the system is also underway in a number of other countries.

SWEDIS uses the Database Management System MIMER developed by the Uppsala University Data Centre. MIMER represents the fourth generation of computer programming tools.

## CONCLUDING REMARKS

Elaborate computer systems in medicine have often failed because of inexperience, mismanagement or lack of appreciation of the complexity of tasks that both the user/initiator of the system, the data-processing group and the computer were required to perform. A systems approach and an analysis plan as described by Bazalo[36,37] can prevent such failures. Clinical, statistical and data-processing staff should work closely together from the very beginning of the design of a project. This co-ordination must continue and each group must maintain responsibility for the tasks that fall within its field of expertise. The clinical staff should realize that standardized terminologies may have to be created and then adhered to for retrieval purposes. It is also the responsibility of the clinical and the statistical staff to specify the objectives of the project and to give detailed instructions for the kind of output desired which should be in a user-oriented manner. Heavy computer printouts should be avoided. Summarized tabulations with proper headings and graphical presentations are preferable. Basic knowledge of the file structures helps the clinician's understanding of the potentials and limitations of the system. Detailed knowledge of hardware and software is not necessary. A well documented computer system is, however, a necessity and the documentation should be prepared by the data-processing group.

It should include procedures for coding, error corrections, updating, retrieval, output presentations and file descriptions. This is particularly important because continuity in systems analysis and programming so highly desirable, is usually not possible. Systems analysts and computer programmers may change jobs during the development of a computer system and proper documentation is, therefore, of vital importance.

Finally we should remember the following words by Feinstein:[4]

> The sooner we relegate the computer to being an ancillary tool, rather than a venerated master, and the sooner we start respecting our own minds rather than bits, bytes, storage modules and central processing units – the sooner will we begin to advance clinical medicine.

## Acknowledgements

The authors wish to thank all former colleagues at the WHO International Monitoring Centre and collaborators in the national centres. Special thanks go to Dr Bruce Royall, former Chief, Drug Evaluation and Monitoring, WHO; to Dr Jan Venulet former Head of the WHO International Monitoring Centre and to Mr Esko Ahlroth, Programmer Analyst, WHO, for valuable suggestions and advice. For supply information on their own national computerized systems, the authors wish to thank: Mr R. E. Wilson, Secretary, Australian Drug Evaluation Committee; Dr E. Napke, Chief, Poison Control and Adverse Reaction Programs Division, Department of National Health and Welfare, Canada; Mr M. Abboud, Head, Adverse Reaction Section, Poison Control and Adverse Reaction Programs Division, Department of National Health and Welfare, Canada; Mr H. O. Andersen, Head of Secretariat, Board on Adverse Reactions to Drugs, Danish National Health Service, Denmark; Professor E. G. McQueen, Medical Assessor, Committee on Adverse Drug Reactions, New Zealand, the staff of the WHO Collaborating Centre for International Drug Monitoring, Mr S. Olsson, Ms C. Biriell and Ms M. Lindqvist.

## Note

This article expresses the views of the authors and does not necessarily represent those of the World Health Organization, or the National Board of Health and Welfare, Sweden.

## References

1. Lasagna, L. (1969). The pharmaceutical revolution: its impact on science and society. *Science*, **166**, 1227
2. Gouveia, W. A. and Hold, E. G. (1982). Computer systems planning, development,

and impact assessment. *Am. J. Hosp. Pharm.*, **39,** 2117

3. Stevens, R. G. and Crabbe, A. M. (1982). What future for the computer? *Pharm. J.*, **20,** 209
4. Feinstein, A. R. (1977). Clinical biostatistics; XXXVIII. Computer malpractice. *Clin. Pharmacol. Ther.*, **1,** 78–88
5. Ducrot, N., Goldberg, M., Hoigné, R. and Middleton P. (eds.) (1978). *Computer Aid to Drug Therapy and Drug Monitoring* IFIP. (Amsterdam: North-Holland Publishing)
6. Manell, P., Johansson, S. (eds.) (1981). *The Impact of Computer Technology on Drug Information.* (Amsterdam: North-Holland Publishing)
7. Gaetano, L. F. and Miller, R. R. (1974). Use of the computer in monitoring drug effects in hospitalized patients. *J. Clin. Comput.*, **3,** 310
8. Jick, H. (1978). In-hospital monitoring of drug effects – past accomplishments and future needs. In Ducrot *et al.* (eds.) *Computer Aid to Drug Therapy and Drug Monitoring.* IFIP. (Amsterdam: North-Holland Publishing)
9. Maronde, R. F. Burks, D., Lee, P. V., Licht, P., McCarron, M. M., McCary, M. and Seibert, S. (1969). Physician prescribing practices, a computer-based study. *Am. J. Hosp. Pharm.*, **26,** 556
10. Maronde, R. F., Lee, P. V., McCarron, M. M. and Seibert, S. (1971). A study of prescribing patterns. *Med. Care*, **IX,** 383
11. Maronde, R. F. (1978). Monitoring for adverse drug reactions, including mutations, in outpatients. In Ducrot, H., Goldberg, M., Hoigné, R. and Middleton, P. (eds.) *Computer Aid to Drug Therapy and Drug Monitoring.* IFIF. pp. 63–7. (Amsterdam: North-Holland Publishing)
12. Royall, B. W. and Venulet, J. (1972). Methodology for international drug monitoring. *Meth. Inform. Med.*, **11,** 75
13. Van der Kuy, A. (1977). ECC survey project on drug data bank systems. In van der Kleijn, E. and Jonkers, E. (eds.). *Clinical Pharmacy.* pp. 133–6. (Amsterdam, Oxford, New York: Elsevier/North-Holland Biomedical Press)
14. Crooks, J. (1978). The prescription, provision and administration of drugs – the contribution of computer technology. In Ducrot *et al.* (eds.) *Computer Aid to Drug Therapy and Drug Monitoring.* IFIP. (Amsterdam: North-Holland Publishing)
15. Beeley, L. (1978). A real-time drug information system to assist prescribing. In Ducrot, H., Goldberg, M., Hoigné, R. and Middleton, P. (eds.) *Computer Aid to Drug Therapy and Drug Monitoring.* IFIP. Amsterdam: North-Holland Publishing)
16. Souder, D. E., Zielstorff, R. D. and Barnett, G. O. (1978). Experience with an automated medication system. In Ducrot *et al.* (eds.) *Computer Aid to Drug Therapy and Drug Monitoring.* IFIP. (Amsterdam: North-Holland Publishing)
17. Morell, J., Podlone, M. and Cohen, S. N. (1977). Receptivity of physicians in a teaching hospital to a computerized drug interaction monitoring and reporting system. *Med. Care*, **XV,** 68
18. Nilsson, S., Dolby, J., Ockander, L., Åstrand, B. (1982). Dataterminal in the physician's office, assistance in issuing prescriptions. *Swed. Med. J.*, **79,** 760
19. (1980). Surgery computers: Prescription monitoring a 'prime requirement' *Pharm. J.* **27,** 341
20. (1980). Computers in Primary Care. *J. R. Coll. Gen. Pract.*, **30,** 387–8
21. Conley, B. E. (1978). Drug consumption and prescribing practices: recent studies in the United States. In Ducrot *et al*, (eds.) *Computer Aid to Drug Therapy and Drug Monitoring.* IFIP. (Amsterdam: North-Holland Publishing)
22. (1978). Bergman, U., Grimsson, A. and Westerholm, B. (eds.) (1978). Drug utilization studies, methods and applications. *WHO Reg. Pub.*, European Series (Copenhagen)
23. Stolley, P. D. (1982). The use of vital and morbidity statistics for the detection of adverse drug reactions and for monitoring of drug safety. *J. Clin. Pharmacol.*, **22,** 499
24. Stainton, M. P., Ehrenzweig, B. A. and Hunt, C. M. (1983). Computerisation of stock and drug use. *Pharm. J.*, **230,** 252
25. Venulet, J. (1977). Methods of monitoring adverse reactions to drugs. In Jucker, E. (ed.) *Progress in Drug Research*, **21,** p. 231. (Basel and Stuttgart: Birkhäuser Verlag)

26. (1977). New strategies for drug monitoring *Br. Med. J.*, **1,** 861
27. (1983). Doctors and the drug industry *Br. Med. J.*, **286,** 579
28. Helling, M. I. and Venulet, J. (1974). Drug recording and classification by the WHO research centre for international monitoring of adverse reactions to drugs. *Meth. Inform. Med.*, **13,** 169
29. Helling, M. I. (1976). Experience with World Health Organization. In Gouveia, W. A., Tognoni, G. and van der Kleijn, E. (eds.) *Clinical Pharmacy and Clinical Pharmacology.* pp. 141–51. (Amsterdam, New York, Oxford: North-Holland Publishing)
30. Biriell, C., Olsson, S. and Liljestrand, Å. (1983). The spontaneous adverse drug reaction reporting system and the WHO drug monitoring system, (1981). In Laporte, J. R. and Tognoni, G. (ed.) *Principios de epidemiologia del medicamento.* pp. 147–65 (Salvat: Barcelona)
31. Biriell, C., Dagerus, B., Johansson, S., Manell, P., Olsson, S. and Östling, B. (1981). INTDIS-database for the WHO drug monitoring program. In Manell, P., Johansson, S. (eds.) *The Impact of Computer Technology on Drug Information*
32. (1974). Adverse Drug Reactions Advisory Committee Report for 1973. *Med. J. Austr.* December 14th, 875
33. (1978). Wilson, R. E., Secretary, Australian Drug Evaluation Committee. Personal communication
34. Manell, P. (1981). Computer technology requirements to design a computerized drug information system. In Manell, P. and Johansson, S. (eds.) *The Impact of Computer Technology on Drug Information*, pp. 63–9 (Amsterdam: North-Holland Publishing)
35. Dagerus, B., Johansson, S. G., Lindgren, K., Manell, P. and Östling, B. (1981). The Swedish Drug Information System, SWEDIS. In Manell, P. and Johansson, S. (eds.) *The Impact of Computer Technology on Drug Information.* pp. 103–13 (Amsterdam: North-Holland Publishing)
36. Bazalo, G. (1977). A system approach to the design and analysis of clinical studies. *Drug Inf. J.*, June, p. 70
37. Bazalo, G. (1976). Data processing coordination in NDA preparation. *Drug Inf. J.*, October/December, p. 115

# 21
# Anaesthetics

J. W. DUNDEE

## INTRODUCTION

There can be few specialties in which the 'pioneer' drugs have stood the test of time so well as in anaesthesia, and where these are still regarded as the standard with which to compare new drugs. In the inhalational field diethyl ether (1846) is the most widely used drug in the world: its flammability has led to its eclipse in Western medicine, yet it is still the standard with which new drugs with a similar clinical use have to be compared. Chloroform (1847) had more than 100 years clinical use before being superseded by halothane. Nitrous oxide (1844) still remains the standard gaseous agent, and is unsurpassed in its lack of toxicity. In the intravenous field, thiopentone (1935) is the least toxic and most widely used induction agent in the world. Although tubocurarine (1947) has been largely replaced by the less toxic pancuronium, suxamethonium (1957) is still the depolarizing relaxant of choice. This generalization does not apply to local anaesthetics.

The excellence of the initial drugs in anaesthesia may be the reason why anaesthetists have until recently been unaware of the necessity of monitoring the safety of drugs. 'Prolonged curarization' introduced this problem,[1] but it was the reports of liver dysfunction following a second administration of halothane which highlighted it, and prompted the first 'official' comment on drug toxicity related to anaesthesia.[2] Ketamine sequelae, high-output renal failure after methoxyflurane or hypersenstivity to intravenous anaesthetics are more recent examples of notable side-effects. The latter of these is an instructive example of collaboration between official and university departmental monitoring of side-effects.[3]

## ANAESTHETIC PROBLEMS

On the surface it would seem to be a simple matter to monitor the side-effects of drugs given by anaesthetists, particularly as many of these occur in hospital practice. Anaesthesia, both general and regional, is an 'acute pharmacological and physiological insult' to the patients, with most toxic effects occurring in a short period of time. Patients with severe reactions will usually stay in hospital, and an appropriate follow-up should be easy.

Clinical experience and an interest in side-effects of drugs over a period of 25 years has shown that this is an over-simplification. Each branch of medicine has problems which are peculiar to the discipline, and this certainly applies to anaesthesia. It is important to look at these problems before suggesting how they may be overcome. The limitations of clinical trials in anaesthesia must also be considered in the light of these problems as must any suggestions for future drug monitoring.

(1) In most instances anaesthesia is a single exposure of a patient to one or, more frequently, a number of drugs, the actual dosage of which, or duration of exposure, may be inadequately recorded.

(2) Current clinical practice favours 'balanced' techniques in which a number of agents contribute to the state of surgical anaesthesia. Known synergisms between different component drugs often play a part in these techniques. It may thus be difficult to attribute a side-effect to a specific agent.

(3) With different techniques employed for different types of operation, what is a desired effect on one occasion may be a side-effect on another occasion. Examples of this are halothane-induced bradycardia and/or hypotension (desirable for middle ear surgery) and buprenorphine-induced respiratory depression (no problem in ventilated patients) which most would generally regard as undesirable.

(4) Side-effects may first appear in the post-operative period when it is difficult to separate the residual effect of anaesthetic drugs from those of the operation and attendant therapy. Jaundice on the 3rd–4th post-operative day could be due as readily to blood transfusion as to the hepatotoxic effects of the anaesthetic, while post-operative (?post-anaesthetic) vomiting can be caused by dilation of the cervix or by morphine. The rare occurrence of respiratory depression after ether in patients who had neomycin insufflated into the peritoneal cavity by the surgeon is another example.

(5) Some effects of drugs used by the anaesthetist may be missed altogether, or their frequency underestimated because of the time taken for these to develop and the resulting difficulty in follow-up. Venous thrombosis after diazepam has been found to be more than twice as frequent on the 7th–10th post-operative days as on the 2nd–3rd days, which is the common time for follow-up.[4]

(6) Certain toxic effects occur so rarely, or only in certain circumstances, that tens of thousands of administrations may be necessary to establish their authenticity and causal relationship to anaesthesia. Outstanding among these is liver dysfunction on the second

administration of halothane and the dose-related, methoxyflurane-induced, high-output renal failure.

(7) Certain hereditary traits occurring in a small percentage of the population may induce sensitivity or other adverse reactions to anaesthetics. It may take some time and many case-reports to establish the all-important relationship. Prolonged apnoea after suxamethonium in patients with an abnormal type of plasma cholinesterase, inducement of an acute attack of intermittent porphyria by thiopentone, greater likelihood of hypersensitivity reactions to intravenous anaesthetics in atopic patients and the occurrence of malignant hyperpyrexia in susceptible patients are examples.

## Documentation problems

There are very real documentation problems for the anaesthetist, particularly if working single-handedly. The critical time for recording data of an adverse reaction is during the induction and recovery periods. Yet it is at these times that the anaesthetist is least able to make detailed notes. Logistics of large operating lists, and the need to minimize the waiting time between cases, gives little opportunity for proper documentation of side-effects. If these occur in a recovery ward the anaesthetist concerned may not be able to leave the operating theatre and see the patient, and a wrong causal relationship may be attributed by an inadequately informed observer. In these circumstances documentation again is poor.

'A yellow card' issued by the Committee on Safety of Medicines is completely unsatisfactory for use by the anaesthetist. It is essentially designed for a less acute reaction perhaps to drugs given on more than one occasion, and the space for describing the type of reaction is of no help because it is not suitable for the anaesthetist. To obtain maximum reporting of reactions during anaesthesia one would need a questionnaire type of record which could be rapidly ticked off, to which could be appended the patient's record chart (probably with the name removed) and any other letters such as a medico-legal report. This would need careful decoding by someone aware of what happens in anaesthesia. Alternatively, with so much sophisticated computer monitoring of the drugs it should be a simple matter to perfect a method where the anaesthetist could use either an existing line or a bench computer, which is being used increasingly in this field of medicine. Here we have a big challenge both to the specialty and to the regulatory drug authorities.

These points are stressed, not to exonerate anaesthetists from all blame for inadequate record-keeping, but to highlight the problems which are present in clinical practice. The complete absence of any recorded data concerning the anaesthetic is inexcusable, but on occasions all that is possible is a simple statement of the drugs given, with doses where possible, and a comment on the smoothness of the anaesthesia. It would be unrealistic to suggest a scheme for monitoring side-effects of drugs given in the para-anaesthetic period which could not be carried out in practice. To make such a scheme mandatory could lead to records being meaningless.

The author has seen examples of this in various North American centres where often detailed questionnaire-type records have to be completed, the anaesthetist collects a large number of these at the end of a busy day and may be so tired that he takes these home to complete. Other demands prevent this, and they are eventually hurriedly completed (often quite inaccurately) a day or so later to beat the deadline demanded by the system. The incidence of drug-induced side-effects will be underestimated by this type of intensive compulsory monitoring which lacks the one thing needed for the accurate recording of data – motivation for the correct reason. One can record data (or at least complete a form) because one is compelled to do so, or one can record it in a genuine attempt to detect side-effects and improve patient care. A less complex system would have given more accurate information and resulted in more realistic data on side-effects of drugs.

## SIDE-EFFECTS

This is not a detailed survey of side-effects of agents used in anaesthetic practice, but rather an outline of the background against which the role of clinical trials and further drug monitoring should be considered. As with all drugs, side-effects can be due either to the parent compound or a breakdown product. In some instances the breakdown product will only lead to an enhancement or prolongation of the action of the parent compound, and this cannot be classed as a side-effect. Examples of this are succinymonocholine prolonging suxamethonium apnoea and n-desmethyl diazepam delaying recovery from diazepam. More sinister is the high-output renal failure attributed to the action of free fluoride ions following large doses of methoxyflurane. It has been suggested that a breakdown product is responsible for the undesirable effects of halothane on liver function, but this is not proven.

Until recently it was believed that inhalational agents differed from intravenous anaesthetics and other adjuvants in that they were exhaled unchanged *in toto*. This is not so, and while breakdown products are fairly innocuous, their concentrations cannot easily be controlled, since there is a great variation in the individual ability to metabolize drugs. It is thus desirable that as far as possible new inhalational agents will not be broken down in the body. This, at least, minimizes one source of drug toxicity.

As far as danger to the patient is concerned, we have to distinguish between three types of reaction:

(1) Known controllable side-effects which an anaesthetist is prepared to accept because of other advantages of the technique. These should be detected in the initial clinical trials. (Regretfully, as will be shown later, this is not always so.) With continuing use one 'learns to live with' such side-effects, and continuing research shows how they can be minimized: furthermore there is no danger to the patient. A good example of this is the extraneous muscle movements which occur with methohexitone. We now know that their incidence and severity is increased with both rapid injection and high total dosage and that they can be minimized by the use of opiate premedication: thus the advantages of more rapid recovery from anaesthesia outweigh the technical problems of induction of anaesthesia. Likewise the respiratory depressant effects of the 'neurolept' drugs or tachypnoea from trichloroethylene are not problems to be considered here.

(2) Toxic effects – usually unsuspected, which only occur very rarely but which may place the life of a patient in jeopardy. These may appear only when the drug has been in use for several years, and there may be several fatalities before the causal relationship to the anaesthetic is considered as a possibility. By virtue of their rarity, one many never be able to establish a definite causal relationship, but the probability is such that either the drug is withdrawn, it is used in safe doses or avoided completely in circumstances where there is a strong likelihood of a dangerous effect. One could classify these toxic effects under various headings, but from the point of view of monitoring for drug safety it is most helpful to consider these in relation to the reason for their rarity.

   (a) Dose-related toxic effects will be rare because of the few occasions on which the 'threshold' dose is exceeded. One can assume that less serious dose-related reactions will have been detected in the initial trials. Here the prime example is the high-output renal failure following methoxyflurane, which has already been referred to. This is produced by a concentration of free fluoride which is only achieved after very prolonged use of low concentrations or after moderate exposure to excessive concentrations. One cannot foresee how often an anaesthetist will give an excessive concentration of a drug: we can assume that this is not a major problem and the number of occasions on which methoxyflurane is given for a sufficiently long time to build up a significant concentration of the toxic ion are very few. The difficulty in establishing a causal relationship is further complicated by the individual response to the toxic metabolite – not every patient exposed to a given concentration will get high-output renal failure – and the enhancement of renal toxicity and concomitant administration of other drugs. One can see that an element of good fortune must be combined with good monitoring to detect this type of side-effect before a considerable number of patients are involved.

(b) Some toxic effects are more common on the second or subsequent administration of a drug. Here, one is dealing presumably with a hypersensitivity type of response in which the first administration induces a state of increased responsiveness in the patient. Since we do not yet know which agents will induce sensitivity to others we cannot rule out a reaction on first exposure falling into this class. The example of this *par excellence* is the effects of a second administration of halothane on liver function. Undoubtedly these occur more frequently after a second administration, particularly when given within a short period of the first, and they do not appear to be related to the dose used. However the frequency of hepatic dysfunction is rare even after a second exposure and such an administration may be given in circumstances where there are other more likely causes of liver dysfunction (sepsis, etc.). It is not the purpose of this chapter to discuss halothane-induced liver dysfunction in depth, but rather to put this into perspective in relation to the monitoring of toxic effects. It does show the need for extremely good records of a degree of excellence which is unachievable in clinical practice. Perhaps it again shows the need for an enquiring mind to probe into the occurrence of unexplained sequelae and try and relate these, not only to the previous administration of an anaesthetic, but to other factors which may be unrelated to anaesthesia.

We now have the results of prospective studies encouraged and partially financed by the Medical Research Council, on liver function following repeated administrations of halothane and enflurane. While these did demonstrate a higher incidence of sequelae after enflurane the results were disappointing from a number of viewpoints. Firstly as regards clearcut evidence incriminating one or the other drug: one was able to highlight some circumstances in which halothane would be likely to cause liver dysfunction, such as repeated administration within 6 weeks or repeated administration in obese patients, but the relationship was not as clear as one would have liked. Considering the effort both in manpower and expense involved in these studies it is unlikely that anyone would ever repeat them. Perhaps the lesson to be learnt is that better monitoring of side-effects with good records of anaesthesia and patient's condition in repeat and previous anaesthetics could probably have produced this information several years earlier than was done by this prospective study.[5–7]

It has been suggested recently that toxic effects, of a hypersensitivity type, are also more likely to occur on the second administration of intravenous agents, but this was not established in the above-mentioned studies.[8]

Before leaving this aspect of drug toxicity it is worth noting that a recent study was aimed at determining, among other factors, the frequency of repeat anaesthetics in an unselected pre-anaesthetic population.[9] The findings in 10 000 patients are shown in Table 1.

**Table 1** Number of patients with a history of 1–8 and 9 or more previous anaesthetics

| No. of exposures | 1 | 2 | 3 | 4 | 5 | 6 | 7 | 8 | 9+ |
|---|---|---|---|---|---|---|---|---|---|
| No. of patients | 2930 | 1539 | 748 | 502 | 239 | 170 | 58 | 37 | 449 |

(c) Thirdly, the toxic effects of anaesthetics may be rare due to the nature of the host. This includes genetically determined reactions such as those in Table 2. The patients under (b) could be included here, but this group is intended to highlight those patients who show hypersensitivity to the intravenous induction agent.

In some instances there is a history of atopy (asthma, hay fever or eczema) or more frequently a history of hypersensitivity to other drugs and the frequency of these in a surgical population and their importance has recently been discussed.[10] However, these do not reveal the underlying pathological state which is responsible for the findings.

**Table 2** Some genetically determined side-effects

| | |
|---|---|
| Suxamethonium | Prolonged response in patients with atypical plasma cholinesterase |
| Halothane<br>suxamethonium | Induced attack of malignant hyperthermia in susceptible patients |
| Barbiturates | Acute porphyria in patients with latent disease |
| Hypoxia and stress | Acute sickling of red cells in susceptible patients |

(3) Sequelae of the ketamine type, which occur during recovery from anaesthesia and may persist for up to 24 hours after operation. These consist of acute delirium during recovery and dream-like experiences which may be unpleasant or have a morbid content. The patient may feel detached from his surroundings and be unaware of his uncontrollable behaviour. It is now clear that these

do not endanger life but they affect a patient's attitude to subsequent anaesthetics and may thus indirectly interfere with health.

There are different standards considered to be acceptable in relation to side-effects of drugs by different investigators, and this poses a problem of comparability. There are also very large differences between the standards and practice of anaesthesia in continental Europe, Britain and North America. As an example, when ketamine was introduced into Britain, without extensive clinical trials in this country it became obvious that many patients had what were declared to be unacceptable side-effects. These had not been recorded in seemingly comparable cases in North American literature. However, it was eventually established that the minor operations in Britain took 2–3 minutes whereas a comparable procedure in North America may have taken 20–30 minutes. Here we certainly have an unknown factor influencing not only the frequency of side-effects but also one that is important irrespective of the nature of the operation since anaesthesia is induced with a standard dose of 1–2 mg $kg^{-1}$ given intravenously. With a relatively short procedure the patient wakens with a high plasma concentration and a resulting high incidence of emergence sequelae. With longer procedures, during which narcotic analgesic and inhalation agents may also be given, the patient wakens up with a much lower concentration and this, together with the residual effects of other drugs, can lead to a low incidence of sequelae.

It is perhaps for this reason that many countries require at least some clinical trials of new drugs to be carried out by their own physicians, and are not prepared to accept that all the clinical studies can be done outside the country in which they are seeking permission to market the drug. This may be more common in anaesthetics than in other forms of medical practice, but it does apply to a lesser extent with suxamethonium. In the UK we often use single doses and rarely an infusion, whereas in North America the reverse applies.

## CLINICAL TRIALS

While at one time one could have implicated clinical trials as a 'bottleneck' holding up the development of new drugs, this no longer applies in anaesthesia. Generally speaking, however, clinical trials are not as good and lack the sophistication shown by other branches of medicine. Perhaps this is not important, since, apart from local anaesthetics, most agents will be part of a sequence of multiple drugs given to the patient. There have been a number of reports of side-effects of drugs given under strictly controlled conditions (minor operations, unpremedicated patients), and while these are of value in indicating fundamental problems which one could expect with a drug, they may be unrelated to clinical practice. There is a need for more widely spread trials, and yet when these are designed by pharmaceutical firms, as is often the case, the degree of sophistication and reduction in variables leaves a lot to be desired. Investigators do not always appear to be aware of potential interactions, and such simple factors as the influence of pre-anaesthetic medication on induction chracteristics of intravenous anaesthetics and post-operative vomiting. Even in the evaluation of drug combinations, such as the neurolept sequence, it is important to look at the individual constituents. More than one anaesthetist has been surprised to find that the action of droperidol was very different from that of a droperidol–narcotic analgesic mixture.

On the other hand controlled trials alone yield data which may not be relevant to everyday practice. Reduction of variables in observers and patients places limitations on the number of cases that can be included in a clinical trial in a reasonable period of time. Research investigators may miss points which are of clinical importance and, strictly speaking, the results of controlled trials are only variable in the circumstances in which they are carried out. Furthermore because of rigid selection of cases for controlled trials interactions may be missed, and the side-effects of drugs in ill patients may be underestimated.

## GROUP TRIALS

The author has organized 'group trials' of several new intravenous anaesthetics and this concept is worth pursuing. It should be the logical sequence to, and not a substitute for, the controlled trial. Ideally it should be organized by the same person as is responsible for the controlled trial, but a full-time 'field worker' is essential for correlation of data and liaison with a group of clinicians.

Our studies aimed to involve all the anaesthetists in one region. A simple data sheet summarized the known information on the drugs, including the results of our own clinical trials. Each participant was visited personally when the nature of the study was explained and cooperation requested. In addition to the data sheet they were given a questionnaire to be completed for each administration. They were asked to use the drug with their routine premedication in consecutive unselected patients, and to form an impression as to how it would compare with their standard technique. They were contacted from time to time by the field worker (who was always available for advice) and questioned in detail at the end of the study.

With periodic prompting we got a 78% and 91% response in two successive studies which involved 1402 administrations of propanidid[11] and 2800 of althesin.[12,13] The most important result of these group studies was to show that new agents with a different duration of action cannot be routinely substituted for thiopentone. Without the results of such a group trial many people might have got into clinical difficulties with propanidid, with its very rapid recovery, and from this point of view it minimized what might have been dangerous clinical conditions. Since drug toxicity must be increased by a stormy clinical administration, group trials at least could circumvent this. More such trials are required to assess their value as a useful part of initial monitoring of drug toxicity. A group trial also detected an unacceptably high incidence of ketamine sequelae when the drug was first used in Britain, and in this case showed a difference from US results.[14]

Group trials did not uncover any cases of hypersensitivity either to propanidid or althesin. This is surprising since the incidence of reactions to the latter has been placed as high as 1:1000, though most feel that this is an overestimate.[15] The finding of no cases of propanidid sensitivity is easier to explain – many of these may be the result of overdosage with a drug which produces marked cardiovascular depression in high doses, yet which is relatively safe in recommended doses. (If one tries to prolong the action of an ultra-short-acting agent by increasing the dosage the possibility of excessive toxicity must be borne in mind.) The group trials may have been too limited in their extent, and a multi-centre trial is worth considering.

## INCREASING PROBLEMS

Perhaps this is the place to mention the possibility that the general patient population may be becoming more prone to hypersensitivity reactions.[16] Thiopentone was in clinical use for 20 years before a definite case of hypersensitivity to it was described, yet a recent survey gave details of 67 such cases.[18] Althesin, which clearly is more likely to cause reactions than thiopentone, was in clinical use for 3–4 years before the first definite case of hypersensitivity to it was reported, yet at least 200 of these have now occurred. Increased drug-taking (tranquillizers, contraceptives, aspirin, etc.) or exposure to drugs in food, etc., may contribute to this increase in hypersensitivity, and it would be instructive to know whether this has occurred with other types of drugs.

There is a problem of the slow publication of a suspicion of side-effects. Leading journals such as the *British Medical Journal* (see Chapter 51) will only take correspondence when this relates to a paper previously published. At present there is no way in which one could put in a letter saying that we have found a distressing incidence of a certain side-effect in a certain number of patients and ask if others have had similar experiences. By the time one prepares a full paper, an excessively large number of patients could have suffered an unnecessary side-effect. This is something which should be resolved, and if there were some simple method of letting the suspicion be known to readers then this would certainly increase the safety of many of the new preparations.

## CONTINUED MONITORING

It is obvious from the above that there is a need for some system of continued monitoring of the side-effects of new anaesthetics once they have become available for general clinical use. As stated earlier the yellow report cards issued by the Committee on Safety of Medicines (CSM) have proved inadequate for this purpose, at least as far as anaesthesia is concerned. Anaesthetists may not only not have the time to report them, but when questioning a number of colleagues recently in relation to whether a side-effect was reported it was noted that many of them did not know where to find the cards: this was particularly awkward when three were required on one morning and there was no information as to where these could be obtained. Much more publicity will have to be given about this by the regulatory authorities.

The importance of direct person to person contact in reporting should be stressed. This is shown by the recent example of reporting of hypersensitivity reactions to intravenous anaesthesia. A letter appeared in two journals requesting details of suspected cases to be sent to one of two addresses with telephone numbers provided for discussion of these. This was most successful and an enormous amount of relevant information was collected. Furthermore the anaesthetists concerned were asked to complete a very detailed questionnaire which was especially designed for this survey. Although this exercise was time-consuming, out of over 200 requests there were only four or five who did not go to the trouble to complete the form. Sometimes there were several telephone calls involved, with much useful discussion. Above all, those anaesthetists who reported cases all felt that there was an interest shown in their problem by those to whom the reports were sent, and they appreciated any advice which was given to them. Three other points emerge from this exercise:

(1) It was only with detailed questioning, and a knowledge of the problem involved, that it was possible to exclude a proven causal relationship in 14% of reported cases.[3] This may seem to be a small percentage but, above all, it did show that some cases of hypersensitivity were due to other drugs given simultaneously to the patients – particularly myoneural blocking drugs which had not previously been suspected.

(2) Although it was requested that all anaesthetists who reported hypersensitivity cases in response to the specific request should also send details to the CSM, less than one-third actually did so. Furthermore there were very few case-reports sent directly to the CSM which were not reported to the organizers of the detailed study.

(3) The collection, correlation and subsequent publication of 100 cases of sensitivity was unexpectedly time-consuming both as regards medical and secretarial time. It was carried out by existing

staff in an academic department with the financial assistance of a drug firm, but if it were to be done again it is suggested that a full-time worker, with back-up facilities, would be necessary. This person could best be located in an existing anaesthetic department with a knowledge of the problems involved. There should be a fixed time for completion of the survey. One would suggest that 2 years are needed for correlation, presentation and publication of the findings, with a possible extension for a third year in exceptional circumstances. Above all, the expenses of such a survey should be borne by an official agent (e.g. CSM, MRC) and with no obligation to the pharmaceutical industry. There may be exceptions to this if one is doing a field study of the complications following a single new drug, in which case the company involved should cover the expenses.

The monitoring of a specific side-effect would yield useful information and increase safety to the patients. It must, however, be initiated as soon as the possibility of the existence of such a side-effect is considered, and therein lies the difficulty in this type of drug monitoring. The organization of such a survey might be considered on a 'multi-centre' basis with a number of academic departments collaborating, and each having someone available for consultation and possibly to visit the anaesthetist involved in case-reports.

Another form of monitoring which is practical to some extent is to limit the use of new drugs to consultants, and to stipulate that juniors only use them under supervision. This was done with ketamine, but the results were not particularly impressive. Not all consultants are interested in new drugs, and they may give the supplies directly to a junior to use and then report the results to the Committee. There is also the very real fact that consultants are not necessarily the most informed as far as new drugs are concerned and may rely on those who have recently acquired the diploma of Fellowship for keeping them up to date on recent advances. Even if one supplies a particular questionnaire to be completed for each administration one wonders how reliable the findings will be. Again there is the question of motivation for completing the form. It can be completed as a necessary chore or as a means of providing useful information. Recently there has been a study in which investigators were paid for completed forms. This certainly is another means of motivation and if continued the sum involved should be purely nominal, and not sufficient to induce anaesthetists to use the drug and complete forms purely for financial reasons.

Attention should be given to the best way of setting up a mechanism for monitoring the side-effects which occur in, say, the first 10 000 administrations of a new drug. This will undoubtedly require completion of a specific form or questionnaire for each administration, and this should include as good a follow-up as it is practicable to obtain. Such a plan is fraught with problems and must not be so rigid as to antagonize those who will use the drug in routine practice. There is a danger of initial use being limited to those of a particular bent who enjoy completing forms, but who do not represent the 'bread and butter' anaesthetists. Could a system be devised in which an already respected investigator in each region has an overall remit for supervising the monitoring in his clinical area? This may involve academic departments and perhaps most of these feel that they already have enough administrative work to do. With goodwill all round it should be possible for one person in each clinical area to be designated as supervisor of drug monitoring and to work closely with the statutory body and academic departments. There must be some means of remuneration of such a person and this may have to be included in his contract. A problem arises from the fact that there will not be a continuous need for monitoring of new drugs – there are frequent lulls in their production – and this must be considered in relation to making specific appointments for this purpose.

One could challenge organizations such as the Association of University Professors of Anaesthesia or the Anaesthetic Research Society to look at the question of continued monitoring of side-effects. This is badly needed, and one hopes that any solution to this will not be forced on the speciality without due consultation with bodies such as these. However, if they themselves do not feel the need for it and do not make any attempt to improve the situation we may finish up with a system which was designed by non-anaesthetists, and which bears little relationship to clinical practice or the needs of the specialty. It is clear that all is not well in this field, and that more thought is required as to where we proceed next.

## References


1. Hunter, A. R. (1956). Neostigmine-resistant curarisation. *Br. Med. J.*, **2**, 919
2. Inman, W. H. W. and Mushin, W. W. (1974). Jaundice after repeated exposure to halothane: an analysis of reports to the Committee on Safety of Medicines. *Br. Med. J.*, **1**, 5
3. Clarke, R. S. J., Dundee, J. W., Garrett, R. T., McArdle, G. K. and Sutton, J. A. (1975). Adverse reactions to intravenous anaesthetics. A survey of 100 reports. *Br. J. Anaesth.*, **47**, 575
4. Hegarty, J. E. and Dundee, J. W. (1977). Sequelae after the intravenous injection of three benzodiazepines – diazepam, lorazepam and flunitrazepam. *Br. Med. J.*, **2**, 1384
5. Fee, J. P. H., Black, G. W., Dundee, J. W., McIlroy, P. D. A., Johnston, H. M. L., Johnston, S. B., Black, I. H. C., McNeill, H. C., Neill, D. W., Doggart, J. R., Merrett, J. D., McDonald, J. R., Bradley, D. S. G., Haire, M. and McMillan, S. A. (1979). A prospective study of liver enzyme and other changes following repeat administration of halothane and enflurane. *Br. J. Anaesth.*, **51**, 1133
6. Fee, J. P. H., Black, G. W., Dundee, J. W., Doggart, J. R., McIlroy, P. D. A. and Neill, D. W. (1980). Hepatotoxicity of repeat inhalation anaesthetics, *Br. J. Anaesth.*, **52**, 839
7. Dundee, J. W., McIlroy, P. D. A., Fee, J. P. H. and Black, G. W. (1981). Prospective study of liver function following repeat halothane and enflurane. *J. R. Soc. Med.*, **74**, 286

8. Clarke, R. S. J. (1978). Hypersensitivity reactions to intravenous anaesthetics. In Dundee, J. W. (ed.) *Current Topics in Anaesthesia: New Intravenous Drugs in Anaesthesia.* (London: Arnold)
9. Fee, J. P. H., McDonald, J. R., Dundee, J. W. and Clarke, R. S. J. (1978). Frequency of previous anaesthesia in an anaesthetic patient population. *Br. J. Anaesth.*, **50,** 917
10. Fee, J .P. H., McDonald, J. R. and Dundee, J. W. (1980). Frequency of atopy, allergy and previous general anaesthesia in surgical specialties. *Ann. R. Coll. Surg.*, **62,** 125
11. Clarke, R. S. and Dundee, J. W. (1966). Group trials of propanidid as an intravenous anaesthetic. *Ulster Med. J.*, **35,** 44
12. Carson, I. W. (1972). Group trials of Althesin as an intravenous anaesthetic. *Postgrad. Med. J.*, **48,** 108
13. Carson, I. W. (1974). Althesin: a group trial as an intravenous anaesthetic. *Ulster Med. J.*, **43,** 151
14. Dundee, J. W. (1978). Editorial. *Anaesthesia*, **33,** 497
15. Evans, J. M. and Keogh, J. A. H. (1977). Adverse reactions to intravenous anaesthetic induction agents. *Br. Med. J.*, **2,** 735
16. Dundee, J. W. (1978). Total intravenous anaesthesia. *Br. J. Anaesth.*, **50,** 9

# 22
# Radiological contrast media

**G. ANSELL, M. C. K. TWEEDIE, C. R. WEST and D. A. PRICE EVANS**

## INTRODUCTION

Contrast media play an essential role in many radiological investigations. Most of them are iodinated derivatives of organic molecules. In this chapter it is proposed to restrict the discussion to the monitoring of adverse reactions following intravenous urography, intravenous cholangiography and computerized axial tomography (CAT). The causes of these reactions are still uncertain. Minor reactions with allergic-like phenomena are not uncommon. Severe and fatal reactions are rare, but mainly unpredictable. In order to study these major reactions, it is necessary to undertake a large-scale survey. Pendergrass and his colleagues analysed 99 urographic deaths occurring in the United States between 1942 and 1956.[1] During this period it was estimated that 11 546 000 urograms had been performed, giving a mortality rate of 8.6 deaths per million examinations (1 in 117 000). In France between the years 1955 and 1965 a mortality rate of approximately 1 in 61 000 was estimated,[2] and in Italy it was estimated that the rate was 1 in 85 000.[3] In a survey carried out amongst radiologists in the UK during the years 1966–9, the mortality rate for intravenous urography was 1 in 40 000, and the rate of severe life-endangering reactions was 1 in 14 000. Although contrast media used during the UK survey were generally considered to be less toxic than those used during the earlier surveys conducted in the United States, the mortality rate had certainly not decreased and, if anything, was somewhat higher. This might have been due to the less restrictive selection of patients for urography and also to the use of higher dosage. In an analysis of 81 278 urograms performed in 30 hospitals the mortality appeared to be as high as 1 in 14 000.[6]

In the interval since the first UK survey, there had generally been a further increase in dosage schedules of urographic contrast media. A second survey was therefore commenced in 1977 under the auspices of the Committee on Safety of Medicines (CSM) to determine whether there was any associated increase in the incidence of reactions.

## DESIGN OF REPORT FORMS

Forms used to report adverse reactions fall into two main categories. In the 'open' type of form, detailed questions are kept to a minimum, and generous blank spaces are provided for a written description of the reaction. This type of form is uncluttered and easy to complete, but it subsequently requires detailed analysis and information may be incomplete. The 'analytical' type of form, on the other hand, consists of a detailed questionnaire covering the known features of reactions to a specific category of drugs or contrast media, and it can also include questions concerning suspected aetiological factors. This latter type of form can, therefore, provide greater accuracy, but it has the disadvantage that there may be less scope for reporting unforeseen types of reactions. In addition, the increased complexity of the form may deter prospective investigators from participating in the survey. This latter problem can be partially overcome by the design of the form. Questions should be grouped in sections in a logical manner, under appropriate subheadings. The various sections and subsections should then be clearly demarcated from one another, using vertical and horizontal rules of varying thickness. By breaking up the form in this manner, the visual impact is improved and relevant sections can be quickly located. The design and layout of the form should also ensure a satisfactory aesthetic appearance. Since adverse reactions occur infrequently, there is a tendency for reporting forms to be mislaid. To help overcome this, it is suggested that they be large, e.g. 30 × 20 cm, supplied either as a tear-off pad or in a distinctive wallet. When the design of the form has been agreed, a small-scale trial should be performed using duplicated copies, to detect any fault before the main print is ordered. Much useful information relevant to the design of forms of inquiry is provided by Bradford Hill.[7]

In the first UK survey 1966–1969[4,5] an open type of form was used. The intention in the second survey was to explore, in depth, some of the problems raised as a result of the earlier survey. Were there any predisposing factors in the individual, such as age, ethnic group, cardiac state or allergy? Was preceding drug therapy relevant and what was the significance of previous reactions to contrast media or other drugs? Of equal interest were questions of contrast media dosage and rate of administration. To collect all this information, it became obvious that an analytical type of form was required. Because of the large numbers of forms involved, it was decided that 'mark sensing' forms should be used. The appropriate answer was marked in pencil, and this was read automatically by an optical scanner. There was also provision in these forms for 'free' information, such as the names of contrast media or drugs, to be encoded during processing. The questions on the front of the form concerned clinical information and details of the contrast medium examination. If an adverse reaction occurred, this was analysed in a questionnaire on the back of the form.

Reserved blocks of digits were also provided on the back of the form for encoding the names of contrast media, drugs, etc. Each form had an individual serial number. This was recorded when the form was issued and could subsequently be used to identify the hospital of origin. Specimens of the forms are available from G. Ansell on request.

In the two US surveys performed in 1942 and 1951, the total number of urograms was estimated by using manufacturer's data on the sales of ampoules after an appropriate correction had been made for alternative use, breakage, etc. At that time, the standard dose of contrast medium for intravenous urography was 20 ml. Since then, however, the use and dosage schedules of contrast media have become so diverse that this approach would now be meaningless. Radiologists participating in the first UK survey submitted annual returns of the number of investigations, types of contrast media used, and dosage schedules. For the second survey a more accurate data-base was required, covering not only contrast media usage, but also information relating to the spectrum of patients undergoing the examination.

The survey was planned to extend over 12 months. Ideally, it would have been desirable for a report form to be completed for each examination. However, this would have created an impossible work load in a busy X-ray department. It would also have caused considerable practical problems for the survey staff. As a compromise, it was decided that the survey would consist of two components: A and B. In component A, each department would, for two sample weeks during the year, complete a form for each intravenous urogram, intravenous cholangiogram, and CAT scan. During these sample weeks, *all* reactions would of course be reported. Sample weeks for each hospital were determined by using a computer-generated list of random weeks with the stipulation that the two sample weeks should be separated by a minimum of 12 weeks. They were otherwise distributed throughout the 12-month period with the exception of a 9-week period covering July and August, when it was anticipated that staff shortages due to holidays might make completion difficult. Sample weeks containing public bank holidays were also included in the survey but, on the rare occasion when both sample weeks included public holidays, the next set of random weeks was selected. In component B, which extended throughout the remainder of the survey year (apart from the two sample weeks in component A), radiologists were asked to complete a form only in the event of a 'moderate', 'life-endangered' or 'fatal' reaction. Grading of reactions was as follows:

*Minor* (reported only in sample week i.e. component A of the survey): transitory reactions which subsided without treatment (however 'loss of consciousness' with spontaneous recovery would be graded 'moderate' or even 'life-endangered' depending on the degree).

*Moderate*: reactions which required some form of treatment, but there was no undue alarm for the patient's safety and response to treatment was usually rapid.

*Life-endangered*: severe reactions threatening life and usually requiring intensive treatment.

*Fatal*: death which appeared to be related to the injection of contrast medium.

To simplify the task of collecting clinical data in the X-ray department during the sample weeks, printed slips were supplied for completion by the ward staff. The information requested included weight, blood-pressure, blood urea, serum bilirubin, history of cardiac disease and the names of all drugs received in the preceding 7 days. For out-patients, similar forms were available for the patient to take to his general practitioner, but the information requested was restricted to drug therapy.

## COMMUNICATIONS

Full support for the survey was given by the Royal College of Radiologists, and a notice to this effect appeared in its journal. During 1976, the names of chairmen of radiological divisions, or alternatively of consultant radiologists in charge of hospital X-ray departments, were obtained by writing to all the Area Health Authorities in England, Wales and Scotland. Personal signed letters were then written to each of these radiologists explaining the nature of the survey and inviting their participation. A reply form was enclosed together with a stamped addressed envelope, and radiologists willing to join the survey were asked to state the approximate number of intravenous urograms (IVU) and intravenous cholangiograms (IVC) performed in each hospital during the previous year (1975). Hospitals performing fewer than 100 urograms annually were excluded. Neurological centres performing CAT scans were added to the survey at a later stage.

Each hospital was allocated an individual seven-digit reference number based on region, area, district and hospital type. Addressograph labels were prepared for each hospital and used for all subsequent documentation and correspondence. The survey was controlled by means of an index ledger arranged in numerical sequence. This ledger contained details of the number of examinations performed in 1975, sample weeks, and serial numbers of report forms issued in respect of each hospital. This information was subsequently put into the computer file store. A diary was also prepared listing the hospitals for each sample week. Although it would have been possible to write a computer program for these control measures, it was considered that conventional methods were more suited to the prevailing circumstances. Prior to the commencement of the survey year each hospital was issued with a labelled cardboard file (SO 23–107, size 35 × 23 cm), made more distinctive by means of a band of red Scotch tape. Each file contained:

(1) A sheet of instructions with the dates of the sample weeks, brief guidance notes on completion of the computer report forms and criteria for grading reactions.

(2) A small supply of computer forms for reporting reactions which might occur before the first sample week.

(3) Special 'ward' and 'GP' forms.

(4) A labelled postcard for ordering additional supplies of forms.

(5) An HB pencil.

(6) An eraser.

The main supply of forms was dispatched 1 month before each sample week together with a reminder notice; the number of forms issued to each hospital varied according to the number of examinations performed in 1975 or to the postcard demands. An additional reminder letter was sent to all hospitals at the mid-stage of the survey, stressing the importance of reporting all major reactions throughout the survey year. Where there was undue delay in receiving the returns of sample weeks, written or telephone reminders were made as appropriate.

## PROCESSING AND COMPUTING

Reports of major reactions were inspected as they arrived, and if there were any unusual features a written request was made for further information. Returns for the individual sample weeks were checked against the diary and the occasional inconsistency in dates or other obvious errors were investigated. Items of free information, such as the names of contrast media or drugs, or details of previous adverse reactions, etc. were converted into numeric code derived from the CSM list, and the numbers were then entered into the reserved blocks on the back of the form. This operation was performed by a part-time pharmacist. At this stage, forms containing items of specific interest, such as reactions, were separated from the routine sample week returns, so that they could be more easily accessible for individual study at a later date.

The optical reading forms were visually checked for marks which the optical scanner might misread before being input to the computer system. Additional information (allocated sample weeks, numbers of 1975 returns and serial numbers of sheets sent to particular hospitals) was input *via* punched cards.

A verification program checked the information before the records were input to the main data-base. Other information, such as the names of drugs and symptoms with particular code numbers (obtained from the DHSS office in Reading), was input to the data-base separately.

The data-base consisting of over 600 000 items, was managed under a system which uniquely identified each case by serial number, and which could deal with a variable number of items (such as drugs given) per case. The management system could produce report listings of particular cases or could output cases in the form of a data file to be input for statistical analysis by SPSS (Statistical Package for the Social Sciences), GLIM (Generalized Linear Interactive Modelling),[8] or other programs (specially written when necessary).

(Further information on the computing aspects of this survey appears in the 1st edition of this book, and is also available from C. R. West).

## SURVEY-RELATED PROBLEMS

In the 1966–69 UK survey, 183 hospitals participated during the year 1966. It was estimated that this represented approximately one half of the radiological work load in the UK. However, there was a progressive decrease in the number of participating hospitals during the ensuing years. Numbers fell by approximately 50% in 1967, 16% in 1968 and 26% in 1969, by which time there were only 82 hospitals in the survey. This illustrates the difficulty in sustaining prolonged interest during monitoring procedures.

As has been mentioned earlier, in the present investigation we limited the survey period of component A to 2 weeks and of component B to 12 months: the intention being to ensure greater compliance. Invitations were sent to 367 radiologists and 251 (69%) representing 312 hospitals agreed to participate. A further 20 hospitals were willing to participate in the survey, but they were not included because of the small numbers of examinations performed. After receiving their survey forms, 26 hospitals withdrew. Although not formally withdrawing, 37 other hospitals did not return any reports during the year. Thus, 63 (20%) of the 312 hospitals were effectively withdrawn from the survey. Of the 249 hospitals continuing in the survey, 2 hospitals returned data only on CAT scans. 31 hospitals completed only 1 sample week; 20 completed their first sample week but not the second week, whilst 11 failed to complete the first week but completed the second week. On occasion, it was necessary to change the randomly allocated sample week for the convenience of the hospital.

In the final allocation, the numbers of departments in any given sample week varied from a minimum of 8 to a maximum of 21. However, two hospitals elected to perform one of their sample weeks during July and August, respectively. In a very few cases, hospitals peformed their sample on the wrong week or transferred survey forms to another hospital without formal notification. These caused some difficulties in the checking procedure when the forms were received.

Altogether, 7616 forms were completed relating to intravenous urograms, intravenous cholangiograms and CAT scans. Detectable errors or omissions were noted on some of the forms, but in the great majority of cases the standard of completion was remarkably high. In retrospect we consider the wording of some questions could have been improved. The forms were usually completed at the time of injection, but some hospitals preferred to make their own special questionnaires and fill in the survey forms from these. In some cases, responsibility for the survey was apparently passed on to the superintendent radiographer, but here again the standard of completion was satisfactory.

In planning the survey, we tried to minimize the effort required to complete the forms, but it must be admitted that an appreciable extra work-load was required during sample weeks, particularly in busy departments which were not infrequently suffering from staff shortages. It is therefore highly creditable that such a large number of radiologists participated.

Most people dislike filling in forms and radiologists are no exception. It is therefore of interest to consider the motivation of those involved. Undoubtedly, an important factor was the still-unsolved problem of contrast media reactions which concern all radiologists and the evident belief that this was a worthwhile investigation. Many drug-monitoring programmes have in the past been based mainly on University teaching hospitals. Our radiological surveys show that there is a considerable potential to be tapped from the more peripheral hospitals. Indeed in the first survey, co-operation from non-teaching hospitals (approximately 55%) was distinctly better than that from the teaching hospitals (approximately 30%). One can only speculate on the reason for this, but it may be that radiologists in the peripheral hospitals felt more isolated and welcomed the opportunity to participate in a research project, whereas the teaching hospital departments were more self-assured. In the second survey, teaching hospitals were more adequately represented. Among the other factors which were presumably encouraged participation in the second survey was the official support of the CSM and the Royal College of Radiologists.

Not least important, was perhaps the personal relationship which was built up with radiologists as a result of the previous survey, and the feedback of information both by publications and by ready availability for telephone consultation on problems affecting contrast media. It is of interest that this service was not infrequently used by radiologists who themselves had declined to take part in the surveys.

In a large-scale survey of this nature there are several possible sources of error. One problem is in grading the severity of reactions. The classification of reactions was derived from the first UK survey where it had proved its practicability. In general there was little difficulty in grading the important severe (life-endangered) reactions, but decisions on the overlapping spectrum between minor and moderate (intermediate) reactions could be subject to greater variation. The original hospital grading of reactions was usually accepted, but in some cases it was altered by G.A. when the forms were received and checked. An important source of error lies in the possible omission to notify some of those reactions which occur outside sample weeks. This would result in falsely low incidence figures. However, there is usually considerable motivation to report severe reactions and it was thought that few of these would have been omitted.

In the non-sample weeks (component B), reactions considered to be 'minor' would not normally be reported and they would, therefore, not be available for up-grading. Thus recoding of reactions from 'moderate' to 'minor' was possible, but recoding in the opposite direction was not, except for a comparatively few cases in which hospitals returned reactions categorized as 'minor' during non-sample weeks. Some of these were recategorized to 'moderate'.

A major problem in any survey is the consistency of reporting. The numbers of reports of intravenous cholangiograms and CAT scans were relatively small, and we shall not discuss them further in this chapter.

Table 1 compares the incidence of urography reactions reported during the sample week in all of the 247 participating hospitals. It is apparent that the incidence of reactions reported in the second sample week was substantially lower than that reported in the first week. The incidence of reactions was also lowered in those hospitals returning only 1 sample week. These results suggest that variations in observer threshold at different times and in different hospitals could be an important factor.

Table 2 compares the incidence of intermediate, severe and fatal reactions after urography reported in all hopsitals during the sample weeks (component A) with the reports received in the remainder of the 12 months survey period (component B). We had expected that there would be a degree of under-reporting in component B of the survey,

**Table 1** IV Urograms. Incidence of reactions reported in sample weeks (247 hospitals)

| | *Total No. IVUs* | *Minor reactions* | *Intermediate reactions* | *Severe reactions* |
|---|---|---|---|---|
| 1st sample week | 3249 | 267<br>1/12.2 | 55<br>1/59.1 | 6<br>1/542 |
| 2nd sample week | 2963 | 163<br>1/18.2 | 28<br>1/106 | 2<br>1/1482 |
| 1 sample week only | 368 | 21<br>1/17.5 | 3<br>1/123 | 1<br>1/368 |
| All sample weeks | 6580 | 451<br>1/14.6 | 86<br>1/76.5 | 9<br>1/731 |

but the difference in the incidence rate was surprisingly high. In the intermediate reactions there was a variation by approximately a factor of 9 and in the severe reactions by a factor of 7. By definition reactions in patients who received treatment were classified at least 'intermediate'. In some of these cases treatment may have been superfluous and this might have tended to artificially raise the incidence level of intermediate reactions in the sample week. Cases of this nature might be less likely to be reported in the non-sample weeks. Nevertheless, although there may have been some over-reporting of intermediate reactions in the sample weeks, it appears that there was a very significant degree of under-reporting of reactions in non-sample weeks. Human nature being what it is, this would not be entirely surprising when one considers the heavy routine work load in the average X-Ray Department if the under-reporting applied only to the

**Table 2** IV Urograms. Incidence of reactions reported in sample and non-sample weeks. (247 hospitals)

| | *Total no. IVUs* | *Minor reactions* | *Intermediate reactions* | *Severe reactions* | *Deaths* |
|---|---|---|---|---|---|
| All sample weeks | 6580 | 451<br>1/14.6 | 86<br>1/76.5 | 9<br>1/731 | 0 |
| All non-sample weeks | 173 700* | — | 249<br>1/698 | 34<br>1/5109 | 4<br>1/43425 |

*Estimated for 50 weeks

**Table 2a** IV Urograms. Incidence of reactions reported in sample and non-sample weeks. (103 hospitals reporting in components A and B)

| | *Total no. IVUs* | *Minor reactions* | *Intermediate reactions* | *Severe reactions* | *Deaths* |
|---|---|---|---|---|---|
| All sample weeks | 3640 | 251<br>1/14.5 | 53<br>1/68.7 | 5<br>1/728 | 0 |
| All non-sample weeks | 93 900* | — | 249<br>1/377 | 34<br>1/2762 | 4<br>1/23475 |

*Estimated for 50 weeks

intermediate reaction. It is more difficult to explain under-reporting of severe reactions.

Although 247 hospitals submitted IVU returns for component A, only 103 of these hospitals reported any IVU reactions for component B. That is to say, 144 hospitals reported on the IVU examinations performed during their respective sample weeks, but failed to report any reactions outside those weeks. Some of these 144 departments were small: 17 reported IVU examinations at the rate of 5 or fewer per 2 sample weeks, but even they should have performed roughly 2000 such examinations in the remainder of the year, and might therefore have been expected to report at least some 'intermediate' reactions. The other 127 departments should, from their sample weekly returns have performed about 80 000 IVU examinations outside their sample weeks. Therefore, assuming an arbitrary rate of one reaction of reportable severity per 100 examinations, about 800 such reactions may have been unrecorded in our survey. In an attempt to allow for the absence of reports being possibly genuine in some cases but not in others, we have explored the use of various statistical models.

The question arises whether under-reporting might have been selective. The 144 hospitals which only submitted IVU returns during sample weeks (component A) reported 2940 such examinations in these weeks. These reports showed four reactions graded as severe (but no deaths). This is a rate of 1 in 735 examinations. The 103 hospitals which contributed to both components of the survey reported 3640 IVU examinations for component A. This included five patients with severe reactions (but no deaths). This is a rate of 1 in 728, which compares favourably with the other group of hospitals. The individual departments varied widely in their reported rates of reactions. This suggests that there were differences in their probabilities of reporting the cases which did occur. The dates of the final reports received from each hospital in non-sample weeks were surprisingly evenly spread over the year. This suggests that a number of departments may have terminated their reporting prematurely, and this might account for some of the under-reporting.

As far as we have been able to detect, under-reporting did not appear to be seriously selective apart from a greater likelihood of preferential reporting in respect of severe reactions.

The 103 hospitals which reported at least one IVU reaction in their non-sample weeks (component B) proved that they had complied at least in part with the requirements of the survey. If we use these hospitals to compare the incidence of reported reactions in sample and non-sample weeks (Table 2a) we find that there is closer agreement, although there still appears to be significant under-reporting of intermediate reactions in the non-sample weeks.

The number of minor and intermediate reactions reported during the sample weeks are sufficient to give a reasonable assessment of the incidence of these two grades of reaction. There is less certainty about the incidence of severe reactions. It would be expected that dramatic events of this nature would be more fully reported. In Table 2a, the difference in incidence rates of severe reactions reported in sample and non-sample weeks is unlikely to be due to chance ($p = 0.020$).

On the other hand, calculations based on data from only the 103 hospitals which reported reactions in the non-sample weeks might overstate the incidence of reactions. We think that this is most likely with fatal reactions and that the rate for these given in Table 2 covering all 247 hospitals might be more appropriate.

Through the courtesy of the Office of Population Censuses and Surveys, we attempted to determine from death certificates whether there had been any relevant deaths due to contrast media during the survey year which were not reported to us, and we did not find any such cases. On the contrary, we found that survey notifications appeared more reliable than death certificates. We obtained copies of death certificates in a small series of 13 contrast media-related deaths which had been reported to us over several years and where the information enabled us to identify the patients concerned. In one death certificate, contrast medium was specified as the primary cause of death and in five cases it was given as a subsidiary cause. In the remaining seven death certificates, there was no mention of the use of contrast medium.

Another problem to be considered is the uniformity of reaction rates among different sections of the population. In recent years, there has been a sizeable degree of immigration into the United Kingdom, and we have taken advantage of this to compare the risk of reactions in different ethnic groups. If the risk ratio of North-Europeans is given a value of 1, the risk for Africans does not differ significantly from North-Europeans. However, there is an increased risk in the Mediterranean group, and an eightfold increased risk of a severe reaction being reported among Indians. At present, the reason for this increased risk is unknown.[9]

Most contrast media reactions usually commence during the course of the examination and are therefore readily apparent. Delayed adverse effects appear to be uncommon, but it is possible that if they should occur once the patient has left the X-ray department they might be taken for granted, or they might not be recognized as being connected with the X-ray examination. For one reason or another, it is rare for delayed adverse effects to be reported back to the radiologist. Occasional cases of this nature have come to light fortuitously, but it is difficult to estimate their true frequency.

We have collected a considerable quantity of clinical data in the second survey which was not available in previous surveys. This has been used to investigate the predisposing factors in severe contrast media reactions, notably the effects of previous reactions to contrast media, asthma, cardiac disease and contrast medium dose. These results have been reported elsewhere.[9] There is also evidence to suggest that there may be a synergic action between beta-blockers and contrast media in causing reactions with bronchospasm.

We have drawn attention to the problems of under-reporting which may occur in a large survey of this nature. Nevertheless, these still compare favourably with the very considerable uncertainties and inaccuracies inherent in other voluntary schemes of drug monitoring. We consider that, in appropriate circumstances, survey techniques can provide an invaluable source of information on specific problems. Moreover, the introduction of departmental micro-computers could provide an opportunity for improved data acquisition.

## Acknowledgements

We should like to acknowledge the co-operation of Dr P. Davies, Mr A. D. Goddard, Mrs L. Couch, Mrs M. Cooper and Mrs B. Rothwell.

We should also like to acknowledge the co-operation of the Committee on Safety of Medicines and its secretariat. The survey was funded by a grant from the Department of Health and Social Security, and the University of Liverpool provided generous computer facilities.

## References

1. Pendergrass, H. P., Tondreau, R. L. *et al.* (1958). Reactions associated with intravenous urography: historical and statistical review. *Radiology*, **71,** 1
2. Wolfromm, R., Dehouve, A. *et al* (1966). Les accidents graves par injection de substances iodées pour urographie. *J. Radiol. Electrol.*, **47,** 346
3. Toniolo, G. and Buia, L. (1966). Risultati di uno ischiesta nazionale sugli incidente mortali da iniezioni di mezzi di contrasto organo-iodata. *Radiol. Med. (Torino)*, **7,** 625
4. Ansell, G. (1968). A national survey of radiological complications: interim report. *Clin. Radiol.*, **19,** 175
5. Ansell, G. (1970). Adverse reactions to contrast agents. Scope of problem. *Invest. Radiol.*, **5,** 374
6. Shehadi, W. H. (1975). Adverse reactions to intravascularly administered contrast media: a comprehensive study based on a prospective survey. *Am. J. Roentgenol.*, **124,** 145
7. Hill, A. B. (1977). *A Short Textbook of Medical Statistics*, pp. 34–42. (London: Hodder and Stoughton)
8. Baker, R. J. and Nelder, J. A. (1978). *Generalised Linear Interactive Modelling (GLIM) Numerical Algoriths Group.* (Oxford: NAG)
9. Ansell, G., Tweedie, M. C. K., West, C. R., Price Evans, D. A. and Couch, L. (1980). The current status of reactions to intravenous contrast media. *Invest. Radiol.*, **15,** S. 32

# 23
# Radiopharmaceuticals

D. H. KEELING

## INTRODUCTION

Radiopharmaceuticals are not specifically mentioned in the Medicines Act of 1968, but since it is clear that they are administered to patients 'for the purpose of diagnosing disease or ascertaining the existence, degree or extent of a physiological condition' they are to be considered as medicinal product within the meaning of the Act and covered by its provisions. The fact that they contain radioactive atoms within their molecules is immaterial from a pharmacological point of view, though clearly important from the question of radiation dosage. These aspects are separately covered by legislation and Codes of Practice[1–3] which are currently under review. Radiopharmaceuticals currently used in medical practice vary enormously in their chemical, physical and pharmacological properties, and include not only true aqueous solutions but macromolecular and colloidal preparations, particulates, aerosols and gases. As indicated above, the only unifying feature is the possession of radioactive atoms for their subsequent recognition. They also differ markedly from most therapeutic, and many diagnostic, medicinal products in the minute quantities of materials involved and pattern of use, in that any individual patient is only likely to receive one or a very few doses of material. Because of this, and their radioactivity, it is obvious that problems with them are likely to be very different from normal medicinal products.

## THE RANGE OF RADIOPHARMACEUTICALS

Diagnostic materials form by far the largest class of radiopharmaceuticals, and include all the scanning and imaging materials used in nuclear medicine plus those given for organ function and blood flow measurements and for studying the lifespan and distribution of blood cells and platelets: other materials are used to study the absorption of nutritional and therapeutic compounds. The therapeutic radiopharmaceuticals are a much smaller group, and would not include the small sealed capsules and wires implanted within the body which simply act as radiation sources (they do not have any pharmacological activity and just irradiate a volume of tissue around them). However, there are some well-known examples of therapeutic radiopharmaceuticals – the commonest being the radioiodine isotope $^{131}I$ used in the treatment of thyrotoxicosis and some forms of thyroid carcinoma. The pharmacological behaviour of a radiopharmaceutical is determined by its physical and chemical form: this can vary from a simple inorganic ion to a complex biochemical molecule or even labelled cells, and will determine the timing and pathway of its metabolism in the body and its subsequent excretion. These in turn are important considerations in determining the radiation dose to tissue.

The earlier radiopharmaceuticals consisted of relatively simple inorganic preparations with a few exceptions, such as those based on the mercurial diuretics and iodinated X-ray contrast agents. At that time almost all radionuclides were produced in reactors in atomic energy establishments, and inevitably the radioisotopes had to have a not-inconsiderable half-life to allow for their preparation, purification and delivery to hospitals. The introduction of radionuclide generators – and later of cyclotrons – has brought about the most significant change in radiopharmaceutical manufacture in the last two decades. Cyclotrons in hospitals have made available some extremely important radionuclides, but their complexity and cost has greatly limited their use. It has been the development of radionuclide generators, in particular the $^{99}Mo-^{99m}Tc$ form which has been responsible for this revolution. In these generators, which are usually sterile chromatography-type columns, the longer-lived parent nuclide is absorbed and the short-lived daughter isotope separated daily by a simple elution process in the hospital ready for use. A peculiarity of radiopharmaceuticals is the excessively small quantity, in chemical terms, of the radionuclidic element involved. A bone scanning dose of $^{99m}Tc$ MDP contains only about 15 ng Tc – at which level there can be no problems with toxicity nor adverse effect. A dose of 100 mCi (3700 MBq) $^{131}I$, sufficient to completely destroy the thyroid gland, would contain no more iodine than is present in the red colouring dye of a single glacé cherry.

Radiopharmaceutical preparations often contain milligram quantities of carrier molecules, bacteriostats, buffers, stabilizers including radiolysis inhibitors and perhaps physiological blocking agents to regulate handling within the body, and pharmacological reactions can and do occur with these materials, though the great majority are hypersensitivity type reactions. However, some radiopharmaceuticals do have pharmacological activity at these concentrations and require *slow* intravenous administration. It is clear from the pattern of use of diagnostic and therapeutic radiopharmaceuticals that chronic toxicity is never a problem.

$^{99m}$Tc generators are available in many hospitals, and with a range of (non-radioactive) 'kits' also readily obtained from commercial sources, short-lived radiopharmaceuticals are now in widespread use. The most recent data on radiopharmaceutical use in the UK[4] shows three quarters of all *in vivo* nuclear medicine investigations involved $^{99m}$Tc compounds. Over 80% of all administrations were of materials that had been in some way or other prepared 'in house', as opposed to straightforward 'bought in' commercial products. It is because of this 'in house' preparation, even though it may involve commercially obtained pretested starting materials, that responsibility for radiopharmaceuticals and their adverse reactions becomes complex.

## HAZARDS OF RADIOPHARMACEUTICALS

Monitoring the safety of radiopharmaceuticals involves many factors, some obvious for all medicinal products, some unique. The problems which might be anticipated with radiopharmaceuticals include both those due to their radiation and those due to their physicochemical properties. Because they are products of the atomic age with all its attendant anxieties, nuclear medicine procedures have evolved with a very conscious realization of the radiation dose being delivered to patients. However, to put these risks in perspective, it is fair to say that most diagnostic nuclear medicine tests involve a tissue irradiation dose less than comparable X-ray diagnostic studies.

The radiation dose to a tissue will be greatly influenced by the effective half-life within that tissue. This is a product of the physical half-life of the radioactive atom and the biological 'half-life' due to its biochemical handling in the body. A long physical half-life will have the attraction of giving the material a useful shelf-life which is both convenient and financially attractive. However, it does mean that to keep the radiation dose within predetermined limits, the biological excretion of the radiopharmaceutical must be rapid and reliably so. Unfortunately many examples exist where this has led to problems, either due to inappropriate administration or to pathological conditions slowing down excretion with resulting high radiation dose. For this reason radionuclides administered for diagnostic purposes should preferably have short physical half-lives; this, together with favourable nuclear decay characteristics, can mean that even with total retention within the body, radiation dosimetry is perfectly acceptable, and has been a major factor accounting for the success of the $^{99m}$Tc generator.

Radiopharmaceutical production 'in house' presents unusual problems, and requires close collaboration of physicists and pharmacists with medical specialists.[5–8] Radiation safety both of staff and patients requires special monitoring, handling techniques and tests. There is no time for the normal full pharmaceutical quality control; the radiopharmaceuticals are usually required the same day. The batch size may be just a single vial containing four or five patient doses in 5–10 ml of fluid. Starting materials may not be obtainable in a pharmaceutical grade, and the standards required must be a matter of judgement. An important factor contributing to the reliability of a safe production method is the design of the laboratory. This is more fully discussed in References 9 and 10, the facilities required depending upon the type of work being done.

For many radiopharmaceuticals prepared by the addition of sterile ingredients via a 'closed' system to pre-sterilized closed containers and used the same day, it is recommended that the manipulations should be performed within a Contained Work Station complying with the requirements of BS 5295. The work station itself should be in a room preferably supplied with filtered air, and monitored to demonstrate its continuing suitability.

Sterile radiopharmaceuticals which are neither terminally sterilized nor prepared by 'closed' procedures, should be prepared in an aseptic room with air filtered to the requirment of Class 1 of BS 5295 *and* a Contained Work Station as described in Section 9 of Reference 7. For many hospitals with a limited requirement for these expensive facilities, it may be quite sufficient to use a totally enclosed work station of the glove-box type with a self-contained air filter/circulation unit. The Medicines Inspectorate will check and advise on particular requirements relating to pharmaceutical aspects of laboratory design.

In the introductory period when an new radiopharmaceutical is under investigation[5,8] its behaviour in animals must be carefully investigated. It is preferable to use at least two species of animal (only one a rodent), and to check on the concentration in every tissue in the body. Even then it has been found that there are many cases where animal experiments have given quite misleading results when extrapolated to man. Subsequently small numbers of human subjects must be studied, including normal and relevant pathological states, distribution and excretion measurements must be rechecked, and radiation dosimetry re-calculated.

The radionuclide to label the pharmaceutical must also meet certain minimum standards. Its nuclear production process must be such that other radioactive atoms – even of the same element – are kept below specified limits. Problems of usable shelf-life can still arise if the radionuclidic impurities are longer-lived than the primary product, as the proportion of the longer-lived isotope will increase with time till it reaches unacceptable levels.

As previously mentioned, radionuclides such as $^{99m}$Tc are likely to be present in only nanogram quantities, and at a concentration of perhaps one millionth that of impurities in analytical grade chemicals. The elution of radionuclide generators must be extremely reliable as it may not be feasible to test for the long-lived parent nuclide coming through in the eluate prior to its use in patients. This must be checked at weekly intervals, allowing the short-lived daughter nuclide to decay, and measuring any leakage of the parent isotope. At the same time eluate sterility should also be checked.

Radiochemical purity is a second problem requiring that the subsequent chemical processes only yield the required chemical form of that isotope. If other chemical compounds, reaction products or residues are present, they again must be kept within specified limits and these need to be checked. Apart from a simple radioactivity assay, only a few quick and simple chemical measurements are possible on most preparations prior to use,[11,12] and batch control assumes less importance than process control. Safety lies in the reliability of a tried and tested production process, helped of course by the fact that the final product is used almost immediately. Few radiopharmaceuticals are potential microbial growth agents, and there will not be time for bacterial or fungal multiplication.[13] Modern radiopharmacy techniques require that a worksheet is kept for each radiopharmaceutical showing that the normal procedure has been followed. Radioactivity measurements are made on the batch itself and then on individual doses. The doses should be calculated from the concentration in the stock material and then individually checked in a calibration meter. Direct reading meters are to be preferred; they can easily be checked daily against a known long-lived standard and there is no subsequent calculation to be made where human error may creep in. In addition, random samples are kept back for subsequent normal quality control of sterility, etc.

## REPORTING ADVERSE REACTIONS

A final aspect of monitoring for safety with radiopharmaceuticals is the collection and collation of reports of adverse reactions. The introductory trials and experience will have weeded out any suspect materials and the incidence of reactions is likely to be very low. Because of this it is not feasible to assess the true incidence in a single hospital, and countrywide reporting is now in practice in the UK, the USA, Australia and elsewhere. Because the great majority of radiopharmaceuticals are, in part at least, prepared 'in house', they were not originally included in the DHSS countrywide 'yellow card' reporting system, and a separate system evolved in the UK through the offices of the professional bodies involved. Originally this was the British Institute of Radiology, the British Nuclear Medicine Society and the Hospital Physicists Association, shortly joined by the Regional Radiopharmacists Sub Committee. An initial report[14] appeared in 1974 with up-dates being published from time to time.[15,16] Recently the European Joint Committee on Radiopharmaceuticals has set up its own scheme to gather reports across Europe, but they gather their information largely via the few established national schemes, and it is clear from their recent reports[17] that without some organization at national level, the system is scarcely workable. In addition to adverse reactions involving patients, a number of the schemes also collate reports on drug defects, including packaging and product information problems.

The present reporting schemes are principally looking for pharmacological reactions rather than radiation dosimetry problems. This is understandable when there is very rarely any immediate radiation effect, merely a statistical risk of some long-term sequela. However, if it served to point out an avoidable problem, it would be sensible to disseminate such information.

The reported adverse reactions to radiopharmaceuticals over the last two decades have shown, as expected, that problems can arise with *in vivo* distribution giving local or generalized over-irradiation. This can occur, for example, with poor clearance of a radiopharmaceutical from its injection site. Investigation of lymphatic clearance in gross lymphoedema has yielded examples where tissue necrosis has occurred owing to complete failure of a relatively long-lived radiocolloid to move from its subcutaneous injection site: Only short-lived radiopharmaceuticals that would still not produce excessive local irradiation should be used.

The published reports of adverse reactions to radiopharmaceuticals which are of a pharmacological nature show an extremely diverse picture with little pattern. It is certain that a significant proportion of the more trivial reactions was unreported. Three main groups of radiopharmaceuticals were seen to make up a majority of the earlier reports; these included several of the particulate preparations and the intrathecal radiopharmaceuticals. In cisternography studies, to follow the movement of cerebrospinal fluid which has proved to be of value for investigating hydrocephalus, there was an alarming number of cases of aseptic meningitis reported. All the preparations involved had passed the standard pharmacopoeial rabbits test for pyrogens and were sterile. Furthermore, they were not confined to a single type of radiopharmaceutical, both iodine and technetium-labelled albumin preparations, colloids and chelated compounds were involved. It was not until the introduction of the *Limulus amoebocyte* test for pyrogens that the classic investigation of Cooper and Harbert[18,19] showed that the presence of bacterial endotoxin insufficient to be detected by the pharmacopoeial test was the cause of the trouble. It was found that phosphate buffers and anion exchange resins could contain large quantities of endotoxin, and although subsequent dilution reduced it below the normal detectable levels, intrathecal injection led to a prompt reaction. Subsequent to the use of the Limulus test, this problem is no longer seen.

In Europe, several cases have been reported of severe neurological sequelae following the (lumbar) intrathecal injection of $^{99m}$Tc-labelled DTPA (diethylene triamine penta acetate).[20] Original work had used the mixed calcium and sodium salt without problems, but with the use of the trisodium salt, permanent saddle anaesthesia and sphincter problems could occur, presumably related to the 'deionization' of the lumbar CSF. On a number of the commercially available DTPA kits, it was not clearly stated which salt was present, with resulting neurological disaster. Particulate radiopharmaceuticals, including the radiocolloids, have accounted for a substantial proportion of reported adverse reactions. The larger macroaggregates and microspheres used for lung perfusion scans and certain blood flow studies embolize in the first capillary bed they reach and thus, by ante-cubital vein injection, give rise to a picture of a normally perfused lung. Haemodynamic problems are now very rarely seen, as these preparations can be accurately sized and counted prior to use, and the number of particles injected carefully controlled. In chronic pulmonary hypertension the additional micro-embolization has very rarely been blamed for right heart failure. and the particles have been used for arterial flow studies. Again the possibility of over-dosage arises and fatal reactions have occurred following intra-coronary artery use. It is clearly particularly vital that the number and sizes of particles used is carefully controlled. Less rarely these human albumin preparations have caused anaphylactoid reactions. These, however, are heat denatured particulates and there has frequently been a history of atopy in these patients. The reactions have usually been of a vasomotor type, often with breathlessness and tightness in the chest, and have often passed off without treatment. More recent data from the North American reporting scheme[21] shows that the microsphere preparations are much more likely to cause this problem than the macroaggregates of albumin.

Radiocolloids have been implicated in a considerable number of reactions, which are seen with both sulphur and antimony sulphide colloids of technetium – both widely used for liver scans. The more frequent type of adverse reaction is again a form of vasomotor upset. Similar reactions have been reported with $^{99m}$Tc-labelled 'phytate colloids'. The most recent UK report[16] shows the largest single cause of reactions is the diphosphonates used for bone scans. These investigations are the commonest nuclear medicine investigation, and a significant number of erythematous itching skin rashes have been reported.

Reliable incidence figures are not available, but if even trivial reactions are included, may be as high as 1:2750. This, however, compares very favourably with X-ray contrast media reaction figures.

In the UK professional bodies are now co-operating in a scheme linked to the CSM and the European Reporting Scheme. A questionnaire is sent to members from time to time, and all reports are subsequently banked in the computer data-files of the CSM Reporting Scheme as a valuable cross-check in case relevant information should become available based on (non-radioactive) medicinal products. From time to time updated articles appear in the medical literature giving details of reported adverse reactions. Similarly warnings are given if any particular formulation appears to be associated with an unduly high number of reactions.

## References

1. *Radioactive substances Act.* Department of the Environment (1960). (London: HMSO)

2. *Code of practice for the protection of persons against ionising radiations arising from medical and dental use.* DHSS. (1972). (London: HMSO)
3. *Health and safety at work Act.* Department of Employment. (1974). (London: HMSO)
4. Wall, B. F., Hillier, M. C., Kendall, G. M. and Shields, R. A. (1985). *Br. J. Radiol.*, **58,** 129–35
5. Guidelines for the preparation of radiopharmaceuticals in hospitals. *Royal Marsden Hospital Conference Working Party.* (1975). *Br. Inst. Radiol. London Spec. Rep.* No. 11
6. The hospital preparation of radiopharmaceuticals. (1977). *Hosp. Physic. Assoc. Sci. Rep. Ser.* 16
7. DHSS (1983). *Guide to Good Pharmaceutical Manufacturing Practice* 3rd Edn and Appendices. (London: HMSO)
8. Larson, S. M., Siegel, B. A. and Robinson, R. G. (1978). Guidelines for the clinical evaluation of radiopharmaceutical drugs. *J. Nucl. Med.*, **19,** 1359
9. Kristensen, K. (1979). Preparation and control of radiopharmaceuticals in hospitals. *Tech. Rep. Ser.* No. 194. Vienna: IAEA)
10. DHSS (1984). *Guidance Notes for Hospitals. Premises and Evironment for the Preparation of Radiopharmaceuticals.* (London: HMSO)
11. Safety and efficacy of radiopharmaceuticals. (1984). In Kristensen, K. and Nørbygoard, E. (eds.) Boston: Martinus Nijhoff
12. Chromatography of Technetium-99m radiopharmaceuticals – A practical guide. (1984). In Robbins, P. J. (ed.) (New York: Society of Nuclear Medicine Inc.)
13. Abra, R.M., Bell, N.D.S. and Horton, P.W. (1980). The growth of microorganisms in some parental radiopharmaceuticals. *Int. J. Pharm.*, **5,** 187
14. Williams, E. S. (1974). Adverse Reactions to Radiopharmaceuticals: a preliminary survey in the United Kingdom. *Br. J. Radiol.*, **47,** 54
15. Keeling, D. H. (1979). Side-effects associated with the use of radiopharmaceuticals. In Gorrod, J. W. (ed.) *Drug Toxicity*, Ch. 16, pp. 285–95. (London: Taylor and Francis)
16. Keeling, D. H. and Sampson, C. B. (1984). Adverse reactions to radiopharmaceuticals: United Kingdom 1977–1983. *Br. J. Radiol.*, **57,** 1091
17. Kristensen, K. (1984). Reporting of adverse reactions and drug defects. Second report 1982–1983. *Eur. J. Nucl. Med.*, **9,** 388
18. Cooper, J. F. and Harbert, J. C. (1973). (Abstract). Bacterial endotoxin as a cause of aseptic meningitis following radionuclide cisternography. *J. Nucl. Med.*, **14,** 387
19. Cooper, J. F. and Harbert, J. C. (1975). Endotoxin as a cause of aseptic meningitis following radionuclide cisternography. *J. Nucl. Med.*, **16,** 809
20. Verbruggen, A., de Roo, M., Dewit, P., Guelinckx, P. and Dom, R. (1982). Complications after intrathecal administration of Tc-99m DTPA In Cox, P. (ed.) *Progress in radiopharmacology*, P. III. pp. 223–35 (Boston: Martinus Nijhoff)
21. Cordova, M. A., Rhodes, B. A., Atkins, H. L., Glen, H.J., Hoogland, D. R. and Soloman, A. C. (1982). Adverse Reactions to Radiopharmaceuticals. *J. Nucl. Med.*, **23,** 550

# 24
# Skin reactions

W. BRUINSMA

## INTRODUCTION

Clinically recognizable adverse drug reactions (ADRs) more often affect the skin than any other organ or system, and an increasing part of dermatological practice consists of their diagnosis and treatment.

There is a tendency for drug-regulatory agencies (DRAs), together with a large segment of the medical community, to regard the common types of skin reaction as of minor consequence. It should be realized, however, that in addition to considerable individual discomfort, they are responsible for a far-from-negligible number of sick days and occupied hospital beds, with their consequent economic effects.

In descending order of frequency, the most common types of drug-induced skin reaction are:

The exanthema (rashes)
Urticaria
Eczematous eruptions (e.g. contact dermatitis)
Purpura

In the following list will be found, in alphabetical order, a selection of rare skin reactions:

acanthosis nigricans; acne; alopecia; chloasma; depigmentation; elastosis perforans serpiginosa; epidermolysis bullosa; erythema multiforme; erythema nodosum; erythrodermia; exacerbation of dermatitis herpetiformis, herpes gestationis, herpes zoster, psoriasis; exfoliative dermatitis; fixed eruption; hypertrichosis; lichenoid eruptions; lupus erythematosus; lymphoproliferative disease; oculomucocutaneous syndrome; oral ulceration; pemphigoid; pemphigus; periarteritis nodosa; photosensitivity; pigmentation; porphyria cutanea tarda; pruritus; skin tumours; toxic epidermal necrolysis; vasculitis.

Some of these rare reactions, such as toxic epidermal necrolysis and erythema exudativum multiforme, are extremely serious and frequently fatal. The latter led to restriction of the use of long-acting sulphonamides in a number of countries. Until recently this was the only example of a skin reaction which had a major effect on drug policy. In 1974, however, skin, ocular and other effects of practolol (oculomucocutaneous syndrome) led to the withdrawal of this drug.

## INVESTIGATIONS OF SKIN REACTIONS

Various drug-monitoring systems are required to investigate skin reactions according to the frequency of their occurrence. Common reactions such as the exanthema and urticaria have an incidence within the range of 0.1% to several per cent for a large proportion of drugs, and it should be possible to estimate their incidence during pre-marketing clinical studies and hospital monitoring. When attempting to obtain precise measurements of their frequency it is important to remember that this depends not only on the drug itself, but also on the characteristics of the population at risk. Factors such as the age, sex and disease being treated account at least partly for differences in frequency quoted in the literature, and the dermatologist can play an important role in this type of monitoring. It is his responsibility to ensure that skin reactions are accurately described and classified, that appropriate laboratory methods are used to evaluate them, and that reactions that are due not to the drug but to colouring agents or preservatives, are excluded. Tartrazine, for example, may induce urticaria; parabens may produce eczematous eruptions. It is important that the pharmaceutical literature should specify the nature of the colouring agents and preservatives included in the formulation of all medicines.

Accurate estimates of frequencies in excess of 0.1% are of great practical importance to clinicians and to DRAs. When a patient is receiving several different drugs concurrently and develops a skin reaction of one of the common types the clinician may, if he has adequate data on their frequency, make a reasonable guess at which of the drugs was the most likely cause.

Rare reactions may be defined as those which occur in fewer than 0.1% of patients treated with a drug, those which occur only after prolonged administration, or after a long lapse of time since the drug was given, or only in a particularly susceptible group of patients or when combined with some other factor such as a particular food. These are unlikely to be detected during pre-marketing studies or in hospital monitoring. Usually they are detected and published by astute clinicians, and later confirmed by similar observations by their colleagues. Indeed it can be argued that it is the medical community as a whole that must carry the burden of responsibility for detection of rare or unexpected reactions. All prescribing physicians should be aware that no biologically active agent is free from risk.

Voluntary reporting systems (VRSs) have been established for the purpose of collecting suspicions of new or unexpected ADRs and have had some successes and some failures (see Section I, Chapters 1–11). Specifically they failed to detect the oculomucocutaneous syndrome of practolol.[1] Many cases had occurred which were not reported to the monitoring agencies, but there is always the danger that even if they had been reported, their significance might have been missed by monitoring staff. Monitoring centres are under-staffed, and must be supported by consultants representing all the various specialities so that potentially important information will not remain unanalysed. Obviously such a group of consultants must include a dermatologist since the most frequently reported ADR is a skin reaction.

Expert analysis of reports of skin reactions may provide information not obtainable elsewhere. Estimates of the relative incidence of particular ADRs affecting the skin may be made by plotting their profiles.[2]

Frequently, reports of suspected ADRs are presented at seminars or hospital meetings or as letters to journals. This method of communication has been and will continue to be important, but unfortunately often introduces considerable delay.

## THE *FILE OF ADVERSE REACTIONS TO THE SKIN*

In 1977 the *File of Adverse Reactions to the Skin* was established at the department of dermatology of the Free University of Amsterdam. Reports of suspected and previously unknown adverse reactions to the skin are accumulated. By sending a report of such a reaction the participating dermatologist automatically receives a copy of similar reports from the File, if available. These data may be freely used for publication. The fact that he can match these data with his suspicion of an adverse reaction may be of considerable assistance to the reporting dermatologist in evaluating his own observation. About once every 4 years the information in the File, supplemented by data from the literature, is made available for a nominal charge in a clear and accessible way in revised editions of the *Guide to Drug Eruptions*.[3] As a rule, the File does not publish reports of suspected unknown adverse reactions to the skin in the interval between two editions of the *Guide*. It is felt that the reporting dermatologist, using his own observation combined with the data in the File, is in a better position to evaluate these combined data, and to publish his findings when appropriate. In this way the *File of Adverse Reactions to the Skin* acts essentially as a communication centre for suspicions and reports of as yet unknown ADRs. The File offers the following advantages:

(1) Great homogeneity and significance of the input data, thanks to the more accurate classification and diagnostic acumen of the participating dermatologists.
(2) Confidence among participants in the professional judgment and

use of the data provided in the course of communication from specialist to specialist.

(3) Provision of the accumulated data in a usable form for practising dermatologists, which will provide tangible proof of the usefulness and permanency of the programme.

(4) The possibility of linkage with similar suspected adverse reactions to the skin without any publication lag.

In addition to providing a procedure for detecting new ADRs to the skin, the File and its publication *A Guide to Drug Eruptions*, which gives a framework for reporting adverse reactions in addition to reporting forms, may in the future also be able to assess the significance of some adverse reactions published in the past. It is not unusual for some adverse reactions to be quoted from one review article to the next, almost attaining 'eternal life', while the original source, in the distant past, may now seem to be of doubtful significance. By inviting dermatologists to report observations on some of the old adverse reactions, it should be possible either to confirm them or, when the File has attained sufficient momentum, to eliminate the adverse reaction concerned, in this way purifying some data of the past.

Reports of suspected favourable reactions to drugs are communicated following the same procedure. The favourable drug reaction, i.e. the improvement or cure of a pre-existing dermatological disease during or after the administration of a drug, given for an unrelated disease, whose effect on that particular disease had not been previously reported, simply represents the sunny side of the endeavours of the File.

Thalidomide, already mentioned elsewhere, equally illustrates the benefits that might be obtained from the favourable side-effect of a drug unknown at the marketing stage. Probably few people are aware of the fact that thalidomide, since this effect was first noticed in 1965,[4] is now the drug of choice for leprosy patients who develop the second type of leprosy reaction. In 1975 a marked therapeutic effect of thalidomide was observed in cases of discoid lupus erythematosus and has subsequently been confirmed by later studies.[5] More recently a possible therapeutic effect of thalidomide has been described in patients with Hailey–Hailey disease, a rare hereditary bullous disease, for which no remedy is yet available.[6]

The favourable drug reaction (FDR) most likely will in the future become as important as the ADR in drug monitoring. Minor unexpected therapeutic effects of drugs might provide important clues in the development of new drugs. Major unexpected therapeutic effects for disease entities, like Hailey–Hailey disease, where the extremely small number of patients makes an extensive major research programme for drugs by pharmaceutical companies unfeasible, might provide new indications for existing drugs, which would remain unknown without drug monitoring for these effects.

Since its introduction at the International Congress of Dermatology, Mexico City, October 1977, several hundred ADRs and FDRs have been communicated among the participating dermatologists. An encouraging number of ADRs have subsequently been confirmed and published in the literature.

A VRS, like the *File of Adverse Reactions to the Skin*, limiting itself to a speciality in medicine, but international in scope, may have an advantage in detecting the unexpected drug effects in its field.

## References

1. Gross, F. H. and Inman, W. H. W. (eds.), *Drug Monitoring* (1977). (London: Academic Press)
2. Bruinsma, W. (1972). Adverse reaction profiles of drug eruptions. *Dermatologica*, **145,** 377
3. *A Guide to Drug Eruptions*, The File of Adverse Reactions to the Skin (Distributed by De Zwaluw, PO Box 21, Oosthuizen, The Netherlands)
4. Sheskin, J. (1965). Thalidomide in the treatment of lepra reactions. *Clin. Pharmacol. Ther.*, **6,** 303–6
5. Samsoen, M., Grosshans, E. and Basset, A. (1980). La thalidomide dans le traitement du lupus érythémateux chronique. *Ann. Dermatol. Venereol.* (Paris), **107,** 515–23
6. Schnitzler, L. (1984). Effet bénéfique de la thalidomide dans un cas de pemphigus de Hailey–Hailey. *Ann. Dermatol. Venereol.*, (Paris), **11,** 285

# 25
# National Registry of Drug-Induced Ocular Side-Effects

F. T. FRAUNFELDER

## INTRODUCTION

While on a sabbatical year at the Institute of Ophthalmology and Moorsfield Eye Hospital in London, England, I became aware that the clinicians in Great Britain were much more interested in post-marketing surveillance of drugs than was true in the United States. I also saw the unfolding of the practolol story[1] by an astute clinician, Mr Peter Wright, who had the privilege of seeing a large group of patients funnelled through the National Health Service to a particular clinic. This was the 'Dry Eye Clinic' at Moorsfield Eye Hospital where persons with a deficiency of tear secretions were sent for evaluation. If these patients had not been referred to a common source so that one physician could examine multiple similar cases, possibly the common denominator for this particular clinical picture would have been missed. If not missed, at least many more years would have been necessary to correlate these extremely devastating drug-induced ocular findings with this drug.

While present-day sophisticated medical systems are highly specialized with their own diagnostic and therapeutic regimens, only occasionally are there clinical settings where a single physician sees a large volume of patients who are on a particular drug. Therefore, it is often difficult for the average clinician to draw a relationship or a clinical impression of drug-induced pathology, due to insufficient sample size. This is probably especially true in the surgical specialities.

Yet, time and time again, medical history shows where an astute isolated clinician has suspected an adverse drug response many years before it was recognized as a possible adverse drug reaction (ADR). Examples of this include the fetal alcohol syndrome, thalidomide-induced birth defects, and clindamycin and lincomycin induction of ulcerative colitis. It seemed reasonable then that suspicions of the practising clinician, if sought, could be pooled to increase the database and could act as a flagging system to decrease the lag-time in recognizing a possible adverse drug response. For example, 20 years of human topical ocular steroid application passed before it was realized that steroids can cause cataracts, and it took 10 years of widespread clinical use before ophthalmologists were aware that topical ocular steroids could cause glaucoma.

I then went to the literature to see how to set up a drug registry for ophthalmology and found to my dismay that all drug registries in the past were doomed to failure. The primary reasons these registries failed seemed to include physician apathy, fear of malpractice, lengthy forms, insufficient number of reports, and incomplete or unreliable data. With these thoughts in mind, I thought that the odds were quite poor that this type of programme in ophthalmology could be developed, so I went no further. However, with time, colleagues became aware that I was interested in human ocular toxicology, so they started to ask me to present papers on this subject at meetings. Soon I was being contacted by physicians in practice to tell me about their various possible drug-induced ocular side-effects. Academic associates, commercial toxicologists, and attorneys were seeking and giving information from which I learned of trends of possible cases. In essence, I found that I was starting my own mini-registry. So the transition from that into the one which I will outline briefly came about easily from having inadvertently already started one on a small scale.

## THE NATIONAL REGISTRY

The National Registry of Drug-Induced Ocular Side-Effects became an official entity in July 1976 after being funded by the United States Food and Drug Administration. Before attempting to set up this registry, we felt we had to have it approved by the American Academy of Ophthalmology so as to have official backing from our National Society. To make this long-term registry feasible, it seemed essential that it must give a service to ophthalmologists or it would have only transitory acceptance. In an attempt to achieve this the registry does the following:

(1) We keep an ongoing file of any report in the world literature of a possible drug-related ocular event. The clinician can call or write to us, and we will then review for him what data are available on that drug and send a bibliography, if requested.

(2) We are available for phone consultations, and often from this are able to get that particular physician's case to add to our files.

(3) We prepare, each year, an annual report listing all cases which were sent to the Registry, and that year's bibliography of possible adverse events which we obtained from the world literature. This is sent to anyone, at cost.

(4) If there is evidence of a possible association, articles are published in the ophthalmic literature. Since this is a flagging system, we cannot really prove a cause-and-effect relationship, and it is more of a question-generating system. Significant cardiovascular effects, including 15 cases of myocardial infarcts and 11 deaths, have been reported primarily in the older age groups secondary to topical 10% phenylephrine.[2] Systemic side-effects secondary to topical ocular administration of timolol have been reported to be essentially the same as those seen from systemically administered beta-blockers.[3,4]

(5) Each person who sends in a case-report gets a personal letter in return from the director of the Registry, often containing recent data that relate to the adverse ocular event he has reported.

(6) Each physician is aware that no files are kept with his or his patients' names, to prevent medico-legal problems for the physician or the Registry. Therefore, there is protection for the physician, which at this point in time in the United States is a major concern from a malpractice point of view. Since the director of this programme is fairly well known within the speciality, there appears to be an easier and more trustworthy interchange than if this were reported to a federal agency or board.

(7) If the physician reports his case to a drug company or to the Food and Drug Administration, he would be contacted with a request for additional data; thus producing far more paper work. This is a mechanism required by federal law. This is not the case if reported to the Registry. The Registry therefore allows more freedom and encourages participation, since the physician knows that rarely is further inquiry to be made.

## DATA COLLECTION

How are data collected?

(1) Advertisements reminding the clinicians that this Registry is available for their use are placed in various journals (Figure 1).

(2) Each ophthalmologist in America is sent FDA Form 1639 from the Registry by mail at least twice each year.

(3) All data sent to the FDA with possible drug-related ocular side-effects are given to the Registry. This also includes the total community studies currently being undertaken in Florida and Massachusetts by the FDA.

(4) An outline of how to send data to the National Registry is placed in a book published by Lea & Febiger, *Drug-Induced Ocular Side Effects and Drug Interactions*, 2nd Edn., by F. T. Fraunfelder, MD (1982). In addition each edition of the *Physicians' Desk Reference for Ophthalmology*, published by Medical Economics Company,

# Drug-Induced Ocular Side Effects

A national registry has been established to collect data on suspected drug-induced ocular side effects. If enough responses suggest a cause and effect relationship, prospective studies will be done. Please send us your ideas of previously unsuspected, rare, severe, or unusual drug-induced ocular side effects. If reporting a specific case, please include the following: suspected drug and reaction, age and sex of patient, route of administration, dosage, course of adverse reaction, other drugs taken at the time, and your opinion as to cause and effect.

Send to: Ms. Martha Meyer, Department of Ophthalmology, University of Oregon Health Sciences Center, 3181 S.W. Sam Jackson Park Road, Portland, Oregon 97201.

**Figure 1** Advertisement of this Registry

contains a chapter on ocular toxicology provided by the National Registry.

(5) In our experience, some of the best cases are given verbally, since some physicians are wary of putting possible legally sensitive cases in writing. These are given over the 'phone or by telling the director in person at various ophthalmic meetings. The Director presents ocular toxicology lectures at a minimum of six to eight major ophthalmic meetings per year; during these 1–2-day meetings, the clinicians are asked to relay their cases and suspicions to him. This has been a highly rewarding method of gathering data.

(6) An unexpected benefit has been to act as intermediary to connect clinicians and basic scientists for toxicological collaboration. Since the Registry, in essence, knows the latest trends and persons working in basic toxicology, we act as a clearing house to join clinicians with similar cases or clinicians and basic scientists. In the first year, six such instances occurred and resulted in toxicology publications.

(7) The Director is frequently asked opinions in legal cases, and these cases are then added to the Registry.

(8) We are in contact with 25 other adverse drug reaction registries

from countries throughout the world. They are sending their annual reports to us for incorporation into our Registry.

(9) Every 2 years, we hold a National Symposium of Drug-Induced Ocular Side Effects. The fourth meeting was held in Augusta, Georgia, April 27–28, 1984. This brings together the academician, the clinician, the drug companies, and the researchers and results in increased interchange, emphasis, and data for the Registry.

During the first nine years of the Registry, we have indeed been pleasantly surprised by the response we have obtained from the ophthalmic community. The reason, we feel, for this excellent response is an increased public and physician awareness of possible adverse drug reactions. The Registry provides a service to the ophthalmologists in practice. The success of the Registry is also in part due to the attempt to take the fear of legal implication or 'harassment' out of the reporting for physicians, the brevity of the forms, and the prompt feedback to the clinicians. It is essential to have a nationally recognized director in the speciality who can continually keep the Registry in front of the clinician, and with whom the clinician can develop trust and with whom he can identify. An important aspect of the Registry is the lay associate director. This person has to be familiar with pharmacology and toxicology and be able to communicate with the clinician. We are most fortunate to have such a person, Mrs Martha Meyer, and she is invaluable to the success of this Registry. The Registry may also be successful in that it has realistic objectives. It is not intended to find cause-and-effect relationships, but it is intended to obtain 'clues' and act primarily as a 'flagging'-system.

## DISCUSSION

Attitudes in drug use have swung from uncritical enthusiasm about benefits to undue pessimism about risks. Surveillance of drugs is indispensable because clinical trials can only include a small, and at times, an atypical fraction of patients with adverse responses. A registry of the type described here is obviously far from ideal, but possibly for many speciality groups, may be the only *economically* feasible system available to us at this point in time. The drawbacks of this system are multiple and cannot be defended on a statistical or purely scientific basis. It is basically a question-generating system. Within the given limitations, this system can only raise questions, although already it has suggested an occasional answer. Interpretation of these data is indeed most difficult, and overviews were published only after a minimum of 3 years' data accumulation.[5,6] Unless there are some fairly obvious trends already set that need to be reported to the medical community, the Registry proceeds cautiously. For example, a case of fatal aplastic anaemia possibly associated with topical ocular chloramphenicol solution was reported as the second fatal case, although two previous reports of reversible bone marrow hypoplasia had also been reported following topical ophthalmic chloramphenicol.[7] This is not to say that rapid detecting of an adverse reaction in medicine has not occurred from a limited number of case-reports without controls. A prime example of this is the vaccines which have caused polio, or other neurological disorders.

An additional problem is the publication of data. Impressions, correct or incorrect, from this Registry could severely damage a particular product; the Director, the funding or sponsoring organization, such as the American Academy of Ophthalmology, could be sued. Attempts have been made to have the data looked at by a larger body, such as the Committee on Drugs and Toxicology of the American Academy of Ophthalmology. However, they felt passage of any recommendations by this body would then constitute official policy of the American Academy of Ophthalmology. At this point in time, they felt it best not to commit the Academy to this. Therefore, it is the responsibility of the director of the National Registry; however, before any overview article is written, it will be reviewed by others interested in ocular toxicology and legal consultants.

While research projects have already become evident by looking at the preliminary data from this Registry, prospective toxicological studies are not always feasible. For example, according to the Registry, there appears to be a higher propensity for terminal myocardial infarcts in the older age-groups in patients placed on topical ocular 10% phenylephrine. A protocol to test this in humans would indeed have difficulty in passing a medical human research committee, let alone that funding be necessarily available.

In summary, to date, the National Registry of Drug-Induced Ocular Side-Effects has had a success beyond our expectations. Few physicians in certain specialities see at large enough number of patients on a particular drug to be able to readily associate a possible cause-and-effect relationship as an adverse drug-related event. If a large number of physicians 'pool' their experiences, possibly trends could become evident. It must be stressed, however, that relevant analysis of data from this type of registry will indeed be most difficult, and that this system is primarily a flagging system or an hypothesis-generating system, and not intended to be a cause-and-effect relationship system. Functions of this Registry have, however, included an increased ophthalmic awareness of human ocular toxicology, stimulation of ocular toxicological research, acted as a clearing house for worldwide drug surveillance of possible adverse drug-related ocular events, acted as a ready data source for ocular toxicological problems for the practising physician, and has published articles on possible ocular toxicological effects. In monitoring systems, seldom are ocular adverse drug reactions reported even with known significant side-effects.[8] However, registries of the type described here, with nationally recognized personnel, can be sensitive to speciality groups' trends or clues of possible ADRs. This is not a scientific system. Much of the value of the data is in serious question; however, at this time, economically this type of programme may be warranted as a stop-gap system for some medical specialities.

## Acknowledgement

This study was funded by Contract No. 223-82-3012 from the Food and Drug Administration.

## References

1. Wright, P. (1975). Untoward effects associated with practolol administration: oculomucocutaneous syndrome. *Br. Med. J.*, **1,** 595
2. Fraunfelder, F. T. and Scafidi, A. F. (1978). Possible adverse effects from topical ocular 10% phenylephrine. *Am. J. Ophthalmol.*, **85,** 447
3. Van Buskirk, E. M. (1980). Adverse reactions from timolol administration. *Ophthalmology*, **87,** 447
4. Van Buskirk, E. M. and Fraunfelder, F. T. (1981). Timolol and glaucoma. *Arch. Ophthalmol.*, **99,** 696
5. Fraunfelder, F. T. (1979). Interim report – National Registry of Drug-Induced Ocular Side-Effects. *Ophthalmology*, **86,** 126
6. Fraunfelder, F. T. (1980). Interim report – National Registry of Drug-Induced Ocular Side-Effects. *Ophthalmology*, **87,** 87
7. Fraunfelder, F. T., Bagby, G. C., Jr. and Kelly, D. J. (1982). Fatal aplastic anemia following topical administration of ophthalmic chloramphenicol. *Am. J. Ophthalmol.*, **93,** 356
8. Stewart, R. B., Cluff, L. E. and Philp, J. R. (1977). *Drug Monitoring: A Requirement for Responsible Drug Use*, pp. 118–21 (Baltimore: Williams & Wilkins)

# 26
# Obstetrics and gynaecology

J. S. SCOTT

## INTRODUCTION

Drug consumption in obstetrics and gynaecology can be regarded both as the *raison d'être* for drug safety monitoring and at the same time its Achilles heel.

The massive surveillance programmes which have developed over the last two decades stem from the tragedy of grossly deformed babies born to mothers given thalidomide. Paradoxically, pregnant women are almost always specifically excluded at the clinical stage of drug testing, and drugs are released on the market without any experience of their use in pregnancy. The difficulties are very great, and neither manufacturing nor drug-regulating authorities are to be blamed. New methods of drug assessment are most urgently needed; the thalidomide disaster could happen again. Practitioners must be taught and re-taught that drug therapy should only be used in pregnancy for the most pressing indications.

Although the thalidomide tragedy had the greatest impact, the most frightening episode from a clinical point of view has been the diethylstilboestrol story. This was not merely a question of a drug, given to a mother, affecting the child; but of that effect being manifest decades after the drug administration, in the form of cancers or pre-cancers in the female offspring.

The contraceptive pill has been the most comprehensively monitored drug in history, but this has led to unfortunate difficulties for the clinician. The oestrogen/progestogen preparations used as contraceptive pills also have important roles in the management of various gynaeological problems. The safety assessment of 'the pill' has been much more critical than that of any other drug or group of drugs, and has been much more widely publicized. Many patients who could benefit from the administration of oestrogen/progestogen preparations prescribed for serious symptomatic reasons are unwilling to take them because of the adverse publicity surrounding their use as contraceptives.

## OBSTETRICS

Pregnancy is the greatest physiological event in human existence, and it is not surprising that during it responses to drugs are different from those in the non-pregnant state; drugs may also cross the placenta and affect the fetus.

Systematic trials of drugs in pregnancy are almost impossible, except for preparations used specifically for obstetric purposes. Prediction of likely effect of drugs must be based largely upon knowledge of physiological changes of pregnancy and how they would be likely to affect their action. In the gastrointestinal tract ingestion and absorption of oral preparations may be impaired. 'Routine' drugs taken in pregnancy, such as iron, may alter drug absorption. The increased plasma, extracellular fluid and fat stores, together with the conceptus mass, usually reduce the effective levels of a given dose of drug.

Altered metabolism, which may occur from increased hydroxylation capacity induced by steroids, may affect drug activity and the placenta may augment hepatic activity. Albumin-binding may be altered and also binding to specific receptors. Drug excretion may be affected by the 40–50% increase in glomerular filtration rate in pregnancy.

All the above effects collectively might be expected to make a given dosage of a drug less effective in the pregnant woman, but with a few outstanding exceptions, such as insulin, the reality of this has not yet been established.

With regard to placental transfer to the fetus, water-soluble, polar compounds are in general poorly transferred while non-polar, lipid-soluble drugs cross relatively easily. The degree of ionization is relevant: the more complete it is, the smaller the tendency for the drug to cross the placenta. Plasma binding is another factor: drugs which are heavily bound tend to stay within the maternal system. When there is a rapid distribution throughout the body, and prompt protein-binding after a single-bolus intravenous injection, the time during which a significant concentration of free drug is available for transfer to the fetus may be insignificant, but with multiple or continuous dosage the situation will of course be different.

Drugs requiring surveillance in pregnancy can be divided into:

(A) Drugs taken at or about the time of conception and in the first trimester:
  (i) Drugs such as insulin or anti-epileptics taken on a long-term basis.
  (ii) Drugs such as antibiotics taken for some temporary condition (including non-prescribed drugs).
  (iii) Drugs taken with the specific object of encouraging or maintaining pregnancy.

(B) Drugs taken in the course of established pregnancy (second and third trimester)

- (i) As in A(i) above
- (ii) as in A(ii) above
- (iii) as in A(iii) above
- (iv) Drugs to correct a specific pregnancy abnormality such as hypertension.

(C) Drugs used to induce or expedite labour, or control pain.

(D) Drugs taken in the puerperium which may be excreted in breast milk or affect lactation.

With regard to A(i) and B(i) the problem is to differentiate the drug effects from those of the disease being treated on a long-term basis. This can be studied through the various specialized clinics (diabetic, epileptic, etc.) which many of these patients attend. Categories A(iii) and B(iii), B(iv) and C, in which the drug is specifically used in relation to pregnancy, are usually well documented in obstetric units and co-operative studies with paediatricians can be arranged to detect any malinfluence on the child. Proving and explaining the mechanism of these effects can be difficult and tedious, as exemplified by the studies of the relationship between oxytocin and neonatal jaundice.

The most difficult categories on which to obtain data are A(ii), B(ii) and D. Here the drugs are given on an *ad hoc* basis, usually for some temporary condition unconnected with the pregnancy. The patients are not usually attending any specialist clinic and the record of drug therapy may not reach the obstetric case-record. Furthermore, it is in this type of situation that drugs released without prior assessment in human pregnancy (though carrying a warning to this effect) are most likely to be used in pregnant patients. There is a need for a system of central notification of such usage which would permit maximal information to be obtained from the relatively small numbers of cases involved. Without such an arrangement it could be many years before an untoward effect is detected.

## Teratology

At the first ante-natal attendance, histories of recent drug consumption are now standard practice and as most confinements in urban areas are in relatively large units, it follows that correlations between drug consumption and gross malformations evident at birth should be easily detected. This is augmented in certain countries, including the United Kingdom, by a system of notification of congenital abnormalities.

## Drug prescribing in pregnancy

Drug consumption in early pregnancy has some similarity to diagnostic radiation in the same period. In the latter, a '10-day rule' has been introduced whereby the doctor requesting examination must state the date of the patient's last menstrual period and the X-ray is only performed at more than 10 days if specific authorization is given. It would be possible to introduce a similar arrangement in drug prescribing. This would not apply to long-term drug use, but it could help reduce unnecessary prescribing and would help to ensure that drug exposures were adequately documented. A willingness to report abnormalities is essential. Unfortunately, in certain countries the legal climate is such that doctors are unwilling to record anything which might possibly be regarded as a harmful consequence of any action by themselves or their colleagues.

It is not only the effects of individual drugs in pregnancy which need to be monitored, but also the general prescribing patterns. Multiple-drug consumption is usual. Throughout the ante-natal period it is routine practice in many units to give vitamins and iron supplements, with or without folic acid, though the justification for this has been questioned.[1] Even with the alternative policy of keeping a close check on the haemoglobin level and precribing haematinics only if it falls below a specific level, a large proportion of pregnant women will still be treated in this way.

An American survey[2] of over 2500 pregnant women indicated that 62% received systemic drug therapy (excluding dietary supplements). This review was conducted through 'Medicaid' files, women being identified retrospectively as claims were made for medical expenses. The 6 months prior to conception was used as a 'control' period, but additionally two other non-pregnant women were studied for each pregnant woman; these gave information on changes in prescribing patterns in pregnancy. The study involved recording pharmacy prescriptions, but no data were produced for 'over-the-counter' medicines.

The study was designed to discover whether the medical profession as a whole was putting into practice the teaching that restraint in prescribing during pregnancy was desirable. It is disappointing that this was generally not so. Tranquillizers, anti-infective agents and narcotics were given just as frequently to the pregnant as to the non-pregnant. The only specific decrease in prescribing noted was that of tetracycline, presumably because of its known risk of interfering with dentition and bone growth. Diazepam was very widely used despite an official label or insert stating that this should almost always be avoided in pregnancy. It was concluded that narcotics, tranquillizers, anti-histamines and anti-infective agents were used without restraint, and that new drugs were often being given to pregnant women.

The results of this US study are very similar to those from studies in the UK[3] in which more than 60% of women received multiple-drug treatments during pregnancy, including between 25% and 40% treated with antimicrobial agents.

## Combined therapy

A good example of a serious hazard with combined drug treatment, which does not occur when the drugs are used individually, is the combination of beta-sympathomimetic preparations, such as ritodrine hydrochloride, salbutamol and orciprenaline sulphate, with corticosteroid agents given in relation to premature labour. Beta-sympathomimetic drugs can, in a high proportion of cases, suppress premature uterine contractions;[4] corticosteroid preparations such as betamethasone or dexamethasone can accelerate maturation of the fetal pulmonary epithelium, making neonatal respiratory distress less likely.[5] While initial studies involved testing these drugs separately it is understandable that when premature labour is threatened clinicians may attempt to postpone this for a few days or a week, while trying to achieve accelerated lung maturation with corticosteroids. The principal side-effect of the beta-sympathomimetic agents is tachycardia, and this is the dose-limiting factor. The corticosteroids, on the other hand, cause fluid retention and it is not surprising that the two drugs given together may lead to cardiac failure.[6,7]

## Drug therapy in concomitant disease

The story of drug therapy in thyrotoxicosis (due to Graves' disease) in pregnancy provides an excellent example of the difficulty of interpreting and reacting in a balanced way to any untoward effects. Changes in maternal physiology in pregnancy have many effects on thyroid function,[8] complicated by the possible thyrotropic activity of gonadotropin or closely related hormones and the presence of the developing fetal thyroid. When antithyroid drugs became available they were used with enthusiasm in pregnancy, but it soon became clear that they could have disastrous effects on the child – severe goitre and frank cretinism.[9] This led to the virtual abandonment of such therapy in pregnancy and its replacement by surgery.[10] However, it later became clear that in moderate dosage drugs such as carbimazole were relatively safe in pregnancy and there was a swing back to them, sometimes combining them with thyroxine with the intention of trying to ensure that thyroid hormone levels were not severely depressed. Now carbimazole is even given with the *deliberate* intention of depressing the fetal thyroid when high levels of thyroid-stimulating immunoglobulins in the maternal serum suggest this is a fetal hazard.[11]

## Use of drugs in labour

In the past, the analgesics used during labour were mostly narcotics;

today, conduction-block analgesia is becoming more general. Careful co-operation between obstetrician and paediatrician is essential for monitoring in this field; perhaps a single individual should fill both roles as a 'perinatologist'. Relatively long-term effects of narcotics have been demonstrated but there is also a need to study the long-term effect of narcotic *antagonists* such as naloxone, which appear to be so effective in countering their immediate effects in the newborn.

It is known that tranquillizers and anti-convulsants such as diazepam may affect the fetus during labour by reducing beat-to-beat variation in fetal heart rate recordings. It is likely that the increased use of ultrasonic and other sophisticated methods of studying fetal heart rate, respiration movements and limb movement will help to give better information on the effect of such drugs upon the child while it is still *in utero*.

Inhalational agents generally achieve rapid transplacental equilibration. With the co-operation of anaesthetists specializing in obstetric anaesthesia, measurements of the concentration of these drugs and assessement of their effects on the child can be expected more frequently. This applies also to neuromuscular relaxants which are mostly fully ionized and only minimally transferred transplacentally. Local anaesthetic agents also require monitoring, but although lipid-soluble, and therefore capable of rapid placental transfer, they are to a large extent protein-bound and this restricts the amount reaching the fetus. There is a need for improved non-invasive techniques to measure uterine blood flow in human pregnancy as this has a major influence on placental transfer of drugs and their metabolism in the placental tissue.

## Lactation

Some drugs may be concentrated to a greater degree in breast milk than in maternal serum while others reach at least as high a concentration[12]. Drug levels can be monitored when a lactating woman has to be given a drug, by arranging for specimens of milk to be collected and sent to the appropriate laboratories for estimation of concentration. The infant's sensitivity to the drug must also be considered. For example, because of increased brain permeability, sedatives may have a more powerful effect, or deficient enzymatic conjugation may increase various drug levels. Co-operative studies of this nature can involve obstetricians and pharmacologists.

## Requirements for a drug monitoring system in relation to pregnancy

The ideal system for drug monitoring in pregnancy does not exist, but various communities have certain advantages. Although it is well recognized that environmental and genetic factors may lead to varying responses to drugs in different populations, there is much to be said for increasing our efforts to develop good-quality, long-term monitoring in places where it is most practical. Factors which should be taken into account include the place of antenatal care and confinement, and the stage of pregnancy at which antenatal care is started. The ideal would be a population in which pre-pregnancy medical consultation is the rule. Comprehensive birth notification and the availability of systems for follow-up must be available.

## GYNAECOLOGY

In many ways monitoring for drug safety in gynaecology is a small-scale variant of that of general medical therapy, though there are a number of important differences.

The most commonly used drugs are oral contraceptives. Fortunately they have been very closely and comprehensively studied; the motivation of the consumers and the arrangements for prescription and dispensing have helped. However, similar or identical preparations are also used for treatment of menstrual disorders. Different standards of safety would apply to the same drugs used to control severe menstrual haemorrhage in a young girl, and thus avoiding the need for a tragic hysterectomy, than when used as a 'convenience' form of contraceptive or to control minor symptomatology.

Much drug use in gynaecology is for relatively minor complaints; for example, pre-menstrual tension or dysmenorrhoea which carry no mortality risk. Usually for the former and sometimes for the latter, patients will commence medication after ovulation but before the start of menstruation, so there is always the risk it will be given in the very earliest stage of pregnancy. The problems which may arise in proving a cause-and-effect relationship are exemplified by the difficulties which arose in relation to hormonal tests for early pregnancy.[13]

Drug action may be affected by ovarian cyclic changes with their consequent alteration in hormonal environment; for example, in the drug control of epilepsy. The same may be true for all forms of drug therapy in females of the menstrual age group, but it is quite rarely considered.

### Monitoring oral contraceptives

Deciding whether drugs taken for non-medical purposes (such as contraception) are safe, involves a very much finer balance of judgement than would, for example, the assessment of a drug which may cure cancer, but there are some factors which facilitate carrying out assessment of drugs taken as oral contrceptives. Women who wish to take 'the pill' have to approach a doctor for a prescription and, if they receive one, they are generally well motivated towards assessing its effects. Many are in the upper social bracket and well aware of the hazards which may be involved; also they have to stay under medical surveillance to obtain repeated prescriptions.

In the UK the Royal College of General Practitioners (RCGP) has proved a particularly good organization for reviewing the risks and benefits.[14–18] The RCGP study involves the comprehensive recording of all doctor-consultations by large numbers of women using various methods of contraception, and the variations in lethal and non-lethal disease states.

Most studies on oral contraceptive usage have concentrated on untoward effects, but unexpected health *benefits* may also occur. It seems that endometrial cancer incidence may be lower in pill users[19,20] and this also may hold for other cancers, especially ovarian cancer.

## Hormone therapy for climacteric problems

A major contemporary problem is the use of hormonal preparations at or after the climacteric to relieve various symptoms and to prevent undesirable sequelae such as osteoporosis. This problem resembles that of oral contraception and the hormones used are in many cases almost identical, although oestrogens are often used alone and dosages are less. The major difference is that with hormone replacement therapy the effects are much less precise and depend (a) upon symptom alleviation, (b) on positive 'well being' and (c) on prevention of such complications as fractured femur in old age. These benefits have to be assessed in relation to long-term consequences of manipulation of the post-climacteric endocrine environment.

Of these effects the one which has caused most concern and controversy is excessive endometrial stimulation possibly proceeding to carcinoma. Many studies have been published but have not been universally accepted as valid; usually because of criticism of the controls. However, a number of cohort and other well-planned studies in the US and the UK[21–25] have shown a variation in the incidence of abnormal endometrial stimulation or cancer. The variation depends upon the precise drug preparation used, whether it is a mixture of oestrogen with a progestogen or an oestrogen alone, and on the dosage and length of therapy, and whether the therapy is given on a sequential or continuous basis. The British study dealt with endometrial biopsy material and changes in the endometrium which fell short of carcinoma. Further elucidation of this difficult, but very important, problem involving drug consumption by a large proportion of the female population should be obtained by studies conducted along the lines of those of the RCGP on the 'pill' but involving the co-operation of gynaecologists.

Unfortunately elderly patients are not always so well motivated to attend clinics for surveillance, and the prescription of preparations is relatively haphazard. Record-linkage studies would be ideal. So far the best data on carcinogenicity have come from those regions of Minnesota, where the Mayo Clinic has had a long-term monopoly of the local medical care, and where, although the numbers are relatively small, there has been continuous high-quality recording.[21]

There is persuasive evidence coming forward to suggest that if a progestogen is prescribed in association with the oestrogen it may be protective against a carcinogenicity risk.[26,27]

## Ovulation stimulation

An important form of therapy is that used to treat infertility. This involves the use of synthetic forms of hypothalamic gonadotrophin-releasing hormones; human pituitary gonadotrophins extracted from pituitaries at autopsy or from the urine of post-menopausal or pregnant women; oestrogen analogues such as clomiphene and dopamine agonists such as bromocriptine. Obviously such drugs present particular problems in relation to teratology. Particularly with regard to the pituitary hormones of human origin, the fact that they are specifically human makes animal testing even less appropriate than usual. Fortunately most of these preparations are only marketed in a restricted way in many countries and most of their usage is in highly specialized centres where strict and well-organized monitoring is possible. In this category of therapy the high level of patient motivation makes for good monitoring while an overwhelming desire to achieve a pregnancy often leads to informed acceptance of a high level of risk, especially that of multiple pregnancy. Monitoring involves measuring the rate of rise of ovarian steroid hormone during therapy to predict the number of follicles ripening. Daily oestrone assays plotted on a log-scale provide a slope which gives a reasonable guide. If the slope is excessively steep it points to a multiple-follicle ripening; by avoiding the administration of a luteinizing preparation ovulation can be prevented and the risk avoided.[28] An alternative physical technique is to monitor follicular development by ultrasound scanning.[29,30]

These patients have inevitably suffered a delay in reproduction pattern, and this in itself is a cause of poor performance when pregnancy does occur. Obtaining control subjects is a major problem.

## Second-generation contraceptive-drugs

Steroid contraceptives are being used on a diminishing scale. This is mainly because careful comparative monitoring has shown that for many categories of women, particularly those in the older age-groups, there is an increased mortality from a number of cardiovascular problems. However, the last 20 years have conditioned a generation of women to expect, as a matter of right, the availability of highly efficient methods of contraception which do not produce side-effects or mortality risk. As the hunt for new methods fulfilling these demands intensifies,[31] it becomes evident that a very high degree of specificity to the human reproductive process is going to be required, and that animal studies of the type used to monitor therapeutic drugs may have very limited application.

One approach in which this applies involves adding active drugs to intrauterine contraceptive devices, aimed to increase efficacy and/or reduce side-effects. Another is the development of immunological techniques utilizing antibodies to various human antigens, e.g. zona pellucida, sperm antigens or human chorionic gonadotrophin.[32,33]

Lest the enormity of the problems apparently involved in trying to introduce specific human preparations to manipulate immune responses seem daunting, it is appropriate to note the outstandingly successful example of anti-D immunoglobulin. The prevention of rhesus iso-immunization by this means is the outstanding success story of modern obstetrics. Despite world-wide use for over a decade there have only been isolated reports of adverse effects in individuals with an IgA deficiency state.[34] It is salutary to appreciate that anti-D immunoglobulin might not have reached the stage of clinical trial if modern criteria for assessment had been rigidly applied.

## References

1. Do all pregnant women need iron? (1978). *Br. Med. J.*, **2,** 1317
2. Brocklebank, J. C., Ray, W. A., Federspiel, C. F. and Schaffner, W. (1978). Drug prescribing during pregnancy. *Am. J. Obstet. Gynecol.*, **132,** 235
3. Forfar, J. O. (1973). 'Drugs and the unborn child'. *Nature*, **242,** 367
4. Wesselius-de Casparis, A., Thiery, M., Yo le Sian, A., Baumgarten, K., Brosens, I., Gamisans, O., Stolk, J. and Vivier, W. (1971). Results of double-blind, multicentre study with Ritodrine in premature labour. *Br. Med. J.*, **3,** 144
5. Howie, R. N. and Liggins, G. C. (1977). Clinical trial of antepartum beta-methasone therapy for prevention of respiratory distress in pre-term infants. In Anderson, A., Beard, R., Brudenell, J. M. and Dunn, P. M. (eds.) *Pre-Term Labour*, pp. 281–289. (London: Royal College of Obstetricians and Gynaecologists)
6. Stubblefield, P. G. (1978). Pulmonary edema occurring after therapy with dexamethasone and terbutaline for premature labor: A case report. *Am. J. Obstet. Gynecol.*, **132,** 341
7. Kubli, F. (1977). Discussion following paper by Beard, R. W. The effect of β-sympathomimetic drugs on carbohydrate metabolism in pregnancy. In Anderson, A., Beard, R., Brudenell, J. M., Dunn, P. M. (eds.) *Pre-Term Labour*, pp. 218–220. (London: Royal College of Obstetricians and Gynaecologists)
8. Ramsay, I. D. (1977). Thyroid therapy in pregnancy. In Lewis, P. J. (ed.) *Therapeutic Problems in Pregnancy*, pp. 93–102. (Lancaster: MTP Press Ltd.)
9. Keynes, G. (1952). Obstetrics and gynaecology in relation to thyrotoxicosis and myasthenia gravis. *J. Obstet. Gynaecol. Br. Emp.*, **59,** 173
10. Hawe, P. and Francis, H. H. (1962). Pregnancy and thyrotoxicosis. *Br. Med. J.*, **2,** 817
11. Scott, J. S. (1980). Immunological diseases occurring in pregnancy. In Sakamoto, S., Tojo, S. and Nakayama, T. (eds.) *Gynecology and Obstetrics – International Series No. 512. Proceedings of IX World Congress of Gynecology and Obstetrics Tokyo*, pp. 225–31 (Amsterdam: Excerpta Medica)
12. Stirrat, G. M. (1976). Prescribing problems in the second half of pregnancy and during lactation. *Obstet. Gynaecol. Surv.*, **31,** 1

13. Ambani, L. M., Joshi, N. J., Vaidya, R. A., *et al.* (1977). Are hormonal contraceptives teratogenic? *Fertil. Steril.*, **28**, 791
14. Royal College of General Practitioners (1974). *Oral Contraceptives and Health.* (London: Pitman Medical)
15. Royal College of General Practitioners (1977). Mortality among oral contraceptive users. *Lancet*, **2**, 727
16. Royal College of General Practitioners (1977). Effect on hypertension and benign breast disease of progestagen component in combined oral contraceptives. *Lancet*, **1**, 624
17. World Health Organization (1978). Steroid contraception and the risk of neoplasia. World Health Organization Technical Report Series No. 619. (Geneva: World Health Organization)
18. Layde, P. M., Beral, V. and Kay, C. R. (1981). Further analyses of mortality in oral contraceptives. RCGP Contraception Study. *Lancet*, **1**, 541–6
19. Weiss, N. S. and Sayvetz, T. A. (1980). Incidence of endometrial cancer in relation to the use of oral contraceptives. *N. Engl. J. Med.*, **302**, 551–4
20. Cole, P. (1980). Oral contraceptives and endometrial cancer. *N. Engl. J. Med.*, **302**, 575–6
21. McDonald, T. W., Annegers, J. F., O'Fallon, W. M., Dockerty, M. B., Malkasian, G. D. and Kurland, L. T. (1977). Exogenous estrogen and endometrial carcinoma: Case-control and incidence study. *Am. J. Obstet. Gynecol.*, **127**, 572
22. Sturdee, D. W., Wade-Evans, T., Paterson, M. E. L., Thom, M. and Studd, J. W. W. (1978). Relations between bleeding pattern, endometrial histology, and oestrogen treatment in menopausal women. *Br. Med. J.*, **1**, 1575
23. Antunes, C. M. F., Stolley, P. D., Rosenshein, N. B. *et al.* (1979). Endometrial cancer and estrogen use. *N. Engl. J. Med.*, **300**, 9–13
24. Jick, H., Watkins, R. N., Hunter, J. R., Dinan, B. J., Madsen, S., Rothamn, K. J. and Walker, A. M. (1979). Replacement estrogens and endometrial cancer. *N. Engl. J. Med.*, **300**, 218–22
25. Shapiro, S., Kaufman, D. W., Slone, D. *et al.* (1980). Recent and past use of conjugated estrogens in relation to adenocarcinoma of the endometrium. *N. Engl. J. Med.*, **303**, 485–9
26. Whitehead, M. I., Townsend, P. T., Pryse-Davies, J., Ryder, T. A. and King, R. J. B. (1981). Effects of estrogens and progestins on the biochemistry and morphology of the postmenopausal endometrium. *N. Engl. J. Med.*, **305**, 1599–1605
27. Macdonald, P. C. (1981). Estrogen plus progestin in postmenopausal women. *N. Engl. J. Med.*, **305**, 1644–5
28. Hancock, K. W., Scott, J. S., Stitch, S. R., Levell, M. J., Oakey, R. E. and Ellis, F. R. (1970). Ovulation stimulation, Problems of prediction of response to gonadotrophins. *Lancet*, **2**, 482
29. Sallam, H. N., Marinho, A. O., Collins, W. P., Rodeck, C. H. and Campbell, S. (1982). Monitoring gonadotrophin therapy by real-time ultrasonic scanning of ovarian follicles. *Br. J. Obstet. Gynaecol.*, **89**, 155–9
30. Fink, R. S., Bowes, L. P., Mackintosh, C. E., Smith, W. I., Georgiades, E. and Ginsburg, J. (1982). The value of ultrasound for monitoring ovarian responses to gonadotrophin stimulant therapy. *Br. J. Obstet. Gynaecol.*, **89**, 856–61
31. World Health Organization (1981). Special programme of research, development and research training in human reproduction. Tenth annual report. (Geneva: World Health Organization)
32. Stevens, V. C. and Crystle, C. D. (1973). Effects of immunization with hapten-coupled hCG on the human menstrual cycle. *Obstet. Gynecol.*, **42**, 485
33. Talwar, G. P., Sharma, N. C., Duby, S. K., Salahuddin, M., Das, C., Ramacrishman, S., Kumar, S. and Hingorani, V. (1976). Isoimmunization against human chorionic gonadotropin with conjugates of processed β-subunit of the hormone and tetanus toxoid. *Proc. Natl. Acad. Sci.*, **73**, 218
34. Bowman, J. M. (1978). Suppression of Rh isoimmunization. *Obstet. Gynecol.*, **52**, 385

# 27
# Drug teratogenicity

R. W. SMITHELLS

## INTRODUCTION

Although the number of children with malformations confidently attributable to drugs pales into insignificance beside the many people who have suffered from other side-effects of drugs, the current and sustained upsurge of concern about drug safety has its roots in thalidomide. Furthermore, the emotive picture of a deformed baby looking at a pharmaceutical juggernaut with wide, reproachful eyes provides constant joy to the media, and is not a matter of total disinterest to the legal profession. It is, therefore, likely that watchfulness for drug teratogenicity will continue to make demands on time and money.

The extensive animal reproductive studies to which all new drugs are now subjected are more in the nature of a public relations exercise than a serious contribution to drug safety. Animal tests can never predict the actions of drugs on humans. In theory these tests might even be doing more harm than good, in that a new drug which shows evidence of teratogenicity in animals will never reach the market, where it might have proved to be therapeutically useful and non-teratogenic in humans. The illogicality of the situation is demonstrated by the continued use of well-established drugs which are known to be teratogenic in some mammalian species (e.g. aspirin[1], penicillin/streptomycin[2], cortisone[3]). Conversely, a new drug which comes through its animal reproductive studies with flying colours may nevertheless be teratogenic in man.

## WHAT IS A TERATOGEN?

At this point it is worth pausing to consider what exactly we mean by a teratogenic drug. In monitoring for teratogenesis what precisely are we looking for? If a pregnant woman takes a single dose of thalidomide on the 40th day of pregnancy she can almost be given a written guarantee that her baby will be deformed. If a pregnant epileptic takes phenobarbitone and phenytoin daily throughout her pregnancy, her baby has an increased chance of being born deformed but will probably be normal.[4] We can describe thalidomide and anti-convulsant drugs as teratogenic if we wish, but not in the same sense. The first is virtually an obligate teratogen, the second is not.

A teratogenic agent is, in everyday usage, an agent which has the capacity to cause malformation. The term is being used more widely to include functional as well as structural disorders, as in behavioural teratology,[5] but a teratogen etymologically refers to the production of monsters in the physical sense rather than the social. A teratogenic drug may, therefore, be regarded as one which, if it reaches a developing embryo, has the capacity to cause malformation.

This sounds simple enough but it is not, the complexity lying in the causal relationship itself. If we consider an agent A and an effect E, a number of possible relationships might exist between them (see Figure 1).

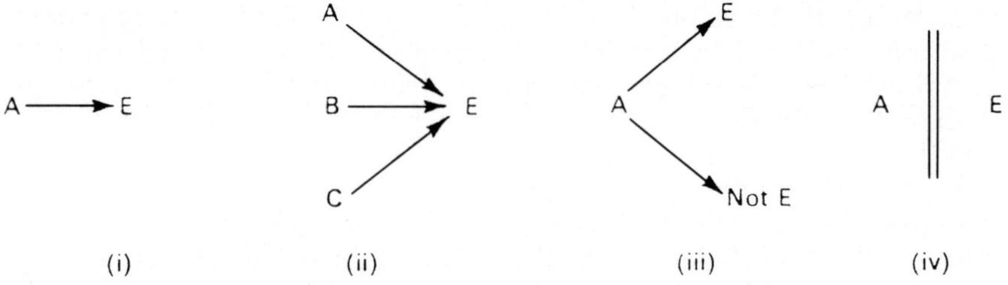


**Figure 1** (i) A is *the* cause of E. A is invariably followed by E: E is invariably preceded by A. (ii) A is *a* cause of E. A is invariably followed by E: E is not always preceded by A. (iii) A causes E sometimes (i.e. under some circumstances). Factors other than A determine whether E will follow. (iv) A never causes E. A is never followed by E: E is never preceded by A.

A moment's reflection reveals that in real life, and especially in clinical medicine rather than in the more controlled circumstances of the laboratory, options (i) and (iv) are almost non-existent, option (ii) is rare, and option (iii) is the one we usually meet. This real-life option has been beautifully analysed by Rothman.[6] He uses the term 'sufficient cause' to describe a factor or (usually) a combination of contributory factors which will invariably lead to a stated effect. If one contributory factor is missing, the remaining factors become collectively insufficient and the effect does not follow. A 'necessary factor' is one which alone may not be a sufficient cause, but which is an indispensable component of a sufficient cause (e.g. the tubercle bacillus in pulmonary tuberculosis).

A century ago Europe was torn by great medical argument as to whether rickets was caused by a dietary deficiency or by a lack of sunshine. In a way both parties were right, but more strictly both were wrong. A vitamin-D deficient diet *plus* a lack of sunshine together made a sufficient cause of rickets, but neither is sufficient on its own.

Returning to teratogenesis and to Figure 1, if A represents a drug and E a malformation, we can interpret the four diagrams as follows:

(i) Drug A is teratogenic and is the only known cause of malformation/syndrome E.
(ii) Drug A is teratogenic and is a cause of malformation/syndrome E, but there are also phenocopies attributable to other causes.
(iii) Drug A is not of itself a sufficient cause of malformation/syndrome E: it is a contributory factor: it may or may not be a necessary factor.
(iv) Drug A does not cause malformation/syndrome E.

It must be emphasized again that options (i) and (iv) are almost fictional: even thalidomide does not completely comply with (i). Option (ii) is possibly seen in the relationship between warfarin and punctate epiphyseal dysplasia.[7] Option (iii), the awkward squad, is the one we have to live and work with. Most common malformations are thought to be multifactorial in causation, the result of the additive effects of many genetic and/or environmental factors, each with a small teratogenic potential. If the total load exceeds a threshold a defect results.

For humans troubles never come singly, and women who take drugs in pregnancy, whether they need them (because they are sick) or not (in which case they are foolish) are likely to be those in whom a multitude of genetic, medical, social and cultural problems can be identified. A marginal correlation between a drug history and a birth defect could be interpreted as suggesting that the drug is teratogenic, but might equally suggest that the drug acts as a biological stress test and identifies those mothers whose fetuses were already trembling on the brink of malformation. When a drug history correlates with a multitude of defects the second interpretation is the more tempting to accept.

## HOW CAN TERATOGENIC DRUGS BE IDENTIFIED?

Links between maternal medication in pregnancy and fetal malformations may be sought or revealed in many different ways, of which the most important are:

(1) The observations of alert clinicians.
(2) Case-control studies.
(3) Cohort studies.
(4) Birth defects monitoring.

## Alert clinicians

Clinicians are likely to be alerted by the occurrence of something unusual or by an unusual frequency of any clinical event. The combination of a receptive mind, ready to be surprised and interested, with an enquiring mind, ready to ask questions, was responsible for associating microcephaly with ionizing radiation,[8] cataracts with rubella,[9] and limb reduction deformities with thalidomide.[10,11] Retrospective enquiries of this kind can bring to light associations which in turn may lead to hypotheses. The hypotheses must then be tested by other techniques which will also quantify the teratogenic risk, if there is one.

When such an observation is made the result may well be a letter or brief report in a medical journal reporting the association, in the present context, between a drug taken in pregnancy and the subsequent birth of a malformed child. It is usually the malformation that triggers the enquiry which is therefore retrospective. Some general principles apply:

(a) If the original enquiry yields no positive associations, it is unlikely to be written up, or, if submitted for publication, less likely to be published. Positive associations are, therefore, over-represented in the literature.
(b) If an interesting association is found in a single case, other examples may be sought in order to yield something more 'publishable'. This is a variation on the theme of stamp-collecting.
(c) After publication of a positive association, people will write either to the same journal or to the original author to report similar examples (the me-too syndrome). This increases the over-representation of positive associations.

## Case-control studies

These compare the drug histories of the mothers of a group of infants suffering from a stated malformation/syndrome with the drug histories of mothers of infants without this defect ('controls') and may demonstrate that one or more drugs were taken by a higher proportion in one category. There are two principal difficulties to be overcome in the design of case-control studies:

(a) As admission to the study is determined by the presence of a malformation, the collection of information about drug intake is largely retrospective. In so far as it is obtained by interviewing the mothers, it will be subject to the errors of memory bias. In so far as it is obtained from written records made during pregnancy, it will be more reliable. Checking maternal recall from medical records can only check the accuracy of that which is recalled.

(b) 'Controls', apart from being the mothers of infants without the defect under study, are conventionally matched for a few humdrum variables such as age, parity and social class and are then accepted as comparable. This is like using a carthorse as a control for a racehorse after matching for age, sex and parity.

### Cohort studies

These follow to delivery a group of pregnant women known to have taken the drug under study, and compare the prevalence of defects in their offspring with the prevalence in a 'control' group, or with the population prevalence in the same place at the same time. Cohort studies avoid the problem of retrospective bias inherent in case-control studies. Such studies can also be initiated *after* the birth of the babies (e.g. by identifying mothers from prescriptions or drug records). Provided the mothers are identified before the status of the infants is known, this is still a prospective technique.

The major difficulty in cohort studies rests with the choice of controls. If the study drug is an antibiotic, the women who took them were presumed to have infections. How do you separate the effects of the illness, the fever and the drug? If the drug is an anti-emetic, should you make comparison with vomiting mothers who took a different anti-emetic, with vomiting mothers who took no drugs, or with mothers who did not vomit? When pregnancy-test drugs (which were used for diagnosis rather than for therapy) were under scrutiny, the choice of controls required answers to the following questions:

(1) Why did the mother go to the doctor for a diagnostic test? (Was it because she hoped that she was not pregnant?)
(2) Why did the doctor think a test was necessary?
(3) Why did he use a hormone test and not a urine test?

## BIRTH DEFECTS MONITORING SYSTEMS

These systems, or registries, count malformations in a defined population and watch for significant changes. An increase in the incidence of one or more malformations *could* indicate the recent arrival of a new environmental teratogen (not necessarily a drug). The principal problems here are to decide what should be regarded as significant (epidemiologically rather than statistically) and how to play hunt-the-teratogen.[12,13] There are many problems in running successful monitoring programmes, including the definition and classification of defects, methods of ascertainment, size of population and analysis of data. So far, in spite of an international proliferation of such organizations, no new teratogen has been identified by this technique. Registries do, however, embody a reliable mass of data on an unselected population, and provide a convenient basis for testing the hypotheses of alert clinicians and for checking the results of case-control and cohort studies. Even the association of spina bifida with the antiepileptic drug sodium valproate (valproic acid), although highlighted by reports from birth defects registries,[14,15] was first reported as a clinical observation.[16]

How effective are surveillance programmes likely to be in detecting an honest-to-badness teratogenic drug in the future? It is to be hoped that post-marketing drug surveillance, which is the logical, direct and quickest way of detecting teratogenic potential, will be sufficiently well established to relegate such programmes to a back-stop role so far as drugs are concerned, though they will still be needed to watch for other environmental teratogens. The Liverpool Congenital Abnormalities Registry functioned from January 1st, 1960[17] and recognized the epidemic of limb reduction deformities in the first year of work. It did not identify the teratogen, but provided a convenient means of quickly confirming the suggestion of Lenz[10] and McBride[11] that thalidomide was responsible. There is every reason to believe that similar programmes would detect similar events.

The thalidomide epidemic was easy to detect because (a) the sales of the drug increased very rapidly, and (b) the most striking defects had previously been excessively rare.

A teratogenic drug used on a smaller scale or increasing in use more slowly would take longer to detect because it would require more *time*. A drug causing a defect which was already common would take longer to detect because it would require larger *numbers*. A drug which caused over 10 years a 5% increase in anencephaly or ventricular septal defect (two of the commonest defects in humans), would probably go undetected by any system monitoring birth defects.

International co-operation will help because new drugs are usually launched initially in one or two countries, not worldwide. Contrasts may therefore appear, comparable to the disparity noted in 1960–61 between the frequency of limb defects in the offspring of Germans in West Germany and their rarity in the babies of American forces families in the same country.[18]

## TERATOGENESIS AND THE EMBRYOLOGICAL TIME-SCALE

Most malformations arise as a consequence of changes in the rate or direction of growth of tissues in the embryo. The period of embryogenesis is usually defined as lasting for 8 weeks after fertilization, and there is detailed information on the timing of key events (e.g. closure of neural tube). Some key events (e.g. closure of the palate) take place more than 8 weeks after fertilization, and some malformations (e.g. congenital dislocation of the hip) appreciably later in pregnancy. If a malformation can be timed with reasonable confidence, a responsible teratogenic agent must have been active at *or before* that time.

Accurate timing of drug consumption is clearly important in teratogenicity studies, but is difficult to achieve in humans. Patient personal interview, seeking to establish links between the symptom or illness requiring the drug and personal or family events can be rewarding. The UK National Health Service provides an excellent opportunity to date *prescriptions* accurately, and repeat prescriptions (e.g. for an anti-nauseant) suggest that the medication is being taken. Such data provide reasonable evidence of the earliest date in pregnancy on which the drug could have been taken.

Many teratogenicity studies refer simply to drugs taken in the first trimester of pregnancy, which is usually from 2 weeks before conception until 10–11 weeks after. This is a very crude measure indeed, although something may be learned by comparing first trimester with second trimester drug consumption.

## CONCLUSION

Considerations of this kind almost certainly underlie the apparent conflicts of evidence about drugs of doubtful, marginal teratogenic potential (e.g. sex hormones) which contrast strikingly with the total unanimity of evidence about thalidomide. Correlations will continue to be found, sometimes statistically significant, between various drugs and various birth defects not only by chance (in 5%), but for the same reasons that correlations will be found (I guess) between football hooliganism and in-growing toenails. This kind of relationship is likely to show up particularly in case-control studies because the controls are so imperfect, but less so in cohort studies.

Post-marketing surveillance of new drugs offers a far better prospect, and similar studies of old drugs, based on the linkage of prescriptions to pregnancies, are certainly feasible.[19,20] Difficulties of interpretation of 'weak teratogens' will continue to provide a diversion for doctors and lawyers alike.

## References


1. Wilson, J. G. (1971). Use of rhesus monkeys in teratological studies. *Fed. Proc.*, **30,** 104
2. Filippi, B. (1967). Antibiotics and congenital malformations: Evaluation of the teratogenicity of antibiotics. In Wollam, D. H. M. (ed.) *Advances in Teratology*, Volume 2 p. 239. (London and New York: Logos Press and Academic Press)
3. Fraser, F. C. and Fainstat, T. D. (1951). Production of congenital defects in offspring of pregnant mice treated with cortisone. *Pediatrics*, **8,** 527
4. Speidel, B. D. and Meadow, S. R. (1974). Epilepsy, anticonvulsants and congenital malformations. *Drugs*, **8,** 354
5. Werboff, J. and Gottleib, J. S. (1963). Drugs in pregnancy; behavioural teratology. *Obstet. Gynaecol. Surv.*, **18,** 420
6. Rothman, K. J. (1976). Causes. *Am. J. Epidemiol.*, **104,** 587
7. DiSaia, P. J. (1966). Pregnancy and delivery of a patient with a Starr–Edwards mitral valve prosthesis: Report of a case. *Obstet. Gynecol.*, **28,** 469

8. Murphy, D. P. (1929). The outcome of 625 pregnancies in women subjected to pelvic radium or roentgen irradiation. *Am. J. Obstet. Gynecol.*, **18,** 179
9. Gregg, N. (1941). Congenital cataracts following German measles in the mother. *Trans. Ophthalmol. Soc. Austr.*, **3,** 35
10. Lenz, W. (1962). Thalidomide and congenital abnormalities. *Lancet*, **1,** 45
11. McBride, W. G. (1961). Thalidomide and congenital abnormalities. *Lancet*, **2,** 1358
12. Klingberg, M. A., Papier, C. M. (1979). Teratoepidemiology. *J. Biosoc. Sci*, **11,** 233–58
13. Källén, B., Winberg, J. (1979). Dealing with suspicions of malformation frequency increase. *Acta Paediatr. Scand, Suppl.*, **275,** 66–74
14. Robert, E. and Guibaud, P. (1982). Maternal valproic acid and congenital neural tube defects. *Lancet*, **2,** 937 (letter)
15. Bjerkedal T. *et al.* (1982). Valproic acid and spina bifida. *Lancet*, **2,** 1096 (letter)
16. Gomez, M. R. (1981). Possible teratogenicity of valproic acid. *J. Pediatr.*, **98,** 508–9 (letter)
17. Smithells, R. W. (1962). The Liverpool Congenital Abnormalities Registry. *Develop. Med. Child Neurol.*, **4,** 320
18. Taussig, H. B. (1962). A study of the German outbreak of phocomelia: the thalidomide syndrome. *J. Am. Med. Assoc.*, **180,** 1106
19. Smithells, R. W. and Chinn, E. R. (1964). Meclozine and foetal malformations: A prospective study. *Br. Med. J.*, **1,** 217–8
20. Smithells, R. W. and Sheppard, S. (1978). Teratogenicity testing in humans: a method demonstrating safety of Bendectin. *Teratology*, **17,** 31

# 28
# The role of the coroner

D. R. CHAMBERS

## INTRODUCTION

Coroners exist in many countries subject to systems of law based on English common law. In this chapter I shall describe the present system in England and Wales which is based on the Coroners Act 1887[1] and the Coroners (Amendment) Act 1926;[2] more detailed regulations are contained in the Coroners Rules 1984.[3] The jurisdiction of a coroner has two elements: the first is geographical, in that the body which is to be the subject of his enquiries is lying within the area for which he is coroner; and the second, that '*there is reasonable cause to suspect that such person has died either a violent or an unnatural death, or has died a sudden death of which the cause is unknown . . .*' (Section 3 of the 1887 Act, as amended).

A coroner must be 'a barrister, solicitor, or legally qualified medical practitioner, of not less than 5 years standing in his profession' (Section 1 of the 1926 Act). The term 'legally qualified' means registered as a medical practitioner and so legally a doctor. There is no formal requirement that the person appointed has had experience as a deputy or assistant deputy to a coroner, but this is almost the universal rule. There are about 160 coroners' juridictions in England and Wales, and these are either counties or parts of counties. The majority of coroners are solicitors and they hold office in a part-time capacity. A certain number of jurisdictions are whole-time appointments and may be held by members of any of the three professions. In the Greater London Council area there are seven coroners; all but one are doctors who are also barristers. Outside London this combination is less often found.

## CRITERIA FOR REPORTING TO CORONER

Deaths thought to be subject to the coroner's authority are variously reported to him by the deceased's own doctor, a doctor of the hospital where he died, or if no doctor has treated the deceased in his last illness, by the police.

Where a doctor has issued a 'medical certificate of cause of death' under Section 22 of the Births and Deaths Registration Act 1953[4] this may be referred to the coroner by the registrar under regulation 51 of the Births, Deaths and Marriage Regulations 1968.[5]

Subsection 1 paragraphs (d), (e) and (f) are particularly relevant and refer to death:

(d) the cause of which appears to be unknown; or
(e) which the registrar has reason to believe to have been unnatural or to have been caused by violence or neglect, or by abortion, or to have been attended by suspicious circumstances; or
(f) which appears to the registrar to have occurred during an operation or before recovery from an anaesthetic.

These categories of death elaborate those in Section 3 of the 1887 Coroners Act, but the essential element of '*unnaturalness*' remains. Conversely a death which is certified by a doctor who has treated the deceased in his last illness as being from a natural cause will be registered without further ado, there being no rule requiring the registrar to do otherwise. In such circumstances the coroner is clearly not involved. Where, however, the certifying doctor considers that the cause of death, although natural, may have occurred as a result of an adverse reaction to therapy, he may so certify on the certificate he issues. More probably he may report his suspicions to a colleague for advice, or report the death to the coroner. He may issue his certificate and report his suspicions to the Committee on Safety of Medicines using a 'yellow card' (see Chapter 1).

So described, the law and practice of death registration and the referral of deaths to the coroner is hardly designed to detect hazards which cause death from 'natural causes'. This point has not escaped the members of the Committee on Death Certification and Coroners whose report appeared in November 1971, and which is known by the name of its chairman as the Brodrick report.[6] No. 4 in the summary of recommendations of this report states:

> A qualified doctor should issue a certificate of the fact and cause of death only if (i) he is confident on reasonable grounds that he can certify the medical cause of death with accuracy and precision; (ii) there are no grounds for supposing that the death was due to or contributed to by any employment followed at any time by the deceased, any drug medicine or poison or any violent or unnatural cause.

In July 1985, as a result of the Industrial Diseases Notification Act 1981 the Medical Certificate of Cause of Death was amended to include a statement for the certifying doctor to tick if it is thought that the deceased's occupation might have been related to the death. The back of the form notes the coroner's concern with the fact that 'the death might have been due to or contributed to by drugs, medicine, abortion or poison.'

## CORONER'S DECISIONS

A coroner to whom a death is reported with the suggestion that it may be related to the use of a medicinal substance will have to consider what steps to take. As a matter of law I think there is no doubt that a report by a competent authority, such as the physician in charge of the deceased, is sufficient to give him jurisdiction. That being so, his next action must be to order a post-mortem examination and to await the report from the pathologist.

Pathologists vary in the degree to which they are prepared to attribute their findings to the adverse effect of a medicine and, in my experience, tend to err on the side of caution. This is hardly surprising since if his view is that a named substance (or substances) has been the cause of the pathological changes then an inquest is a very likely consequence, an inquest moreover at which this view might be challenged. The pathological findings are not the only ones which the coroner will have to consider for the attending physician's observations during life also have relevance. A fatal cardiac arrhythmia leaves little even for the most experienced pathologist to demonstrate in the mortuary – although he may find a condition in the heart which itself might have been a cause, in whole or part, of the cardiological findings in life. It is at this point, when his pathologist has given his report, that the coroner has to decide whether the death is one which he can sign up on pink form B where no inquest is necessary (Section 21(2) Coroners (Amendment) Act 1926), or to hold an inquest. The factors which influence this decision are almost entirely medical, so coroners without medical qualifications are very much in the hands of their medical advisers, particularly their pathologists. In my view, the advent of the 'yellow card' has helped coroners in cases where the evidence of a definite adverse reaction is doubtful. If there is enough natural disease present to account for death it is possible for him to issue his pink form B, and without an inquest, report the death and the circumstances which raised the possibility of an adverse reaction to the Committee on Safety of Medicines. This indeed is my practice in those deaths which appear to be drug-related, but for which my pathologist can find no supporting evidence; reporting my suspicion to the Committee may help to uncover a definite relationship.

Where the consensus of medical opinion is that a suspected adverse effect has substance, this is still not the end of the coroner's decision-making process. In the case of a person, for example, with malignant disease who had been treated by substances known to possess toxic properties, he might well consider that the adverse effect has not affected the outcome, and certify death as due to the disease. No general rules can be drawn up to meet every possible combination of circumstances, but many coroners may share my view that an inquest in the case of a person whose death was inevitable is of little benefit. On the other hand, an inquest into a death arising out of an adverse effect from a medicine used for a disease which did not threaten life, plainly has value. Where coroners can legitimately differ is in deaths from well-known adverse effects of long-term administration with drugs used in chronic diseases, such as arthritis.

## ILLUSTRATIVE CASES

The accounts of inquests which follow illustrate the problems a coroner has to face when a death is reported to him and the cause appears to be an adverse reaction. These deaths have been reported to me either because the death or collapse has followed rapidly after administration of the drug or the manner of the patient's death suggested that a drug reaction may have been the cause, in whole or in part.

An 18-year-old schoolgirl had suffered from asthma for which she had been treated with steroids. Later the decision had been made to use synthetic ACTH instead. Because she was worried that her condition might worsen during her 'A' level examinations, she arranged with the out-patients department of the hospital to have an injection of this substance. An intramuscular injection of 1 mg was given, and the patient left the hospital immediately, driving herself in her car accompanied by her mother. She collapsed while still in the car and was driven to a neighbouring hospital where she died. The post-mortem examination findings were not remarkable save for the presence of some mucus plugs in the bronchi; zinc, a component of the injected substance, was found in the injection site. Professor Camps suggested that the substance might have been massaged into the circulation whilst driving the car. Clinically the death was due to an anaphylactic reaction.

Collapse and death following an injection may not always be so easily explained. A 26-year-old male who died very unusually was suffering from chronic schizophrenia and had recently developed fits. His current treatment included depot injections of long-acting fluphenazine. Shortly after returning home after such an injection he retired to bed and was found by his mother dead in opisthotonos. At post-mortem material was found in the alveoli which might have been aspirated stomach contents or other foreign matter. Sudden fatal collapse following immediately upon an intravenous injection raises the question whether the substance administered was the cause. In one death following a diagnostic dye injection it became obvious that it was not the dye which had been the cause of death, but the 'shock' of its injection into a patient whose heart muscle was infiltrated with lymphomatous tissue and much fibrosed.

As a coroner I seldom find that an ADR is alleged when the evidence of it is flimsy. However, death following an anaesthetic, even if long delayed, will be reported either by the hospital or by the registrar under the regulations described earlier. As anaesthetic deaths are considered elsewhere I will not elaborate on them here. Death following a diagnostic procedure has always excited my concern as I consider that such procedures should rarely be lethal. As an example of a long-delayed death from the adverse reaction the following is of interest. A lady of 55 years with a long history of heart disease underwent cardiac catheterization, following which she collapsed and remained in coma for some $2\frac{1}{2}$ years, eventually dying from a urinary tract infection secondary to stone in the bladder. From the history as understood at the time of death, the collapse had been attributed to sensitivity to an iodine-containing radio-opaque agent. When, however, the original notes of the catheterization were produced, there was no written evidence that such an agent had been administered.

On the other hand, the doctor may have no doubt that death has followed the administration of a drug. Such was the case of a 71-year-old man who had a long history of chronic bronchitis and emphysema. He had been treated by conventional means and some time before death had also been given an anabolic steroid. In part II of the death certificate the doctor had written 'Drug-induced jaundice' and so the registrar referred the death to me. At post-mortem there was no doubt that the liver showed a pattern of necrosis more in keeping with a direct action of toxic chemical than with naturally occurring liver disease, and the doctor who had issued the certificate was adamant that the steroid had been responsible.

Another problem arises when the deceased has taken a number of drugs and has died from a cause which is often drug-related. I recall an example where a man who was receiving a number of drugs developed a fatal bone marrow depression 3 months after phenylbutazone was added to his regime.

A recent jury inquest illustrates many of the problems which a coroner may face in investigating a death in which a number of drugs have been used. A 29-year-old male had been compulsorily admitted to hospital under the Mental Health Act 1959.[8] During his admission his behaviour was disturbed and he frequently absconded and assaulted staff. Initially his condition was controlled by administration of chlorpromazine and sodium amytal. After a few days the sodium amytal was no longer given and haloperidol and occasional paraldehyde were added to the chlorpromazine. The maximum possible daily dose of chlorpromazine under a regime of regular and as-required dosage could have been 4000 mg. Under this regime his behaviour was far less disturbed, but some hours after oral administration of his evening medication he collapsed and died. A post-mortem toxicological examination revealed very high levels of chlorpromazine to which death was attributed by the toxicologist. This view of the matter was disputed by the legal representatives of the deceased who had obtained sight of the in-patient records, and had had an opinion obtained from an expert in the clinical pharmacology of the class of compounds concerned. One of the coroner's legal problems is whether this opinion is legally receivable in a coroner's court. After legal argument I decided to admit this evidence at the adjourned hearing on the grounds that the toxicologist had considered the hypotheses put to him by counsel for the family based on their expert's views. These were that the high levels of chlorpromazine were not solely the result of high dosage with that compound, but of an interaction with the concurrently administered haloperidol. (A suggestion that the prior administration of sodium amytal and its discontinuance might have affected the metabolism of chlorpromazine was not as energetically pursued.) The view that chlorpromazine in the high doses used might have interfered with its own metabolism as advanced by the toxicologist was discounted by the expert. In the event I did my best to put the conflicting views to the jury and invited them to alter the cause of death to chlorpromazine and haloperidol overdosage, an invitation they declined. At the hearing I made it clear that the jury may not be the best method of settling problems like this and I reported all the facts to the Committee on Safety of Medicines. In the course of the inquest, which lasted 3 full days every nurse who could be traced and all the doctors involved in his management gave evidence and were minutely cross-examined. A request that the matter be referred by me for enquiry by the DHSS was declined.

## DISCUSSION

The future of the Coroner system in England and Wales is still much under discussion; what was proposed in the 'Brodrick' recommendations[6] was not only a tighter system of death certification, but also a greater degree of discretion for the coroner to decide if an inquest is necessary. Under such a system where a certifying doctor would specifically have to state that he believed the death not to have been influenced by *inter alia* drug therapy it may be that more drug-related deaths might be reported. Without the legal necessity to hold an inquest the coroner would still be able to pursue his investigations and then decide if holding the inquest was in the best interests of all. In practice this is what happens when a coroner decides that the evidence does not warrant an inquest, but there is nothing in the present law which requires him to notify the Committee on Safety of Medicines.

The 'Brodrick' Committee[6] recommended that the Secretary of State for Social Services should have power to introduce regulations which would make certain categories of death '*reportable deaths*'. The report clearly implied deaths following the use of specific drugs (Report: paragraph 6.20). Among coroners who have written books, interest in ADRs is a relatively recent phenomenon; *Jervis on Coroners*,[9] which is now over 20 years old, makes no mention of them under the general discussion of unnatural disease, although drug overdose, poisoning and drug addiction are discussed. Dr Gavin Thurston in his book *Coronership*[10] has some doubts regarding the publicity which inquests into adverse reactions attracts. In Chapter 4 entitled 'Coroner's choice of procedure after report', of his book, he plainly regards reporting the death to the Committee of Safety of Medicines as a better procedure than inquest. In his view an inquest into a death following the use of a contraceptive pill 'may do more harm than good'. As I know myself, such an inquest in the case of a single girl may distress the parents – as indeed would an inquest into a death following a therapeutic abortion, on which most coroners would believe they were bound to order an inquest.

In my own series of inquests, those into ADRs are far fewer in number than other categories of therapeutic misadventure or hospital deaths which are unrelated to therapy following falls or other accidents. The reason is not that such deaths are so infrequent, but that the present Coroners' system is probably not best designed to look into them. There may well be unknown drug hazards yet to be detected. In my more contemplative moments I have reflected on what might happen if, in addition to certifying the cause of death, the deceased's doctor also had to note all the medical conditions from which the patient had suffered in the year preceding death and the treatment given. Who knows what lethal combinations of disease and drug might not be revelaed by such a requirement. To my knowledge, although there is a body concerned with discussing changes in the law relating to coroners, I do not know that it, or any other authority, is much concerned with remedying the deficiencies I have indicated in the reporting of ADRs. I do not anticipate much progress on the problem in my professional lifetime.

## CONCLUSIONS

Historically the role of the Coroner has been the immediate investigation of sudden death and others which appeared to have been violent or unnatural. Looking at those inquests in which an ADR has been suspected it is clear that the very suddenness is the factor which has led to the report to me, and to the subsequent investigation culminating in an inquest. This may have excluded the suspected reaction as a cause. In other cases, such as unexplained jaundice it has needed the conviction of the reporting doctor to bring the death to my notice. The system does not provide for this to happen in every case of doubt. Some of the measures proposed by the Brodrick Committee would help greatly to remedy this, but this is plainly only one facet of the general problem surrounding the reporting of ADRs.

### Acknowledgement

It would not have been possible for me to have written this without the help of John Harvey, Esq, BSc, by whose labours and the willing assistance of Messrs Sterling Winthrop a card index and computer records of my inquest material has been constructed.

## References


1. Coroners Act 1887 50 & 51 Vict. c. 71
2. Coroners (Amendment) Act 1926 16 & 17 Geo. 5 c. 59
3. The Coroners Rules 1984 Statutory Instrument No. 552
4. The Births and Deaths Registration Act 1953 1 & 2 Eliz. 2 c. 20
5. Births, Deaths and Marriage Regulations 1968 Statutory Instrument No. 2049
6. Report of the Committee on Death Certification and Coroners MTP, (Brodrick report) Cmnd 4810
7. Industrial Diseases Notification Act 1981.
8. Mental Health Act 1959
9. Purchase, W. B. and Wollaston, H. W. (eds.) (1957) *Jervis on the Office and Duties of Coroners*, 9th Edn. (London: Sweet & Maxwell)
10. Thurston, G. (1980). *Coronership*, 3rd Edn. (Chichester and London: Barry Rose)

# 29
# The role of the pathologist

DAVID HALER

## INTRODUCTION

The role of the Coroner has been fully discussed in the previous chapter, and the purpose of this short article is to outline the differing role of the pathologist and to emphasize, particularly, the techniques for the collection and preservation of samples required for the investigation of suspected drug reactions.

In view of the rapid advance in immunology and particularly as it is being applied to therapeutics, the morbid anatomist is most likely to recognize potential dangers.

Pathologists who carry out tests on living patients may encounter the results of untoward reactions, and should report their suspicions to the prescribing doctor or doctors and, in the United Kingdom, to the Area Community Physician and to the Committee on Safety of Medicines (see Chapter 1). Hospital pathologists, especially morbid anatomists, who conduct routine post-mortem examinations may also suspect adverse reactions to medicines, in which case they have the additional duty to notify the Coroner and, if necessary, the Medical Committee at the hospital. It is also desirable to pass on early information to the manufacturers of the 'suspect' drug.

Many doctors, particularly pathologists, may feel diffident about their role in the investigation of ADRs, and especially when it comes to reporting the unfortunate results of a colleague's treatment. It is rare; but it does happen. Nevertheless, it is the plain duty of any pathologist when called upon to investigate the death of a patient, or to investigate an untoward reaction, to report any suspicion that he may have that a drug may have been responsible. There is no place for diffidence in science, just as in the post-mortem room there is neither modesty nor inhibition about what is done to the body in the course of scientific investigation of the cause of death.

## COLLECTION OF SAMPLES

This often presents problems to people who are not accustomed to transmitting samples. It must be emphasized that the techniques of investigation of deaths that may have been caused by an ADR following normal therapeutic doses does not differ appreciably from those used when there has been overdosage. There is no need for highly specialized techniques, at least during the initial stages of investigation. The essential rule is to collect adequate samples of tissues and body fluids and to store them under proper conditions. All tissues should be tightly sealed and deep frozen: in this way they may be stored indefinitely. As much of the body fluids as is available should be collected and tightly sealed. Blood, urine, bile and cerebrospinal fluid should all be dated for reference and be refrigerated.

### Blood samples

If there is a suspicion that a drug may have played a part in a patient's death, heart and portal blood samples should be taken. These should be withdrawn from an auricle using a sterile needle and syringe, and should immediately be placed in a sterile container. Note that puncture of the auricles may present difficulties, as such specimens are often clotted. Blood from the left ventricle or ascending aorta is less likely to be clotted. Always detach the needle from the syringe when transferring to the sterile container, as haemolysis may well occur from forcing blood through a fine needle, and remember to exercise caution against contamination of the outside of the container or of personnel.

Whole blood should never be frozen. Normally it is best stored at 4° C, but should it have to be deep-frozen the plasma and formed elements should be separated before freezing. As with all specimens these samples should be adequately labelled and indexed with the records of the time, date, name and age of the patient.

If possible a sample of portal blood should also be taken (although it is unusual to obtain much more than, at the most, 5 ml). Portal blood is usually not clotted and often contains unexpectedly large concentrations of any drugs the patient may have taken, together with other sometimes unexpected substances, such as large quantities of insulin, even in non-diabetics. Portal blood is unfortunately little examined but is very rewarding in the elucidation of the fate of drugs prior to detoxification in the liver. (Remember that it is an afferent vessel to the liver c.f. the German term '*Pfortader*'.)

### Urine

The largest possible samples should be obtained, using an aseptic technique, preferably by puncturing the bladder with a large-bore needle, and decanting into a sterile container. Urine should also be stored at 4° C, taking great care not to use a sampling bottle containing inhibitors.

### Other body fluids

A specimen of bile should be collected by needle and syringe puncture as in the case of urine, and also stored at 4° C. It is noteworthy that many of the alkaloids and quite a number of other drugs can be isolated from bile, even when they cannot be obtained from other specimens.

Cerebrospinal fluid deserves a special mention, and should be collected by the following recommended technique. The fluid should be taken from the lateral ventricles, rather than by any other route, after removal and laying open of the brain. Lay open the lateral ventricles with a sterile scalpel by reflecting the Corpus Callosum bilaterally and posteriorly.

Stomach contents should be measured, and an aliquot taken and stored at 4° C. It may be desirable to freeze them. It is best to preserve the stomach in a deep-frozen state because it arrests further autolysis of the organ and the contents.

It is important when collecting specimens in the course of the autopsy to examine carefully the gullet and stomach walls and the rest of the alimentary tract for evidence of possibly more or less intact residues of drug or capsules which may throw light upon a possible ADR.

### Tissues

Organs should be taken for chemical analysis, noting the weight of the whole organ and the weight of the portion taken for analyses to be made, elsewhere, for drugs. Tissues required for histological study are usually stored in formol–saline.

### General considerations

It must be mentioned that fluid and tissue samples are a potential source of danger (e.g. hepatitis). The pathologist is *personally* responsible for safe handling, storage, collection and transport of samples.

Transfer to other laboratories, particularly in warm countries, may call for some ingenuity. Deep-frozen specimens at −20° C may be transported in vacuum flasks, or in suitable 'freezer' containers packed with dry ice.

Details of the technique for drug identification and assay are beyond the scope of this article. They include thin layer and gas chromatography and studies of immunofluorescence. For the latter, pathological material should not be fixed, and should be handled in conditions of temperate refrigeration rather than deep-freeze.

In many countries embalming is very primitive and is often done using very poor techniques which leave a gross excess of formaldehyde and crude alcohols in the 'preserved' body.

## POST-MORTEM OBSERVATIONS

Many clues to possible drug reactions are more obvious in death than in life. Skin eruptions, jaundice, muscle-wasting, enlargement or contraction of various organs are commonplace. Ecchymoses or petechiae are often present. Pharyngeal ulceration may lead to the diagnosis of agranulocytosis. Haemorrhages into the brain or skin may suggest a thrombocytopenia. These and other signs should lead the pathologist to search the patient's history carefully for possibly relevant drugs and to consult with hospital colleagues, if possible, or the patient's general practitioner. It is worth remembering that patients who have recently been abroad, or who have been transported in the emblamed state, may have been exposed to drugs obtained overseas. In many countries with less stringent drug regulations amidopyrone and/or chloramphenicol may be freely purchased. In South America there is practically no restriction on the purchase of any drug. These drugs are not an infrequent cause of fatal blood dyscrasia in recently returned travellers.

## THE PATHOLOGIST'S RESPONSIBILITY

The procedure for reporting deaths to the Coroner is dealt with in the previous chapter. Where there is strong suspicion that death has resulted from a drug reaction the pathologist will send a report of his observations to the Coroner. Usually, also, as a courtesy, he will inform the manufacturer of the drug and, of course, discreetly the patient's physician. He should also be encouraged to notify the Committee on Safety of Medicines, with whom most pathologists are on good terms and receive nothing but help in return for their reports.

Although many drug reactions are indistinguishable from conditions which occur spontaneously, the pathologist can often provide the final confirmation of a diagnosis of drug toxicity. By communication in a helpful rather than an accusatory manner with his medical colleagues, and others involved with the care of the community, he can play an important role in the continuance of drug safety and its surveillance.

# 30
# Poisons information services

G. N. VOLANS

## POISONS INFORMATION SERVICES – THE CONCEPT

The origin of Poisons Information, or Poisons Control, Centres dates back little more than 25 years. Retrospectively it is difficult to believe that the pioneers of this movement, which has now assumed almost world-wide coverage, ever contemplated drug monitoring as being among their objectives, at least at the outset. Instead, they were prompted much more by expediency. 'Following World War II', wrote Crotty and Verhulst,[1] 'there seemed to be a proliferation of new chemicals and new common household products. The names, characteristics and toxicity of these new chemicals were unfamiliar to practising physicians. Even the medicines which were their tools had unknown facets when they were ingested in an acute overdose.' At the same time the incidence of misadventures with these materials, whether accidentally (notably in children), or deliberately (with adults), especially with the growing vogue for self-poisoning, seemed to be increasing. Doctors, whether working in hospitals or engaged elsewhere, were being confronted more and more by patients who might, or might not, be poisoned. Professional ignorance or inability properly to diagnose and manage these problems clinically could be rectified adequately neither by expanded professional education, before or after qualification, nor by turning to text-books or current works of reference. So to meet this need a novel system was inaugurated. An entirely separate advisory service was established, to operate throughout the 24 hours and, on an emergency basis, to answer queries arising in this way. Further, in the beginning and still commonly in many countries, this facility was available not only to doctors but to members of the public as well. Setting the pattern in 1953, the Poisons Control Centre, which came into being in Chicago, Illinois, USA, was designed in a way that immediately 'provided information on and treatment for poisonings', though subsequently it proceeded by 'establishing a program of prevention'.[2] These two principles, with the former predominating, have remained virtually intrinsic to the corresponding information and control services for poisoning that have since come into effect in numerous other countries throughout the world.

Two features should, perhaps, be borne in mind: first the scope of operations in this field has not been confined to drugs. Indeed, it might be averred that they often occupied a lesser role, on the assumption that generally there was at least some understanding about their toxicity. Far more enigmatic in the sense of hazard were the household products, the industrial chemicals, the pesticides and even the wild and domestic plants, for which toxicological data were commonly lacking. Secondly, the primary purpose at the start was to provide information and not to gather it. Thus it was only later that any efforts were mobilized to collect data, usually by some manner of follow-up procedure. In the United States this took the form of standard returns from the various control centres throughout the country, by then numbering some hundreds, and furnishing them to the official Clearing House, which functioned under the Government Department of Health, Education and Welfare, where they were collated. Similar arrangements were set up in Canada. In this manner national statistics could be compiled, with subdivisions under various headings – types of product, sex and age of patients, symptoms, etc. From an epidemiological point of view, however, the figures were somewhat unrepresentative, for they referred only to incidents which provoked enquiries. Poisoning could still occur and be treated without any reference to control centres and not all centres managed to complete their returns. Secondly, as a majority of the calls emanated not from doctors but from the public, it was often far from easy to obtain all the requisite particulars. A categorical definition of 'poisoning' had not been propounded and this type of illness was not formally notifiable.

In the United Kingdom a follow-up operation was instituted from the very beginning, for no other reason than to meet an immediate need.[3] In compiling the index, constructed as a reference from which enquiries could be answered, it became disconcertingly obvious that, for most of the items, toxicological characterization was lacking, sometimes totally. Extrapolation, analogy and guesswork – hopefully inspired, had therefore to be substituted for facts. In order to remedy this deplorable state of affairs it was decided that a record of actual cases, contributed by the doctor personally dealing with them, would put the whole index on a firmer footing and suffuse greater medical authenticity and authority into the answers and guidance subsequently extended.

The mechanics of the process were simple enough. Within 7–10 days of handling each call the doctor making it received a simple form embracing seven questions: the sex and age of the patient, the product involved, the quantity believed to be implicated, the symptoms, the treatment and outcome. A stamped-and-addressed envelope was also supplied to facilitate posting the reply. The response was gratifying in that the overall rate was in excess of 60% and, furthermore, the answers proved most informative. One reason for this, no doubt, was the principle by which the British service catered only for the medical profession and did not entertain calls from the rest of the community. Essentially, too, confidentiality was strictly observed. Co-operation and cohesion were, moreover, enhanced because of the existence of only four centres in the United Kingdom and one in Eire, all subject to unified co-ordination. By this means it proved possible, within 2–3 years, fundamentally and fairly comprehensively to revise and update the whole index in relation to this recently constructed corpus of case records. Henceforth the features of poisoning and suspected poisoning in Britain could be presented on a foundation of fact in place of belief. By this method of working, though, all classes of products were surveyed and not drugs alone. At the same time it was revealed, as a generalization, that medicines and drugs were responsible for the more serious poisonings and that, within this simplification, substances such as barbiturates and aspirin could prove devastating, whereas the oral contraceptives, in the acute sense, were virtually innocuous. From there it became but a short step to plan and conduct a more specific type of monitoring for certain selected drugs (and, incidentally, for other particular products as well), even if the full implementation of the scheme had to be delayed pending the expansion of staff in the service to undertake this further work.

## DATA BASE

For the older and traditional drugs the experimental data on their toxicology are commonly incomplete. That omission has nevertheless been made good over the years, sometimes over a course of centuries, by the substitution of clinical experience. Yet, ever since the Committee of Safety of Drugs in the United Kingdom first came into being in 1963, being superseded under the Medicines Act 1968 by the Committee on Safety of Medicines, all bodies submitting applications for approval to market new drugs have been obliged to appraise systematically beforehand the pharmacological and toxicological properties of each of the agents concerned. The idea has been to advance towards use in man only against a background of knowledge derived from animals. Valuable though this has been in arriving at therapeutic indications, dosages, the avoidance of side-effects and the catastrophes of overdosage, there is the sobering constraint that animal toxicology, after all, cannot yet be exalted to the status of a truly predictive science. Nevertheless, if acute toxicity tests are properly conducted and are not confined just to arriving at a mathematical LD50, but extended to the observation of the time, the course and the mode of death, then they can point the way to anticipating what may happen to man. Even if these data are not always published it is the fortunate experience of the National Poisons

Information Service in the United Kingdom that manufacturers are prepared to disclose their findings in this respect to the Service as well as to the Committee on Safety of Medicines and, within the limitations to which reference has already been made, this as-it-were lateral communication has proved invaluable.

In addition, the Statutory Committee nowadays requires an insight into pharmacokinetics, including that applied to man, together in many instances with methods for measuring the levels of the drug in the blood and other tissues. These findings can be of great assistance, too, in deducing what might happen with an overdose in a patient, its diagnosis and management. Once more it can be said that most commercial firms are forthcoming with the National Poisons Information Service in this regard. Nonetheless, an accepted and agreed procedure for this interchange would be preferable and might with advantage be discussed with the Committee itself and the Association of the British Pharmaceutical Industry.

Similarly, the outcome of the official clinical trials leading up to a Product Licence could be helpful to the Poisons Information Service, with the reservation that, by the very design of these studies, frank overdoses are very seldom encountered during the course of these exercises.

This is not to imply that the exchange of knowledge should be entirely in one direction. No responsible manufacturer can afford to dismiss incidents of overdose with a proprietary medicine. By contrast, they are nearly always on the alert for such eventualities, if only to devise measures for avoiding them, or mitigating them, in the future. Sometimes they may learn of these events from the physician directly responsible for the patient. Yet the majority of these cases come promptly and inevitably to the notice of the National Poisons Information Service, and, so long as confidentiality is always respected, it would seem very worthwhile for the Service to relay the details to the firm concerned, having obtained the agreement of the physician beforehand and not divulging his name or that of the patient or the hospital without his prior acquiescence.

## MONITORING DRUG OVERDOSE IN PRACTICE

By contrast to the objectivity and exactness that are the concomitants of toxicological experiments in animals the study of drug overdosage in man would seem beset by so many variables and occasionally imponderables, e.g. reliable knowledge of the amount taken, time, age, interaction of other drugs, influence of disease, so that very little reliability could be placed on the findings. In fact this is not so, provided the various factors are accurately noted and allowance is made for them.

Questionnaires are essential and, although they can impose an undesirable element of rigidity on the data collected, this can be minimized by careful design and by pilot runs. This attention to design should ensure that the recipient clinician will find the questionnaire acceptable, and the response rate can be further improved if the accompanying letter provides an adequate explanation as to why the data are being collected. This approach, backed up, where necessary, with telephone calls and even personal visits, consistently produces a 50–60% return of the data being sought. For some intensive studies, much greater returns (even 80–90%) have been achieved. The clinical observations obtained in this way may then be supplemented, if possible, by laboratory checks such as drug levels in body fluids, the presence or absence of other drugs, etc. Given a good understanding and rapport with the clinicians whose assistance is sought it is remarkable just how instructive these surveys can prove; a belief that may best be illustrated by recent examples undertaken by the National Poisons Information Service, covering a range of drugs, some of them long-standing and others newly introduced.

As a start one can consider the monitoring of the incidence of drug overdosage where the toxicity is already known:

*'Lomotil' (Searle)*: This preparation, advocated for the symptomatic control of diarrhoea, contains a non-analgesic narcotic, diphenoxylate hydrochloride, along with atropine sulphate as an anti-spasmodic. Reports have been published of a number of overdoses, some of them culminating fatally.[4]

Since a number of cases had come to the notice of the National Poisons Information Service it was decided in 1976 to embark on a prospective survey collecting details about the supposed quantity taken, the symptoms, the treatment and the outcome, the conclusions being published by Penfold and Volans in 1979.[5]

Briefly, 86 episodes of 'Lomotil' overdose were reviewed, 71 of them afflicting children under the age of 5 (see Table 1). No less than 26 of the patients had exhibited pronounced symptoms, 7 of the children being profoundly ill (see Table 2). One, indeed, a youngster of 2½ years, swallowed about twenty tablets, suffered a cardiac arrest and died in

**Table 1** Age and sex of patients reported to be suffering from overdose of Lomotil

| | *Age (years)* | | | *Total* |
|---|---|---|---|---|
| | $\leqslant 5$ | *6–12* | $\geqslant 12$ | |
| Males | 34 | 1 | 5 | 40 |
| Females | 30 | 3 | 6 | 39 |
| Not known | 7 | 0 | 0 | 7 |
| TOTAL | 71 | 4 | 11 | 86 |

**Table 2** Relation between age and symptoms associated with overdose due to Lomotil (in cases where adequate follow-up information was received)

| | *Age (years)* | | | *Total* |
|---|---|---|---|---|
| | *⩽5* | *6–12* | *⩾12* | |
| Group 1 | 21 | 0 | 1 | 22 |
| Group 2 | 16 | 2 | 1 | 19 |
| Group 3 | 6 | 1 | 0 | 7 |
| TOTAL | 43 | 3 | 2 | 48 |

**Definition of Groups**
Group 1, No definite symptoms; Group 2, Definite symptoms of drowsiness, flushing, dry mouth, tachycardia, dilated pupils, rash and nausea; Group 3, Severe symptoms of Grade IV coma, respiratory depression, respiratory arrest, cardiac arrest

spite of energetic treatment, including the administration of naloxone. From these results it is clear that 'Lomotil' can give rise to serious poisoning, notably in young children, some of them developing marked symptoms after only one to five tablets, depending on age. The frequency and severity of these episodes could suggest that doctors should be more impressively alerted to the dangers attendant upon the misuse of this preparation, warnings to parents should be reinforced and insistence on dispensing this product only in child-resistant containers should be adopted, the more so as, to date, there appears to be no decline in the incidence of this type of poisoning with 24 cases reported in the first 6 months of 1983.

*Clonidine:* This drug was initially introduced into Britain in 1971 as a treatment for hypertension under the proprietary name of 'Catapres' (Boehringer, Ingelheim), the white uncoated tablets each containing 0.1 mg or 0.3 mg clonidine hydrochloride. Later, another preparation reached the market under the trade name of 'Dixarit' (WB Pharmaceuticals Ltd.), the presentation taking the form of attractive, blue, sugar-coated tablets each containing 0.025 mg clonidine hydrochloride intended for the relief of migraine and menopausal flushing. Publications on the subject of clonidine overdose indicated that the reactions might be serious, but there was no consistency about the clinical picture, nor was there unanimity about effective treatment.[6]

Accordingly, the National Poisons Information Service launched a 2-year prospective survey, covering 305 enquiries in all and obtained follow-up reports on 170 of these.[7] From these it emerged that the major problem was the ingestion of 'Dixarit' by young children (see Table 3), probably owing to their attractive appearance. The clinical features were then more clearly defined, the time-course of the symptoms became evident (see Table 4) and the indications for

**Table 3** Total enquiries and cases of clonidine overdosage in children and adults notified to the National Poisons Information Service during 1976 and 1977

| *Age-group* | *No. of calls received* | *No. of cases involved* | *Follow-ups received* | *No. of cases for which follow-ups received* |
|---|---|---|---|---|
| *1976* | | | | |
| Children (1–10 years) | 97 | 105 | 60 | 66 |
| Adults (14–72 years) | 49 | 49 | 21 | 21 |
| Age unknown | 6 | 6 | 0 | 0 |
| TOTALS FOR 1976 | 152 | 160 | 81 | 87 |
| *1977* | | | | |
| Children (1–9 years) | 100 | 109 | 61 | 67 |
| Adults (14–64 years) | 35 | 35 | 16 | 16 |
| Age unknown | 1 | 1 | 0 | 0 |
| TOTALS FOR 1977 | 136 | 145 | 77 | 83 |

**Table 4** Clinical features of acute clonidine overdosage in 133 children aged under 10 years (mean age 2 years 8 months) and in 37 adults (mean age 29). Mean clonidine dosage: children 0.509 mg (range 0.025–3.000 mg); adults 2.096 mg (range 0.250–7.000 mg)

| *Signs and symptoms* | *No. (%) of children* | *No. (%) of adults* |
|---|---|---|
| Impaired consciousness | 113 (85) | 29 (78) |
| Pallor | 36 (27) | 6 (16) |
| Bradycardia* | 32 (24) | 18 (49) |
| Cardiac arrhythmias | 6 (5) | — |
| Cardiac arrest | — | 1 (3) |
| Hypotension† | 28 (21) | 12 (32) |
| Depressed respiration | 20 (15) | 2 (5) |
| Apnoea | 3 (2) | — |
| Miosis | 18 (14) | 3 (8) |
| Unreactive pupils | 7 (5) | — |
| Hypotonia | 14 (11) | 2 (5) |
| Irritability | 14 (11) | 1 (3) |
| Hyporeflexia | 5 (4) | 1 (3) |
| Extensor plantar reflex | 4 (3) | — |
| Hypertension | 3 (2) | 4 (11) |
| Dry mouth | 3 (2) | 4 (11) |
| Mean duration of effects (h) | 16.2 (range 3.5–48.0) | 15–95 |
| Mean duration of hospitalization (h) | 32.5 (range 1.0–72.0) | 24–>96 |

* Bradycardia defined as a pulse of <80/min age 1–4 years; <75/min age 4–6 years; <70/min age 6–10 years; <60/min age >10 years.

† Hypotension defined as a systolic blood pressure of: <75 mmHg age 1–2 years; <80 mmHg age 2–40 years; <90 mmHg age >40 years.

treatment were clarified. Once acquainted with these findings, the manufacturers of the preparation alerted all pharmacists, incorporated a special warning on the container label and, as a safety measure, from January 1980, this product has been available only in an opaque blister pack. Monitoring of this product continues, and it is hoped it will be possible to report on the influence of the new packaging, taking into account both the time needed to clear supplies of the original packs already distributed before January 1980 and changes in the product sales.

*Paracetamol overdose in children:* The nature and intensity of acute overdose of paracetamol first came to medical attention in 1966, and since that time the incidence of this form of hepatotoxic poisoning has steadily increased in the United Kingdom and elsewhere, leading to extensive research in the subject, both from the biochemical and the clinical point of view.[8] Impressively, the patients always seemed to be adults who had resorted to this drug for self-poisoning and while, by analogy with aspirin poisoning in children, fears were expressed about the dangers of paracetamol for youngsters (particularly because of its extensive usage in the home), no one could say anything about the scale of the paediatric hazard. For this reason Meredith *et al.*[9] scrutinized and followed up the calls about paracetamol and children directed to the National Poisons Information Service of a period of 3 years. From this it became clear that serious cases in the young age-group were not encountered, the only children coming to harm in this way being those approaching adolescence who were emulating the adults and indulging in deliberate self-poisoning. From that report in 1978, to this date, we have received no reports of serious cases of poisoning from paracetamol alone in young children. There have been fatalities, however, following overdose of benorylate[10] (an aspirin salicylate ester) and Safapryn (personal communication) – a sustained-release tablet consisting of an aspirin core surrounded by paracetamol. In both cases, post-mortems revealed extensive centrilobular necrosis in the liver. This is characteristic of damage due to paracetamol hepatotoxicity. In the case of the Safapryn overdose, the aspirin also made a significant contribution to the child's death.

While these three examples have been cited to indicate the potentialities of a Poisons Information Service, they are by no means exhaustive. Corresponding exercises have covered poisoning due to hypnotics in general,[11] chloral hydrate and its cardiac actions,[12] chlormethiazole,[13] tricyclic antidepressants,[14] non-barbiturate anticonvulsants,[15] salbutamol,[16] theophylline derivatives[17] and methionine as a treatment for paracetamol poisoning.[18] No less can the same resources be deployed to monitor drugs as soon as they are released for medical use generally. Thus some of those that are acccorded a Product Licence are well-nigh automatic candidates for overdose; e.g. antidepressants and hypnotics. Others are likely to qualify on account of their expected scale of use, e.g. $H_2$-receptor antagonists. Finally, there are some that, *prima facie*, might be disregarded in this respect, e.g. cardiac anti-dysrhythmics. Whatever the predictions arrived at in this way, prudence demands that overdoses of any new drugs, into whatever category they may ultimately fall, should give cause for alert and should be meticulously recorded. Only in this way will the clinical features become recognised and appropriate treatment be devised. That a Poisons Information Service lends itself to this monitoring role may be demonstrated by recent experiences.

*New antidepressants:* Recent additions to the catalogue of antidepressants have included maprotiline (with its bridged tricyclic molecule), nomifensine (with a simple tricyclic molecule), mianserin (with a tetracyclic molecule) and trazodone (a triazolopyridine derivative). To judge from the biochemistry and pharmacology of these compounds, an overdose of maprotiline would be expected to resemble that of the other and older tricyclics (e.g. amitriptyline, imipramine), whilst the other three might well be less toxic owing to an absence of anticholinergic activity. These similarities and disparities have been borne out in practice by monitoring organized by the National Poisons Information Service.[19–21]

*Cimetidine:* This drug, the prototype $H_2$-receptor antagonist marketed for clinical use, has rapidly gained widespread acceptance, and since its introduction in 1977 now enjoys prescribing on an enormous scale. Under these circumstances, overdoses would surely be unavoidable and, as only to be expected, 24 such cases were reported to the National Poisons Information Service within a short time. The so-far unpublished follow-ups on these and subsequent patients have confirmed what was foreseen from the animal toxicity testing in that the sequelae are relatively insignificant, even after verified doses of up to 19.2 g.

*Disopyramide:* This cardiac anti-dysrhythmic agent of the Class 1 type, has electrophysiological properties akin to those of quinidine. Four oral preparations are now marketed, Rythmodan, Rythmodan Retard [sustained-release formulation] (Roussel) containing the disopyramide base and Dirythmin, Dirythmin SA [sustained-release formulation] (Astra) containing the phosphate. All four of these are employed prophylactically, principally after myocardial infarction, and they have a wider therapeutic dose-range than most of the other anti-dysrhythmics. Within a period of a few months, the National Poisons Information Service was asked about five cases of deliberate overdose arising in the United Kingdom. All died, notwithstanding prompt referral to hospital and the mobilization of full resuscitation facilities. It was deemed timely, therefore, to warn doctors of this danger, and an account of these cases was published in *The Lancet* on 6 May 1978.[22] Subsequently, we have elucidated the sequence of events following

**Table 5** Disopyramide overdosage – recommended treatment

(1) Monitor arterial blood pressure closely – preferably with an indwelling cannula;
(2) Establish intravenous infusion with isoprenaline available: dose 0.04–0.1 $\mu g\ kg^{-1}\ min^{-1}$;
(3) Avoid anti-arrhythmic drugs;
(4) Cardiac muscle may be refractory to pacing (high threshold);
(5) Correct acidosis and $K^+$;
(6) Consider haemoperfusion for high plasma disopyramide (*in vivo* clearance 95–122 ml/min).

disopyramide overdosage by means of an animal model.[23,24] Based on these observations, a scheme for management of disopyramide overdosage was proposed (Table 5) which has been shown to be effective in man, although there remains doubt as to the value of haemoperfusion.[25]

## LIMITATIONS OF DRUG MONITORING BY POISONS INFORMATION SERVICES

Although the procedures and surveys described here have been regarded as impressive, they suffer from intrinsic deficiencies. Firstly, the nature of the calls directed at a Poisons Information Service cannot

**Table 6** Sources of analgesic drugs in 878 cases of acute poisoning

| *Source* | *Drug* Aspirin | Paracetamol | Narcotic | Other | Total |
|---|---|---|---|---|---|
| *Prescription* | | | | | |
| Chemist | 22 | 39 | 155 | 20 | 236 |
| Other | 3 | 0 | 5 | 0 | 8 |
| *Non-prescription* | | | | | |
| Chemist | 214 | 130 | 0 | 5 | 349 |
| Other | 107 | 42 | 0 | 0 | 149 |
| Not known | 116 | 78 | 59 | 7 | 260 |
| TOTAL | 462 | 289 | 219 | 32 | 1002 |

*Totals:* Prescription 24%; Non-prescription 50%; Not known 26%.
All analgesics classified as 'not known' could have been obtained without prescription
Reproduced by the kind permission of the Editor of *Human Toxicology*

escape being biased. Emphasis will fall on the exceptional case, and the uncommon drugs, whereas queries are less likely to be prompted over those drugs with the vagaries of which doctors are already more familiar. Secondly, certain hospitals tend to make more use of the Information Service than others, so that geographically and, possibly, socially as well, the clientele is not truly representative. Thirdly, the quality of this clinical reporting is far from uniform and, allied to this, the extent to which different hospitals seek to verify their findings by analysis in the laboratory is very variable.

To some extent these defects can be overcome by devising modified monitoring techniques, and by the provision of supra-regional laboratory facilities such as those at the Guy's Hospital Poisons Unit. Thus, having selected a particular drug or group of drugs for surveillance, a designated series of hospitals could be enlisted along the lines of the Boston Scheme.[26] In this manner a survey has been made in which the Poisons Information Service co-ordinated the collection of special detailed records on every case of analgesic poisoning seen in five major accident and emergency departments.[27] That study yielded a great deal of useful information not only on the incidence of poisoning but also on the source of the drugs, their formulations, the frequency of multiple drug ingestion, the methods of treatment used and the fatalities. Notable amongst these observations was the severity and frequency of salicylate poisoning (9 deaths in 453 cases out of a total of 878 patients) and the finding that between 50–76% of the analgesics were obtained without prescription (Table 6).

The success of this scheme has opened the way for further studies into other aspects and other types of poisoning. Currently, work is in progress to assess the effectiveness of child-resistant closures for drugs, and other surveys are planned. None of these projects would be feasible without computer assistance, and the Information Service has been fortunate to have access to a powerful database management system previously used in post-marketing surveillance.[28] Experience with this system led to the realization that a similar but less powerful program, if used to store data on all cases referred to the Information Service, would be invaluable as an adjunct to the monitoring function.

From December 1982, all enquiries have, therefore, been input to a microcomputer[29] and, for the first time in the history of the Service, it is an easy matter to answer in detail the unexpected enquiries on the incidence or severity of cases reported.[30] For the future, therefore, the monitoring capabilities of the Poisons Information Service are much improved and it should be possible to study both established problems and new developments such as the change in status of ibuprofen to permit pharmacy-only over-the-counter sales.[31] The latter exercises can, indeed, be considered a part of post-marketing surveillance, and it would seem prudent to advise reporting to the Poisons Information Service of overdosage with all new products in much the same way as adverse reactions are reported to the CSM

## Acknowledgements

We are grateful to the Editors for permission to reproduce the tables, previously published in the *British Medical Journal* and *Human Toxicology*. In updating this chapter, I would like to acknowledge the work of Dr Roy Goulding who directed the National Poisons Information Service from its inception until his retirement in 1980, and who built the monitoring system which we are continuing to develop. Thanks are also due to my many colleagues, whose work is quoted in this review, and to Heather Wiseman in particular for helping me to review the new work which has been added for the second edition.

## References

1. Crotty, J. J. and Verhulst, H. L. (1970). Organisation and delivery of poison information in the United States. *Pediat. Clin. N. Am.*, **17,** 741
2. Goulding, R. (1975). Poisons Control Centers – an essay on information and prevention. *Ess. Toxicol.*, **6,** 79
3. Goulding, R. and Watkin, R. R. (1965). National Poisons Information Service. *Mon. Bull. Min. Health.*, **24,** 26
4. Harries, J. T. and Rossiter, M. (1969). Fatal Lomotil poisoning. *Lancet*, **1,** 150
5. Penfold, D. and Volans, G. N. (1979). Overdose from Lomotil. *Br. Med. J.*, **2,** 1401–2
6. Wing, L. M. H., Davies, D. S., Reid, J. L. and Dollery, C. T. (1975). Clonidine overdose. *Br. Med. J.*, **4,** 408–9
7. Stein, B. and Volans, G. N. (1978). Dixarit overdose: the problem of attractive tablets. *Br. Med. J.*, **2,** 667–8
8. Symposium on Paracetamol and the Liver. (1976). Overdosage and its Management. *J. Int. Med. Res.*, **4,** (Suppl. 4)
9. Meredith, T. J., Newman, B. and Goulding, R. (1978). Paracetamol poisoning in children. *Br. Med. J.*, **2,** 478–9
10. Symon, D. N. K., Gray, E. S., Hanmer, O. T. and Russell, G. (1982). Fatal paracetamol poisoning from benorylate therapy in child with cystic fibrosis. *Lancet*, **2,** 1153–4
11. Hampel, G., Wiseman, H. and Widdop, B. (1979). Acute poisoning due to hypnotics. The role of haemoperfusion in clinical perspective. *J. Hum. Vet. Toxicol.*, (Suppl. 121) 4–6
12. Wiseman, H. M. and Hampel, G. (1978). Cardiac arrhythmias due to chloral hydrate poisoning. *Br. Med. J.*, **2,** 960
13. Houston, A., Essex, E. G., Wiseman, H. M. and Flanagan, R. J. (1983). Acute chlormethiazole poisoning. *Hum. Toxicol.*, **2,** (2) 361–9
14. Crome, P. and Newman, B. (1979). The problem of tricyclic antidepressant poisoning. *Postgrad. Med. J.*, **55,** 528–32
15. Berry, D. J., Wiseman, H. M. and Volans, G. N. (1983). A survey of non-barbiturate anticonvulsant drug overdose. *Hum. Toxicol.*, **2,** (2) 357–60
16. Prior, J. G., Raper, S. M., Ali, C., Cochrane, G. M. and Volans, G. N., (1981). Self-poisoning with oral salbutamol. *Br. Med. J.*, **282,** 1932
17. Jefferys, D. B., Raper, S. M., Helliwell, M., Berry, D. and Crome, P. (1980). Haemoperfusion for theophylline overdose. *Br. Med. J.*, **1,** 1167
18. Crome, P., Volans, G. N., Vale, J. A., Widdop, B. and Goulding, R. (1976). Oral methionine in the treatment of severe paracetamol (acetaminophen) overdose. *Lancet*, **2,** 829–30
19. Crome, P. and Newman, B. (1977). Poisoning with maprotiline and mianserin. *Br. Med. J.*, **2,** 260
20. Montgomery, S., Crome, P. and Braithwaite, R. A. (1978). Nomifensine overdosage. *Lancet*, **1,** 828–9

21. Henry, J. A. and Ali, C. J. (1983). Trazodone overdosage. *Hum. Toxicol.* **2,** 353–6
22. Hayler, A. M., Holt, D. W. and Volans, G. N. (1978). Fatal overdosage with disopyramide. *Lancet,* **1,** 968–9
23. Hayler, A. M., Medd, R. K., Holt, D. W. and O'Keeffe, B. D. (1979). Experimental disopyramide poisoning: treatment by cardiovascular support and with charcoal haemoperfusion. *J. Pharmacol. Exp. Ther.,* **211,** 491–5
24. Hayler, A. M., Holt, D. W., O'Keeffe, B. and Medd, R. K. (1979). Treatment of disopyramide overdosage. *Med. J. Austr.,* **1,** 234
25. Holt, D. W., Helliwell, M., O'Keefe, B., Hayler, A. M., Marshall, C. B. and Cook, G. (1980). Successful management of serious disopyramide poisoning. *Postgrad. Med. J.,* **56,** 256–60
26. Miller, R. R. and Greenblatt, D. J. (eds.) (1976). Drug Effects in Hospitalised Patients. (London: John Wiley Biomedical)
27. Volans, G. N., Wiseman, H. M., Newman, B. C., Guest, K., Rose, D. B., Adams, R. H., Dallos, V., Daniels, R. G., Helps, P. J. and Rogers, N. C. (1981). Analgesic Poisoning; a Multi-Centre, Prospective Survey. *Hum. Toxicol.,* **1,** 7–23
28. Harcus, A. W., Ward, A. E. and Smith, D. W. (1979). Methodology of monitored release of a new prescription: buprenophine. *Br. Med. J.,* **2,** 163–5
29. Edwards, J. N. and Madge, B. E. (1983). Computer application in Poisons Information and Library Services. *Hum. Toxicol.,* **2,** 420
30. Edwards, J. N., Volans, G. N. and Wiseman, H. M. (1984). Poisons information processing: The development of a computer database for case records. In Kostrewski, B. (ed.) *Current Perspectives in Health Computing.* (Cambridge: Cambridge University Press)
31. Court, H. and Volans, G. N. (1984). Poisoning after overdose with non-steroidal anti-inflammatory drugs. *Adv. Drug React. Acc. Pois. Rev.,* **3,** 1–21

# Section 3:
# EPIDEMIOLOGY, COMPLIANCE AND JUDGEMENT

# Editor's Introduction and Commentary

In this third section of the book we consider the scientific basis of drug monitoring, and some of the epidemiological problems frequently encountered. We consider the use that can be made of morbidity and mortality statistics and the importance of doctor and patient compliance, and we look into the problems of decision-making and those associated with establishing causal relationships between drug exposures and adverse drug reaction.

Through the courtesy of the Editor of *Methods of Information in Medicine* we once again reproduce Professor Finney's chapter on the statistical logic of drug monitoring, first published in 1971 together with his comments in 1979 which appeared in the first edition of this book. Had Finney's guidelines been followed many misleading studies would have remained unpublished.

He shows how an investigator may apply statistical tests and reach conclusions without ensuring that the group of patients he is studying is truly representative of all patients treated with that drug. He reminds us of the importance of ensuring that the choice of a drug is not related to a patient's susceptibility to a reaction, and shows why it is unsatisfactory to compare the incidence of events in patients treated with a particular drug for a certain disease with the incidence in patients not using the drug who do not suffer from that disease. He also stresses the importance of unbiased reporting. Publicity surrounding the first suspicion about a new event will lead to more complete reporting than for patients taking older drugs with which the new one will be compared.

Finney draws on the study by the Editor and his colleagues which showed that oral contraceptives containing larger doses of oestrogen probably carried an increased risk of thromboembolism. This was the study that led to the 'Mini-pill', in which it was possible to apply statistical tests to uncontrolled data in the form of spontaneous reports (see Chapter 1). This is one of the only two occasions over a period of more than 20 years when it was justifiable to apply statistical tests to data collected by the Committee on Safety of Medicines. On another occasion it was possible to show a relation between the number of exposures to the anaesthetic halothane and the speed of onset of jaundice, also referred to in Chapter 1.

Mann (Chapter 32) makes the important point that the more studies that are undertaken the greater the chance that one or other of them will show statistically significant differences by *chance alone*. He also highlights the dangers of jumping to conclusions when small relative risks (e.g. less than 2) have been demonstrated in one or two studies. He lists eight common sources of bias, including the vitally important 'recall' bias where patients' memories of drug exposures may be enhanced by the media or perhaps influenced by successful lawsuits. This reminded the Editor of a story recently retold by Bondi,[1] of the opinion polster who predicted a Republican landslide in a forthcoming election. There was in fact a landslide victory for the Democrats! He had used the telephone interview technique at a time when only rich people could afford telephones!

Doctor Adelstein (Chapter 33) takes us through the various registries available in the United Kingdom for obtaining data on morbidity and mortality. He cites a number of examples of correlations between drug utilization figures and trends in vital statistics, including the relationship that was demonstrated between pressurized aerosol bronchodilating drugs and sudden deaths of young asthmatics. This particular incident was remarkable in several ways. Although more than 3000 deaths were involved, there was almost no publicity to what must have been the largest number of fatalities ever recorded in a comparatively short period for a single group of drugs. It is very unlikely, in fact, that many of the deaths were actually caused by overdoses of these drugs. The probable explanation for the 'epidemic' was that a normally very effective treatment was relied on too much by both patients and doctors. As a consequence, the danger of an asthma attack which failed to respond to treatment was not appreciated. The death rate rose and fell in line with the sales of the aerosol before and after the potential danger was recognized. Admissions to hospital, however, rose and then remained at a high level. This suggests that, once the danger of treatment-resistant asthma was fully appreciated, patients were being admitted to hospital at an earlier stage in their attack and were being effectively resuscitated. It is likely, therefore, that this fairly large 'drug accident' was actually not a drug accident at all but a problem related to the introduction of a preparation which was much more effective than anything previously available, but which lulled doctors and patients into a false sense of security.

Sackett and his colleagues (Chapter 34) have expanded the word 'compliance' to include not only its usual meaning in terms of whether the patient takes his medicine, but also whether the doctor complies with the manufacturers instructions when prescribing the drug, whether the patient complies with requests to report side-effects to the doctor, and whether the latter in turn reports them to the authorities.

Some appalling examples of poor compliance in the treatment of serious diseases suggest that ineffective therapy from this cause may be a more important problem than adverse drug reactions.

In chapter 35, Robin Hogarth takes doctors into unfamiliar territory. He asks how much of that most precious commodity – time – do we consciously allocate to reflecting on the scientific basis of our intuitive decisions? In an area of public-decision making, to what extent are groups of experts influenced by the ability of members of the group to remember facts, by the status of their leader or the length of their agenda?

The biases that can affect decision-making can be subjected to scientific analysis. Individual clinicians make their own judgements and operate on their patients surgically or chemically on the basis of personal experience and the knowledge they have gained mostly from what they have heard or read. Those who provide the information cannot play both the roles of scientific adviser and law-maker. They must transmit information about efficacy and safety of drugs so that the clinician can make a risk/benefit decision to suit the individual patient, but they must do so in such a way that the clinician will not find himself in court if he decides the advice is not appropriate in an individual case. In extreme cases the reasons for decisions to withdraw drugs from the market must be explicit and acceptable to the profession.

Hogarth reminds us that most people look for evidence which agrees with their ideas; most admit to bad memory, but nobody to bad judgement. Since much of our decision making is based on published evidence, it is worth remembering that negative results are much less frequently published than positive ones. Accounts of suspected ADRs abound, and reviews of the literature may lead us to the impression that a drug may be more dangerous than it really is; we are more often biased against a drug than in favour of it. The issues are complex and further research into the application of behavioural science in monitoring and drug regulatory decision making is clearly essential.

Finally, Jan Venulet contributes a new chapter to this work dealing with the problems of assessing causality in individual drug reaction reports. Obviously, when epidemiological or other evidence suggests that drugs may be causing problems it is always necessary to examine individual case histories, in order to assess the probability that factors other than the administered drug might have been responsible. This is not simply a question of checking that the patient took the drug and that the reaction actually occurred or that the temporal relationships between the various events were as stated in the original report. Many ADRs defy attempts to establish a cause–effect relationship in individual patients because the events are of a kind that may have occurred spontaneously. These include all the type C and many of the type B events described in the first commentary. The only exception is the event which is normally very rare, but which has been shown to occur many times more commonly in patients treated with a particular drug. Here it would be reasonable to say that the probability that the event was caused by the drug was very high. Otherwise probabilities can only be estimated on the basis of the results of epidemiological studies. With type A effects, which can be explained on the basis of knowledge of the drug's pharmacology, and with some type B reactions, which have, for example recurred on rechallenge with the drug or been closely related in time to challenge and dechallenge, it may then be reasonable to attempt to assign causality to an individual experience.

Various algorithms have been devised to assist in this task, and Professor Venulet's algorithm developed for Ciba includes 27 different questions. Clearly it is impractical to use them routinely for all ADR reports, but they may be very useful when following up clusters of reports of serious ADRs.

## References

1. Bondi, H. (1985). Risk of Perspective. In Cooper, M. G. (ed.) *Risk, man-made hazards to man*, pp. 8–17. (Oxford: Oxford University Press)

# 31
# Statistical logic in the monitoring of reactions to therapeutic drugs

D. J. FINNEY

## 1. INTRODUCTION

Recent years have seen the development of systems for monitoring adverse reactions to therapeutic drugs, first independently in several countries and now increasingly co-ordinated through the World Health Organization. These involve arrangements for reporting to a national centre instances of adverse reactions, suspected adverse reactions, or even adverse experiences not obviously related to drugs. The exact nature of what is reported differs from one system to another, but the essential components for any one patient are a statement of drug or drugs administered and a statement of one or more 'reactions' exhibited; these will usually be supplemented by other information, at least the sex and age of the patient and possibly further details about his life and medical history.

The records obtained may have superficial resemblance to those from a plannned clinical trial, but they are not capable of the same interpretation. Provided that proper randomizations have been used in a clinical trial, the records (of therapeutic benefit or of adverse side-effects) can be used for inference in a strict probabilistic manner. The theory and techniques of statistical analysis are well-documented and need not be discussed further here.

## 2. THE NATURE OF A MONITOR

The records obtained during monitoring of adverse reactions are in some degree necessarily voluntary and spontaneous. One essential feature of monitoring is that large numbers of subjects should be capable of contributing information, far more than could be included within the plan of detailed observation appropriate to a clinical trial.[1,2]

The instructions for a particular monitor will doubtless ask that 'all patients in certain hospitals who receive any of a specified list of drugs and manifest any of a specified set of reactions be reported', or that 'general practitioners report every instance of a suspected adverse reaction among their patients', but performance will not match the ideal. Even in hospital, imperfect definition of categories, emphasis on more immediately urgent aspects of patient care, or simple lack of interest by some key persons will reduce reporting. In the experience of the UK Committee on Safety of Drugs, the intensity of reporting by general practitioners varies widely, only a few doctors ever submit, and the threshold of suspicion at which an individual is moved to make a report is not the same for all physicians.[3,4]

In the following sections, the inferences that can be drawn from monitoring, and the assumptions essential to their validity, are examined. These assumptions derive from the uncertainties of reporting, and also from the fact that the drugs recorded were administered in the course of ordinary therapeutic practice without any randomization of allocation to patients. Discussion of monitoring must distinguish clearly between three types of ascertainment of records:

(1) *Ascertainment by Patient*, in which the intention is to follow the history of all patients, in categories specified without reference to the drugs, and to record for each the drugs administered and all events experienced that could conceivably be harmful consequences of drugs;
(2) *Ascertainment by Drug*, in which the intention is to record all instances of use of any of a specified set of drugs, together with all events experienced by the recipients that could conceivably be harmful consequences of these drugs;
(3) *Ascertainment by Event*, in which the intention is to record all events of specified categories (e.g. all birth abnormalities, all thromboses, all sudden deaths) and to attach to each record information on the patient and the drugs he has received.

Ascertainment by patient involves essentially a cohort study as used for many medical and sociological investigations. All individuals satisfying a pre-condition not directly determining the matters under investigation are identified, and subsequent relevant features of their history and experience are recorded. Here the pre-condition is that of being a patient, qualified perhaps by additions such as 'in certain hospitals' or 'between 20 and 50 years of age'. A cohort study is commonly prospective, but sometimes its members are identified later than the events to be investigated and information must be obtained retrospectively. By its nature, the cohort includes its own controls, though the comparability of different groups within the cohort may need careful checking.

Ascertainment by event has much in common with retrospective clinical studies: these often involve 'case-control' by matching of the subjects reported with others as like as possible in important factors, and the same ideas have been adopted for monitoring purposes. Ascertainment by drug has aspects of both the cohort and the case-control approaches. Because adverse reactions of any one kind are rare, a pure cohort study directed at a particular situation would yield very few reactions and would usually be inordinately expensive. Restriction to patients receiving specified drugs concentrates effort on more relevant subjects, and enables an appropriate subsection of a cohort to be followed; however, retrospective case-control methods may also be required as a basis of comparison. Cornfield and Haenszel[5] have made important comments on this situation.

## 3. CLINICAL TRIALS

In a clinical trial for assessment of the value of a particular therapeutic regime, or for comparison between two or more drugs for treatment of the same disease, the necessity that final choice of the treatment received by a patient be *randomly* determined is now generally conceded.[6] Some constraints on total randomness are permissible features of a good experimental design; a rigorously defined random element, however, is a prerequisite of any inference that an observed difference between the experiences of two treatment categories can reasonably be attributed to effects of the drugs under trial rather than to inherent differences in the groups of patients.

A further requirement imposed in the design of a clinical trial is *Independence* of allocation. Apart from constraints built into the structure of the randomization (such as matching of pairs of patients), each patient must be allocated to treatment independently of all others. To assign all patients in one ward, or all patients of one physician, to one drug would offend against this principle by confounding a difference between drugs with a difference in the character of patient care. With a number of wards or a number of physicians for each drug (and appropriate randomization), offence against the principle of independence becomes logically less objectionable; the obvious statistical analyses and tests of significance may still be wholly misleading, as in some respects the single patient is no longer the unit.

When a clinical trial has been completed, the applicability of its results is logically limited by a condition of *Representativeness*. The patients in the trial may have been chosen from those in certain hospitals or those under the care of certain medical practitioners. If a drug is demonstrated to have a particular beneficial (or adverse) effect on patients in a Birmingham hospital, an assertion that the same consequences will follow its administration in Belfast or Bergen implicitly assumes that in some sense the original patients were representative of a super-population. If the trial was conducted on young adult males with a specific disease, to apply its findings to elderly females or primary school children calls on a similar assumption. There can perhaps be no complete way of escape, but medical investigators should not ignore the existence of this difficulty of practical inference merely because the fact is inconvenient.

## 4. ASCERTAINMENT BY PATIENT

When ascertainment is by patient, as is sometimes possible in a monitoring study based upon hospitals,[7] the aim will be to include all persons within certain categories defined without reference to drug administration. These might be all patients in certain hospitals, all female patients over the age of 45 in certain hospitals, or all patients who consult certain general practitioners. In practice, some persons will be omitted because, for one of many reasons, information was unobtainable. The information sought on each person could be the complete drug history for a period and all events experienced that conceivably might be adverse reactions. Alternatively it can be limited to drugs and possible reactions specified in accordance with the interests of a particular investigation. For example, the study might be limited to anaesthetics (or even to three named anaesthetics) and the reactions might be limited to those related to the liver. Table 1 shows the form in which the records might be summarized.

Of course the table could be more complicated; it could include a greater number of drugs and more than one class of reaction. One important feature of its construction is that each person must enter only once. If a patient may receive more than one of the set of drugs, possible combinations must be placed in further columns; if a patient may manifest more than one of the reactions, either further rows of the table must be added to accommodate such cases or conventions must be established such as always classifying under the more serious reaction.

Interpretation of Table 1 requires reference to the population from which its members come. As already emphasized, reporting is inevitably less than complete and may be far below 100% of the cases eligible for inclusion. Table 2 shows the population numbers corresponding to Table 1, each symbol being at least as great as, and possibly much greater than, the corresponding symbol in Table 1.

Several conditions must be fulfilled if Table 1 is to be a trustworthy basis for inference. In practice, these are unlikely to hold at all exactly, and one task for an investigator is to satisfy himself that deviation

**Table 1 Summary of records from ascertainment by patient**

| | *No drug* | *Drug I* | *Drug II* | *Drug III* | *Total* |
|---|---|---|---|---|---|
| Unaffected | $u_0$ | $u_1$ | $u_2$ | $u_3$ | $u$ |
| Affected | $a_0$ | $a_1$ | $a_2$ | $a_3$ | $a$ |
| TOTAL | $n_0$ | $n_1$ | $n_2$ | $n_3$ | $n$ |

**Table 2 Population classification corresponding to Table 1**

| | *No drug* | *Drug I* | *Drug II* | *Drug III* | *Total* |
|---|---|---|---|---|---|
| Unaffected | $U_0$ | $U_1$ | $U_2$ | $U_3$ | $U$ |
| Affected | $A_0$ | $A_1$ | $A_2$ | $A_3$ | $A$ |
| TOTAL | $N_0$ | $N_1$ | $N_2$ | $N_3$ | $N$ |

from them is so small as not to invalidate the qualitative truth of his inferences. An investigator who has data in the form of Table 1 will commonly apply statistical tests of significance, either based on $\chi^2$ or using some logically similar assessment of probabilities. Too often he neglects the requirement without which no such tests are valid, that of:

*Independence.* The persons in Table 1 must enter the records independently of one another. This consideration is essentially as for clinical trials. Randomness alone is not enough, for this could be taken to mean random selection of groups of patients (by ward, by physician, by locality) and any heterogeneity between groups would reduce the weight that ought to be attached to the evidence: lack of independence does not of itself introduce bias, but it does cause $\chi^2$ and other tests to exaggerate the degree of statistical significance.

A second major requirement is that of:

*Representativeness.* The $n_0$, $n_1$, $n_2$, $n_3$ persons in Table 1 need to be fully representative of the $N_0$, $N_1$, $N_2$, $N_3$ in the population. In fact, the only trustworthy way of securing fair representation is by random selection (though there are many different ways of conducting a proper randomization), and the question to be considered is whether each $n$ can be regarded as effectively a random sample from the corresponding $N$. The implications should be examined carefully. If monitoring is undertaken within certain hospitals, reporting of a representative sample of their patients will provide sound data from the set of hospitals, but any attempt to extend inference to a wider hospital population introduces the same problems as have been discussed above in respect of clinical trials.

These two conditions have their counterparts in clinical trials. Others that are automatically ensured in a well-conducted clinical trial require very careful attention in the interpretation of monitoring records. First is:

*Susceptibility Equivalence.* If the reason for prescribing drug II rather than drug I for a patient is related to his inherent suceptibility to a reaction, the records will tend to suggest a relation between drug and reaction. For example, if renal damage were to be observed frequently in patients receiving a particular hypotensive drug, causation by the drug could not easily be distinguished from a secondary result of the hypertension for which patients were being treated. Comparison of incidence with that in non-hypertensive patients not receiving the drug could be seriously misleading. Comparison with hypertensive patients receiving different drugs might show more clearly whether the one suspected was associated with an exceptional frequency of renal damage; even then, the possibility remains that patients with a form of hypertension that made them peculiarly prone to renal damage tended to have this drug prescribed for them. Herein lies a major difficulty in monitoring: how can one be sure that a difference between two drugs in frequency of an undesirable reactions is not an inherent property of the two groups of patients rather than a consequence of differences in therapy? Statistical tests cannot discriminate, and the only useful procedure is a careful medico-logical elimination of alternatives.

A somewhat analogous condition is that of:

*Background Equivalence.* A relative frequency of occurrence of a certain reaction after drug II, as compared with drug I or with the 'control' of no drug, naturally suggests that drug II may cause the reaction. Such an interpretation supposes no relevant differences between groups of patients in respect of other drugs or other aspects of their management and care. One must beware of attributing harmful effects to an analgesic merely because it happens to be that usually prescribed in association with another drug.

Although logically included within the conditions of representativeness, another condition is so important to the interpretation of monitoring that it needs separate mention:

*Unbiased Reporting.* The chances of a reaction being reported must not depend upon the drug. If ascertainment by patient is properly conducted, so that attention is concentrated on the experiences of specific patients, no trouble should arise. However, publicity given to a first suspicion of adverse reactions with drug II may cause those in charge of patients to be more assiduous in reporting new instances than they are for patients on drug I. Only 100% intensity of monitoring of specified patients guards fully against the danger: if the average proportion of patients whose reports are submitted is of the order of 20%, drugs that are being compared may differ appreciably in this percentage.

An attractive feature of ascertainment by patient is that rates of incidence of adverse reactions can be estimated and compared in a way that assists quantitative evaluation of risks. For the population under study, the risks are (from Table 2)

$$P_i = A_i/N_i \qquad \text{for } i = 0, 1, 2, 3, \tag{1}$$

the relative frequencies of reactions in the four drug classes. If the conditions specified above are satisfied, each $P_i$ will be estimated, without bias, by the corresponding

$$p_i = a_i/n_i \qquad \text{for } i = 0, 1, 2, 3, \tag{2}$$

The statistical significance of differences between the $p_i$ can be based upon $\chi^2$ or similar tests, at least when the $n_1$ are small relative to the $N_1$ as will normally be true. Such tests should not be trusted uncritically, because even when all other conditions are strictly satisfied a small amount of heterogeneity that constitutes an unsuspected lack of independence of selection can permit a true significance level of, say, 0.15, to masquerade as 0.03. Perhaps more important is the fact that the $p_i$, as estimators of the $P_i$, permit the risk of adverse reactions to a drug to be compared with the risk of the same events in the absence of the drug, as a basis for balanced assessment of whether and in what circumstances the drug should be used.

## 5. ASCERTAINMENT BY DRUG

If ascertainment is by drug, the immediate difference from ascertainment by patient is that the column 'No drug' disappears from Tables 1 and 2. For trustworthy inference, the conditions of Independence, Representativeness, Susceptibility Equivalence, Background Equivalence, and Unbiased Reporting are required as before. The records on a patient begin only when one of the monitored drugs is prescribed for him. Although information may be obtainable retrospectively, the investigator may have additional difficulty in being satisfied of equivalence. In addition, emphasis on the drug instead of the patient may increase the danger of bias in reporting in relation to a drug of topical interest or of special concern to some physicians.

In equations (1) and (2), $P_0$ and $p_0$ are no longer available. Consequently the incidence of a particular event in patients receiving a stated drug cannot be compared with a control incidence. In some circumstances this may be important; in others, chief interest may lie in comparing a new drug with an older one used for similar purposes.

## 6. ASCERTAINMENT BY EVENT, WITH CONTROLS

A situation involving ascertainment by event that at first glance can look like a clinical trial is well illustrated by the study of Vessey *et al.*[8] on oral contraceptives and thromboembolism. The description below is grossly over-simplified, but shows the main statistical structure; for reassurance that proper precautions have been taken to exclude appropriate operations, to check non-responding subjects to allow for differences between two hospitals, and so on, the original paper should be read.

The essential features of the study are that hospital records were searched for married women who suffered venous thrombosis or pulmonary embolism within one month after a non-obstetric surgical operation. Before enquiry into contraceptive practice, cases of certain

**Table 3** Summary of records from Vessey's study of oral contraceptives (OC)

| | *No OC* | *OC* | *Total* |
|---|---|---|---|
| No thromboembolism | $u_0 = 51$ | $u_1 = 9$ | $u = 60$ |
| Thromboembolism | $a_0 = 18$ | $a_1 = 12$ | $a = 30$ |
| TOTAL | $n_0 = 69$ | $n_1 = 21$ | $n_1 = 90$ |

gynaecological operations and of operations for conditions that might have influenced contraceptive practice were excluded. From the same hospital, patients having had the same operations without thromboembolism were selected as controls. Information was then obtained from all the patients on whether or not they had been using oral contraceptives during the month before admission to hospital.

Although the manner of acquiring data is quite different from that with the other forms of ascertainment, a simple summary of the data (Table 3) looks very much like Table 1. The difference is best seen by again referring to the population from which the records come (Table 4), 'population' here implying all married women who have one of the operations deemed acceptable for the study. In their investigation, Vessey *et al.* sought to improve the comparability of classes by matching controls with thromboembolic patients. For each affected patient they chose two unaffected patients who corresponded closely in age, parity and year of admission to hospital. This is analogous to stratifying the population of $N$ into sub-populations defined by the matching factors and sampling separately from each. The essential features of the argument that follows are not altered by this complication, as long as the sub-populations behave similarly, and details will not be pursued here. The standard significance tests, however, are no longer appropriate, and alternative forms that take account of the matching should replace them.[9–14]

From Table 4, the risks of thromboembolism in women without and with the contraceptive are

$$\left.\begin{aligned} P_0 &= A_0/N_0 \\ P_1 &= A_1/N_1 \end{aligned}\right\} \tag{3}$$

**Table 4** Population classification corresponding to Table 3

| | *No OC* | *OC* | *Total* |
|---|---|---|---|
| No thromboembolism | $U_0$ | $U_1$ | $U$ |
| Thromboembolism | $A_0$ | $A_1$ | $A$ |
| TOTAL | $N_0$ | $N_1$ | $N$ |

respectively. However, corresponding quantities calculated from Table 3 no longer directly estimate these, because selection is now in terms of the $u$ and the $a$ persons, not the $n_0$ and the $n_1$. The conditions for valid inference need to be re-examined.

*Independence* is almost automatically taken account of in the Vessey study. The emphasis on matching should remove any fear that unaffected women are chosen in groups rather than independently of one another.

*Representativeness* now means that the two classes of patients $U$ and $A$ must be fairly represented by the samples $u$ and $a$. Vessey took *all* records of affected women in the agreed surgical categories, for four consecutive years in two hospital regions, so that the only question relates to whether these years and hospitals adequately represent a wider population. Had only a sample been taken from the hospitals, the method of selection of the samples would have needed discussion. The matching procedure should have gone far to ensure representativeness of the $u$ patients.

*Susceptibility Equivalence and Background Equivalence* need very thorough consideration. Those women who were taking oral contraceptives were doing so of their own choice: is it likely that women with certain conditions conducive to development of thromboembolism tend to use oral contraceptives? Even were no reason for such an association evident, it might exist. In fact, a hypertensive, multiparous, obese woman aged 40 might be prescribed the 'pill' precisely because another pregnancy is highly undesirable; she clearly has four strong reasons for a greater risk of spontaneous thrombosis than a normotensive, nulliparous, thin 20-year-old. Vessey *et al.* excluded gynaecological, varicose vein, and certain other operations that might disturb the equivalence of medical background for the $n_0$ and $n_1$ women. This and their matching should go far to avoid confusion entering because of interaction between the reason for surgery and the side-effects of the contraceptive. Whether they have also successfully eliminated inequalities of susceptibility might be debated; here the need is only to emphasize the general point that in each new situation the issue needs discussion.

*Unbiased Reporting* should have been secured because all patients had passed through hospital, the reaction under discussion was severe, and once a patient was identified attention was strongly focused on her. Nevertheless, important information had to be obtained retrospectively, and the possibility that recording or memory was biased by the occurrence of thromboembolism cannot be entirely dismissed. The authors looked specially at this.

On the assumption that the conditions are satisfied, analysis and interpretation of Table 3 is needed. As a first method, simple and appropriate to many sets of data, ignore the matching constraint. Suppose that the sampling from the populations of $U$ and $A$ women were of fractions $\theta$, $\varphi$ respectively, so that

$$\begin{aligned} \theta &= u/U \\ \varphi &= a/A \end{aligned} \tag{4}$$

If the sampling could be repeated many times in an unbiased manner, the average frequencies would be those shown in Table 5. Evidently no quantities calculatable from Table 3 can estimate $P_0$, $P_1$ (unless, as could rarely be true, $\theta$ and $\varphi$ are known). Vessey *et al.* had to be content with discussing the quantitative comparison in terms of a measure of relative risk. This they defined as

$$D_{01} = \frac{A_1 U_0}{A_0 U_1} \tag{5}$$

the ratio of $A_1/U_1$ to $A_0/U_0$. The authors had good reason for choosing this measure, but their name is perhaps misleading: *relative risk* would better refer to

$$R_{01} = \frac{P_1}{P_0} = \frac{A_1 N_0}{A_0 N_1}, \tag{6}$$

whereas $D_{01}$ can more appropriately be termed the *relative odds* in favour of thromboembolism. In interpretation of results, the distinction between $R_{01}$ and $D_{01}$ can be important, though when $P_0$ and $P_1$ are both small $R_{01}$ and $D_{01}$ are almost equal.

**Table 5** Expected frequencies for Table 3

| | *No OC* | *OC* | *Total* |
|---|---|---|---|
| No thromboembolism | $\theta U_0$ | $\theta U_1$ | $\theta A$ |
| Thromboembolism | $\varphi A_0$ | $\varphi A_1$ | $\varphi A$ |
| TOTAL | $\theta U_0 + \varphi A_0$ | $\theta U_1 + \varphi A_1$ | $\theta U + \varphi A$ |

As may be deduced from Table 5, $a_0/n_0$ and $a_1/n_1$ are no guides to $P_0$ and $P_1$; nevertheless, the ratio

$$d_{01} = \frac{a_1 u_0}{a_0 u_1} = \frac{12 \times 51}{18 \times 9} = 3.8 \tag{7}$$

is a consistent estimator of $D_{01}$ since it estimates

$$\frac{\varphi A_1 \, , \theta U_0}{\varphi A_0 \, , \theta U_1} = D_{01}$$

On the other hand, an attempt to estimate the true relative risk from Table 3 would correspond to

$$\frac{\varphi A_1}{\varphi A_0} \cdot \frac{\theta U_0 + \varphi A_0}{\theta U_1 + \varphi A_1} = \frac{A_1(U_0 + \varphi A_0/\theta)}{A_0(U_1 + \varphi A_1/\theta)} \tag{8}$$

which is in general equal to $R_{01}$ if and only if $\theta = \varphi$, a condition that cannot be imposed in this type of sampling. Indeed, if the sampling is regarded as being from a large population in space or time, $\theta$ and $\varphi$ are likely to be unknown, but rather small quantities with $\theta$ much less than $\varphi$. Vessey's preference for the relative odds instead of the true relative risk is thus well-founded. As Cornfield and Haenszel[5] emphasize, when $P_0$, $P_1$ are sufficiently small to make the economy of a retrospective study particularly advantageous, the relative odds and risks, $D_{01}$ and $R_{01}$, will be practically equal.

In the simplest sampling situation, the null hypothesis that the risk of thromboembolism is unaffected by oral contraceptives can be tested by any standard test of proportionality in the contingency table, Table 3. For example, a $\chi^2$ test or, if $a_0$, $a_1$ are small, the so-called 'exact' test can be used to examine the deviation of $d_{01}$ from unity. As already mentioned, Vessey's matching modifies the appropriate significance test. Moreover, $d_{01}$ as defined by equation (7) can now only estimate some form of weighted average of $D_{01}$ for all sub-populations, unless (somewhat surprisingly) all have the same value of $D_{01}$ (cf. Cox[10]).

The extent to which the conditions stated above limit interpretation of any significance test must be kept in mind. Briefly, they are primarily concerned with ensuring that any difference found between the patients in the two classes may reasonably be attributed to the oral contraceptives and not to differences in age distribution, standard of living, medical history, or any other fact that distinguishes the classes. Independence of selection, however, is primarily an insurance that a test of significance will not have its probability level distorted by heterogeneities.

## 7. ASCERTAINMENT BY EVENT, WITHOUT CONTROLS

The study discussed in Section 6 was of unusual quality, but it indicates what can be achieved by careful planning of a retrospective study based upon hospital records. Spontaneous reporting of adverse reactions to a central register, such as has been organized by the United Kingdom Committee on Safety of Drugs and by similar bodies in other countries, gives less refined but more abundant information that is interpretable only with the aid of further assumptions. Nevertheless, this monitoring may be the only channel by which

**Table 6** Classification of spontaneously reported thromboembolisms in women taking one of three oral contraceptives

| | *OC I* | *OC II* | *OC III* | *Total* |
|---|---|---|---|---|
| Number of reports | $a_1$ | $a_2$ | $a_3$ | $a$ |

suspicion of a pattern of adverse reactions can accumulate. The logic of interpretation therefore deserves examination, even though any confident assertion of a causal relation between reaction and drug may require additional planned research.

Another paper on oral contraceptives[15] illustrates problems and methods. Here the concern was that the risks of adverse reactions might depend upon steroid content, with particular emphasis on total oestrogen dosage. Again the original paper should be read for an account of the authors' careful examination of their data and exhaustive discussion of possible explanations. For the present purpose, a simplified formal presentation will suffice.

Table 6 shows the only type of data directly available from the monitor, simply numbers of reports that refer to the several drugs. These reports are voluntary, and few of the total number of events that occur will find their way to the monitor. Corresponding to Table 6 is the population classification specified in Table 7.

In themselves, the numbers in Table 6 tell nothing. Yet undoubtedly records that showed $a_1 = 6, a_2 = 47, a_3 = 1$ would arouse comment and further enquiry. Why? The frequencies immediately suggest that adverse reactions are more likely with II than with I or III, but of course other explanations are possible. Once again the conditions for valid inference must be examined, and in addition account must be taken of differences in the usage rates of I, II, and III. The conditions are as follows:

*Independence.* Selection of each individual for reporting must be independent of that of other individuals. If the data can include groups of records with a common origin, the expected frequencies need not be affected, but large discrepancies have much greater probabilities than the standard tests of significance imply. For example, if one physician contributed records of 10 patients on drug II, these may have qualities in common that make them worth less as evidence than an equal number of reports from independent sources. Under normal circumstances of spontaneous monitoring, almost inevitably the reports will

**Table 7** Population classification of thromboembolism corresponding to Table 6

| | *OC I* | *OC II* | *OC III* | *Total* |
|---|---|---|---|---|
| Numbers in population | $A_1$ | $A_2$ | $A_3$ | $A$ |

include some large contributions from enthusiastic collaborators, and the extent to which these could interfere with inference must be examined in detail.

*Representativeness.* The women reported in $a_1$, $a_2$, $a_3$ must be fully representative of the totals $A_1$, $A_2$, $A_3$ in the population.

*Susceptibility Equivalence.* The assortment of the population at risk (from which come the $A_1$, $A_2$, $A_3$) into users of the different oral contraceptives must have been made independently of any differences in inherent liability to thromboembolisms or of any factor that happens to be correlated with such liability. This is essential in order to dispose of the possibility that, for example, women with certain conditions conducive to development of thromboembolisms may tend to use one oral contraceptive rather than another. The nature of any predisposition to thromboembolism may be totally unknown, yet an association could come about because, perhaps, I tends to be recommended for young women but II for older; even more complex is a possibility that women in industrial areas differ from those in non-industrial in their liabilities to thromboembolisms and that the prescribing habits of doctors in industrial areas tend to favour II, but those in non-industrial areas favour I.

*Background Equivalence.* Similarly the assortment of the population into users of different contraceptives must have been made independently of other medical considerations relating to individuals. Any tendency to recommend II rather than I or III for women who are regularly taking a certain anti-depressant, or for women who have recently experienced a particular form of surgery, could lead to an impression that II was responsible for adverse reactions really due to another cause. In the present context, disturbance from failure of this condition is perhaps unlikely to be large. Uncritical survey of monitoring records, however, could attribute disastrous consequences to some analgesics or sedatives merely because of their common therapeutic association with other drugs. Again evidently each new problem needs examining on its own merits.

*Unbiased Reporting.* The probability that a particular instance of thromboembolism from the total of $(A_1 + A_2 + A_3)$ enters the records as one of the $(a_1 + a_2 + a_3)$ must be independent of the drug used. If an instance of adverse reaction to III is more likely to be reported than one of reaction to I or II, perhaps because of recent publicity given to III in the medical or general press, all inference will be distorted.

Unless the investigator is satisfied that these conditions are fulfilled, or at least can set upper limits to the consequences of deviations from them, he cannot safely draw any inference from Table 6. If he is satisfied, he can seek to combine with Table 6 information on usage of the drugs. On seeing the (hypothetical) values of $a_1$, $a_2$, $a_3$ stated above, any investigator is likely to have his interest aroused by the large $a_2$. He should realize that his immediate response to the data rests heavily upon an instinctive assumption that the three drugs will not have differed greatly in total usage. For such an assumption, the monitor itself gives no support; the only merit in his response is that it arouses a suspicion and initiates a fuller study. Suppose that, of a total of $N$ users of one or other of the contraceptives, proportions $q_1$, $q_2$, $q_3$ are on the three types ($q_1 + q_2 + q_3 = 1$). Consequently the risks of a thromboembolism are respectively

$$P_i = \frac{A_i}{q_i N} \qquad \text{for } i = 1, 2, 3, \tag{9}$$

equations which correspond with equation (1). If $\varphi$ is the proportion of thromboembolisms reported to the monitor, now assumed constant for the three drugs, the expected numbers of reports are

$$E(a_i) = \varphi A_i \qquad \textit{for } i = 1, 2, 3. \tag{10}$$

Nothing can be said about the risk of thromboembolism in the absence of all drugs, and therefore neither the risk ratio $R_{01}$ not the relative odds $D_{01}$can be estimated. However, ratios of risks (not relative odds) for any pair of drugs can be estimated, by expressions such as

$$r_{12} = \frac{a_2 q_1}{a_1 q_2}. \tag{11}$$

This is essentially how Inman *et al.*[15] analysed their data. From a commercial bureau, they were able to obtain estimates of the share of the market attributable to each oral contraceptive for each of five years. (In other circumstances, prescription records might suppy such information.) If the total number of thromboembolic events of a particular type in 1965 were $a$, the values of $q_1$ for that year could be used to calculate an expected frequency

$$\hat{a}_i = a q_i \tag{12}$$

representing a division of the reported events in proportion to the market figures. This step was necessary because of the rapidly changing market; it was repeated for each year separately, and the observed and expected frequencies were then totalled over years.

Table 8 has been obtained from Inman's paper as an illustration. The authors showed there to be no differences between products, or between mestranol and ethinyloestradiol, that could not be explained

**Table 8** Reports of pulmonary embolism, fatal and non-fatal, among women taking oral contraceptives (British data, 1965–69, Inman *et al.*)

| *Doses of oestrogen* (µg) | | *50* | *75–80* | *100* | *150* | *Total* |
|---|---|---|---|---|---|---|
| Reports | ($a_i$) | 94 | 33 | 140 | 26 | 293 |
| Expectation | ($\hat{a}_i$) | 137.52 | 36.15 | 108.53 | 10.80 | 293.00 |
| $a_i/\hat{a}_i$ | | 0.68 | 0.91 | 1.29 | 2.41 | — |

solely in terms of total oestrogen content of the pill; therefore, at least for illustrative purposes, this simple condensation of records of pulmonary embolism (fatal and non-fatal) seems adequate. The ratio of observed to expected has no absolute meaning for a particular oestrogen dose, but from (11) and (12) one may see that the ratio of two such quantities is the ratio of risks. For example, the risk associated with 100 μg relative to that with 50 μg is

$$r_{13} = 1.29/0.68 = 1.9.$$

This corresponds exactly to the definition in (11), except for the more complicated analysis for separate years.

If the association of risk with dose were less obvious, a $\chi^2$ test might be used to compare the observed and expected frequencies. Here

$$\chi^2 = 44.6 \text{ with 3 d.f.},$$

leaving no doubt of statistical significance. The strict basis for calculating $\chi^2$ is perhaps undermined a little by the complicated construction of the expectations, but a more serious concern is the validity of the conditions of independence, equivalence, and so on already stated. Because interest lay in the ascending scale of oestrogen dosage, and not merely in any differences between columns of Table 8, Inman *et al.* chose to use the more sensitive form of $\chi^2$ test[16] that concentrates on a linear trend of association.

## ADDITIONAL FACTORS

The type of argument used in Section 7 becomes harder to sustain if an additional factor of classification is introduced. For example, one might have drugs I, II, III (not necessarily oral contraceptives) yielding data like those of Table 6, but cross-classified according to presence or absence of a further factor *F*, as shown in Table 9. Here '*F*–no *F*' might correspond to a blood group classification, presence or absence of another specified drug in the current or past treatment of the patient, two age-groups, two regions of the country, or any other subdivision of the population. The question of interest is whether occurrence of adverse reactions is affected by the factor *F*, and in particular whether a danger that is negligible in the absence of *F* becomes appreciable in the presence of *F*. If those with *F* are only a small proportion of the general population, such a phenomenon may easily be missed in scrutiny of data that make no classification for *F*. Here only the simple dichotomy for *F* is discussed, but obviously the ideas can be generalized.

A table of the same form as Table 9 can be specified for the population total of events occurring, *A*, but it is not shown here. The five conditions for inference stated in Section 7 can then be re-examined. To be satisfied of their approximate correctness is perhaps more difficult than before, but does not involve intrinsically new

**Table 9** Classification of reports similar to Table 6 but with additional factor

| | *Drug I* | *Drug II* | *Drug III* | *Total* |
|---|---|---|---|---|
| Without *F* | $a_{10}$ | $a_{20}$ | $a_{30}$ | $a_0$ |
| With *F* | $a_{1F}$ | $a_{2F}$ | $a_{3F}$ | $a_F$ |
| TOTAL | $a_1$ | $a_2$ | $a_3$ | $a$ |

arguments. If reporting is unbiased, the generalized form of equation (10) will apply; $\varphi$ being the proportion of reactions reported to the monitor, the same for all drugs and unaffected by *F*, the expected frequencies of reports for drug II will be

$$\left.\begin{aligned} E(a_{20}) &= \varphi A_{20} \\ E(a_{2F}) &= \varphi A_{2F} \end{aligned}\right\} \qquad (13)$$

In some circumstances, of course, there will be doubts to whether $\varphi$ can safely be assumed unaffected by *F*: for blood groups the assumption could be reasonable, but perhaps not for age groups.

**Table 10** Proportions of patients falling within the classes of Table 9

| | *Drug I* | *Drug II* | *Drug III* | *Total* |
|---|---|---|---|---|
| Without *F* | $q_{10}$ | $q_{20}$ | $q_{30}$ | $q_0$ |
| With *F* | $q_{1F}$ | $q_{2F}$ | $q_{3F}$ | $q_F$ |
| TOTAL | $q_1$ | $q_2$ | $q_3$ | 1 |

Trouble enters with the information on drug usage. As in Section 7, one may have values for the proportionate usage of each drug, but this represents only the lower margin of Table 10. For some factors, one might be prepared to assume the further subdivision of usage between 'Without *F*' and 'With *F*' patients to be in proportion to the total numbers of these, totals that may be obtainable from other sources; this assumption would scarcely be reasonable if *F* corresponded to the elderly or to those in receipt of another specified drug. Even for blood groups, the well-known differences between regions in respect of frequencies could conflict with an assumption that national usage figures divided in proportion to national blood-group frequencies will give a fair basis for assessment of the $q$. If factor *F* is something that can fairly easily be collated with prescription records, the $q$ might be more satisfactorily assessed from analysis of a sample of these than from manufacturers' sales, but except for common drugs the sample would have to be large. If $q_0$, $q_F$ can be assessed adequately and also proportionality holds throughout Table 10, the relations

$$\frac{q_{10}}{q_{1F}} = \frac{q_{20}}{q_{2F}} = \frac{q_{30}}{q_{3F}} = \frac{q_0}{q_F}, \tag{14}$$

enable relative risks to be estimates as in Section 7. For example, the risk of drug II with $F$ relative to drug I without $F$ is

$$r_{10,2F} = \frac{q_{10}\, a_{2F}}{q_{2F}\, a_{10}} \tag{15}$$

Moreover, from (14),

$$\left.\begin{aligned} q_{10} &= q_1 \cdot q_o \\ q_{2F} &= q_1 \cdot q_F \end{aligned}\right\} \tag{16}$$

are easily proved. Hence, with the obvious meaning of symbols

$$r_{10,2F} = r_{12} \cdot r_{0F} \tag{17}$$

This justifies the taking of products of relative risks to give a composite value, as was done by Inman,[17] but even small deviations from (14) and (16) could seriously distort the estimation.

Under the conditions of proportionality of usage expressed by equations (14) and (16), and of course on the assumption that the reporting rate, $\varphi$, is constant, a test of significance of disproportionality in Table 9 is appropriate as a test of whether relative risks are affected by $F$. If an ordinary $\chi^2$ test is used, independence of reporting is essential, and the interpretation in terms of drug effects requires all the usual conditions of representativeness and equivalence.

Jick *et al.*[18] presented data showing a higher incidence of thromboembolic events in persons of blood groups A, B, AB than in those of blood group O; they found the ratio of risks to be still higher in women who are taking the pill. Their method of evaluation was essentially as here, although displayed a little differently. In particular, the assumption that relative frequencies of the blood groups in the general population will also describe the women on the pill and the other special categories of person discussed was an integral part of the argument, as of course was the assumption of unbiased reporting.

## 9. GENERAL IMPLICATIONS

The investigations described in Sections 6 and 7 were good logical approaches to the elucidation of problems made difficult because of the necessity of relying on observation unsupported by experimental planning. They do not have the status of the logic applicable to an experiment on animals, in which treatments can be allocated *at random* to subjects, and conditions can be controlled in ways that prevent the effect of a treatment being confused with the effect of fortuitous differences in the environment and management of subjects. As argued elsewhere,[2] clinical trial in man is valuable for study of drug efficacy but usually inadequate for demonstrating adverse reactions. Although animal experiments could involve adequate numbers, they may be unreliable predictors of adverse reactions in man. The attempt to draw trustworthy inferences from monitoring drug experiences in man is therefore essential. This paper in no way intends destructive criticism of the methods described, but recognition of logical weaknesses and of implicit assumptions is important; these may point to interpretations of data other than the most obvious, which need to be examined critically before any causal connection between a drug and an adverse reaction can be confidently asserted.

Because the interpretation of monitoring data requires assessment of how the records were acquired, in a manner that cannot be made entirely quantitative and objective, analysis of the data cannot rest upon statistical techniques alone. Studies of two different sets of drugs might produce tables like Table 6 with identical frequencies of reports. Even if it were known (and this could scarcely ever be) that the corresponding populations (like Table 7) and the usage proportions ($q_i$) were also identical, the inferences drawn might differ because of different assessments of the evidence for *Susceptibility Equivalence* or *Unbiased Reporting*.

As has been argued elsewhere,[2] the function of monitoring is to keep a continuing watch on all reports relating to adverse reactions and to use these to generate suspicions. The monitoring operation has analogies with the work of a detective agency; it seeks for any indications of unexpected differences in the incidence of adverse phenomena. Formal tests of statistical significance can be regarded as establishing that certain differences in rates or frequencies are unlikely to have occurred by chance, provided that assertions of independence are true, but they cannot of themselves determine that one factor rather than another caused the differences. In a planned experiment, all causes but one are disposed of by the experimental design; in monitoring, each must be the subject of informed medical discussion. The conditions for valid inference discussed in this paper are part of the machinery for eliminating explanations of a difference. Those stated are not necessarily the complete set or mutually exclusive: they are presented more as examples of a type of argument that must be constructed anew for each problem than as a blueprint for research. Compliance with the conditions will scarcely ever be exact, for lack of information even if for no other reasons. Moreover, even compliance with all conditions that have been made explicit is no guarantee that an assertion of causation for an adverse reactions is correct. Often the most that can be said is that a good *prima facie* case has been established for new research planned with a better-defined purpose from the start, and that until its completion extreme caution is required in the care of patients receiving certain forms of drug therapy.

## A Comment in 1979

I am indebted to Professor Dr G. Wagner for permission to reproduce the above paper from *Methods of Information in Medicine*, volume 10, pages 237–245. Looking back on this paper after 8 years, I am aware that it has much in common with the more formal theory of retrospective case-control studies, to which epidemiologists have recently given much attention. In particular, the requirements and conditions presented in Section 4 are equivalent to much that has been said, often with greater detail and exactness, by those who have helped to establish the case-control method; indeed, analogues of some of these conditions are very relevant to prospective clinical trials. Statistical analysis can never bring interpretation of spontaneous reporting of adverse reactions to the logical status of good case-control studies. Despite apparent similarities, the procedures described in this chapter aim more at systematic arousal of suspicions of causal relations than at conclusions: they are *hypothesis-generating*, not *hypothesis-testing*. More recently, interest has grown in methods specifically directed at detecting patterns in monitor files. Mandel and his colleagues[19,20] have offered an entirely new approach, but adequate trial of this on data is likely to be delayed by the computing costs.

## Acknowledgement

I am indebted to Dr W. H. W. Inman for a long series of discussions over several years that has helped the development of the ideas of this paper, and also for his valuable comments on a first draft of the paper.

## References

1. Finney, D. J. (1965). The design and logic of a monitor of drug use. *J. Chron. Dis.*, **18,** 77
2. Finney, D. J. (1971). Statistical aspects of monitoring for dangers in drug therapy. *Meth. Inform. Med.*, **10,** 1
3. Inman, W. H. W. and Adelstein, A. M. (1969). Rise and fall of asthma mortality in England and Wales in relation to use of pressurised aerosols. *Lancet*, **2,** 279
4. Inman, W. H. W. and Vessey, M. P. (1968). Investigation of deaths from pulmonary, coronary, and cerebral thrombosis and embolism in women of child-bearing age. *Br. Med. J.*, **2,** 193
5. Cornfield, J. and Haenszel, W. (1970). Some aspects of retrospective studies. *J. Chron. Dis.*, **11,** 523
6. Hill, A. B. (1963). Medical ethics and controlled trials. *Br. Med. J.*, **1,** 1043
7. WHO (1969). International drug monitoring – The role of the hospital. (Report of a WHO meeting). *WHO Technical Report Series*, No. 425 (Geneva)
8. Vessey, M. P., Doll, R., Fairbairn, A. S. and Glober, G. (1970). Postoperative thromboembolism and the use of oral contraceptives. *Br. Med. J.*, **3,** 123
9. Cochran, W. G. (1950). The comparison of percentages in matched samples. *Biometrika*, **37,** 256

10. Cox, D. R. (1970). *Analysis of Binary Data.* (London: Methuen)
11. Finney, D. J. (1961). Symmetry in contingency tables. In *Studi in Onore di Corrado Gini*, Vol. 1, pp. 115–132
12. McNemar, Q. (1947). Note on the sampling error of the differences between correlated proportions or percentages. *Psychometrika*, **12,** 153
13. Pike, M. C. and Morrow, R. H. (1970). Statistical analysis of patient-control studies in epidemiology. *Br. J. Prev. Soc. Med.*, **24,** 42
14. Stuart, A. (1957). The comparison of frequencies in matched samples. *Br. J. Statist. Psychol.*, **10,** 29
15. Inman, W. H. W., Vessey, M. P., Westerholm, B. and Engelund, A. (1970). Thromboembolic disease and the steroidal content of oral contraceptives. *Br. Med. J.*, **2,** 203
16. Armitage, P. (1955). Tests for linear trends in proportions and frequencies. *Biometrics*, **11,** 375
17. Inman, W. H. W. (1970). Role of drug-reaction monitoring in the investigation of thrombosis and the 'pill'. *Br. Med. Bull.*, **26,** 248
18. Jick, H., Slone, D., Westerholm, B., Inman, W. H. W., Vessey, M. P., Shapiro, S., Lewis, G. P. and Worcester, J. (1969). Venous thromboembolic disease and ABO blood type. *Lancet*, **1,** 539
19. Mandel, S. P. H., Levine, A. and Beleño, G. E. (1976). Signalling increases in reporting in international monitoring of adverse reactions to therapeutic drugs. *Meth. Inform. Med.*, **15,** 1
20. Levine, A., Mandel, S. P. H. and Santamaria, A. (1977). Pattern signalling in health information monitoring. *Meth. Inform. Med.*, **16,** 138

# 32
# Principles and pitfalls in drug epidemiology

J. I. MANN

## THE NATURE OF THE PROBLEM

Occasionally an adverse reaction may present as a dramatic increase in frequency of a very uncommon condition (for example sclerosing peritonitis and practolol,[1] phocomelia and thalidomide[2] and pulmonary hypertension and aminorex fumarate).[3] The major problem in drug epidemiology stems from the fact that the vast majority of adverse reactions are not unique clinical entities. Oral contraceptives may increase the risk of myocardial infarction in young women, but the adverse reaction there is clinically indistinguishable from the condition which can occur in women who have never used hormonal preparations. Consequently in individual cases it may be virtually impossible to decide whether an adverse reaction has taken place. Other difficulties include the facts that most serious adverse reactions represent a relatively small increase in risk of a relatively uncommon condition, and also that drugs are prescribed because of some medical need. Hence, one always needs to consider whether the reason for prescribing the drug, rather than the drug itself, may be responsible for the adverse reaction. This chapter will attempt to describe the various epidemiological approaches used in detecting adverse effects of drugs once they have become widely introduced, and the problems of deciding whether an association between drug and disease is causal.

## TRENDS IN DISEASE FREQUENCY

The study of trends in disease frequency as a means of detecting or confirming an adverse drug reaction has been discussed in detail elsewhere. There is however one point which needs to be made in this chapter concerning epidemiological principles. A change in disease frequency (whether detected on the basis of morbidity or mortality data) will only be apparent if an appreciable proportion of the disease is drug-induced. For example even if a drug greatly increases the risk of a common disease, but only a small proportion of the at-risk population is exposed to the drug, one is unlikely to detect a trend in the disease rate in the population.

## CASE-CONTROL STUDIES

Case-control studies are most frequently undertaken after the suggestion of an adverse reaction has been made on the basis of individual clinical observations, signals from voluntary reporting systems or trends in disease frequency. The chief advantage of the classical case-control investigation is that such studies may be undertaken quickly and at relatively low cost. The principle underlying this approach is essentially simple: patients developing a particular disease are identified and the frequency of prior drug exposure ascertained. The frequency of exposure in these people, 'the cases' is compared with that of a 'control' series of subjects who do not have the disease under investigation. The exposure rate amongst the controls provides an estimate of the rate which might be expected amongst the cases if no association existed between the exposure and the disease of interest.

There are essentially three different types of case-control study: one, in which all cases that have occurred during a specified interval in the past are identified and investigated at a particular time; a second in which there is ongoing identification and investigation of cases and controls; and finally case-control drug surveillance. The first two approaches are intended specifically for hypothesis-testing, whereas the last approach also generates hypotheses. The first approach is certainly the most quickly executed, but has the disadvantage that clinical and historical information required may not have been adequately recorded and it may not be possible to trace individual patients diagnosed some years previously. This approach was used in several of the British Studies which first showed the association between oral contraceptives and idiopathic venous thrombosis, pulmonary embolism, stroke and myocardial infarction.[4–7] On the other hand, the North American Collaborative Study for Stroke in Young Women, which strikingly confirmed the association between oral contraceptives and both thrombotic and haemorrhagic stroke, used the ongoing case and control identification procedure,[8] thus enabling comprehensive clinical information, including angiography where this was necessary for diagnosis, to be collected.

Some of the misunderstanding of case-control studies derives from the confusion about terminology. They have also been described as 'case-referent', 'case-comparison', 'retrospective' and 'trohoc' studies. The term 'retrospective' has been found to be confusing because some case-control studies are in fact ongoing. The term however refers to the

Case-control studies

| | Exposure | Adverse reaction | |
|---|---|---|---|
| | | Present (cases) | Absent (controls) |
| Cohort studies | Present | *a* | *b* |
| | Absent | *c* | *d* |

**Figure 1** The principles underlying the case-control and cohort approaches to the detection of adverse reactions to drugs

fact that the method involves collecting exposure data relating to events which have already occurred (Figure 1). The term 'trohoc' (cohort spelled backwards) was introduced by Feinstein[9] and was almost certainly intended to be derogatory.

There are two principal disadvantages of the case-control approach. One has already been mentioned; namely that data concerning events which have already occurred may be inadequate. The second is the fact that these studies may be subject to a number of biases (discussed in more detail later). Careful study design, however, along the lines suggested below will help to eliminate at least some of these sources of bias.

## The cases

### *Description of disease*

It may sound trite to suggest that the condition under study should be clearly defined. It is, however, essential to stress the necessity for clear diagnostic criteria. In the case of diseases which can be readily proven histologically, this rarely presents as a problem, but in a condition such as myocardial infarction the situation is much more difficult. If rigid diagnostic criteria (e.g. those laid down by the World Health Organization)[10] are not followed, it is very likely that at least some cases labelled by clinicians as myocardial infarction could include cases of severe angina in whom no infarction had occurred. This is more important than might seem at first glance, since angina and myocardial infarction do not have an identical aetiology: for example, both cigarette smoking and the use of oral contraceptives seem to be far less relevant in increasing the risk of angina than that of myocardial infarction.

*Selection of cases*

'Selection bias', one of the most important sources of bias in case-control studies, is largely avoidable if it is possible to study all cases of the disease in a defined area, region or country such as was done in the study of all deaths from myocardial infarction occurring in young women in England and Wales in 1973 in an attempt to examine the relationship between oral contraceptives and this disease.[6] In this study all death certificates on which the principal cause of death was ascribed to ICD Code 410 (acute myocardial infarction) in the appropriate age-group, were provided by the Office of Population Censuses and Surveys. Cases were included in the study only if a post-mortem had been carried out or if detailed ante-mortem clinical data were available. More frequently, however, cases are identified from hospital diagnostic indexes or some locally available computerized system of recording hospital discharges (e.g. hospital activity analysis). It is extremely important that cases are not limited to those being admitted to one hospital since referral to hospital may be determined by the known special interests of certain consultants, and the most satisfactory compromise is usually to study all cases admitted to hospitals in a particular region. If, however, the hypothesis being tested is widely known, an unmeasurable degree of bias could be introduced by a tendency to admit patients exposed to a particular drug. A very obvious example here would be a study of oral contraceptives and thromboembolic disease in which general practitioners may be more likely to admit to hospital a woman using oral contraceptives who develops deep venous thrombosis than one not using these preparations.

It is also of importance to note that the disease being investigated should in no way influence the likelihood of the drug being prescribed. This usually means studying newly diagnosed cases (incident cases) rather than prevalent cases. In the example already given, women with recurrent myocardial infarction or indeed any other form of ischaemic heart disease are less likely to be prescribed oral contraceptives, and a study including such cases could well miss a true association between the drug and the disease. It is, of course, obvious that the disease should have a reasonable possibility of having been induced by the drug concerned. There would be little point in looking for an association between oral contraceptives and thromboembolic disease in post-menopausal women or indeed in women immediately after delivery.

*Selection of controls*

Many definitions have been suggested for control subjects. Perhaps the most useful is that they should be representative of the population from which the cases are drawn. They should, assuming no association exists, be as likely to be users of the drug under investigation as the cases. Neighbourhood or community controls randomly drawn from sources such as electoral rolls, or simply by finding the first house in the same street containing an appropriate subject, have been regarded by many as the optimal sources of a control population. However this method is costly, the response rate is often low and the method by no means guarantees that they are likely to be comparable with the cases in respect of likelihood of being a drug user. Experience of case-control studies of drug-induced disease has shown that the use of hospital controls can in many circumstances be a satisfactory method provided certain rules are followed.

The controls should be randomly drawn from a wide range of conditions, excluding those which are known to be caused or prevented by the drug being investigated. In studying the relationship between myocardial infarction and oral contraceptives it was essential to exclude cases of pulmonary embolism where an association with the drug had already been demonstrated[4,5] and similarly cases of ovarian cysts, which were known to be less common amongst users of oral contraceptives.[11] Patients admitted for conditions in which the drug is known to be contraindicated should also be eliminated from the control group (e.g. in the example given above, other thromboembolic disease) since inclusion of an appreciable number of any such patients would result in an unrepresentative estimate of drug exposure. It is also important that likelihood of hospital admission for cases and controls be similar. Thus in a case-control study of myocardial infarction the controls should ideally be patients admitted as other acute medical or surgical emergencies. However Smith and Jick have shown in a large series of hospitalized patients that regular drug use was rather similar in acute and elective admissions[12] so that this rule may be of more theoretical than practical consequence. The use of a wide range of control diagnoses eliminates the possibility that an unknown association between the drug and one of the control diagnoses could mask the association being investigated. For example gall-bladder disease is now known to be associated with oral contraceptive use;[13] if patients with this condition comprised a large proportion of the control population in a study of myocardial infarction and the pill, conducted before this was known, a true association might have been missed.

Controls may also be selected from general practitioners' records, as was done in the studies relating fatal thromboembolic disease to oral contraceptive use.[4,6] The doctor in whose practice a 'case' was found was asked to provide two controls as follows: he located in his files the position which would have been occupied by the late patient's records. Moving first forwards and then backwards from that position, the doctor selected the first two sets of case notes encountered relating to women who matched the cases for the criteria which had been laid down in these particular studies.

Much has been written concerning the criteria for which controls should be matched with the cases. Age and sex are almost always the two most important factors associated with drug use and the disease under study, and controls should nearly always be matched for these two variables, though they can also be controlled by stratification in the analysis. Year of study and geographic area might also be important, and it is usually as well to match also for these factors. Matching is undertaken to eliminate the possibility that a confounding factor (a factor associated with both the drug exposure and the disease) is responsible for an association which is demonstrated between drug and disease. Factors other than those mentioned above may also cause confounding, but as a general rule they are better coped with in the analysis of the results rather than by matching.

Usually one control is selected for each case, but when it is possible to study only a limited number of cases of a rare disease it may be an advantage to study two or even three controls for each case in order to obtain a more reliable estimate of exposure in the control series. In many studies it is possible to identify cases and controls randomly by means of computerized data systems of hospital discharge, but this has often also been done using manual hospital diagnostic indexes.

## Data collection

Information concerning drug exposure is usually obtained either by means of an interview with the patient or from case records kept by doctors – either by general practitioners or hospital physicians. In order to avoid bias it is essential for the method of data collection to be the same for cases and controls. Ideally a 'double-blind' technique should be used when subjects are interviewed; that is neither the interviewer nor the patient knows whether he or she is a case or control. In practice this is often very difficult since during the course of an interview the patient may mention the reason for his hospital admission. A 'blind' approach may be more feasible when data concerning exposure are being abstracted from records.

It is obviously wise to obtain as much information as possible concerning the drug exposure (e.g. duration, dose), but in a case-control study where the event under consideration has taken place at some time in the past this may be very difficult. In studies of drug epidemiology it is wise wherever possible to collect information about use of drugs other than the specific one under investigation, and also about any other factors which could possibly be confounding variables. It is not always possible to know what these factors are when designing a study, but as a general rule it is essential to enquire about any other factors known to be associated with the disease. In the case of myocardial infarction, for example, it would be essential to know about the other risk factors for ischaemic heart disease.

It has now been shown that oral contraceptives are independently associated with an increased risk of myocardial infarction, but this risk is very much greater when the pill is used in the presence of other risk factors, especially cigarette smoking. This synergistic effect of risk factors has great clinical application and would not have been discovered had the studies not included detailed information concerning other risk factors.[7]

The importance of as near as possible to complete ascertainment of all identified cases and controls is obvious. It is not possible to lay down rigid criteria concerning the precise proportion of cases and controls which need to be followed for a study to be valid, but one might well be dubious of the findings of any study where fewer than 90% of identified subjects were followed.

## Interpretation of results

The methods of data analysis have recently been reviewed and are beyond the scope of this chapter.[14] Exposure rates amongst cases and controls are compared and the results are very often expressed as relative risks. Relative risk is defined as the ratio of the risk of a particular disease in users of a drug to the risk in unexposed individuals, and gives an indication of the strength of the association. This is estimated indirectly in a case-control study as follows: *ad*/*bc* (see Figure 1). The derivation of this formula is given in standard textbooks of epidemiology, e.g. MacMahon and Pugh: *Epidemiology: Principles and Methods.*[25] It is also possible in studies which have included all cases in a known geographic area to make estimates of attributable risk[7] as well as relative risk. Attributable risk gives an indication of the impact of the drug-induced disease, and is an important consideration since a small relative risk of a common condition may be associated with a far greater degree of overall morbidity than a condition which is associated with a high relative risk but occurs only very infrequently. The first consideration, having found a difference in exposure between cases and controls, is to know whether or not chance could have explained the observed increase in risk. The level of statistical significance (the $p$ value) which is acceptable as a reasonable indication that chance alone is unlikely to have accounted for the increase in risk will depend upon the type of case-control study. In hypothesis-generating studies (such as ongoing case-control surveillance) where numerous associations are being tested, it is likely that some association will achieve traditional levels of statistical significance ($p < 0.05$) by chance alone and much more stringent criteria are required, whereas when the study has been designed to test a plausible hypothesis the same level of statistical significance implies far greater confidence.

The analysis will include an attempt to examine whether the confounding factors, for which matching has not been carried out, could explain any observed association. The possibility that bias could invalidate the results of many case-control studies has been suggested by some workers, and Sackett has indicated eight different biases which might operate.[15] More recently[16] he has described another 27 and I list some of these below:

(1) *Neyman bias* (prevalence incidence bias): 'a late look at those exposed (or affected) early will miss fatal and other short episodes, plus mild or "silent" cases in which evidence of exposure disappears with disease onset'. This Sackett regards as one of the most important potential sources of bias. However, when case ascertainment is complete, with the diagnosis clearly defined and when the study is limited to newly presenting cases, this bias should not present major difficulties.
(2) *Berkson bias* (admission rate bias): 'if the hospitalization rates of exposed and unexposed cases and controls differ, their relative odds of prior drug exposure will be distorted in hospital-based studies'. This is potentially of considerable importance in hospital-based studies where the condition being studied is insufficiently severe to render hospital admission mandatory.
(3) *Non-respondent bias:* 'non-respondents (or "late-comers") from a specified sample may exhibit exposures or outcomes which differ from those of respondents (or "early-comers")'. This bias is self-explanatory and should not present a problem in studies where virtually all cases and controls are followed up.
(4) *Popularity bias:* 'the admission of patients to some practices, institutions or procedures is influenced by the interest aroused by the presenting illness and its possible causes'. This source of bias once again only applies when case ascertainment is undertaken from special care units and not when a defined population is studied.
(5) *Exposure suspicion bias:* 'a knowledge of the patient's disease status may influence both the intensity and the outcome of a search for exposure to the putative cause. This can be best overcome by 'blind' assessment as described above.
(6) *Recall bias:* 'questions about specific exposures may be asked several times of cases but only once of controls'. Patients may remember previously forgotten events and exposures upon repeated interrogation, an opportunity which may be lost to control subjects.
(7) *Unmasking (detection signal) bias:* 'an innocent exposure may become suspect if, rather than causing a disease, it causes a sign or symptom which precipitates a search for the disease'. The particular example which is quoted here is the consideration of the relationship between post-menopausal oestrogens and endometrial cancer. The possibility has been suggested that oestrogens might cause the *search* for endometrial cancer (by causing the symptomless patient to bleed) rather than the cancer itself.
(8) *Diagnostic suspicion bias:* 'a knowledge of the patient's prior exposure may influence both the intensity and the outcome of the diagnostic process'. This bias is particularly important in

observational cohort studies undertaken to test a hypothesis suggested by case-control studies, but it could also affect a case-control study where there has been widespread publicity concerning the possible association between a drug and the disease under investigation.

(For more detailed discussion of these biases, the reader is referred to the publications of Sackett).[15,16]

Thus it can be seen that whilst case-control studies are potentially subject to an appreciable number of biases, most of these are eliminated in a well-designed study, taking into account the principles described earlier in the chapter. Whilst a single case-control study rarely provides conclusive evidence of causality (this subject will be considered in more detail later) well-designed case-control studies have an impressive reputation. There must be few instances of case-control studies which have been designed to test a specific hypothesis where the association demonstrated has not been confirmed subsequently in other studies. This is not always true of studies where associations have been demonstrated as part of a multiple-comparison exercise, and the association between breast cancer and reserpine preparations first detected in 1974[17] by such a technique remains unresolved. Furthermore the case-control approach may be the *only* means by which an association between a particular drug and a very rare disease (e.g. oral contraceptives and tumours of the liver) can be studied, since the cohort which would be required to find a sufficient number of cases would be totally unmanageable and prohibitively expensive.

There are situations in which a case-control approach cannot be applied with confidence, and these occur when it is not possible to find a situation where cases and controls have an equal chance of being exposed to the drug of interest; for example where a drug may be indicated for the treatment of the early manifestations of the illness or predisposing cause, or where use of the drug is contraindicated by early manifestations of the illness.

The terms cohort and prospective studies are often used interchangeably though this is not, strictly speaking, accurate. The main feature of such studies is that the group, or groups of individuals to be studied (the cohorts), are defined in terms of characteristics manifest prior to the appearance of the disease under investigation. The study groups so defined are then observed over a period of time to determine the frequency of the disease among them. Cohort studies may be prospective or retrospective, the distinction depending upon whether or not the cases of the disease have occurred in the cohort at the time when study is begun. In a retrospective cohort study all the relevant events (causes and effects) have already occurred when the study is initiated. In a prospective study the cases of disease will not have occurred, and following selection of the study cohort the investigator must wait for the disease to appear in its members.

Cohort studies have a number of advantages over case-control studies. The various biases described are not as likely to distort the findings, and it is possible to anticipate and overcome most of them. It has been mentioned that it is possible in a case-control study, which has included all cases in a defined geographic area over a specified time-interval, to estimate the absolute as well as the relative risk. In a cohort study this can be done with a greater degree of accuracy, and it is often also possible to derive a risk–benefit analysis. Finally they permit a number of adverse effects to be studied simultaneously, and include the possibility of unsuspected risks and benefits being discovered. There are, however, also disadvantages. Most serious adverse effects of drugs occur relatively infrequently. This means that the cohort which needs to be studied nearly always needs to be large, and to be followed for a long period of time, usually at least 5 years. (Furthermore if the disease is sufficiently rare it may not sometimes be feasible to use this approach at all.) Consequently such studies require a great deal of effort and are very costly. There are a number of different prospective cohort approaches which may be used in evaluating the safety of drugs:

## Intensive hospital monitoring

This approach, such as has been used in the Boston Collaborative Drug Surveillance Program,[18] provides extremely useful information concerning drug epidemiology: the frequency of known adverse drug reactions and drug interactions. New serious untoward effects of drugs are rarely discovered because the follow-up period is too short and the number of patients not large enough. The possibilities and problems of monitoring adverse effects in hospital outpatients and general practice are discussed elsewhere in this book.

## Experimental cohort studies (randomized clinical trials)

These studies are usually set up to examine which of a number of different treatment regimens is the most effective in treating a particular condition, or whether indeed treatment is better than no treatment at all in a particular setting. Since any untoward effect of the drug being tested is not usually suspected it is essential that all events be recorded in such a study, so that overall morbidity and mortality can be compared in the different treatment groups. The principles and the conduct of clinical trials have been described in detail elsewhere,[19] but perhaps a few main points could be enumerated here. Allocation to the different treatment groups should always be made randomly and if at all possible the trial should be conducted under 'double-blind' conditions. In order to recruit sufficient subjects such studies are nearly always conducted in a number of centres, and it is essential that all procedures be standardized in the various centres. The problems of follow-up in such studies are enormous since incomplete follow-up can completely invalidate the results. It is quite conceivable that subjects lost to follow-up may have behaved differently from those who are prepared to attend for regular follow-up. Once again it is not possible to lay down a minimal percentage which needs to be followed up for the results to be valid, but where it is not possible to follow-up over 95% of those initially recruited, it may be possible to go to great lengths to follow a randomly selected proportion of the non-responders in each group, to ensure that they are not appreciably different from those who have been followed.

Even some of the most carefully conducted clinical trials can produce results which are extremely difficult to interpret. The recently conducted World Health Organization-sponsored multi-centre trial of clofibrate versus placebo capsules in the management of hypercholesterolaemia affords a good example of this.[20] Some 30 000 men in five cities were screened and divided into three sub-groups on the basis of their cholesterol levels. Those with cholesterol levels in the upper third of the distribution curve were randomized into clofibrate treatment and placebo control groups, and a randomly selected group in the lower third of the distribution curve provided an additional control group, who were also given the placebo control. The principles of a good clinical trial were rigidly followed. The study showed a beneficial effect of the drug with regard to non-fatal, though not to fatal, ischaemic cardiac events, but of more interest from the point of this chapter is the fact that the study confirmed a two-fold increase in risk of gall-bladder disease in the clofibrate-treated group, an association first suggested in another collaborative clinical trial – The Coronary Drug Project (CDP),[21] which investigated five regimens in the long-term management of middle-aged men who had had a myocardial infarction. The main problem of the clofibrate study is shown in Table 1. The difference in total mortality between the active treatment group and the high cholesterol controls, together with the difference in gall-bladder disease, led an editorial writer in *Lancet*[22] to suggest that perhaps the untoward effects of the drug outweighed any possible advantage of a reduced frequency of non-fatal ischaemic cardiac episodes. However, the writer of the editorial overlooked the fact that the death rates for all causes of death other than ischaemic heart disease for the low cholesterol control group were virtually identical to the clofibrate-treated subjects with high cholesterol levels. This observation is extremely difficult to explain, but taken into account might lead to totally different conclusions, especially if one added the rider that clofibrate should not be used in an individual who might be particularly prone to gall-bladder disease (e.g. obese subjects).

It is clear that these studies are beset with enormous difficulties and can only be undertaken and indeed interpreted by specialists. Despite the problems, though, they clearly need to be carried out.

It has often been said that in order to be valid such studies need to

**Table 1** Deaths in the trial and within 1 year of leaving it. Main cause groups. Numbers of deaths and rates at ages 30–59, and age-standardized rates per 1000 per annum at ages 40–59

| *Cause of death* | *Group I (Clofibrate)* | | | *Group II (High cholesterol control)* | | | *Group III (Low cholesterol control)* | | |
|---|---|---|---|---|---|---|---|---|---|
| | *No.* (*All* | *Rate* *ages)* | *St. Rate 40–59* | *No.* (*All* | *Rate* *ages)* | *St. Rate 40–59* | *No.* (*All* | *Rate* *ages)* | *St. Rate 40–59* |
| Ischaemic heart disease | 54 | 1.6 | 2.1 | 48 | 1.4 | 2.1 | 20 | 0.6 | 0.8 |
| Other vascular | 14 | 0.4 | 0.5 | 14 | 0.4 | 0.6 | 9 | 0.3 | 0.5 |
| Neoplasm: malignant | 58 | 1.7 | 2.2 | 42 | 1.3 | 1.7 | 41 | 1.3 | 2.5 |
| Neoplasm: benign | 3 | — | — | — | — | — | 1 | — | — |
| Other medical causes | 16* | 0.5* | 0.8* | 5* | 0.2* | 0.2* | 7 | 0.2 | 0.4 |
| Accidents and violence | 17 | 0.5 | 0.6 | 18 | 0.5 | 0.6 | 15 | 0.5 | 0.6 |
| All causes other than IHD | 108* | 3.1* | 4.1* | 79* | 2.4* | 3.1 | 73 | 2.3 | 4.0 |
| All causes other than IHD, vascular accidents and violence | 77† | 2.2† | 3.0* | 47† | 1.5† | 1.9* | 49 | 1.5 | 2.9 |
| TOTAL ALL CAUSES | 162* | 4.7* | 6.2 | 127* | 3.8* | 5.2 | 93 | 2.9 | 4.8 |

*Significant difference between Group I and II ($p < 0.05$)
† Significant difference between Groups I and II ($p < 0.01$)

be carried out on representative groups. This statement is, of course, strictly speaking, correct but the possibilities of undertaking such studies on groups of subjects with special facilities for follow-up (e.g. doctors) should not necessarily be rejected. Although the results of such studies are theoretically only applicable to the group which has been investigated, provided randomization and the other principles elucidated have been adhered to, the results are valid and are almost certain to have wider applicability. Doll and Peto are currently investigating the hypothesis that daily use of aspirin is protective against ischaemic heart disease by recruiting doctors as participants, since they had earlier shown that it is possible in this select group to achieve something like a 99% follow-up over a 25-year period.[23]

It is not always possible to randomly allocate subjects to treated and control groups. An example of this situation is provided by the two prospective studies set up to evaluate the long-term safety of oral contraceptives.[11,24] The disease experience of oral contraceptive users was compared with that of women using other methods of contraception. It is essential in such a study that detailed information be available concerning the health status of the subjects at the outset of the investigation, since it is always conceivable that particular characteristics could determine which method of contraception is chosen or recommended; this aspect needs to be examined in the analysis. Oral contraceptive users were shown to have a higher overall mortality than users of other methods of contraception, even though they appeared to be healthier at the outset. An important potential source of bias in these studies is the diagnostic suspicion bias. Since 'blind' assessment is virtually impossible it is conceivable that certain conditions are more likely to be diagnosed in users of a particular method of contraception. This can even apply when the endpoints are 'general practice consultations' or 'hospital referral' for particular conditions. However, the hardest of all end-points, death, cannot be affected this way and it is of great interest that using this end-point, the cohort studies of users of different methods of contraception have confirmed virtually all the findings of the retrospective studies and have uncovered no new serious untoward effects.

## Methods of follow-up and analysis in cohort studies

It has already been mentioned that the proportion of subjects followed is of crucial importance. The methods of follow-up will naturally vary from study to study and from country to country. Follow-up is usually co-ordinated from one centre, and attempts to trace individuals may be made through general practitioners, relatives, neighbours or through central registers in areas such as the United Kingdom, with a National Health Service where records are kept showing with which doctors all patients are registered. Where cancer registers maintain a high ascertainment rate these are a useful source of identifying such cases, but perhaps most useful of all epidemiological methods is the ability to flag the individual health records kept at the central registry in the United Kingdom. This system results in the patient's death certificate being sent to the investigator immediately a participant in a study dies.

Once again, detailed considerations of the analysis are beyond the scope of this chapter and have been described in detail elsewhere,[25] but it is important to point out that in cohort studies relative risk may be directly calculated as follows:

$$\frac{a}{a+b} \div \frac{c}{c+d}$$

(see Figure 1) and the attributable risk can always be calculated

$$\frac{a}{a+b} - \frac{c}{c+d}$$

Most sources of bias can be overcome and the diagnostic suspicion bias in observational cohort studies is the principal one which needs to be borne in mind.

## THE DIAGNOSIS OF CAUSATION

Whether or not an association between drug use and adverse event is truly causal is of such crucial importance that the 'diagnosis of causation' will be discussed in some detail here even though it has been touched upon earlier in this chapter. A number of points are particularly relevant.

A demonstration of an adverse event in a carefully conducted randomized control clinical trial is the best evidence of all that an association is causal. Most of the biases applicable to other methods of investigation are eliminated. However even well-planned human experiments such as the University Group Diabetes Program[26] and the clofibrate study, described earlier, have produced confusing answers.

Where it is not possible to perform human experiments in the form of randomized trials, observational prospective studies can provide very strong support for causal association. They are theoretically liable to biases such as the volunteer bias, the diagnostic suspicion bias and the popularity bias, but quite often these are of greater importance in theory than in practice, as has been for instance shown in the prospective studies of women using different methods of contraception. Experimental and observational prospective studies have a great advantage in that the strength of the association (relative risk) can be directly calculated from the data

$$\frac{a}{a+b} \div \frac{c}{c+d}$$

(see Figure 1), and the attributable risk

$$\frac{a}{a+b} - \frac{c}{c+d}$$

can always be estimated. Relative risk is calculated indirectly from case-control studies and attributable risk can only be calculated when all cases in a defined geographic area have been included. The strength of the association is naturally an important consideration in the diagnosis of causality, though it should be remembered that, in terms of attributable risk, a small increase in risk of a common condition can cause a much greater amount of disease than a high relative risk associated with a very rare disease. It has been argued that findings from case-control studies on their own can never be used to be confident of a causal association. In my opinion they can, under certain circumstances, provide very strong evidence and the arterial thrombotic complications of oral contraceptives, demonstrated first in case-control studies and confirmed in prospective cohort studies, provide excellent examples. A number of important criteria do, however, need to be fulfilled when suggesting a causal association on the bases of such studies.

Case-control studies designed to test a specific hypothesis are much more meaningful than those scanning existing data bases which are chiefly useful for hypothesis-generating unless they are specifically used to test a hypothesis generated elsewhere. The demonstration of a biological gradient provides strong evidence for a causal association, even when this is available only for case-control studies (e.g. the data for myocardial infarction and cigarette smoking shown in Table 2).[27]

**Table 2** The relative risk of developing myocardial infarction associated with different categories of cigarette smoking in young women[28]

| *No. of cigarettes smoked daily at onset of episode* | *Relative risk in smokers in comparison with non-smokers and ex-smokers* |
|---|---|
| $<$15 cigarettes | 1.9:1 |
| 15–24 cigarettes | 4.4:1 |
| 25 or more cigarettes | 19.1:1 |

$\chi^2$ test for linear trend = 35.9; $p > 0.001$.

Biological plausibility (e.g. oral contraceptives cause abnormalities of lipid and carbohydrate metabolism and coagulation mechanisms and it is therefore quite conceivable that they could increase the risk of arterial thrombosis) and consistency (the demonstration of an adverse effect in different settings and using different techniques) provide further support for causality. Additional evidence comes from the association making 'epidemiological sense'. The best example of this is the association between rise and fall of asthma deaths and the number of bronchodilator aerosols sold over the counter.[28] The fit between these two data sets represent a major source of credibility for the proposed link. Though as discussed earlier in the case of a relatively low exposure rate in the at-risk population, even quite a large relative risk may not be accompanied by a change in mortality rate. It is naturally also of importance that the correct temporal sequence has taken place: the adverse event should follow exposure to the drug after a reasonable time-interval has elapsed. This test may be more difficult to apply than is immediately apparent wherever it is conceivable that a predisposing factor or very early stage of the adverse disease is responsible both for exposure to the drug and for the adverse event.

Unfortunately the diagnosis of causation does not in the end depend upon a mathematical formula, and official bodies are often forced to make decisions on the basis of inconclusive evidence.

## References


1. Brown, P., Badderley, H., Read, A. E. *et al.* (1974). Sclerosing peritonitis, an unusual reaction to a β-adrenergic-blocking drug (Practolol). *Lancet*, **2,** 1477
2. McBride, W. G. (1961). Thalidomide and congenital abnormalities. *Lancet*, **2,** 1358
3. Editorial (1971). An epidemic of pulmonary hypertension, *Lancet*, **2,** 252
4. Inman, W. H. W. and Vessey, M. P. (1968). Investigation of deaths from pulmonary, coronary and cerebral thrombosis and embolism in women of childbearing age. *Br. Med. J.*, **2,** 193
5. Vessey, M. P. and Doll, R. (1968). Investigation of relation between use of oral contraception and thromboembolic disease. *Br. Med. J.*, **2,** 199
6. Mann, J. I. and Inman, W. H. W. (1975). Oral contraceptives and death from myocardial infarction in young women. *Br. Med. J.*, **2,** 245
7. Mann, J. I., Vessey, M. P., Thorogood, M. and Doll, R. (1975). Myocardial infarction in young women with special reference to oral contraceptive practice. *Br. Med. J.*, **2,** 241
8. Collaborative Group for the Study of Stroke in Young Women (1975). Oral contraceptives and stroke in young women. *J. Am. Med. Assoc.*, **231,** 718
9. Feinstein, A. R. (1973). Clinical biostatistics: the epidemiologic trohoc, the ablative risk ratio and retrospective research, *Clin. Pharmacol. Ther.*, **14,** 291
10. World Health Organization (1971). Criteria for myocardial infarction. *Ischaemic Heart Disease Register* (Copenhagen: WHO)
11. Royal College of General Practitioners (1974). *Oral Contraceptives and Health* (London: Pitman Medical)
12. Smith, P. G. and Jick, H. (1977). Regular drug use and cancer. *J. Nat. Cancer Inst.* **59,** Part 5, 1387–91
13. Boston Collaborative Drug Surveillance Scheme (1973). *Lancet*, **1,** 1399
14. Miettinen, O. S. (1976). Estimability and estimation in case-referent studies. *Am. J. Epidemiol.*, **103,** 226
15. Sackett, D. L. (1978). Drug withdrawal, drug blame and drug house suits: the admissibility of scientific evidence. In Gent, M. and Schigematsu, I. (eds.) *Epidemiological Issues in Reported Drug-Induced Illnesses – S.M.O.N. and other examples.* (Hamilton, Ontario, Canada: McMaster University Library Press)
16. Sackett, D. L. (1979). Bias in analytic research. *J. Chron. Dis.*, **32,** 51–63
17. Editorial (1975). Rauwolfia and breast cancer. *Lancet*, **2,** 312
18. Jick, H. (1972). The Boston Collaborative Drug Surveillance Program. In Richards, D. J. and Rondel, R. K. (eds.) *Adverse Drug Reactions. Their Prediction, Detection and Assessment*, p. 61. (Edinburgh: Churchill Livingstone)
19. Peto, R., Pike, M. C., Armitage, P. *et al.* (1976). Design and analysis of randomized clinical trials requiring prolonged observation of each patient. *Br. J. Cancer*, **34,** 585
20. Committee of Principal Investigations (1978). *Br. Heart J.*, **40,** 1069
21. Coronary Drug Project Research Group (1975). The coronary drug project. Clofibrate and niacin in coronary heart disease. *J. Am. Med. Assoc.*, **231,** 360
22. Editorial (1978). Clofibrate: a final verdict? *Lancet*, **2,** 1131
23. Doll, R. and Peto, R. (1976). Mortality in relation to smoking: 20 years observations on male British doctors. *Br. Med. J.*, **2,** 1525
24. Vessey, M. P. *et al.* (1976). A long-term follow-up study of women using different methods of contraception. An interim report. *J. Biosoc. Sci.*, **8,** 373
25. MacMahon, B. and Pugh, T. F. (1970). *Epidemiology: Principles and methods.* (Boston: Little, Brown and Co.)
26. The University Group Diabetes Program (1970). *Diabetes* (Suppl. 2) vol. 19
27. Mann, J. I. (1977). Oral contraceptives and myocardial infarction. In Sciarra, J. J., Zatuchni, G. I. and Speidel, J. J. *Risks, Benefits and Controversies in Fertility Control* pp. 129–37. PARFR Series on Fertility Regulation (New York: Harper & Row)
28. Inman, W. H. W. and Adelstein, A. M. (1969). Rise and fall of asthma mortality in England and Wales in relation to use of pressurised aerosols. *Lancet*, **2,** 279

# 33 Vital statistics, censuses and surveys

A. M. ADELSTEIN

## INTRODUCTION

This chapter will describe the main national systems of records used for monitoring trends in disease and in mortality described in more detail elsewhere.[1] In this context monitoring includes both continuous surveillance and testing of hypotheses. A clue that something is amiss may be noted by a clinician during the course of his everyday work; but because of the very nature of small samples there will be many false alarms. It is therefore necessary to have large-scale back-up systems in order to check suspicions and then, usually, to verify them by more formally designed tests of hypotheses, based on appropriate selection of cases and controls.

## SOURCES OF HAZARDS: WHO AND HOW EFFECTED

National systems of records used for analysing adverse effects of drugs are of course also used when considering adverse effects from sources other than medicines, e.g. toxic substances in general, or in the work environment, or from any adverse behaviour, for example, smoking. Adverse effects may involve any physiological system, at any age, in any part of the population. They may affect the person directly or may act on the fetus. The effects could be indicated in various ways: first by syndromes specific to the drug, e.g. the effect of poisoning by mercury (e.g. pink disease); secondly, by syndromes not specific to the drug (e.g. blood dyscrasias, thromboembolism); thirdly by aggravating the condition treated (e.g. treatment of asthma by misuse of aerosols).

## RECORD SYSTEMS

Much epidemiology (whether of adverse effects or otherwise) depends on routine systems of records from health services and registrations of death and births. These systems of records are designed for the day-to-day functioning of a health service, not for research. As such, some items do not reach standards of accuracy expected in studies designed for research. However, these general systems of records, because they are universal and quickly available, covering a wide range of diagnoses, remain the backbone of national epidemiological research. Their limitations should not obscure their great value.

These general systems should not be seen in isolation. Even when they provide information for studies without additional research, interpretation must be related to the general body of knowledge of the particular topic. In addition to analysing records confined to a particular system of records, a second, higher level of specificity is formed when records of an individual are linked for what are known as prospective, or alternatively retrospective, studies. A prospective study begins with individuals' records, each showing how much exposure there has been to a particular hazard. These persons are then, as it were, followed up by linking records to find out about diseases and deaths which occurred over the years. The way this is done through the National Health Service Central Register (NHSCR) is explained later in this chapter.

Retrospective studies begin with records showing that the subjects had (or died from) a particular disorder (for example, thromboembolism) and other records are then sought (for example from general practice or hospitals) to indicate how much, if any, of a particular drug had been prescribed. Both types of study require controls; records at one level – say death certificates – may be checked against other records, for example, the clinical file. The national systems are so important because they are well indexed in standard form and can be linked together, so they are available for the sample of affected persons in a retrospective study or the outcome recorded of a prospective study.

## NHSCR

This is the clearing house for the patient records of general practitioners, and it holds the names of virtually everyone in the UK. Deaths, births and movements of patients between family practitioners' committees are noted. Since 1970 records of cancers have also been noted, but less consistently, as yet, than are records of deaths.

The system enables prospective studies. Records of study-persons are marked in the NHSCR and later, if death or cancer supervenes, the relevant records can be found and linked.

## CERTIFICATION OF CAUSE OF DEATH

Since the event of death is unique, professionally certified, and registered universally and promptly these certificates consitute an unrivalled history of the nation's health for nearly 150 years. In the UK we use the certificate recommended by WHO, completed by a physician who attended the last illness or by a coroner.[2,3] Part I requests a causal sequence of events, line by line showing in the *last* line the disease which started the sequence (the so-called underlying condition). In Part II other significant conditions are shown. The Registrar-General may write for more information when a diagnosis is not detailed enough for precise classification, or when the certifier has indicated that he may be able to give additional information (for example, after autopsy). Registrars of births and deaths copy the medical information and record personal characteristics; for example, sex, date and place of birth, marital state and occupation of a deceased man, of the husband of a married woman, and of the father of a child. After coding, the information is entered on computers. Copies of the registrar's original record have been stored since 1839; since 1959 computer tapes excluding names are cross-indexed to copies of the written records; and since 1939 (with some minor exceptions) the fact and date of death is marked on the relevant record of each person in the NHSCR; this enables research workers to have death certificates required, for example, in prospective studies.

## ANALYSING GENERAL RECORD SYSTEMS (e.g. TIME SERIES)

Inman and Adelstein[4] analysed the rise and decline of mortality attributed to asthma in young persons. They correlated trends over time with the sales of aerosol inhalers, and concluded that the rise in mortality was the result of misuse of aerosol inhalers (see Figure 1).

A second example of the uses of mortality records is from the Decennial Supplement of Occupational Mortality (1970–2).[5] Table 1 shows occupations in which men (aged 15–64) had high standardized mortality ratios (SMR) attributed both to blood diseases and rheumatoid arthritis. (SMR is the percentage ratio of observed deaths to the number expected in the population as a whole, taking account of the age structure).

The first clue to this observation was noticed in a standard tabulation showing that in one of 27 occupation orders (clothing workers) the relative mortality of males was considerably higher than that of married women for disorders of blood and of musculoskeletal systems. Inspection within this and other orders suggested that the specific occupations involved, as shown in Table 1, involve sustained fine handwork. Although there were not many deaths from these causes in each occupation, together they seem to tell a story of possible adverse effects of anti-rheumatic drugs among men who use their

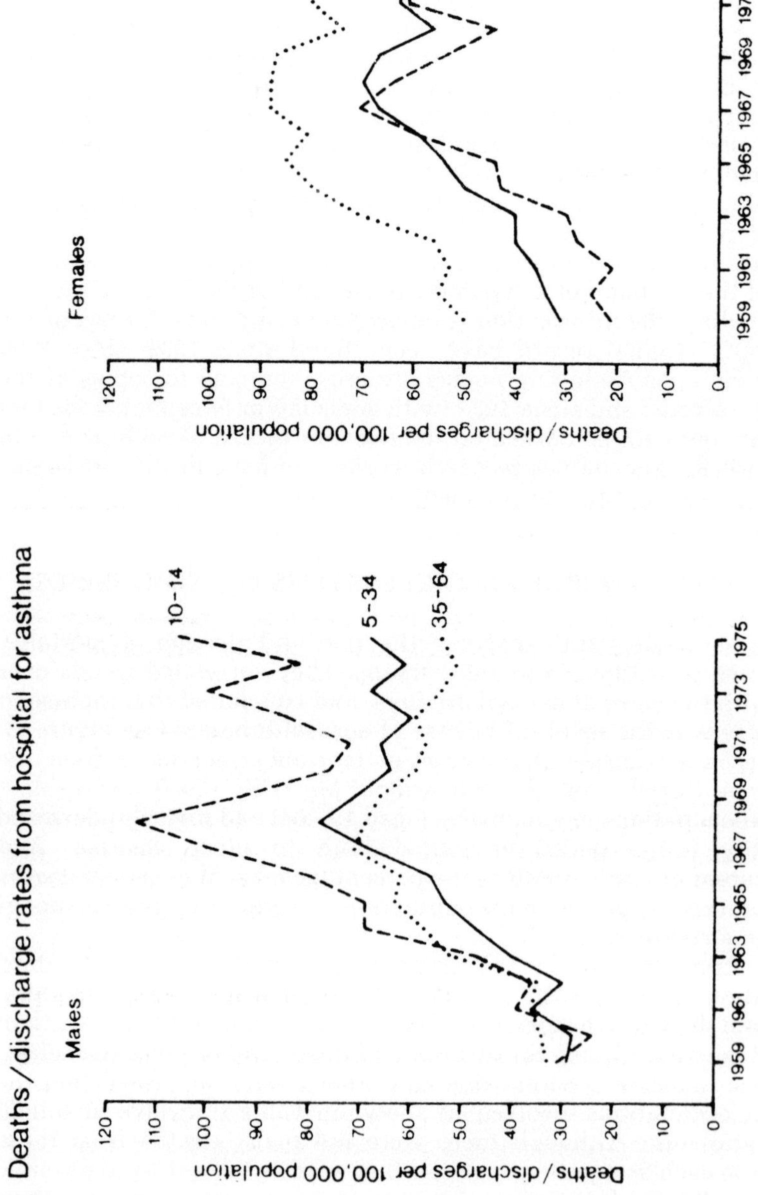


**Figure 1** Deaths/discharge rates from hospital for asthma

**Table 1** Some occupations* with high SMRs for blood diseases or rheumatoid arthritis (numbers of deaths in parentheses)

| *Occupation* | *Blood diseases* | *Rheumatoid arthritis* |
|---|---|---|
| | *SMR* | *SMR* |
| Glass-formers, finishers, decorators | 162 | 275 |
| Smiths, forgemen | 272 | 625 |
| Radio and radar mechanics | 281 | 288 |
| Electric welders | 158 | 144 |
| Watchmakers | — | 1225 |
| Precision instrument makers | — | 403 |
| Goldsmiths | 590 | 1069 |
| Cabinet-makers | 155 | 247 |
| Shoe-makers | 671 | — |
| Spinners | 284 | 489 |
| Tailors | 382 | 862 |
| Upholsterers | 473 | — |
| Hand and machine sewers | 881 | — |
| Clothing and related product makers (n.e.c.) | — | 874 |
| Athletes | — | 1396 |
| Authors | 424 | — |
| Painters, sculptors | — | 307 |
| All occupations listed | 277 (25) | 416 (25) |

*SMRs based on ages 15–64, but supportive evidence is also available at ages 65–74

hands for sustained delicate work, who would readily seek treatment for affected hands. Among the men in these occupations as a group there were 25 deaths attributed to blood diseases and 25 attributed to rheumatoid arthritis; the numbers expected were 9 and 6 respectively, based on the rates for all men in England and Wales, allowing for the age distributions. Thus the SMRs were 277 for blood dyscrasias and 416 for rheumatoid arthritis. It is well to note that inferences (such as these) made from searching through masses of observations, plausible as they may appear, should be regarded as only suggestive until further studies confirm the findings, or at least another set of figures becomes available: For example, a test of our hypothesis about treatment of arthritis will appear in the next study of occupations around the 1981 census.

Formerly we would say that this observation was made after the event, the next will be prior.

The fact that the increased mortality was in two categories of disease illustrates an important point in the use of the International Classification of Diseases for analysing causes of death; one aim is to identify the 'underlying' cause; that is, the disease which initiated the sequence of events leading to death. But this depends on how much is known and how described by the doctor: if a full description is written; for example:

1(a) aplastic anaemia
1(b) (due to) sensitivity to phenyl butazone
1(c) (due to) painful rheumatoid arthritis

the last, rheumatoid arthritis, should be selected; but if this sequence was not recognized by the doctor, perhaps only aplastic anaemia might appear with or without mention of a drug. It follows that in this situation three alternative categories of disease may be coded as underlying cause. This example – assuming that our interpretation of the table is correct – shows an apparent weakness of general statistical systems: they are not designed as research projects would be – focused on one particular question. This leads to a lot of agonizing about the inaccuracy of death certificates, and many papers have been written on the subject. This approach is, however, negative. The system of records when properly organized is robust for a wide variety of analyses and research. Of course death certificates alone could not be useful for analysing every topic or category of disease. Critics seem to want all or none of it. It may be useful to repeat the point that information from these records is not used in isolation. First it is interpreted against a background of knowledge; secondly, further studies may be designed with control groups to allow for errors. Studies may be pursued at different levels, moving from death certificates to other records (e.g. clinical or pathological), as in the analysis of prospective or retrospective surveys. The important point is that clues are thrown up by the records, or more probably by clinicians, and in either event the routine records are available for further studies.

## CANCER REGISTRATION

This system of records has two levels, regional and national. All known cases of cancer should be registered. Cancer registries at local levels are free to organize their records and methods in their own way so long as they include the items asked for by the national scheme. These are kept to a minimum; for example, name, place of residence, date of birth, sex, primary site of cancer, histology or clinical state, date when diagnosis was confirmed.

Some local registries gather more information for their own research, for example, therapy. From 1971 for each person registered as a cancer patient a note is made in his corresponding NHSCR records. This enables us to carry out prospective studies in the same way as we do for deaths; thus in each case the researcher will be informed of each death (and cause) and each cancer (whether the patient is still alive or has died). In the context of this chapter, at national level these records are dealt with by the same method as are death records; that is, they are regularly analysed for trends and associations, and they are indexed so as to be available for retrospective and prospective studies; the latter with the aid of the NHSCR described earlier.

## SURVEILLANCE OF CONGENITAL MALFORMATIONS[6]

Until April 1982 the Area Medical Officer (AMO) collected information on each malformed child notified in his area, and forwarded reports, one per child, to OPCS monthly. Since the National Health Service was reorganized in April 1982 this duty falls to the District Medical Officer. The form provides details concerning the child (date and place of birth, birth-weight, sex, gestation, whether born alive or dead, all malformations detected), and age and parity of the mother. The malformations present are indicated on a check-list of 66 categories of malformations arranged in groups suitable for recording visible or easily detectable malformations present at birth. In processing the data the 66 categories are further grouped to form 28 groups, some of which include babies with two or more malformations. Thus babies with both cleft lip and cleft palate, or with either of these malformations, are grouped into 'babies with facial clefts'.

Monthly tabulations are produced about 5–6 months after the babies were born, giving the numbers of each type of malformation and numbers of babies with combined malformations: these tables are sent as a return to DMOs. In order to investigate increases or decreases in the large numbers of individual series of data, they are analysed with the aid of two types of statistical test: first the current observations (for each of 66 categories of malformations) are added for a trend analysis: secondly, the rate is compared with the national rate. So far there has been only one alarm and it proved to be false, following a notice on how to look for dislocated hips.

The information is stored on computer tapes, and although no names are sent to OPCS, they are available, through reference numbers, at district level. This system is used for a retrospective study of the relationship of drugs in pregnancy to congenital anomalies. Investigators from the Committee on Safety of Medicines searched through relevant records of general practitioners who cared for the mothers during their pregnancies.[7]

## HOSPITAL RECORDS

Since 1957 a 10% sample of the records of every discharge (or death) of acute hospitals (non-psychiatric) have been analysed by OPCS in the system known as the Hospital In-Patient Enquiry (HIPE).[8] Unlike records of deaths, names are absent, but hospital reference numbers are available so that retrospective investigations are possible. Its main weakness is that records of a person's successive spells in hospital are not linked.

At regional level, and in Scotland, analyses are made of all spells (not 10% as for HIPE which is now taken as a sample). Furthermore in Scotland an individual's hospital and vital records are linked.[9]

Two examples show the use of HIPE data in relation to therapy. Figure 2 shows rates of admission of asthma cases over the years 1959–75. Since the rise in admissions after 1959 occurred at about the same time as the rise in mortality, and before this rise was generally known, it is unlikely that the increased admission rate could have been caused by increased sensitivity of doctors. This suggests that many more patients were adversely affected than were shown by the increased number of deaths. Although the rate of mortality has declined to previous levels, admissions to hospital remain higher possibly because clinicians are now more aware of the hazard of unexpected death.

The second example of the use of routine (hospital) records concerns diseases of the ear and mastoid process. Numbers of admissions rose from 35 000 in 1962 to over 68 000 in 1967. Much of this was in the category of otitis media – from 13 000 to over 27 000; but the greatest proportional rise was classified as 'other deafness' which increased from 3200 to over 18 000, the increase being mainly in children. This example highlights questions which need answering when dealing with routine records based on services (especially hospitals), for example whether the increase is real or simply the result of different criteria for admission, and whether it affects relatively fewer children, each with many admissions? Finally, if the increased admission rate reflects a real increase in disease, has therapy been at fault?

This increase is considered to be almost entirely from non-suppurative otitis media, known as 'glue ear'. Although this condition cannot be described as an adverse effect of therapy, it is at least a failure or wrong use of therapy, possibly antibiotics, and is described here mainly to indicate difficulties in interpreting reasons for changing trends in hospital admissions.

## RECORDS IN GENERAL PRACTICE

Three nationwide surveys have been carried out, the most recent being for a period of one year beginning in August 1981. Reports on the previous survey in the 2 years 1971 and 1972 have been published.[10] It was based on the records of about 100 general practices whose doctors were members of the Royal College of General Practitioners and who volunteered to do this work.

At this point it is convenient to mention a study which uses a number of national record systems, even though the study is confined to only one relatively small sample of subjects. In Chapter 19 Skegg describes how, in the Oxford region, for each person he linked

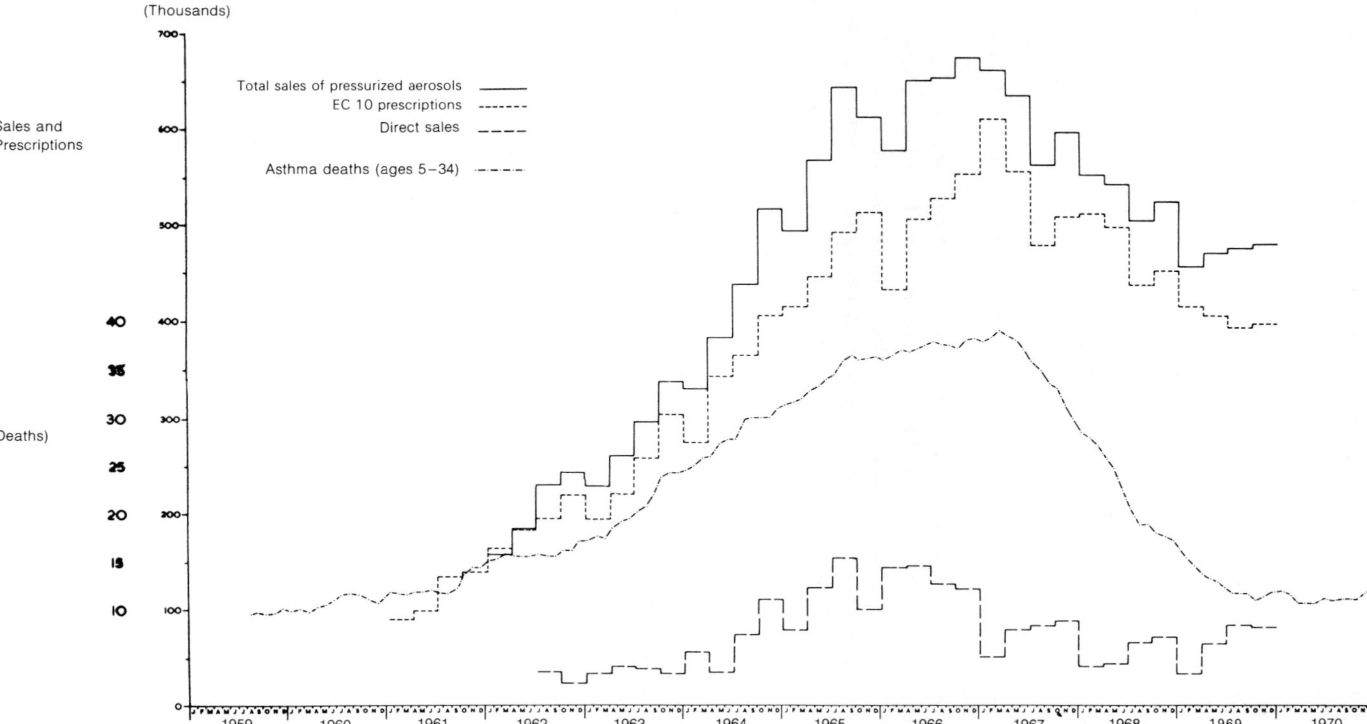


**Figure 2** Sales and prescriptions of pressurized aerosols (actual quarterly figures) compared with deaths from asthma, ages 5–34 (exponentially weighted monthly moving averages), England and Wales, 1959–70

separate records made in various medical services and, if death occurred, to the record of cause of death. The records of one general practice (from the National Morbidity Study) were linked with records of prescriptions (FPC. 10), records of hospital spells and of deaths. It is one of the great advantages of the National Health Service that this and other examples of linkage are feasible. As far as possible linkage is carried out on anonymous records (by substituting numbers for names) and great care is taken to guard the privacy of persons involved.

## OTHER NATIONAL RECORD SYSTEMS

*Surveys:* OPCS carries out surveys on specific topics usually by arrangement with government departments; the General Household Survey (GHS) is continuous with many topics including health and medical care. Questions on the use of medicines have been included. Published analyses and annual computer tape records are available.[11]

It goes without saying that, for these and other personal records, the strictest care is taken to guard their confidential nature and the privacy of the individuals concerned.

## SUMMARY AND CONCLUSIONS

National general-purpose medical records suitably indexed extend the everyday work of physicians with individual patients to the community as a whole. Methods include monitoring trends, correlating trends with other events, organizing surveys prospectively and retrospectively. Sometimes they indicate clues to an adverse effect; mostly they are used to test an hypothesis based on suspected hazards noted by physicians.

### References

1. Adelstein, A. M. (1976). Policies of the Office of Population Censuses and Surveys. Philosophy and constraints. *Br. J. Prev. Soc. Med.*, **30**, 1
2. Graham, A. B. (1977). Death registration in England and Wales. *Health Trends*, **9**, 4
3. Adelstein, A. M. (1977). Certifying cause of death. *Health Trends*, **9**, 4
4. Inman, W. H. W. and Adelstein, A. M. (1969). Rise and fall of asthma mortality in England and Wales in relation to the use of pressurised aerosols. *Lancet*, **2**, 279
5. Occupational mortality 1970–72 (1978). *OPCS Series*, DS No. 1 (London: HMSO)
6. Weatherall, J. A. C. and Haskey, J. C. (1976). Surveillance of malformations. *Br. Med. Bull.*, **32**, 1 (39)
7. Greenberg, G., Inman, W. H. W., Weatherall, J .A. C., Adelstein, A. M. and Haskey, J. C. (1977). Maternal drug histories and congenital abnormalities. *Br. Med. J.*, **2**, 853
8. *Hospital In-Patient Enquiry (published annually)*. OPCS/DHSS. (London: HMSO)

9. *Scottish Hospital In-Patient Statistics* (published annually). Scottish Health Service (Edinburgh: HMSO)
10. Morbidity statistics from general practice, 1970–71 (1974). *Studies on Medical and Population Subjects*, **26** (London: HMSO)
11. General household survey. OPCS (London: HMSO)

# 34
# Compliance

D. L. SACKETT, R. B. HAYNES, M. GENT and D. W. TAYLOR

---

## INTRODUCTION

In this chapter we we shall use the term 'compliance' in a more global fashion than in our most recent publications on this topic.[1] Here, the term will simply mean 'behaviour consistent with health advice', and will encompass the four types of compliance shown in Figure 1:

(1) The extent to which the clinician, when prescribing a drug, complies with the manufacturer's advice about its use.
(2) The extent to which the patient, when taking the drug, complies with the clinician's advice on the regimen.
(3) The extent to which the patient, having attributed an unwanted symptom or sign to the regimen, complies with an actual or implied request to inform the clinician.
(4) The extent to which the clinician, having identified a putative adverse drug reaction, reports it to the proper authority.

As is clear from the other chapters in this book, the pathway between occurrence of an adverse drug reaction (ADR) and its submission to the monitoring authority is strewn with dead ends, false trails and pitfalls. Furthermore, it comes as no surprise that a review of even the limited issue of compliance is further complicated by the dearth of data on most issues. Nonetheless, such a review may permit useful conclusions about the link between compliance and adverse reactions and should, at the least, identify fruitful areas for further research.

Finally, most 'facts' are short-lived, and the up-to-date reader of this book will recognize that portions of it became obsolete before its publication. In an effort to minimize obsolescence, this chapter will focus more on general principles and methods of assessing evidence than on data, and will pay more attention to the theoretical effect of non-compliance on the reporting of adverse reactions than upon the very few instances in which this effect has been measured.

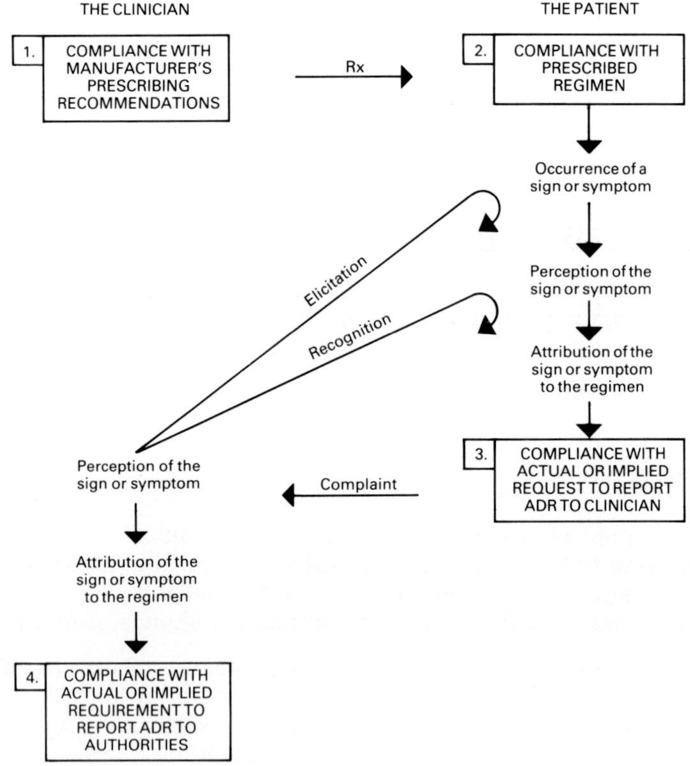


**Figure 1** Some compliance factors in ascertainment of ADRs

## A PROBLEM OF NUMBERS

The competent study of ADRs demands an understanding of the numbers of patients and drug exposures required to permit (under circumstances of perfect compliance) the observation of these adverse reactions. How many patients must be followed to be certain that a new drug will not produce a serious ADR in one of every 500 users? If a clinician uses a drug in 30 patients and notes no ADRs, how safe is the drug? If one compares the ADR rates of 100 patients on a new drug and 100 on an older drug, what conclusions about their relative safety are possible? The answers to these questions can be calculated from the subsequent tables and discussion; see footnote below.*

*The answers to the questions posed are as follows: To be 95% likely of observing one or more ADRs having a true frequency of 1/500, follow 3 $(1/500)^{-1}$ or 1500 patients; if none are observed among these 1500 patients you can be confident that the ADR rate for this drug is less than 1/500 (provided, of course, that you are generalizing to similar patients). Similarly, if no ADRs are noted among 30 patients treated with a drug, the true frequency of ADRs for the drug is probably less than can be detected with samples of size 100.

**Table 1** The likelihood of observing an adverse drug reaction (ADR)

| | *Threshold for an ADR* | | | | | |
|---|---|---|---|---|---|---|
| | *1/100* | *1/500 (e.g. lymphoma from azathioprine)* | *1/1000 (e.g. eye damage from practolol)* | *1/5000 (e.g. myocardial infarction in older women from oral contraceptives)* | *1/10 000 (e.g. anaphylaxis from penicillin, halothane hepatitis)* | *1/50 000 (e.g. aplastic anaemia from chloramphenicol)* |
| No. of patients in ADR study | | | | | | |
| 100 | 0.63 | 0.18 | 0.10 | 0.02 | 0.01 | 0.002 |
| 200 | 0.86 | 0.33 | 0.18 | 0.04 | 0.02 | 0.004 |
| 500 | 0.99 | 0.63 | 0.39 | 0.10 | 0.05 | 0.01 |
| 1000 | 0.99 | 0.86 | 0.63 | 0.18 | 0.10 | 0.02 |
| 2000 | 0.99 | 0.98 | 0.86 | 0.33 | 0.18 | 0.04 |
| 5000 | 0.99 | 0.99 | 0.99 | 0.63 | 0.39 | 0.10 |
| 10000 | 0.99 | 0.99 | 0.99 | 0.86 | 0.63 | 0.18 |
| Number of patients required to be 95% likely to observe = ADR | 300 | 1500 | 3000 | 15 000 | 30 000 | 150 000 |

To the extent that ADRs are rare events, it is reasonable to assume that their occurrence will follow a Poisson distribution. Accordingly, the likelihood (*Pr*) of observing an ADR is:

$$Pr = 1 - e^{-xy}$$

Where e is the natural log; x is the probability of an ADR in an individual patient and y is the number of patients who have been observed for possible ADRs.

This relationship is put in practical form in Table 1. The body of the table shows the likelihood of observing one or more ADRs whose true frequencies are shown at the top of each column when various numbers of patients (by rows) are studied. Thus, if one looked for a rare ADR whose true rate of occurrence was 1 in 1000 in a group of 500 patients, the likelihood of observing one or more instances of the ADR is only 0.39.

The bottom row of the table presents the same relationship in a different fashion and gives the number of patients who would have to be observed in order to be 95% sure of finding one or more ADRs of various true frequencies. It should be noted that an interesting relation emerges: the required number of patients is equal to three times the reciprocal of the true ADR rate.

Because some publications report, and some licensing bodies require, comparisons in the ADR rates of new drugs and the drugs they are replacing, Table 2 has been prepared. It shows, for samples of about 100 patients per group, the degree of difference in ADR rates that must be observed before one can confidently state that they are truly different. In addition to providing specific values, Table 2 also illustrates that, as ADRs become rarer, the relative (but not the absolute) difference in ADR rates must become greater to provide statistically significant results.

**Table 2** The degree of increase in the rate of ADRs that can be detected with 100 patients per treatment (with one-sided $\alpha = 0.05$ and $\beta = 0.10$)

| If the lower ADR rate is: | 1% | 2% | 3% | 4% | 5% |
|---|---|---|---|---|---|
| Then the higher ADR rate must be: | 9% | 12% | 14% | 16% | 18% |
| Difference | 9 times | 6 times | 4.7 times | 4 times | 3.6 times |

The entries in Tables 1 and 2 assume perfect compliance for all of the stages shown in Figure 1. The rest of this chapter will consider what happens when compliance is less than perfect.

## CLINICIANS' COMPLIANCE WITH MANUFACTURERS' PRESCRIBING RECOMMENDATIONS

Increasing failure to comply with manufacturers' prescribing recommendations will tend to increase the occurrence of ADRs. A drug may be prescribed in too high a dose or for too long; or for the wrong diagnosis or to the wrong patient; or with a second, incompatible drug; or without a search for early signs of drug toxicity. Some of these behaviours (dosing too high or for too long) will spuriously raise the *rate* of dose-dependent ADRs, whereas others (dosing the wrong patient or for the wrong disorders) merely increase their overall occurrence. Of course, non-compliance with manufacturers' prescribing recommendations can also occur in the reverse direction when clinicians prescribe too low a dose, or for too short a period of time. The rates of dose-related ADRs will correspondingly drop when such prescribing non-compliance occurs.

The frequency of prescribing non-compliance varies widely from regimen to regimen and drug to drug, and its effects depend upon whether the ADR in question is dose-related. Fottrell *et al.* reviewed 200 psychiatric in-patients in London, UK, and decided that roughly half were receiving unnecessary or excessive medication.[2] Whether such over-prescribing is responsible for increased ADRs is another matter, however, and Koch-Weser *et al.* have convincingly demonstrated the marked variation in opinions of seasoned clinical pharmacologists as to whether a given event in a given patient represented an ADR.[3]

With respect to the 'problem of numbers' and non-compliance prescribing, it follows that excessive doses for excessive periods of time will increase the rates of dose-related ADRs above those observed when proper regimens were prescribed, and that when non-compliance takes the form of prescribing for incorrect diagnoses that cannot benefit from the regimen, the question: does the treatment do more good than harm? will tend to be answered in the negative.

Can prescribing non-compliance be improved? Although we remain largely ignorant in this field, and although some investigators provide evidence that neither the embracing of new drugs nor the relinquishing of old ones is highly rational,[4] there is cause for hope. Achong *et al.* demonstrated that vigorous clinical teaching by clinical pharmacologists was able to reduce prescribing non-compliance for in-patient antibiotic use to one-half of its former level.[5] It thus appears likely that, as new knowledge about the extent and nature of prescribing non-compliance is generated, it can be translated directly into actions which will increase the benefit:risk ratio for our patients.

## PATIENT COMPLIANCE WITH MEDICATION REGIMENS

The writing of a prescription initiates a therapeutic adventure, the outcome of which can be profoundly influenced by the extent to which the patient's behaviour coincides with the health advice summarized in the prescription.

Knowledge of patient compliance with prescribed medical regimens has grown exponentially during the 1970s, and it is clear the low compliance must be considered in all aspects of medical endeavour, from the earliest testing of new drugs in human volunteers to their regular prescription in the provision of medical care.[1]

In usual ambulatory care settings, less than half of the patients will consume a full course of medication.[6] This figure applies both to acute and chronic treatments. For example, for 10-day courses of antibiotics, evidence of medication in the urine will be found in about 60% of patients from 3 to 6 days after prescription and as few as 8% at 9 days post-precription.[7] For long-term regimens such as those for hypertension, over half of the patients drop out of care entirely within a year of diagnosis[8] and of those who stay under medical supervision only about 50% take at least 80% of their prescribed medications.[9]

In clinical trials of new drugs, such levels of non-compliance can vastly increase the number of patients required to demonstrate a benefit of given magnitude, as is shown in Goldsmith's work, reproduced in Table 3.[10] Furthermore, differing compliance rates among the various treatment and control groups can seriously distort the outcome and interpretation of such trials.[11]

Various strategies can be utilized to overcome low compliance. In the ambulatory care sphere, these include instructional techniques,[12] and special forms of pill packaging designed to aid memory.[13] These are effective for short-term treatment,[14] but for chronic conditions other strategies must be adopted. Worthwhile interventions include increased supervision,[15] behaviour modification,[16] serum drug level monitoring,[17,18] and supervised parenteral drug administration.[19]

**Table 3** The effect of compliance on sample size*

| *Mean % compliance* | $\alpha =$ 0.05 | | 0.01 | |
|---|---|---|---|---|
| | $\beta = 0.15$ | 0.10 | 0.05 | 0.10 |
| 100 | 23† | 18 | 33 | 28 |
| 90 | 28 | 22 | 41 | 34 |
| 80 | 35 | 28 | 51 | 43 |
| 70 | 45 | 36 | 66 | 55 |
| 60 | 61 | 49 | 90 | 74 |
| 50 | 88 | 70 | — | 106 |
| 40 | — | 180 | — | — |

*Reproduced from Goldsmith.[10]

†Numbers refer to the required sample size for each of two groups of hypertensive patients where the standard deviation of blood-pressure reduction was 10 mmHg ($\sigma$) and the minimum clinically significant difference in mean blood-pressures between the two groups was 10 mmHg ($\delta$).

In clinical trials in which the efficacy of a drug is at issue, one or more of the above may be applied to advantage or an entirely different tactic can be applied: barring entry of low compliers to the trial. The Veterans Administration trial of antihypertensive therapy[20] provides a notable example of this tactic. In this study, half of the potential participants were excluded for evidence of low compliance during a pre-trial 'faintness-of-heart' period in which compliance was assessed by attendance, pill counts and urinary determinations of riboflavin which had been incorporated into placebo tablets as a compliance marker. The advantages of screening out non-compliers in the pre-trial phase of an investigation are obvious: the efficacy of a new agent can be tested efficiently and without confounding non-response with non-compliance. The disadvantages of this manoeuvre is obvious as well: the results of the trial will not apply to non-compliers who, as we have stated may well be the majority of patients.

In the stages of drug investigation prior to approval for general use, the likelihood of detecting an undesirable effect of a drug depends upon several factors, such as the nature of the side-effect, the vigour of the search for it, the type of subjects or patients selected for the studies of the drug, and so on. Compliance can interfere with the detection of side-effects in other important ways as well. First, patients who consume more of the drug than prescribed may develop toxic effects without it being apparent that they have exceeded the effective and safe dose. It might well be argued, however, that drugs with high therapeutic-toxic ratios are not desirable, and that such patients have unwittingly performed a service for the investigator. Furthermore, 'over-compliance' seldom occurs in non-psychiatric circumstances. Thus, this form of non-compliance is, for practical purposes, not an important problem.

Second, low compliance, a very common problem, can reduce the frequency of an ADR so that the opportunity for detecting it in a clinical trial will be reduced. Simply stated, if an ADR occurs less frequently than the intended effect of a drug, and if only sufficient numbers of patients are recruited to detect the intended effect, then the ADR may bear the label of 'not statistically' significantly more frequent in the treated than in the control group, no matter how clinically important it might be. However, because low compliance will also reduce the frequency of occurrence of the intended effect of the drug, it will not alter the *relative* likelihood of the detection of the ADR compared with that of the intended effect. Thus, while low compliance can play havoc with the number of subjects required for an investigation it does not alter the ability to uncover an ADR any more than it does the ability to determine the intended effect of the drug.

Once the drug has been approved for use, having passed all stages of testing, the need to continue to assess the drug for infrequent but important ADRs can be realized only by surmounting formidable barriers. These include: lack of the ability to control patient selection, lack of appropriate control groups and lack of control of confounding variables (such as other interacting drugs or co-morbid medical conditions). All of these barriers are familiar to those involved in drug monitoring. However, because of the recent and rapid development of knowledge about patient compliance, the role of compliance in raising and lowering these barriers may not be so familiar.

Taking as a reference point the amount of drug required to achieve a therapeutic response, patients can be classified as over-compliers, irregular compliers and under-compliers. Over-compliers can exhibit toxic effects of a drug which would not be apparent at the recommended therapeutic dose. Some irregular compliers could also suffer such effects if they double-up on doses after they have missed a dose, or increase their dose when they are feeling symptoms from their illness. On the other hand, low or non-compliers would be subject to fewer or no side-effects from the medication, but might have intercurrent complaints which could be misinterpreted as side-effects. Adverse events during over-compliance certainly can be regarded as toxic effects – but the contribution of excess dosage to their occurrence will not be apparent unless compliance is known. Similarly, events during undercompliance might be misinterpreted as ADRs but have nothing at all to do with the drug; again a point which may be missed if compliance is unknown. The only way to make the necessary distinction here is to measure compliance when a suspicious event occurs; this is rarely done.

The relationships between patient compliance and the occurrence of ADRs are largely theoretical because studies bearing directly on these relationships have not been reported. However, some pertinent and interesting indirect evidence is available. First, as all those who are familiar with ADR monitoring in placebo-controlled trials will know, 'side-effects' often occur as frequently among those taking placebo as those prescribed the active drug. Table 4 illustrates the results of a search for side-effects in the Veteran's Administration study of antihypertensive agents. Virtually all 'side-effects' with the exception of orthostatic hypotension occurred as frequently among placebo-takers as among actively treated patients.[21]

The second evidence is derived from our own study of compliance among hypertensive steelworkers. Figure 2 shows a slight increase in the frequency of side-effect reports with increased compliance, but there is no level of compliance at which 'side-effects' cease. In this same study we measured absenteeism following the screening and labelling of individuals as hypertensive, and were astonished to find that absenteeism rose dramatically among non-compliant patients, but not at all among those who were compliant.[22] Thus it would appear that simply labelling a person as having a disease can affect their self-perception and behaviour and can result in actions which, on the surface, might be attributed to medications which have been prescribed but which, in fact, are more common among those not actually taking the medication.

The foregoing considerations tend to lead to over-statement of the

**Table 4** Frequency of specific side-effects in the Veterans Administration placebo-controlled trial of antihypertensive therapy*

| | *Placebo-treated group* (%) | *Actively treated group* (%) |
|---|---|---|
| Nightmares | 8 | 3 |
| Depression | 9 | 7 |
| Skin rash | 7 | 8 |
| Arthritis | 32 | 24 |
| Impotence | 22 | 21 |
| Angina | 18 | 9 |
| Headache | 21 | 8 |
| Ulcer symptoms | 9 | 8 |
| Lethargy or weakness | 17 | 20 |
| Nasal stuffiness | 21 | 16 |
| Orthostatic hypotension | 16 | 53 |
| Other complaints | 34 | 31 |
| Any complaints | 63 | 78 |

*Adapted from Veterans Administration.[21]

role of drugs in reported ADRs. However, many drugs do cause important side-effects and another development in the area of compliance is of great importance in this respect. The recent interest in, and concern about, poor compliance has led to the development of a variety of successful strategies for improving it, as enumerated earlier.

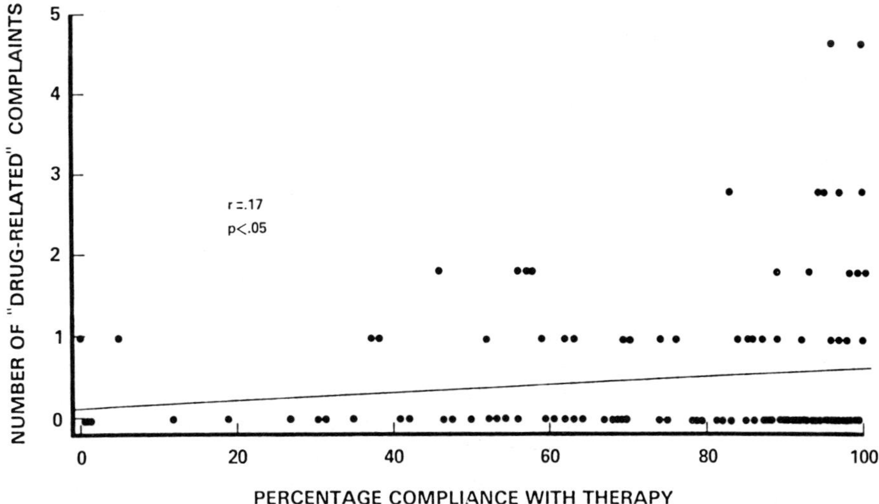


**Figure 2**

To the extent that these strategies improve compliance and are utilized by practitioners, the incidence of ADRs can be expected to rise. Three issues related to this are germane to the current discussion. First, while it might seem undesirable to have more ADRs, these should be outweighed by increased benefits when the drugs are efficacious. Second, unacceptable ADRs from a drug, which are not detected before marketing, will be found earlier in the post-marketing phase when compliance is improved; the 'problem of numbers' declines. Third, if we ever achieve full compliance with ambulatory medication programmes (an unlikely prospect) compliance will cease to require extensive and expensive attention in monitoring drugs for ADRs in the early marketing phase of drug development.

While it is obvious that information about compliance can be of vital importance to the generation and correct interpretation of adverse effect claims, at least one major barrier stands in the way of realization of the benefits of this information. Since the marketing of a new drug precedes the availability of methods of measuring the concentration of the drug in body fluids, the clinician reporting adverse effects has no direct way of measuring compliance. The indirect methods available to the clinician are, unfortunately, inferior or unsatisfactory in many respects.[23] To compound the difficulty, clinicians themselves consistently overrate the compliance of their patients and despite confidence in their assessments, are unable to estimate compliance with better than chance accuracy.[24]

Useful information can be gained, however, from a variety of alternative sources. One simple method is to ask patients themselves. It has been repeatedly shown that about half of non-compliant patients will admit to low compliance on direct questioning, and that this information is virtually never false.[25] Thus, apparent ADRs occurring among confessed non-compliers can be appropriately disregarded at the outset as drug-related.

Other methods can be applied to determine compliance among patients who deny non-compliance on questioning. One method is to have the patient return all remaining medications and compare these with the amount of medication prescribed since the time of dispensing. This method is probably not much more reliable than simply asking the patient, however, as the patient who wishes to conceal his non-compliance can easily remove the appropriate amount of medications without actually consuming them. A third method of measurement is to assess the patient's response to some known physiological or chemical effect of the drug (such as lowered heart rate for propranolol or reduced uric acid for sulphinpyrazone). Frequently, however, these efforts have not proven even as reliable as a verbal reports or pill counts.[26] The inevitable suggestion arising from this litany of measurement woes is that drug manufacturers, at the time of marketing a new drug, publish techniques for measuring the drug in body fluid levels. This could even extend to alerting local labs and clinical pharmacologists as to how and where to send body fluid specimens when ADRs are suspected. The resulting information would obviously need to be interpreted in the context of the clinical situation and last time of claimed drug intake, but could greatly improve our understanding of adverse drug effects.

## PATIENT COMPLIANCE WITH REQUESTS TO REPORT ADRs TO THEIR CLINICIANS

Although much of the foregoing section applies here, the reporting of ADRs by patients to their clinicians deserves special comment. For this portion of the ascertainment sequence to be successfully completed, three preliminary stages must transpire, as shown in Figure 1: first, the ADR must occur in the form of a sign or symptom; second, the sign of symptom must be perceived by the patient (if not, it is up to the clinician to elicit the former and recognize the latter); finally, the patient must attribute the sign or symptom to the drug: it is only then that reporting can occur.

Viewed from these perspectives it can be seen that variations in patient-reporting compliance can profoundly affect the ascertainment of ADRs in either direction. If patients incorrectly attribute signs or symptoms due to disease progression, co-morbidity or labelling to the drug being taken, a false positive rise in the apparent risk of ADRs may follow. Conversely, if true ADRs are not perceived by patients or are incorrectly attributed to co-morbidity or any other extraneous source, a false negative decrease in the apparent risk of ADR will result.

It is clear that compliance with actual or implied requests to patients to report ADRs to their clinicians can be profoundly influenced by the fashion in which this information is requested. For example, Bulpitt *et al.* compared direct interviews with home-completed questionnaires and found that in only 28% of the former, as opposed to 47% of the latter, did patients on various antihypertensive regimens admit to impotence;[27] moreover, it is reasonable to suggest that such a symptom would be rarely volunteered without solicitation. Thus, one can anticipate sharp differences in the rates of reported ADRs (and in the numbers of patients required to establish their occurrence), depending on whether patients were required to volunteer their symptoms, on the one hand, or had specific symptoms elicited from them by interview or by questionnaire, on the other.

## CLINICIAN COMPLIANCE WITH REQUIREMENTS TO REPORT ADRs

In common with the foregoing reporting-compliance for patients, clinicians must both perceive that an adverse event has occurred and attribute the event to a drug before they are even 'at risk' of complying with the requirement that the ADR be reported. As with patients, misconceptions and misperceptions can distort the reporting of ADRs by clinicians, and can therefore produce both false positive elevations and false negative decreases in apparent ADR risks. In view of this, and recalling that Koch-Weser *et al.* demonstrated substantial disagreement about the attribution of possible ADRs among seasoned clinical pharmacologists,[3] it is not surprising that some authorities have suggested that clinical participants in randomized trials record *all* events and use the subsequent data analysis to identify and attribute ADRs.[28]

Even if clinicians were both accurate and compliant in reporting ADRs, however, the resulting information would be seriously deficient because it would be confined to numerators (ADRs) without denominators (the numbers of patients who had received the drug in question). It is for this reason, as well as the realization that both the accuracy and reporting-compliance of clinicians is low, that other basically different approaches have been proposed for obtaining incidence data on ADRs. These approaches, including hospital-based drug surveillance and the 'recorded release' of new drugs,[29] are described in detail elsewhere in this book. Such systems offer substantial promise for overcoming both patient-and clinician-based compliance problems in the detection and reporting of ADRs.

## References

1. Haynes, R. B., Taylor, D. W. and Sackett, D. L. (eds.) (1979). *Compliance in Health Care* (Baltimore: Johns Hopkins University Press)
2. Fottrell, E., Sheikh, M. and Kothari, R. (1976). Long-stay patients with long-stay drugs: a case for review: a cause for concern, *Lancet*, **1**, 81
3. Koch-Weser, J., Sellers, E. M., and Zacest, R. (1977). The ambiguity of adverse drug reactions, *Eur. J. Clin. Pharmacol.*, **11**, 75
4. Mapes, R. E. A. (1977). Physician's drug innovation and relinquishment. *Soc. Sci. Med.*, **11**, 619
5. Achong, M. R., Wood, J., Theal, H. K., Goldberg, R. and Thompson, D. A. (1977). *Lancet*, **2**, 1118
6. Sackett, D. L. and Snow, J. C. (1979). The magnitude of compliance and noncompliance. In Haynes, R. B., Taylor, D. W. and Sackett, D. L. (eds.) *Compliance in Health Care*, pp. 11–22. (Baltimore: Johns Hopkins University Press).
7. Bergman, A. B. and Werner, R. J. (1963). Failure of children to receive penicillin by mouth. *N. Engl. J. Med.*, **268**, 1334
8. Wilber, J. A. and Barrow, J. G. (1969). Reducing elevated blood pressure: experience found in a community. *Minn. Med.*, **52**, 1303
9. Sackett, D. L. Haynes, R. B., Gibson, E. S., Hackett, B. C., Taylor, D. W., Roberts, R. S. and Johnson, A. L. (1975). Randomized clinical trial of strategies for improving medication compliance in primary hypertension. *Lancet*, **1**, 1205
10. Goldsmith, C. H. (1979). The effect of compliance distributions on therapeutic trials. In Haynes, R. B., Taylor, D. W. and Sackett, D. L. (eds.) *Compliance in Health Care*, pp. 297–308. (Baltimore: Johns Hopkins University Press)
11. Feinstein, A. L. (1979). Compliance bias and the interpretation of therapeutic trials. In Haynes, R. B., Taylor, D. W. and Sackett, D. L. (eds.) *Compliance in Health Care*, pp. 309–22. (Baltimore: Johns Hopkins University Press)

12. Colcher, I. S. and Bass, J. W. (1972). Penicillin treatment in streptococcal pharyngitis: a comparison of schedules and the role of specific counselling. *J. Am. Med. Assoc.*, **222,** 657
13. Linkewich, J. A., Cataland, R. B. and Flack, H. L. (1974). The effect of packaging and instruction on outpatient compliance with medication regimens. *Drug Intell. Clin. Pharmacy*, **8,** 10
14. Haynes, R. B. (1979). Strategies to improve compliance with referrals, appointment and prescribed medical regimens. In Haynes, R. B., Taylor, D. W. and Sackett, D. L. (eds.) *Compliance in Health Care* (Baltimore: Johns Hopkins University Press)
15. McKenney, J. M., Slining, J. M., Henderson, H .R., Devins, D. and Barr, M. (1973). The effect of clinical pharmacy services on patients with essential hypertension. *Circulation*, **48,** 1104
16. Haynes, R. B., Sackett, D. L., Gibson, E. S., Taylor, D. W., Hackett, B. C., Roberts, R. S. and Johnson, A. L. (1976). Improvement of medication compliance in uncontrolled hypertension. *Lancet*, **1,** 1265
17. Lund, M., Jorgenson, R. S. and Kuhl, V. (1964). Serum diphenylhydantoin (phenytoin) in ambulant patients with epilepsy. *Epilepsia*, **5,** 51
18. Eney, R. D. and Goldstein, E. O. (1976). Compliance of chronic asthmatics with oral administration of theophylline as measured by serum and salivary levels. *Pediatrics*, **57,** 513
19. Johnson, D. and Freeman, H. (1972). Long-acting tranquillizers. *Practitioner*, **208,** 395
20. Veterans Administration Co-operative Study Group on Antihypertensive Agents (1967). Effects of treatment on morbidity in hypertension: Results in patients with diastolic pressure averaging 115 through 129 mm Hg. *J. Am. Med. Assoc.*, **202,** 1028
21. Veterans Administration Cooperative Study Group on Antihypertensive Agents (1972). Effects of treatment on morbidity in hypertension: influence of age, diastolic pressure, and prior cardiovascular disease: further analysis of side effects. *Circulation*, **45,** 991
22. Haynes, R. B., Sackett, D. L., Taylor, D. W., Gibson, E. S. and Johnson, A. L. (1978). Increased absenteeism from work following detection and labelling of hypertension. *N. Engl. J. Med.* **299,** 741–4
23. Gordis, L. (1979). Conceptual and methodologic problems in measuring patient compliance. In Haynes, R. B., Taylor, D. W. and Sackett, D. L. (eds.) *Compliance in Health Care*, pp. 23–45. (Baltimore: Johns Hopkins University Press)
24. Muchlin, A. I. (1972). A study of physicians ability to predict patient compliance. *Masters thesis*. Johns Hopkins University, Baltimore, Md
25. Sackett, D. L., Haynes, R. B., Gibson, E. S. and Johnson, A. L. (1976). The problem of compliance with antihypertensive therapy. *Pract. Cardiol.*, **1,** 35
26. Sackett, D. L., Taylor, D. W., Haynes, R. B., Gibson, E. S. and Johnson, A. L. (1978). Can simple clinical measurements detect non-compliance? Abstract. *Clin. Res.*, **26,** 487A
27. Bulpitt, C. J., Dollery, C. T. and Carne, S. (1974). A symptom questionnaire for hypertensive patients. *J. Chron. Dis.*, **27,** 309
28. Skegg, D. C. G. and Doll, R. (1977). The case for recording events in clinical trials. *Br. Med. J.*, **1523**
29. Inman, W. H. W. (1977). Recorded release. In Gross, F. H. and Inman, W. H. W. (eds.) *Drug Monitoring*, pp. 65–78. (London: Academic Press)

# 35
# Judgement, drug monitoring and decision aids

R. M. HOGARTH

---

*Neither hand nor mind, left to themselves, amounts to much; instruments and aids are the means to perfection.* Francis Bacon

## INTRODUCTION

Judgement is a pervasive, indeed inescapable, human activity. For instance, as you read this chapter you are probably making three kinds of implicit judgement. First, you are making a prediction concerning, for example, how long it will take you to read the chapter or whether you might learn something in doing so. Second, you are making an evaluative judgement, for instance in respect of your interest in the subject-matter. And third, you will be making a decision, based on your prediction and evaluation, as to whether you will go on to read the rest of this chapter, now, later, or perhaps never.

This example of a decision to read this chapter now, later or never, illustrates two key aspects of decision processes. First, decisions depend – or at least should depend – on the answers to two questions:[1] (1) What is at stake? (In the example here knowledge or ideas from the chapter relative to other uses of your time): and (2) What are the uncertainties? (In this instance, perhaps how long it will take you to read the chapter and/or whether you believe, *a priori*, that the effort of reading will be rewarded.) Second, your decision will be reached by balancing your judgements of the 'stakes' and the uncertainties – usually in some intuitive manner. Indeed, in most decisions, both important and trivial, all three operations – predictive judgements, evaluative judgements and operations on them – are performed intuitively.

The purpose of this chapter is to consider the role of intuitive judgement in drug monitoring by providing an overview of relevant work in the psychology of judgement. The chapter will be primarily concerned with the quality of judgement and seek to exploit findings pertinent to the above questions, namely: How good are people at making intuitive predictions and evaluations? How well can they balance these elements in making decisions? And how can they be helped to perform these tasks better?

It should be emphasized, however, that the chapter is not an exhaustive review of the judgemental literature related to medicine and problems of drug monitoring in particular. There are several useful discussions of judgement in medicine;[2–7] and a number of pertinent reviews of the judgemental literature.[8–11]

The chapter is organized as follows: in the second section I discuss, in quite general terms, the nature and context of human judgement. This is followed in the third section by a discussion of the literature relating to how people select, weigh and combine information for judgemental purposes. The source of the discussion is provided by studies which have examined how people make intuitive judgements in situations where judgements can be compared with normative standards. Analysis of errors people make reveal systematic biases in judgement as well as some understanding of the underlying judgemental process itself. In the fourth section, I shall argue that judgemental processes should be made both explicit and public – in so far as this is possible. I further discuss and provide examples of the concepts underlying a number of judgemental aids which have been used successfully in many diverse fields, including medicine. The final section of the paper summarizes conclusions and makes suggestions concerning the use of judgemental aids in the field of drug monitoring.

The underlying thesis of this chapter is the following: The intuitive processes involved in judgement are amenable to scientific study. Furthermore, it is incumbent upon such study to assess human capabilities in order to find ways of improving judgement (see the quote from Bacon above).

## THE CONTEXT OF JUDGEMENT

Judgements are operations on information. It is therefore appropriate to consider the nature of the human information-processing system. Extensive work in this area over recent decades has produced at least two firm conclusions:[9] first, people have limited information-processing capacity; and second, they are adaptive. That is, the nature of the judgemental task with which a person is faced determines to a large extent how the person can deal with the task (this notion will be explained below). Consequently, to understand the bases of judgement, it is necessary to have a clear notion of human possibilities and limitations relative to judgemental tasks.

There are four major consequences of limited human information-processing capacity. First, perception of information is limited. It has been estimated, for instance, that about only one-seventieth of what is present in the visual field can be perceived at one time. We are literally bombarded with information and have to select; however, to select it is necessary to know what to select. *Anticipations* therefore play a large role in what we actually do see.

Second, since people cannot simultaneously integrate a great deal of information, processing is mainly done in a *sequential* manner. This can, of course, be misleading in the sense that the actual sequence in which information is processed may bias a person's judgement. Furthermore, since we receive most of our information across time, temporal contiguity of information is often an important clue used to infer causality[12] – for example, observation of a reaction following the administration of a drug.

Third, limited processing capacity means that people lack the mental capacity to make what might be termed 'optimal' intuitive calculations. They, therefore, resort to simpler mental strategies, some of which will be illustrated below.

Fourth, people have limited memory capacity. Although there is uncertainty concerning how memory processes actually work, current theorizing supports the notion that memory works by a process of associations which reconstruct past events. That is, unlike a computer which can assess information intact in its original form (i.e. as input), human memory actively reconstructs on the basis of fragments of information. Memory can, therefore, change, depending upon what and how reconstruction takes place.

It would be misleading, however, to think of humans simply as inefficient computers. People have emotions, they can reverse thought-chains in ways that computers cannot and have powers of imagination and creativity that computers lack. People also strive to go beyond the information they receive; they are inquisitive and they experiment. On the other hand, limited information-processing capacity forces people to simplify and structure their environment in order to make sense of it. This is particularly the case when making judgements in the form of predictions or anticipations. People seek to give meaning to what they observe and to impose patterns which may be useful for prediction. As will be illustrated below, they also frequently have a tendency to believe that a pattern exists even when there is none. This can lead both to judgemental errors and illusions of judgemental ability.

The importance of the task in judgement can be illustrated by the following, admittedly simplified situation. Imagine that you use an information source, for example a test of some kind, to predict the safety of a drug and you wish to determine the relationship between results of the test and actual safety. If you were free to experiment and to apply both the test and the drug to a wide range of patients, then the relationship between test results and safety could be represented by the ellipse shown in Figure 1. First, it should be noted that the accuracy of your judgement (based on the test) is represented by the

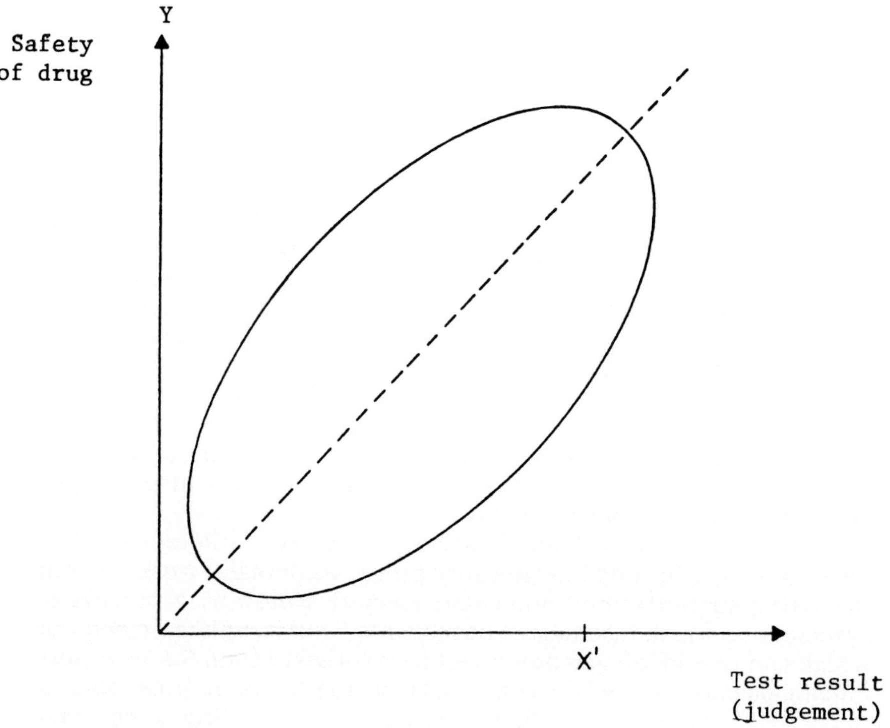


**Figure 1** Relationship between test result (judgement) and safety of drug

shape and size of the ellipse. If the test were 100% accurate, the relationship would be represented by a straight line (the dotted line in the figure). If it were less accurate than shown here, the ellipse would be wider; and indeed, if there were no relationship between the test and actual safety the ellipse would be circular in appearance.

Two factors affect the shape of the ellipse and thus determine the predictive ability of the test. First, there is the inherent predictive validity of the test; second, its reliability, by which is operationally meant the extent to which the test yields the same results on independent occasions under identical circumstances (in other words lack of reliability implies random error in the test).

The fact that cues and outcomes (e.g. test results and actual drug safety) are not perfectly related has the following implications. Consider the point X′ on the axis representing the test result in Figure 1, and ask yourself what the actual level of safety associated with this test score is likely to be. The situation is illustrated in Figure 2. If the predictive ability of the test were 100% accurate, the outcome would be the point Y′ on the axis representing actual safety. However, note that outcomes associated with a score of X′ or more on the test must fall in either the area marked A or B. Furthermore the area A is smaller

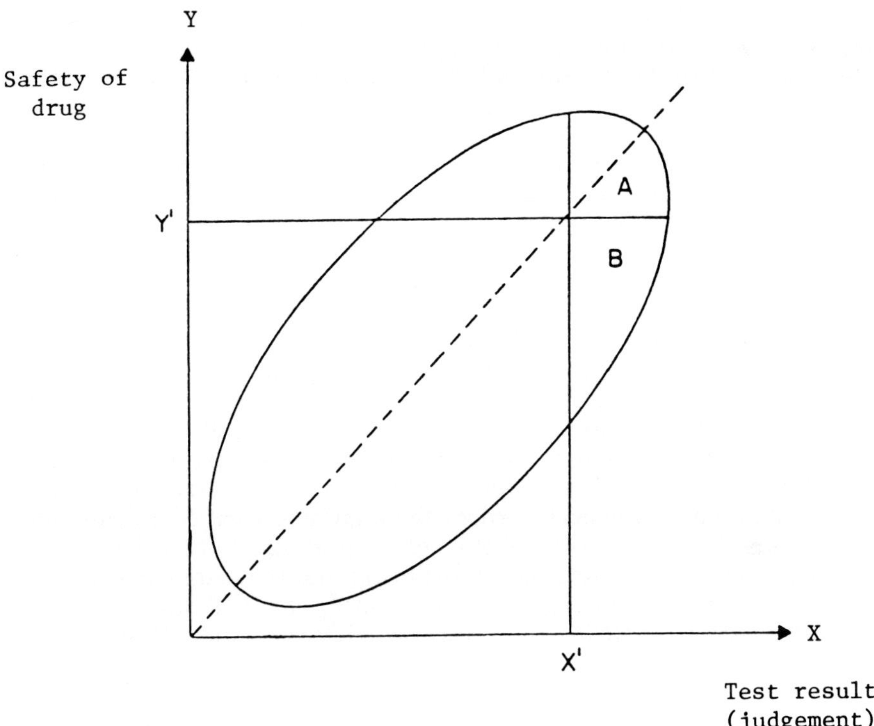


**Figure 2** Illustration of 'regression phenomenon'. Outcomes associated with test results of X′ or greater are more likely to be below Y′ than above it (i.e. B > A)

than B. Thus there is a greater chance that the actual outcome will be below Y′ (i.e. *less* safe) than above it.

The situation depicted here is technically known as the 'regression phenomenon'. Extreme values of cues used for prediction will usually be accompanied by less extreme outcomes, and this is particularly the case when cues (e.g. tests) lack reliability. Although predictions should clearly be moderated by such considerations, empiricial evidence indicates that people often fail to make the necessary adjustments. In particular, they tend to overlook issues of data reliability.[11] Furthermore, people exhibit considerably more certainty when predicting on the basis of extreme test scores than they should.[13] A related issue concerns how people react to and interpret data which are observed across time, for example responses of patients to treatment, readings from medical instruments, performance by doctors or nurses, numbers of incidents of diseases or accidents in specified intervals of time, etc. Such data can often be characterized by random fluctuations around trends of varying complexity. However, trends and random fluctuations are difficult to distinguish by intuitive judgement, and people frequently misinterpret the nature and extent of random fluctuations. In one study for example, surgeons were found to be subject to the 'gambler's fallacy' in respect of rates of a certain post-operative complication.[14] Because the rate reported in the first 6 months of a year was 14%, as opposed to the usual annual average of about 20%, roughly half of 38 surgeons predicted a compensating 25% or 26% rate for the next 6 months. However, given the numbers of cases involved, a 14% rate in 6 months would not have been unusual for an annual average rate of about 20%.

Unnecessary errors can be committed when people base actions on erroneous causal explanations attributed to random fluctuations. This is particularly likely to be the case after the observation of an extreme value of a series. For example, consider that a patient's blood-pressure can be thought to oscillate irregularly around some average level. If blood-pressure is monitored regularly, occasional high or low levels will be observed. What is likely to happen after a patient exhibits exceptionally low (or high) blood-pressure on a particular occasion?

Assume that a physician orders the administration of a drug and subsequently observes the level of blood-pressure to be close to the normal average. Is he justified in believing that the drug has brought about the observed change? Not necessarily, for if fluctuations are indeed random, the next observation is highly likely to be closer to the average level anyway (i.e. low blood-pressure will probably increase, and high blood-pressure decrease). Although this is a contrived example, evidence of such misinterpretations in other fields suggests that medical analogues may well exist.[13,15] The implications concerning unnecessary use of drugs are evident.

A further point concerns the interpretation of results based on sample evidence. People have difficulty in understanding the degree of random fluctuations in samples and tend to believe that samples, and particularly small samples, are more representative of the populations they are drawn from than statistical theory prescribes.[16] Mathematically trained scientists have also been found to consider experimental results to have greater generality than should be the case,[17] and one study shows evidence of apprentice lab technicians being required by their instructors to show greater accuracy in blood-cell counts than was feasible given the amount of sampling variation.[18] Similarly, several instances of misinterpretation and abuse of laboratory test results by physicians have been documented.[19]

It is important to emphasize that judgement leads to actions.[3,20] Consider Figure 3 which reproduces the test-drug safety situation described above. However, on this occasion the diagram has been modified to allow for the fact that the drug is only administered to patients for whom the test indicates that it is safe. This is shown by drawing a vertical line through the point X′ on the test-axis to mark the cut-off point on the test result. That is, patients whose test results exceed X′ are administered the drug, those with scores lower than X′ do not receive it. Similarly, a horizontal line has been drawn through

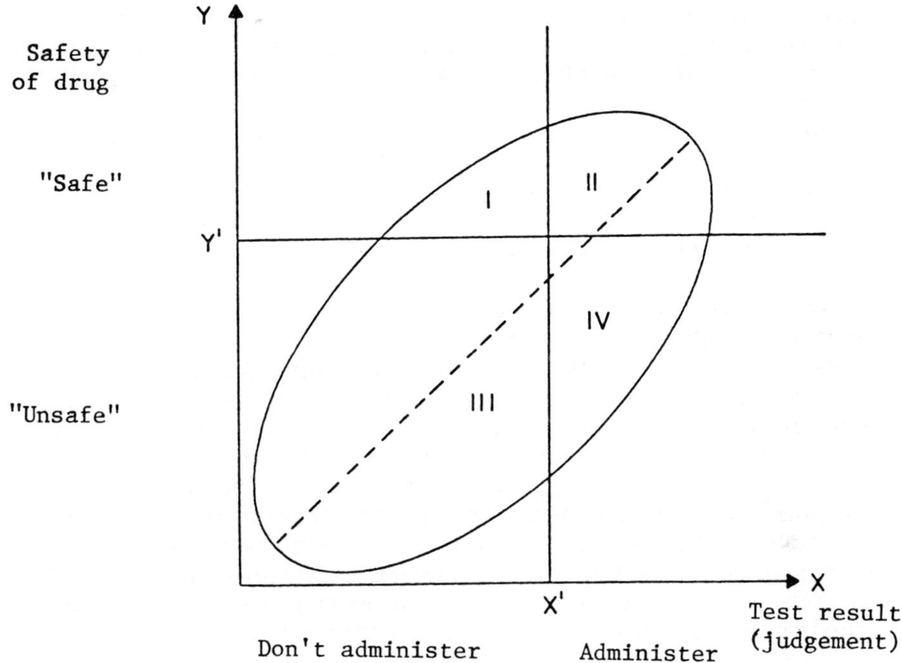


**Figure 3** Effects on test–safety relationship by choice of a cut-off on the test, X′. Quadrants I and III are unobservable

the point Y′ to indicate the point at which the drug actually proves to be safe or unsafe. The horizontal and vertical lines divide the ellipse into four quadrants and these are now discussed from the viewpoints of assessing the test–safety relationship and the physician's ability to understand and learn from the judgemental situation.

The effect of actions being dependent on judgements is that test–outcome combinations to the left of X′ (i.e. quadrants I and III) are not observable. Consequently the only feedback the physician can have concerning the predictive ability of the test is from quadrants II and IV – for example a comparison of II with IV, or II relative to II and IV, etc.

A second point concerns the positions of the cut-off points on both axes, i.e. X′ and Y′. If the cut-off on the test is made more stringent by moving it to the right, this increases the size of quadrant II relative to quadrant IV and the physician will see *relatively* more successful outcomes. The contrary will occur if the cut-off on the test is moved to the left (i.e. when it becomes less stringent). Similarly, movements of the criterion of safe *vs.* unsafe outcomes, i.e. Y′, will change the nature of what the physician will be able to observe. The above situation can, of course, be further complicated when something occurs subsequent to the test but prior to the outcome. For example, the fact that a patient is given treatment may by itself affect the outcome irrespective of the therapeutic properties of the drug. In this event, the observable relationship between test and outcome is complicated even further.[21]

A number of points made above need to be emphasized. First, assuming that the action of giving a drug to a patient does not by itself induce effects unrelated to the drug, the true relationship between test and outcomes can only be ascertained by having information on all four quadrants in Figure 3. However, the physician is only able to make an assessment of the relationship by considering quadrants II and IV. This kind of situation is not, however, uncommon in judgement, and laboratory experiments have shown that even when people receive information on all four quadrants (sequentially as in most realistic situations) they judge the strength of relationship by the frequency of 'positive hits', i.e. the number of observations in quadrant II[22–25]. Furthermore some studies document instances of ignoring the negative feedback implicit in quadrant IV.[26,27] The judgemental literature has also indicated several instances of people having erroneous notions of the extent to which variables covary – the phenomenon of so-called 'illusory correlation'.[28] Given the nature of the task, as illustrated here, this is not surprising. People do not learn from information they do not observe; furthermore, they are not used to seeking information which they do not have the habit of observing. An additional point is that people frequently seek evidence to support their ideas (e.g. hypotheses concerning relationships) rather than attempting to find data that could disconfirm them.[29]

A further issue concerns the location of the cut-offs, Y′ and X′. The physician is often able to control X′ and where he places this should depend on his attitude towards two kinds of errors (assuming he is aware of the situation!): first, observations in quadrant I – people for whom the drug would have been safe but did not receive it – and second, quadrant IV. Unless there is experience with outcomes associated with the whole range of test results, it is difficult to estimate this trade-off of errors. On the other hand, Y′, the cut-off on actual safety, is usually not under the control of the physician (subject to changes of definition) nor is it usually known to him. However, this is crucial, for irrespective of the predictive ability of the test it has a direct bearing on the number of 'successes' the physician will observe. When the effects of drugs are not well known, and particularly in early stages of monitoring, the above considerations are particularly important.

Above, I have tried to indicate some of the factors that affect learning relationships for judgemental purposes and, concurrently, learning about one's own judgemental ability. Although the description made of the task situation was essentially static, it is important to realize that judgement takes place in a dynamic environment. That is, in the situation depicted in Figure 3, it should be noted that the initial judgement of the level at which the drug is supposed to be safe in itself sets off a series of events which eventually affect subsequent judgements. Consider the following sequence: A physician assesses a drug to be safe at a particular dose for a particular class of patients. That judgement leads to an action which is to administer (or perhaps not administer) the drug; the subsequent outcome of the treatment on the patient – *as perceived and interpreted by the physician* – leads to an assessment of the effectiveness of the drug which, in turn, leads to it being either prescribed again or not, which again leads to feedback, etc. In other words, judgements are made in dynamic environments and both affect, and are affected by, the setting in which they occur.

This point is nicely illustrated by the case of Benjamin Rush, a highly respected physician and professor at the first medical school in America. Rush believed in the theory that febrile illnesses resulted from an excess stimulation and excitement of the blood and he advocated and practised blood-letting as a cure.[30] When he fell ill with yellow fever, he instructed that he be bled plentifully.

> From illness and treatment combined, he almost died; his convalescence was prolonged. That he did recover persuaded him that his methods were correct . . . Neither dedication so great that he risked his life to minister to others, nor willingness to treat himself as he treated others, nor yet the best education to be had in his day was sufficient to prevent Rush from committing grievous harm in the name of good. Convinced of the correctness of his theory of medicine and lacking a means for the systematic study of treatment outcome, he attributed each new instance of improvement to the efficacy of his treatment and each new death that occurred despite it to the severity of the disease (p. 1106).

To summarize this section, the picture of human judgemental activity I have depicted is the following: The context of judgement is one of a three-element system involved in mutual interaction. There is the person; actions that result from judgements made by the person; and the environment in which judgements, actions and their outcomes take place and are intepreted by the individual.[31] That is, each of the elements affects and is affected by the others, a good example of this being the case of Benjamin Rush discussed above.

When one considers the information-processing capacity of the person within the three-element system, the picture is one of a selective, essentially sequential information processor with limited powers of 'computation' and memory. Although people have the ability to be creative and do seek to understand, control and master their environment, unaided intuitive judgement is a relatively weak form of comprehending many judgemental situations. Indeed, the potential weakness of unaided judgement has recently been emphasized by Hammond who has distinguished 'six modes of inquiry' people use to learn about the world.[32] These vary from formal experimentation to 'quasi-experiments' to unaided judgement, and can be evaluated on six dimensions as illustrated in Figure 4: (1) type of thought; (2) degree

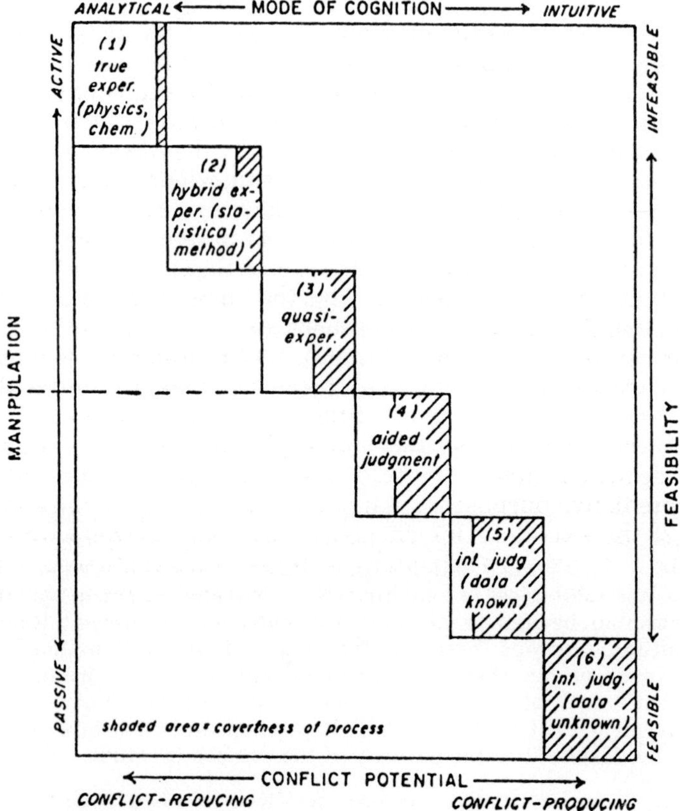


**Figure 4** Matrix of 'modes of thought' (From Ref. 4)

of manipulation of variables; (3) feasibility of such manipulation; (4) potential for evoking interpersonal conflict; (5) covertness; and (6) difficulty of interpersonal learning.[4] As can be seen from this diagram, although intuitive judgement is the most feasible (it can be applied in all circumstances) it also allows for the least possible manipulation of variables and has the greatest potential for conflict (an issue to be discussed below). To this should be added the point that not only does intuitive judgement lack the ability to manipulate variables, it may often lack awareness of important variables.[21]

## SELECTING, WEIGHTING AND COMBINING INFORMATION IN JUDGEMENT

Predictive and evaluative judgements are usually based on a combination of different information sources. For example, the initial impression of the possibility of an adverse drug reaction (ADR) could be moderated by an assessment of a particular patient's condition. A judgement about one drug might be made by comparing it to another drug with which the physician is familiar.

As should be expected from the preceding discussion of limitations of the human information-processing system, combination of different sources of information is difficult. Consider what needs to be done. Information from the environment and/or the individual's memory needs to be selected. Meaning is given to the information and, indeed, such meaning may even guide the search process in the first instance. The different sources of information selected then have to be weighted and combined to form a final judgement. It is clear that in many instances people do not have the mental capacity to perform these operations in the manner of a computer. Consequently they employ mental strategies to simplify the judgemental task and to be able to deal with several information sources. In this section, some of these strategies and their consequences are explored. The following aspects are specifically considered: (1) evidence on how people select information for predictive purposes – that is the 'cues' on which judgement is based; (2) the extent to which people are able to weight different information sources appropriately in judgement; and (3) biases due to memory. In much of what follows, the efficacy of intuitive human judgement will be compared to normative standards based on statistical reasoning.

## Information selection

Judgement is not made in a vacuum. Rather, predictions, for example of whether a particular drug will have an adverse reaction, are based on operations (e.g. comparisons) with other information, either observable or imaginary. Consequently, it is important to consider how these cues for prediction are generated.

A dimension which has been suggested as important in this process is the extent to which cues are *available*.[33] Specifically, if you can imagine or see several instances of one kind of an event as opposed to another, this can lead you to believe that the former is more frequent than the latter. For example, if you were asked to estimate the divorce rate in your city, your estimate would probably be influenced by the number of people you know who are divorced. Indeed, in many instances judgement by availability will be quite effective in that frequently occurring events are more easily recalled than rare events. However, in some instances, the 'availability' strategy can lead to systematic biases.

For example, in experiments designed to test this judgemental strategy, people's intuitive notions of the relative frequency of various diseases or causes of death have been tested. Results indicate that the relative frequency of diseases or causes which are much publicized, such as homicide, cancer or tornadoes are over-estimated; whereas others, such as asthma, emphysema and diabetes are underestimated.[34]

Lest you think that physicians are immune to availability bias concerning medical judgements, they are not. In a particular hospital, surgeons working in different specialities characterized by high (2.42%) and low (0.44%) mortality rates were asked to assess different mortality rates. Whereas surgeons from both specialities correctly estimated that the mortality rate was higher in one group than in the other, assessments of the overall service mortality rate was biased by group membership. Specifically, surgeons in the high-mortality group estimated the overall rate to be double that estimated by the low-mortality surgeons.[14] A further study indicates a strong relationship between the order in which physicians generate diagnostic hypotheses and the probabilities attached to such hypotheses.[35]

These findings are particularly pertinent to problems of drug monitoring where the estimation of low-frequency events is prevalent and important. To the extent that judgement by availability is a common strategy, it suggests that physicians need to think very carefully about the specific instances they recall when making assessments of possible adverse reactions. To what extent are these specific instances representative of the class of drug-patient combinations about which a judgement needs to be made? This point is particularly relevant when one is aware of the non-representative manner in which reports of ADRs become available to physicians.[36]

An important factor in the selection of information is the causal framework within which a person is thinking.[37] For example, a physician examining a patient can reason in a number of ways. He can observe a symptom and then ask what the likelihood is that the patient has a particular disease. Alternatively, the physician can formulate a hypothesis about a particular disease and then ask what the probability is that the patient does or does not have the disease given observation, or non-observation of a specific symptom. Indeed, physicians probably use both forms of reasoning. For example, a patient presents symptoms and the physician reasons from symptoms to hypothesis of a disease; from hypothesis of the disease reasoning then leads to a search for further symptoms and so on.[38]

There are several elements involved in the inferential process described above. There are hypotheses (of particular diseases), and there are likelihoods that specific symptoms will be observed when certain diseases are present. Statistical theory provides a normative framework within which such aspects can be combined in an optimal manner (see Section 4 below). However, empirical evidence indicates that people's intuitive judgements tend to ignore certain information in such problems and even when it is known to be available to them.[13,39,40]

Tversky and Kahneman argue, and provide evidence consistent with their hypothesis, that people will differentially select and use information in judgement to the extent that they perceive it to be *causal, diagnostic* or *incidental*.[41] For example, consider you are investigating the observation of a reaction conditional upon a specific treatment. There are a number of ways you might think about this. First, you might consider a *causal* relationship: the patient suffered a reaction because of the treatment. Second, you could consider the treatment as *indicative* or *diagnostic* of the reaction; i.e. the administration of the treatment increases the probability that the observed reaction was related to it. And third, you might consider the evidence as *incidental*, that is neither as a cause nor even possible cause (i.e. indicative) of the adverse effect. Whereas human judgement selects and weights information according to the meaning given to it, normative statistical procedures do not. In probability theory, data are judged strictly on their *informativeness*. These biases and findings argue strongly for the policy of recording *incidents* in drug monitoring in order to avoid the vagaries of shades of meaning attributed by the human element.[36]

A related issue is the finding that information that is *concrete* (e.g. personal experience or observation of a treatment on a patient) can dominate information that is *abstract* (e.g. statistical reports of drug effectiveness) even though the latter may have greater predictive validity (i.e. reports are based on a greater number of cases)[42]. Knafl and Burkett document incidents of precisely this type of bias in medical judgement.[5]

An additional problem related to selection of information and the physician's beliefs is the following. If a physician believes that symptom Y implies disease X, he is unlikely to consider disease X when Y is absent.[43] There are usually just too many possible hypotheses to consider, and the initial observation of a symptom will automatically exclude a number of hypotheses.

Additional evidence pertinent to information-selection concerns how people tend to seek information to confirm hypotheses, even redundantly, rather than to seek information that could disprove their hypotheses and thus help them to seek more adequate explanations.[29,44] In many situations feedback from the environment is also inadequate – see for example the structure of some judgemental tasks discussed above (p. 487) and thus illusions can continue to exist about the hypotheses of interest, for example concerning a symptom–disease relationship[28] as well as the person's own judgemental ability.[21]

The different sources of information on which judgement is based can vary in the extent to which they are consistent. Statistical principles indicate that consistency of different information-sources is a valid cue for prediction in so far as the different information-sources are not redundant. Nonetheless, people do not seem to have a good intuitive notion of this principle and use consistency of data-sources – whether redundant or not – as a clue for determining confidence in judgement. A good example of this is provided in a study in which the judgements of clinical psychologists were studied as a function of information presented to them.[45] The psychologists were required to make predictions on the basis of a case-study. In addition, they were asked to state their degree of confidence in their judgements under different conditions of amount of information. Results indicated that as the amount of information about the case increased, so did the psychologists' confidence in their judgements. However, there was no corresponding increase in predictive accuracy.

How do people handle inconsistent information? One way is to downplay or ignore the inconsistent information, a finding that has been noted in several studies.[10,11,46] Consistency of information-sources is related to pattern and, as noted above (p. 487), pattern is an important clue in predictive activity.

The subjective salience of information can also be affected by the context in which judgement is made. For example, order of information presentation can produce so-called 'primacy' or 'recency' effects. That is, when being presented with a number of items of information, sometimes the earlier items dominate the individual's final opinion (a 'primacy' effect) and sometimes the latter (a 'recency' effect). From a normative viewpoint, however, it is clear that one should finish with the same opinion at the end of a series of data irrespective of the order of presentation. Furthermore, it appears that primacy and recency effects can be manipulated according to task characteristics.[10]

In addition to 'primacy' and 'recency' effects, too much information can reduce the consistency of a person's judgement;[47] simultaneous presentation of concrete data, e.g. figures, together with qualitative information causes difficulty with people tending to prefer one source to the exclusion of the other;[48] people find information presented with the use of negatives (e.g. 'not', 'no', etc.) instead of positive statements more difficult to process and understand;[29] seemingly complete presentations can blind people to the fact that important aspects of a problem have been omitted;[49] even if people do have appropriate statistical information they can be misled by the labels attached to cues.[50] The list of possible sources of judgemental biases seems interminable.

One commonly used judgemental strategy which is highly dependent on information presented or available to a person has been named 'adjustment and anchoring'.[51] An example will illustrate: Imagine that you wish to anticipate the effects of a drug on a particular person. How would you do it? A common strategy would be to use a cue such as another person who has been given the drug, or a similar drug, as a starting-point – or 'anchor' – and then to make adjustments from the anchor related to specific circumstances of the case under consideration. The dangers of the 'adjustment and anchoring' strategy lie both in the way the original anchor is generated, and people's reluctance to make sufficient adjustments away from the starting-point. This has been dramatically demonstrated in a number of experiments involving judgements about uncertain quantities.[51] The experimenter artificially generated an anchor point by spinning a random device (a so-called 'wheel of fortune') and then asked subjects to make judgements relative to the number generated by the 'wheel of fortune'. Results indicated quite significant effects in subjects' judgements due to the anchor.

Adjustment and anchoring seems to be a judgemental strategy that is almost as necessary as 'availability'. Predictions are made by reference to cues that are 'available', adjustments are then made concerning the particular case to be predicted relative to the available cues. Furthermore, availability and adjustment and anchoring are strategies that both depend heavily upon the initial point in the judgemental process: the information that is available and which forms the anchor. In drug monitoring, where physicians are frequently involved in assessing small probabilities (i.e. for infrequent events), 'available' information is scarce. Consequently, biases in judgement due to the processes discussed here could well be quite prevalent.

## Weighting and combining information sources

Given that people have limited information-processing ability, it should be no great surprise that studies have documented human fallibilities in the combination of information in prediction and choice.

In predictive judgement, combination of different information-sources requires attention to two features of the data; first, the predictive accuracy of each data-source; and second, the extent to which the different data-sources are redundant (that is overlap). Above, problems associated with each of these tasks were mentioned. People have difficulty in assessing the predictive ability of single data-sources and, in particular, tend to overlook questions of source reliability (which reduce predictive accuracy). Cues which exhibit high variability tend to attract attention.[10] However, lack of reliability may contribute to high variability. Data-sources which are redundant are, by definition, consistent. People use consistency of data-sources as a clue to the confidence they can attach to prediction; however, they frequently fail to consider the extent to which data sources are redundant.[11]

An important aspect of predictive activity is the updating of opinions. For example, a physician's opinion of the probability of a patient having a particular disease should be changed when new information, for example results of laboratory tests, is received. Extensive evidence of people's ability to perform this task intuitively indicates consistent fallibilities.[10,52] When the data to be combined are not redundant, people are conservative in the revision of their opinions in the sense that they do not extract as much information from the data as is available (i.e. they fail to revise their opinions sufficiently). Secondly, when the data to be combined exhibit redundancy, revision of opinion can be too extreme.[53]

Given the above findings, it should come as no surprise that statistical means of combining data for prediction out-perform intuitive judgement. Indeed, statistical models of the judgements of individuals often out-perform the individuals from whom the models have been derived.[54] Statistical methods can handle inter-cue redundancies as well as assess predictive accuracy. They are not subject to the random vagaries of human performance such as tiredness, boredom and inconsistency. They can also handle greater quantities of information. In addition, such models are *explicit*: one knows what the input is and what operations are performed on the input. Studies of expert decision-makers, on the other hand, indicate inconsistencies in judgemental strategies,[54,55] lack of awareness of relative weights given to cues for prediction[56] and illusions as to the number of cues people believe they use in judgement.[10,57]

However, the above awareness was not evident when the first studies of statistical *vs.* clinical prediction were undertaken – initially concerning the prediction of academic success and, more extensively, in clinical psychology.[58,59] To quote Dawes:

> The statistical analysis was thought to provide a floor to which the judgment of the experienced clinician could be compared. The floor turned out to be a ceiling.[60]

Since the earlier findings, many studies have replicated the superiority of statistical prediction and this includes applications in medicine.[2,61]

Two immediate objections can be raised against such statistical prediction methods. First, data are often of a qualitative nature and cannot be quantified. Second, good historical data which are necessary to build statistical models are often simply not available. Furthermore, it must be assumed that 'rules' that applied in the past will apply in the future.

These objections can be readily dismissed. First, qualitative data can be scaled and represented in numerical form. Such transformations clearly misrepresent the data. However, the issue to be faced is the extent of the misrepresentation and the degree to which predictive power is reduced. Einhorn, for example, suggests in a medical context (prediction of severity of disease) that the appropriate role for people in judgement is as a 'measuring instrument' for data that are to be combined subsequently by mechanical means.[62] What is lost in the transformation of data from a meaningful, but loose, qualitative form (in Einhorn's study impressions of traits present in biopsy slides) to a rough, but overly precise quantitative form (e.g. a point on a rating scale) can be more than compensated by the ability to combine the data consistently with other sources – be they quantitative or (transformed) qualitative.

To build statistical models for prediction, one needs adequate data-sources. However, even when data-sources are not rich, combinations of judgemental inputs and mechanical combination – for example by taking averages – have been shown to yield relatively accurate predictions.[63,64]

A third, and often emotional, resistance to the use of statistical prediction is the apparently inhuman aspect of mechanical rigidity. People feel averse to having 'machines' predict or make decisions for them. However, the counter-argument has been made by Dawes. He states that the advantage of such rules is that to create them you have to determine a *policy*; you therefore do not treat each case on an *ad hoc* basis.[65] According to Dawes:

> Such procedures follow the categorical imperative of Immanuel Kant: Make each decision as if it were a policy for everyone, or at least as if it were a policy for yourself across time (p. 357).

Rules can, of course, be updated by new data and indeed statistical procedures do precisely this.

The above discussion has focused on prediction. Choices and decisions, however, also require considerations of what is at 'stake', e.g. costs, benefits, patient preferences, attitudes to risk, etc. However, as noted by Slovic, Fischhoff and Lichtenstein: 'In general, people appear to prefer strategies that are easy to justify and do not involve reliance on relative weights, trade-off functions, or other numerical computations'.[11] In a study by Slovic, for example, where subjects were required to choose between two-dimensional alternatives that they had previously equated in value, choices were not made at random: rather, subjects followed the strategy of choosing the alternative that was superior on the more important dimension.[66]

The argument made here is that such choice-processes should also be made explicit, and mechanical weighting and balancing used in arriving at a decision. Some specific examples are given in Section 4 below. In addition to the more evident aspects of making the issues *explicit*, emphasizing the distinction between evaluative and predictive judgements is necessary to avoid tendencies for 'wishful thinking', i.e. letting one's preferences for outcomes influence assessments of uncertainty. Such tendencies are particularly prevalent when 'stakes' are high, for example an individual's life in surgery or vast sums of money when marketing a drug; however, they have also been documented in laboratory experiments involving quite low-valued outcomes.[67]

Sjöberg makes the point that interaction between beliefs and preferences may not only affect the evaluation of alternative sources of action but also the manner in which information is sought to conceptualize a situation.[68] Anticipations of what one does or does not want to see can affect what one does see.

Risk is an important issue in medical decision-making, but unfortunately knowledge of risk perception is not well-developed. However, such psychological knowledge as does exist tends to run counter to 'accepted' economic thinking on these matters.[69–71] Individuals have extraordinary difficulty in perceiving differences between small probabilities, e.g. 0.001, 0.0001 or 0.00001, and if purchase of insurance is a good measure of attitudes to risk, people tend not to insure themselves against high-loss–low-probability events.[69,71] Most individuals have almost no experience of high-loss events, e.g. death or severe side-effects from medical treatment, and thus are ill-prepared to conceptualize such issues. However, from a societal viewpoint, aggregating across both individuals and situations, low-probability –high-loss events occur with alarming frequency.[71] There is an urgent need for work in this area.

## Memory

La Rochefoucauld once said 'Everybody complains about the badness of his memory, nobody about his judgement'. Modern research certainly points to the crucial link between memory and judgement.

In judging the strength of relationship between two variables, for example, an important issue is how people encode the relative strength of relationships observed. In a series of studies, Estes demonstrated that strength of relationships is more likely to be determined by the absolute number of outcomes observed rather than some measure of *relative* frequency which would be a more appropriate statistical measure.[26,27] The significance of this finding is that it suggests an important bias in the manner that intuitive judgement builds up, through memory, notions of relationships – see also p. 487. Successful outcomes, incidentally, also tend to be more easily remembered than unsuccessful outcomes.[26,27,72]

Two well-documented findings concerning judgement and memory are that, first, people have often been found to be over-confident relative to the actual occurrence of subsequent events;[73] and secondly, they over-estimate the extent of their knowledge;[74] people indicate less surprise about past circumstances than their previous behaviour would warrant. This latter finding, known as 'hindsight' bias, corresponds to the well-known phenomenon of the occurrence of events seeming inevitable with hindsight although people did not predict them ahead of time.[75–77] Neither the hindsight bias nor over-confidence are necessarily caused by motivational factors, for instance people selectively remembering or forgetting certain events or incidents. Situational factors and human cognitive limitations appear to play an important role.[21,77]

For example, at the time one makes a prediction, so many different incidents could be relevant to so many different hypotheses, it is difficult to distinguish the important from the unimportant. After the fact, however, the meaning and relevance of certain incidents leading up to an event are far clearer. Indeed, certain events subsequently appear to have become inevitable. How can one avoid such judgemental difficulties? Fischhoff found that telling people of such biases had little effect.[78] On the other hand, Slovic and Fischhoff have shown that in the context of results of scientific experiments, forcing people to consider how results of research might have differed, tends to reduce 'hindsight' bias.[79]

The above experiments and findings are particularly relevant to problems of drug monitoring in that they indicate specific human limitations concerning both the anticipation of future events and the interpretation of the past – for example, were certain mishaps really as inevitable as they seem afterwards? They also point to the need to increase powers of imagination to be able to conceive of future contingencies as well as the need to bolster memory by good record-keeping.

## DECISION AIDS

The evidence reviewed so far suggests several weaknesses in judgement, for example: susceptibilities to selecting certain types of information and ignoring others; lack of ability to aggregate different sources of information; difficulties of learning from experience; problems of balancing differential costs of errors, etc. In this section, I shall argue that several of these difficulties can be alleviated, although not necessarily overcome, by adopting a decision-theoretic approach to medical decision-making and problems of drug monitoring in particular. It should be pointed out, however, that these notions are not new in medicine *per se*. For example, Lusted has written an introductory text on medical decision-making inspired by decision-theoretic notions[80] and *The New England Journal of Medicine* had a special issue on this topic in 1975. Consequently, the experience accumulated to date means that practical examples can be indicated.[81]

Decision theory[82] explicitly recognizes the issues raised at the beginning of this chapter, namely that decisions depend on the answers to two questions: '(i) What is at stake? and (ii) What are the uncertainties?' However, it goes beyond these questions and provides operational concepts to measure 'stakes' and uncertainties, and a set of axioms which prescribe the actions a person must take to be coherent with the expression of his or her beliefs concerning the uncertainties, and preferences (or values) concerning the 'stakes'. Probabilities measure beliefs, and the concept of utility covers preferences. The fundamental operational rule of decision analysis is to decompose a problem into manageable parts, and then to 'recompose' according to normative rules. This does not however mean that the decision-maker, e.g. the physician, has any lesser role to play. On the contrary, the decision-maker must recognize and structure the problem, and provide the subjective inputs necessary for the analysis. In that sense, decision analysis should be considered a mental 'crutch' which allows operations which are often lost in intuitive processes to be made explicit. This does not, of course, mean that no part of the analysis will be intuitive; much will inevitably remain so. However, it does mean that certain intuitive processes can be avoided; furthermore, it implies that the decision-maker probably has to think a lot harder about many of the issues involved.

To give the flavour of this approach, two applications will be described. The first is the analysis of a problem involving the choice between coronary by-pass surgery and medical therapy in patients with angiographically documented coronary artery disease;[83] the second concerns possible side-effects of the use of cortisone drugs.[84]

Pauker structured the coronary problem by considering three main variables which determine the value of by-pass surgery: (1) the prognosis with medical therapy which depended mainly upon the severity of the coronary disease and upon the patient's ventricular function. Data for such prognoses were obtained from a variety of published sources as well as from experienced cardiologists and expressed in probabilistic form. Pauker notes that much data were not available in the literature and thus subjective opinions had to be encoded in probabilistic form together with historical data (see discussion below). Patients were incidentally classified into four groups indicating differential severity of disease in respect of which prognoses differed; (2) assessments of the short-term and long-term surgical results derived from published data and dependent upon both the extent of the patient's disease and results of the *prospective surgical team*; and (3) patient preferences. Pauker considered two dimensions of patient preferences concerning length and quality of life, and classified patients into four groups on this basis. This classification was based on the establishment of a *utility* scale for each class of patients on which *relative* preferences for outcomes could be expressed. Note that the first two steps were used to make explicit and quantify the uncertainties in the problem, the third to specify the 'stakes'.

Next Pauker represented his problem in the form of a decision tree as illustrated in Figure 5. This diagram is, in fact, a simplified version of the full 'tree' used by Pauker but contains the essentials of the problem.

Decision theory states that one should choose the action for which *expected* utility is greatest. That is, each action can be evaluated by weighting the numerical expression of preferences (i.e utility) by their probability of occurrence. Pauker did this for the patients with different levels of severity of disease and so determined the optimal action (surgery or conventional medical therapy) for the different kinds of patient.

The output of an analysis of this kind can clearly only be as good as the input. Consequently, Pauker used the technique of *sensitivity analysis* to assess the importance of the inputs to the decisions for each 'kind' of patient. This involved making changes to the inputs – in terms of both probabilities and utilities – and observing the points at which changes in the inputs would change the decision originally determined by the model.

Results of Pauker's model were summarized by him as follows:

> Coronary by-pass surgery was, in general, found preferable in severely disabled patients, but medical therapy seemed preferable in asymptomatic

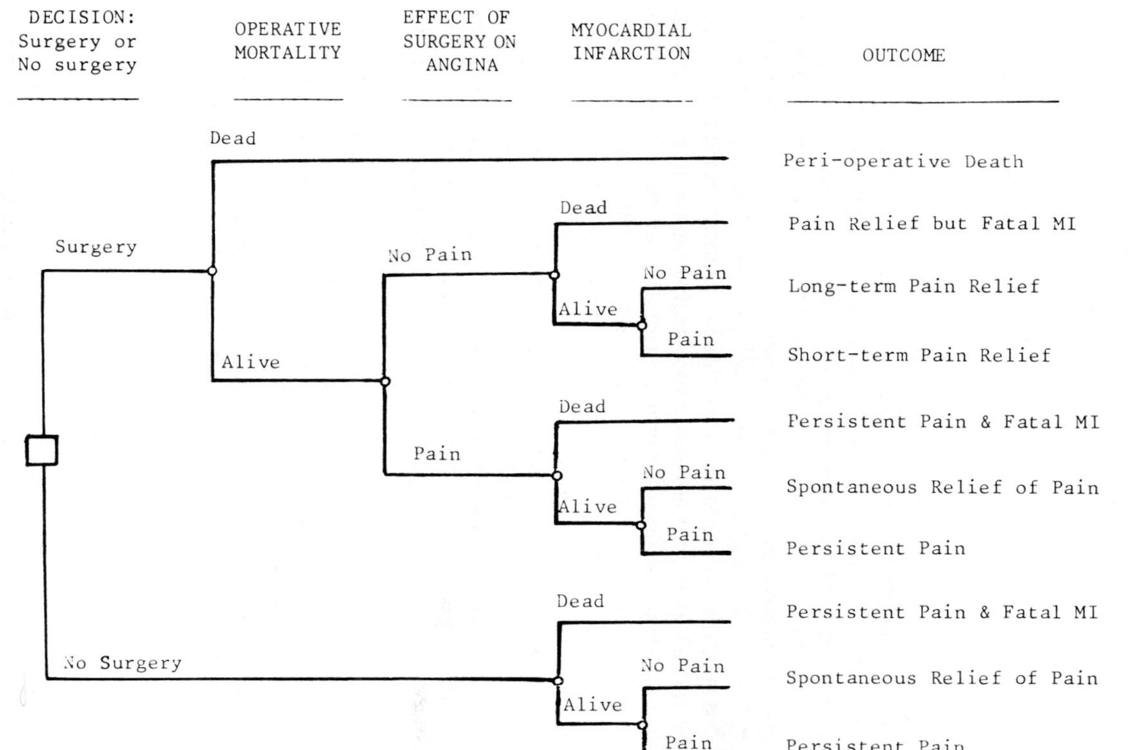


**Figure 5** Decision tree for chronic coronary artery disease. The decision between surgical and medical therapy is denoted by a square node. The circular nodes denote chance occurrences. Fatal MI refers to the occurrence of a fatal myocardial infarction during the time horizon under consideration (From Ref. 83)

> patients. The decision between medical and surgical therapy was sensitive to patient attitudes and to the quality of surgery available. This sensitivity depended on the strong relation, assumed in this model, between operative mortality and long-term graft potency rates. Variation in disease severity and patient preferences influenced the decision more strongly than did variation on operative statistics.

Pauker also counters several possible objections to the decision model. First he admits that the model used and represented in Figure 5 is oversimplified. For example:

> The time horizon can be longer than 5 years; more than one 'event' can occur each year; coronary and myocardial function fall into more classes than those considered here; other factors, such as serum lipids, smoking and blood pressure, are involved in determining prognosis; disability is not a discrete two-valued function (Pain and No Pain); the cost of surgery is not really equivalent to the loss of 1 year of pain free survival; monetary costs should not be neglected.

However, despite these imperfections, Pauker points out that, first, the prognostic model used was a reasonable approximation of the major factors that physicians actually considered at the time of the study. Furthermore, sensitivity analyses had shown that many added complexities did not affect the decision. Second, whereas the model does make several assumptions, physicians' intuitive processes, which are based largely on consideration of the same factors, must make a similar number of *implicit* assumptions. The decision analysis model, however, has the advantage of making factors and assumptions *explicit*. Third, Pauker admits deficiencies in the data base used for prognoses. However, he points out that it was the best available at the time the study was done and, as he puts it, 'today's clinician must make decisions concerning today's patients; he cannot defer such decisions until better data become available'. Faced with such problems, however, the use of sensitivity analysis is particularly useful, i.e. by what amounts would the probabilities of the prognostic model need to be changed to alter the decisions? Finally, Pauker points out that it is illusory to believe that decision analysis can 'improve' the data for therapeutic choices. If anything, it probably highlights their deficiencies, but at least it makes them explicit.

Pauker's decision model was derived by considering four general classes of patient. However, he also demonstrates how it can be tailored to individuals, and an Appendix to his paper discusses three case-studies. In applications of the methodology Pauker reports that patients readily accept the procedure used to elicit their different preferences for outcomes. He states: 'Such debriefing can usually be accomplished within 30 minutes. In addition, explicit questioning of the type described here increases the patient's understanding of his disease and of the thereapeutic options involved.'

The study by Aschenbrenner and Kasubek[84] was directly concerned with possibilities of side-effects resulting from drugs. Specifically, they investigated the assessments by five physicians of the possible side-effects of various cortisone treatments.

Five experienced physicians, who were interviewed individually, participated in the study which examined the comparison of intuitive judgements of the dangerousness of possible side-effects with those derived from a formal decision model. The physicians were told to imagine that they were treating an 'average' patient of 50 years of age. They were then asked to rank order the seven drugs listed in Table 1 as to their relative dangerousness (in terms of adverse side-effects). These rank-orders therefore represented the physician's intuitive judgements of relative undesirability of possible side-effects and were based on whatever information they deemed appropriate.

Second, the physicians were shown a table indicating the incidence of the relative frequencies of side-effects for the different drugs – as in Table 1. These relative frequencies were derived from medical statistics and, after examining the table, the physicians were invited to change their intuitive rank orders of the dangerousness of the drugs if they desired to do so. None of the physicians chose to alter the intuitive rankings.

The next stage of the procedure was to build a formal model based on decision-theoretic principles to evaluate the relative dangerousness of the drugs. The general form of the model was the following: dangerousness of the drugs was conceptualized as a weighted additive function of each of the side-effects, i.e.:

$$u(A_j) = w_i u_i (a_{ij}) + w_2 u_2 (a_{2j}) + \ldots + w_n u_n (a_{nj}) \quad (1)$$

where $u(A_j)$ is the overall dangerousness of drug $A_j$, $u_i(a_{ij})$ is the evaluation of drug $A_j$'s level on the $i$th side-effect, and $w_i$ is the relative importance of the $i$th side-effect. In technical terms, the different drugs are considered as alternatives, and the side-effects as attributes.

The objective of the exercise is thus to characterize each alternative as a function of its attributes. In this study a linear function was found to be appropriate; however, procedures do exist for more complicated schemes.[85,86] Two different methods were used to elicit the physicians' assessments of the relative importance of the attributes (i.e. side-effects) with the interesting and significant result that the simpler and more direct procedure was found to give more consistent results. Measures of the alternatives on each of the attributes were, of course, available from the relative frequency data given in Table 1.

The results of this study can be considered from several viewpoints: differences in assessments of dangerousness between intuitive judgements and those provided by the model; level of agreement between the physicians; and potential applications of the methodology used.

Table 2 indicates the rank orders and average evaluations of the seven cortisone drugs for both the intuitive global judgements and the model assessments implied by the two judgement elicitation methods. As can be observed, across all methods dexamethasone and 6-α-

**Table 1** Relative frequencies of six side-effects of cortisone drugs

| Drug | *Efficiency equivalent* dose (mg) | *Side-effect* | | | | | |
|---|---|---|---|---|---|---|---|
| | | *Increased weight* (%) | *Increased blood-pressure* (%) | *Cushing face* (%) | *Ulcus, hyper-acidity* (%) | *Hyper-trichosis, hirsuitism* (%) | *Myopathy* (%) |
| Cortisone | 50 | 58 | 49 | 78 | 30 | 65 | 4 |
| Dexamethasone | 1.5 | 64 | 2 | 70 | 9 | 8 | 6 |
| Hydrocortisone | 40 | 24 | 18 | 76 | 10 | 58 | 4 |
| Prednisolone | 8–10 | 20 | 11 | 86 | 36 | 68 | 1 |
| Prednisone | 10 | 20 | 11 | 86 | 36 | 68 | 1 |
| Triamcinolone | 8 | 40 | 2 | 70 | 12 | 19 | 20 |
| 6-α-Methylprednisolone | 8 | 30 | 5 | 78 | 5 | 47 | 62 |

From Aschenbrenner and Kasubek[84]

**Table 2** Rank orders and average evaluations of the seven cortisone drugs. The difference between alternatives that are connected by braces are less than the critical difference ($\alpha = 5\%$)

| *Model 1* | | *Model 2* | | *Global intuitive* | |
|---|---|---|---|---|---|
| Dexamethasone | 0.189 | 6-α-Methylprednisolone | 0.082 | 6-α-Methylprednisolone | 1.2 |
| 6-α-Methylprednisolone | 0.191 | Dexamethasone | 0.125 | Dexamethasone | 3.3 |
| Hydrocortisone | 0.246 | Hydrocortisone | 0.190 | Prednisone | 3.9 |
| Triamcinolone | 0.314 | Triamcinolone | 0.281 | Prednisolone | 4.0 |
| Prednisolone | 0.399 | Prednisolone | 0.687 | Triamcinolone | 4.3 |
| Prednisone | 0.431 | Cortisone | 0.707 | Cortisone | 5.5 |
| Cortisone | 0.474 | Prednisone | 0.736 | Hydrocortisone | 5.8 |
| $d_{crit}$ | 0.0498 | | 0.0688 | | 1.608 |

From Aschenbrenner and Kasubek[84]

methylprednisolone are ranked as the least dangerous, although it is interesting to note that both models indicate little or no difference between these two drugs. Overall, the two model-generated rank orders are remarkably similar, but both are different from the intuitive rankings. In particular, whereas hydrocortisone ranks last (i.e. most dangerous) on the intuitive judgements, it is third in both model assessments.

Agreement between the physicians can be considered at two levels – global judgements of dangerousness, and the relative weights given to the different attributes, i.e. side-effects. Inter-judge agreement on relative dangerousness of the seven drugs was high for the two model-induced rankings with only 4.8% and 13.1% of the variance in judgements being attributable to divergent evaluations by the physicians. This was not, however, the case for the intuitive global rankings where the comparable figure was 56.6%. Since no component or part-judgements were available with the intuitive global assessments, comparison at this level can only be made between judgements for the two models. As noted above, the more direct and simpler assessment method indicated considerable agreement concerning the relevant weights given to the attributes.

The above results are consistent with a study by Einhorn, who also showed that although physicians may have divergent opinions concerning overall severity of a disease (specifically, estimates of severity of Hodgkin's disease based on examination of biopsy slides), they can show considerable agreement concerning the components, i.e. relative presence/absence of traits on which assessments of severity are based.[62] Both these studies, therefore, attest to the notion that disagreement amongst physicians does not necessarily repose in the identification and assessment of the elements of judgement, but rather in how those elements are combined. A further example of this was documented by Slovic, Rorer and Hoffman in a study of the judgemental processes of radiologists,[87] although Hammond and Joyce report interesting data of physicians who, when assessing severity of degenerative joint disease, expected *a priori* that there would be little differences in the relative weights they attached to cues they had selected. In fact, the physicians varied widely both in the relative weights and consistency of their assessments.[4]

The Aschenbrenner and Kasubek study was, of course, limited by the fact that it concerned a hypothetical 50-year-old 'average' patient and the relative frequency data were taken from a wide statistical base. However, the methodology suggested is most significant. First, these base-rate relative frequencies could be adjusted for particular cases on a judgemental basis. Second, the fact that the simpler method developed for assessing importance weights worked so well led Aschenbrenner and Kasubek to state:

> . . . other specific cases may occur where a change in importance weights would make some other drug more appropriate. For such cases we would suggest the self-application of the conditional importance rating by the attending physician – or even by the patient himself. The procedure is so simple and fast that every physician should be capable of doing it in five minutes or so.

A further suggestion by Aschenbrenner and Kasubek concerns the use of sensitivity analysis. Specifically, they suggest determining the importance weight *ranges* for each drug which would lead to its choice.

The studies by Pauker, and Aschenbrenner and Kasubek, illustrate several key features of the decision-theoretic approach: structuring the problem by decomposing it into parts that can be meaningfully analysed, and which can be dealt with within limited human information-processing capacity; assessment of probabilities; assessment of preferences; consistent recombination of the parts of the problem by mechanical means; and finally sensitivity analysis to assess the importance of decisions prescribed by the model to data input. We now reconsider each of these aspects.

According to Sir William Osler, 'Medicine is a science of uncertainty and an art of probability'.[88] Consequently it is appropriate to use the language of probability in expressing feelings of uncertainty in both diagnosis and prognosis. In the decision-theoretic approach to decision-making, probabilities are recognized to be subjective and to measure an individual's 'degree of belief'.[82] This does not, however, mean that they are arbitrary for, as de Finetti[89] has shown, subjective probabilities can be operationally measured. There are several advantages of expressing uncertainties of diagnosis or prognosis in probabilistic form: first, quantification of the level of uncertainty is made precise and can be easily communicated. Words like 'likely', 'highly certain', 'unsure', etc. can have different meanings for different people;[90] second, the logic of probability theory can be a great help in structuring data and judgements involved in diagnosis and prognosis (for example, by indicating the necessity to use base-rate data – see pages 494/503); third, it provides a means whereby historical data, usually relative frequencies, can be combined with subjective opinions; and fourth, mechanical means can be used to aggregate subjective data inputs and used in formal models. Another important point is that if opinions are expressed precisely, e.g. in probabilistic form, over a number of cases it is possible to assess a person's predictive 'track record'. Feedback from such records can subsequently help the person refine his opinions more appropriately.

The fact should not be hidden, however, that the expression of uncertainty in probabilistic form is not necessarily easily achieved.[9] A consistent finding, for example, is that probabilistic expressions of belief tend to exhibit over-confidence relative to subsequent events.[73] Spetzler and Staël von Holstein, however provide a useful review of experience of probability encoding procedures which should be required reading for persons seriously interested in probability assessment.[91] Human deficiencies in probability assessment are primarily the result of human judgemental deficiencies rather than any problems inherent in the notion of subjective probability *per se*. Various biases in probability judgements have been conveniently summarized and discussed by Tversky and Kahneman.[51] The explicit use of probabilistic thinking in medical diagnosis and prognosis goes back at least to Gini.[92] It received considerable impetus as a result of a paper by Ledley and Lusted[93] and a growing number of applications were reported in the 1960s and 1970s. Examples of use of the subjective probability concept include: assessing the diagnostic value of X-rays;[94] predicting length of stay of patients in hospital;[95] and problems concerned with acute renal failure.[96,97] Comprehensive and critical reviews of this work have been provided by Beach,[2] and Mai and Hachmann.[61] Of particular interest to drug monitoring are the problems involved in assessing small probabilities. Although not effected within a medical context, Selvidge has made a useful contribution towards developing methodology for this kind of problem[98] although Sjöberg notes that this is not without its problems.[68]

Decisions require the balancing of costs and benefits as well as considerations of risk. These issues are currently best conceptualized through multi-attribute utility theory, a limited example of which was illustrated by the Aschenbrenner and Kasubek study discussed above. Simply stated, multi-attribute utility theory recognizes that the outcomes of decisions involve multiple consequences (i.e. costs and benefits). It provides a systematic manner of eliciting the decision-maker's preferences towards these consequences and of representing them in a form that allows the determination of relative preferences. The recent book by Keeney and Raiffa outlines the theory as well as quoting numerous examples.[85] See also Humphreys[99] and Johnson and

Huber.[100] Further examples are provided in Bell, Keeney and Raiffa.[101] In addition to references cited above, some interesting medical examples have involved developing an index for severity of illness[102] and measuring the desirability of outcomes of cleft lip and palate treatment.[103] Useful expository papers in this area include those by McNeil *et al.*,[104] Pauker and Kassirer,[105] and Thornbury and Fryback.[106]

The underlying rationale of the decision-theoretic approach is to structure the problem in such a manner that all the elements are made explicit. This may, of course, be done in several ways. Above, the methodology of decision trees and multi-attribute utility theory were briefly illustrated. Lusted, on the other hand, has pioneered the use of 'receiver operating characteristic' curves in radiology which can be formulated within the decision-theory framework.[6,107,108] Neuhauser and Lewicki provide an analysis of the costs of sequential tests which could be particularly pertinent to problems of drug monitoring.[109] It is clear that the cost structure and discriminatory ability of sequential tests is not evident to intuition.[6]

A number of objections can be raised against the decision analysis approach as discussed here. First, whereas it provides a framework within which judgements concerning uncertainties and outcomes (i.e. values) can be combined, it does not provide an explicit methodology for structuring problems and identifying alternatives. Second, whereas the methodology allows for the incorporation of personal beliefs and preferences in the model, the underlying theory is comparatively underdeveloped in terms of dealing with beliefs and values of groups of people or indeed communities – as might be the case, for example, in problems of drug monitoring. Third, decision analysis provides no guarantee of good outcomes and particularly in individual cases.

The third objection can be dealt with most easily. In the presence of uncertainty, no methodology can guarantee good outcomes. Decision analysis, however, can provide a systematic procedure as illustrated above, and this should be compared with the *status quo*. If decision analysis is deficient in this respect, what is the alternative? Unaided intuitive judgement, as noted in preceding sections of this chapter, is clearly deficient. On the other hand, one must be aware of substituting naivety for scepticism. Decision analysis is no panacea and apparently complete and 'rational' analyses can often be deficient.[110] Indeed, they may blind people to the omission of important aspects of a problem.[49,111,112]

It is certainly true that decision analysis offers no formal help in inventing solutions and alternatives to problems, as well as in certain aspects of problem structuring. Indeed, this is an area in great need of research. However, the mere act of a systematic approach to a problem can in itself be most revealing and lead to the consideration of alternatives that might otherwise have been overlooked. Finally, although decision analysis has an emphasis on quantification, it is not quantification *per se* which is important. As was noted above, the importance of the quantitative elements can always be assessed through the use of sensitivity analysis.

The issues of 'public' decision-making are fascinating. Although no formal model exists which satisfies all theoretical objections,[113] adaptations of decision-theoretic principles can be most illuminating. First, the methodology involves separating beliefs (i.e. probabilities) from values (i.e. preferences for different outcomes). Consequently, these can be explicitly stated by all parties and the extent of agreement or disagreement assessed at the level of items. Experience indicates that whereas different parties to a decision may disagree as to values or preferences, when confronted with the same evidence, opinions are liable to be fairly similar.[1,114] However, this would not be evident if one only compared global judgements. Second, when problems are suitably decomposed, it is possible to consult experts on aspects relating to their expertise and to incorporate their judgements explicitly in the formal analysis. Third, on the issue of disagreement of values, it is important to ascertain the degree of disagreement and the extent to which this affects the decision. Sensitivity analysis may well reveal that certain value disagreements are not as important relative to a specific problem as the different parties believe. However, unless the problem has been decomposed, it is not possible for the parties to realize this. Considerable evidence attests to the fact that disagreements at the aggregate level of intuitive judgement are heightened by people's inability to process and combine different information-sources consistently, but that people are unaware of this.[115]

An illuminating study of community decision-making involving the above principles has been reported by Hammond and Adelman.[114] The problem involved the selection of a bullet to be used by Denver police force. This was a highly emotional issue involving different interest groups: the police, the city of Denver as represented by its mayor and council, and various civil liberty and other groups. By defining a methodology which, (a) decomposed the problem, (b) made social value judgements explicit, (c) allowed for the incorporation of expert judgements into the analysis (i.e. ballistic experts) and (d) aggregated the components of judgement mechanically, it was possible to help the various protagonists reach a well-reasoned decision. Hammond and Adelman compare the procedure used with a growing tendency to resolve disputes by appeal to scientific experts as partisan witnesses in 'science courts'. As Hammond and Adelman point out, such 'science courts' are indefensible in that they involve partisan testimony by scientists on questions involving both values and scientific judgements (in decision theory terms 'preferences' and 'beliefs') which are pronounced upon at a global level without making the bases of judgement explicit. Hammond and Adelman further claim that the process they initiated was scientifically defensible. However, not because it was flawless – they make no such claim – but rather because it is readily subject to scientific criticism.

## IMPLICATIONS FOR DRUG MONITORING

Good clinical judgement has been noted as the foremost attribute desired in physicians.[116] With this in mind, this chapter has pursued two themes: first, at a descriptive level I have indicated the nature of human judgement, the general context in which it takes place as well as some specific evidence concerning strengths and weaknesses of unaided intuitive judgement. I have also indicated the existence of certain decision aids which, although far from a panacea, can help considerably in judgemental activity. The essence of these methods is to eliminate intuitive judgement as far as possible from decision situations and to make explicit the bases of judgement.

Although many implications of judgemental research for problems of drug monitoring were indicated above, a recent book on drug monitoring[36] emphasizes several areas where ideas discussed in this chapter are relevant: choice of a drug monitoring system for a country; reporting of ADRs; concordance of judgements concerning ADRs; and decisions to administer drugs.

For example, in advocating the system of *recorded release* in drug monitoring. Inman proposes 12 objectives and then attempts to evaluate how his suggestions meet these objectives.[117] Although this is a laudable attempt to evaluate recorded release, it does not go far enough. A full decision analysis would involve comparison of several alternatives to recorded release on all 12 objectives, weighting the objectives relative to their importance and then observing how each of the alternatives fared when subjected to this more rigorous analysis. As indicated in the Aschenbrenner and Kasubek study discussed above, differences between intuitive rankings of alternatives and rankings implied by decomposed judgements can occur and are important. Furthermore, studies of different schemes for drug monitoring should be subjected to sensitivity analysis to assess the relative importance of weights accorded by different parties to the components of such decisions.

To amplify the preceding paragraph, it is important to realize that drug monitoring involves different types of judgements by different parties and a corresponding variety of actions. These are schematically illustrated in Figure 6. First, *scientific* judgements have to be made concerning the risks inherent in the decision to market a drug. Second, both *scientific and administrative* judgement has to be exercised concerning extent of use of a drug and whether and how warnings of possible adverse reactions should be made. Third, largely *administrative* judgement is to be made on issues determining the type of action required. At each of the nodes (i.e. points of judgement/decision) indicated in Figure 6 an 'open' or 'public' decision analysis is called for since (a) different parties have different interests in the outcomes, and (b) the various types of judgement required demand different types of expertise (e.g. scientific *vs.* administrative judgements).

When people with different interests face a common decision it is

SCIENTIFIC JUDGEMENTS
SCIENTIFIC AND ADMINISTRATIVE JUDGEMENTS
MAINLY ADMINISTRATIVE JUDGEMENTS ON TYPE OF ACTION REQUIRED
Identification and measurement of risk
Risk accepted
Risk not accepted
Alternative treatments have better risk/benefit ratio
Alternative treatments have similar risk/benefit ratio
In all cases
In some cases
No danger that public warning will cause serious alarm
Risk that alarm will damage reputation of useful drug
Advise use of alternatives
Limit use to some patients (e.g., in hospitals)
Issue public warning
"Low-key" warning (e.g., in medical product literature)
No warning required
Remove from market

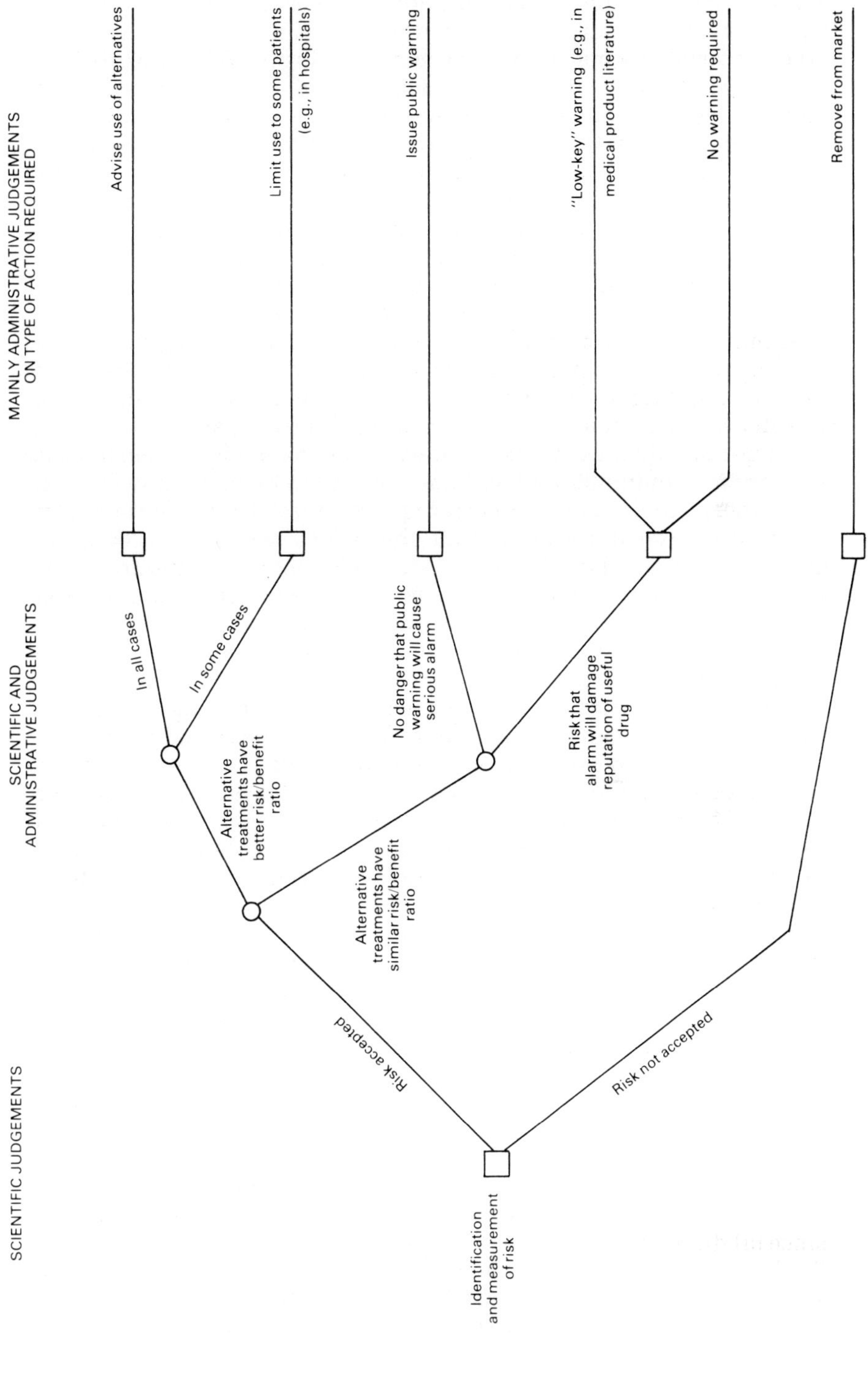

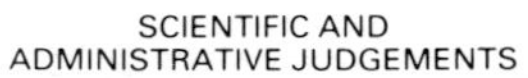

**Figure 6** Schematic (decision tree) representation of the interface between scientific and administrative judgements inherent in drug monitoring. At different stages of the total process, different types of judgements and considerations must be weighed. Without a global, but decomposed, view of the process, unnecessary conflict and lack of communication are inevitable

often implicitly assumed by the different parties that varying interests imply different actions. However, this is not necessarily the case. Experience with formal 'public' decision-making models indicates that actions can often accommodate a wide range of apparently conflicting interests. However, unless alternative actions are explicitly evaluated against the interests of different parties, advantage cannot be taken of the 'insensitivity' implicit in the structure of many decisions.[1,114] If, on the other hand, *real* disagreement about action exists, it is important that the *real* (but not apparent) source of disagreement be identified. Second, when many people are involved in a decision process ineffective communication between groups or sub-cultures invariably results. For example, scientists who express judgements at the first stage may find administrative judgements at subsequent stages to be 'unjustified'. Administrators may fail to understand the basis of scientific judgements – and so on. Lack of understanding leads to lack of co-operation and, as a consequence, ineffective systems. There are two major advantages of having public decision models at each stage of Figure 6: (1) opinions of experts can be limited to their bailiwicks; (2) each expert can see how his or her opinion fits into the total process and obtain a clearer overview of the issues involved at different decision points in the total process. For example, from Figure 6 it is quite clear that several judgements have to be made between the first and last stages concerning a drug with an acceptable risk. Furthermore, different experts (i.e. scientists and administrators) will intervene at different stages.

A public evaluation of different schemes also highlights another important problem in drug monitoring. If agencies produce regulations, who does and can 'regulate the regulators'? The answer to this, I would argue, depends upon the extent to which the regulators' policies are made explicit. Formal judgemental models of the type discussed above are consequently one way of 'controlling' regulatory agencies in the sense that in formulating the models the agencies must make their policies explicit in operational terms. However this does not necessarily mean that such policies must be fixed for all time. But it does mean that when an agency introduces a policy change this is made explicit at the operational level. A good example of this is the study by Hammond and Adelman, discussed above, concerning the choice of bullet for the Denver police force. In that case judgements about both social values and scientific opinions were clearly distinguished and externalized. Consequently criticism of the final choice of bullet could be made on grounds that made clear the nature and source of disagreement and its effect on the final decision.

In the reporting of ADRs the work reported here would certainly support the suggestion made by Finney to report 'events' rather than recording suspicions that events are drug-related.[36] The brief review of the judgemental literature provided here showed that humans show a tendency to over-react to events in the sense of wishing to attribute causal explanations. However, such causal explanations are often spurious. Given that reports of incidents arise across time and that the sequence of reports can distort subjective judgement, the use of statistical time-series analysis could be an important aid to separate random fluctuations from underlying trends. Makridakis and Wheelwright have produced an easy-to-use interactive computer package that could be of considerable help in this respect.[118]

Another important issue to consider here is the manner in which 'events' or reports of ADRs are transmitted to practising physicians. If physicians primarily become aware of possible ADRs through selected channels of communication, e.g. specialized medical journals, they are liable to receive a false impression of the incidence of certain types of reactions relative to others – a point noted in the discussion of 'availability bias' in judgement. How such a problem might be alleviated is, of course, problematical in that the original report of an ADR might itself be motivated by the fact that it is exceptional and thus has a high interest value (e.g. it is more 'publishable' in a prestigious medical journal). A related point concerns the reliability of reports. As indicated above, intuitive judgement tends to overlook data-source reliability although this can be of crucial importance. Estimates of reliability, however, should and could be incorporated in reporting schemes and methods used for aggregating reports. Some normative models and applications are discussed in Peterson[119] and Schum.[120,121]

A further issue raised by both Koch-Weser[122] and Hammond and Joyce[4] is the extent to which physicians' judgements agree with each other. There are two issues involved here: first, the extent to which a physician's judgements are consistent. (That is, does a physician give the same judgement on independent occasions?); second, inter-physician agreement. Few judgements are uni-dimensional. Consequently, the suggestion made here is to decompose judgements as far as possible. Decomposed judgements which are subsequently mechanically aggregated show both greater consistency and greater inter-judge agreement.[62,84] Hammond and Joyce have made a detailed proposal concerning drug monitoring and also listed some further suggestions.[4]

The elements of decisions concerning whether one should administer a particular drug were implicitly discussed in the decision situations described in the preceding section. Probably the biggest difficulty here is not the technical difficulty of actually eliciting judgements concerning probabilities, risks, costs and benefits but the emotional aspects of medicine. The medical profession is jealous of its preserve in society (whether rightly so or not). However, the procedures I have advocated in this chapter might appear to indict one of its most cherished qualities – judgement. When judgements are made 'public', the normal fear of 'accountability' is clearly magnified. Furthermore, 'public' judgements not only require an understanding of the issues as well as acceptance of uncertainty by those making the judgements, but also by the public at large. However, in a very real sense professions absorb public uncertainty in their areas of expertise and thus the expression of probabilistic opinions is by its nature problematical.

Emotional resistances to the introduction of the kinds of decision aids discussed above are inevitable. A further reason is that it is not always evident from subsequent events that judgement has been erroneous, or at least not quite as good as it might have been (recall the case of Benjamin Rush). There is a widespread belief that one can learn from experience, but conversely few people realize that learning is not necessarily possible.[32] Too often it would seem that extreme emotional experiences or catastrophes have to occur before people are willing to take action – a fact evidenced by events that led to the creation of several drug monitoring agencies.

A number of successful applications of decision theory principles clearly need to be effected in the field of drug monitoring to establish credibility.

Finally, one of the major implications of this chapter is educational in nature. Physicians are taught knowledge, they learn to recognize symptoms and they interiorize quite complex causal schemes concerning the nature of the human body, effects of chemistry, etc. However, they are rarely, if ever, taught how to manipulate knowledge in the formation of judgement. Judgement is not supposed to be a skill that can be learned; rather one that the physician acquires through experience.[5] Nonetheless, as indicated above, experience not only teaches good habits, but bad ones too, and learning from judgemental experience is not always evident. Judgement, it has been argued in this chapter, consists largely of performing operations with information. Furthermore, appropriate principles and aids can be taught. However, until such time as they become part of a regular medical syllabus, the introduction of judgemental aids as discussed in this chapter will take longer than their merit deserves.

## Acknowledgements

This chapter was mainly written while the author held a visiting appointment at the London Graduate School of Business Studies. Helpful comments on the manuscript were provided by Michael Aschenbrenner, Hillel Einhorn, Ken Hammond, Bill Inman and Lee Lusted. Bill Inman suggested the framework for considering the process of drug monitoring decisions presented in Figure 6.

## References

1. Edwards, W. (1977). Use of multiattribute utility measurement for social decision making. In Bell, D. E., Keeney, R. L. and Raiffa, H. (eds.) *Conflicting Objectives in Decisions*. pp. 247–275. (Chichester, England: John Wiley & Sons)

2. Beach, B. H. (1975). Expert judgment about uncertainty: Bayesian decision making in realistic settings. *Org. Behav. Hum. Perform.*, **14,** 10
3. Elstein, A. S. (1976). Clinical judgment: Psychological research and medical practice. *Science*, **194,** 696
4. Hammond, K. R. and Joyce, C. R. B. (1977). Psychological influences on human judgment, especially of adverse reactions. In Gross, F. H. and Inman, W. H. W. (eds.) *Drug Monitoring*, pp. 269–287. (London: Academic Press)
5. Knafl, K. and Burkett, G. (1975). Professional socialization in a surgical specialty: Acquiring medical judgment. *Soc. Sci. Med.*, **9,** 397
6. Lusted, L. B. (1976). Clinical decision making. In de Dombal, F. T. and Grémy, F. (eds.) *Decision Making and Medical Care. Can Information Science Help?* pp. 77–98. (Amsterdam: North-Holland)
7. Schwartz, W. B., Gorry, G. A., Kassirer, J. P. and Essig, A. (1973). Decision analysis and clinical judgment. *Am. J. Med.*, **55,** 459
8. Brehmer, B. (1976). Social judgment theory and the analysis of interpersonal conflict. *Psychol. Bull.*, **83,** 985
9. Hogarth, R. M. (1975). Cognitive processes and the assessment of subjective probability distributions. *J. Am. Stat. Assoc.*, **70,** 271
10. Slovic, P. and Lichtenstein, S. (1971). Comparison of Bayesian and regression approaches to the study of information processing in judgment. *Org. Behav. Hum. Perform.*, **6,** 649
11. Slovic, P., Fischhoff, B. and Lichtenstein, S. (1977). Behavioral decision theory. *Ann. Rev. Psychol.*, **28,** 1
12. Michotte, A. (1963). *The Perception of Causality*. (London: Methuen)
13. Kahneman, D. and Tversky, A. (1973). On the psychology of prediction. *Psychol. Rev.*, **80,** 237
14. Detmer, D. E., Fryback, D. G. and Gassner, K. (1978). Heuristics and biases in medical decision making. *J. Med. Educ.*, **53,** 682
15. Campbell, D. T. (1969). Reforms as experiments. *Am. Psychol.*, **24,** 409
16. Kahneman, D. and Tversky, A. (1972). Subjective probability: A judgment of representativeness. *Cogn. Psychol.*, **3,** 430
17. Tversky, A. and Kahneman, D. (1971). Belief in the law of small numbers. *Psychol. Bull.*, **76,** 105
18. Berkson, J., Magath, T. B. and Hurn, M. (1940). The error of estimate of the blood cell count as made with the hemocytometer. *Am. J. Physiol.*, **128,** 309
19. Zieve, L. (1966). Misinterpretation and abuse of laboratory tests by clinicians. *Ann. N.Y. Acad. Sci.*, **134,** 563
20. Einhorn, H. J. and Schacht, S. (1977). Decisions based on fallible clinical judgment. In Kaplan, M. and Schwartz, S. (eds.) *Human Judgment and Decision Processes in Applied Settings*. pp. 125–144. (New York: Academic Press)
21. Einhorn, H. J. and Hogarth, R. M. (1978). Confidence in judgment: persistence of the illusion of validity. *Psychol. Rev.*, **85,** 395
22. Jenkins, H. M. and Ward, W. C. (1965). Judgment of contingency between responses and outcomes. *Psychol. Monographs: Gen. Applied*, **79,** (Whole No. 594)
23. Smedslund, J. (1963). The concept of correlation in adults. *Scand. J. Psychol.*, **4,** 165
24. Smedslund, J. (1966). Note on learning, contingency, and clinical experience. *Scand. J. Psychol.*, **7,** 265
25. Ward, W. C. and Jenkins, H. M. (1965). The display of information and the judgment of contingency. *Canad. J. Psychol.*, **19,** 231
26. Estes, W. K. (1976). The cognitive side of probability learning. *Psychol. Rev.*, **83,** 37
27. Estes, W. K. (1976). Some functions of memory in probability learning and choice behavior. In Bower, G. H. (ed.) *The Psychology of Learning and Motivation* (Vol. 10), pp. 1–45. (New York: Academic Press)
28. Chapman, L. J. and Chapman, J. P. (1969). Illusory correlation as an obstacle to the use of valid pyschodiagnostic signs. *J. Abnorm. Psychol.*, **74,** 271

29. Wason, P. C. and Johnson-Laird, P. N. (1972). *Psychology of Reasoning: Structure and Content*, p. 264. (London: Batsford)
30. Eisenberg, L. (1977). The social imperatives of medical research. *Science*, **198,** 1105
31. Bandura, A. (1978). The self system in reciprocal determinism. *Am. Psychol.*, **33,** 344
32. Hammond, K. R. (1978). Toward increasing competence of thought in public policy formation. In Hammond, K. R. (ed.) *Judgment and Decision in Public Policy Formation.* (Denver, Colorado: Westview Press)
33. Tversky, A. and Kahneman, D. (1973). Availability: a heuristic for judging frequency and probability. *Cogn. Psychol.*, **5,** 207
34. Slovic, P., Fischhoff, B., Lichtenstein, S., Combs, B. and Layman, M. (1976). Misperceived frequencies of low probability lethal events. *ORI Res. Monogr.*, **16,** No. 2. (Eugene: Ore. Res. Inst.)
35. Schiffmann, A., Cohen, S., Nowik, R. and Selinger, D. (1978). Initial diagnostic hypotheses: factors which may distort physicians' judgment. *Org. Behav. Hum. Perform.*, **21,** 305
36. Gross, F. H. and Inman, W. H. W. (eds.) (1977). *Drug Monitoring*, p. 311. (London: Academic Press)
37. Ajzen, I. (1977). Intuitive theories of events and the effects of base-rate information on prediction. *J. Pers. Soc. Psychol.*, **35,** 303
38. Kleinmuntz, B. (1968). The processing of clinical information by man and machine. In Kleinmuntz, B. (ed.) *Formal Representation of Human Judgment.* pp. 149–186. (New York: John Wiley & Sons)
39. Lyon, D. and Slovic, P. (1976). Dominance of accuracy information and neglect of base rates in probability estimation. *Acta Psychol.*, **40,** 287
40. Nisbett, R. E., Borgida, E., Crandall, R. and Reed, H. (1976). Popular induction: information is not necessarily informative. In Carroll, J. S. and Payne, J. W. (eds.) *Cognition and Social Behaviour.* (Hillsdale, N.J.: Erlbaum)
41. Tversky, A. and Kahneman, D. (1980). Causal schemas in judgments under uncertainty. In Fishbein, M. (ed.) *Progress in Social Psychology* pp. 49–72. (Hillsdale, N.J.: Erlbaum)
42. Ross, L. (1977). The intuitive psychologist and his shortcomings: Distortions in the attribution process. In Berkowitz, L. (ed.) *Advances in Experimental Social Psychology*, Vol. 10, pp. 173–220. (New York: Academic Press)
43. Golding, S. L. and Rorer, L. G. (1972). Illusory correlation and subjective judgment. *J. Abnorm. Psychol.*, **80,** 249
44. Bruner, J. S., Goodnow, J. J. and Austin, G. A. (1956). *A Study of Thinking.* (New York: John Wiley & Sons)
45. Oskamp, S. (1965). Overconfidence in case-study judgments. *J. Consult. Psychol.*, **29,** 261
46. Slovic, P. (1966). Cue consistency and cue utilization in judgment. *Am. J. Psychol.*, **79,** 427
47. Einhorn, H. J. (1971). Use of nonlinear, noncompensatory models as a function of task and amount of information. *Org. Behav. Hum. Perform.*, **6,** 1
48. Slovic, P. (1972). From Shakespeare to Simon: Speculations – and some evidence – about man's ability to process information. *ORI Res. Monogr.*, **12,** No. 2. (Eugene: Ore. Res. Inst.)
49. Fischhoff, B., Slovic, P. and Lichtenstein, S. (1978). Fault trees: sensitivity of estimated probabilities to problem representation. *J. Exp. Psychol. Hum. Percept. Perform.*, **4,** 342
50. Miller, P. M. (1971). Do labels mislead? A multiple cue study within the framework of Brunswik's probabilistic functionalism. *Organ. Beh. Hum. Perform.*, **6,** 480
51. Tversky, A. and Kahneman, D. (1974). Judgment under certainty: heuristics and biases. *Science*, **185,** 1124
52. Edwards, W. (1968). Conservatism in human information processing. In Kleinmuntz, B. (ed.) *Formal Representation of Human Judgment*, pp. 17–52. (New York: John Wiley & Sons)

53. Youssef, Z. I. and Peterson, C. R. (1973). Intuitive cascaded inferences. *Org. Behav. Hum. Perform.*, **10,** 349
54. Goldberg, L. R. (1970). Man versus model of man: a rationale, plus some evidence, for a method of improving on clinical inferences. *Psychol. Bull.*, **73,** 422
55. Dawes, R. M. (1971). A case study of graduate admissions: Applications of three principles of human decision making. *Am. Psychol.*, **26,** 180
56. Slovic, P. (1969). Analyzing the expert judge: A descriptive study of a stockbroker's decision processes. *J. Appl. Psychol.*, **53,** 255
57. Shepard, R. N. (1964). On subjectively optimum selection among multiattribute alternatives. In Shelly, M. W. and Bryan, G. L. (eds.) pp. 257–81. *Human Judgments and Optimality* (New York: John Wiley & Sons)
58. Meehl, P. E. (1954). *Clinical versus Statistical Prediction.* (Minneapolis: University of Minnesota Press)
59. Sawyer, J. (1966). Measurement *and* prediction: Clinical *and* statistical. *Psychol. Bull.*, **66,** 178
60. Dawes, R. M. (1976). Shallow psychology. In Carroll, J. S. and Payne, J. W. (eds.) *Cognition and Social Behaviour* pp. 5–11. (Hillsdale, N.J.: Erlbaum)
61. Mai, N. and Hachmann, E. (1977). Anwendung des Bayes-Theorems in der medizinischen Diagnostik-eine Literaturübersicht. *Metamed.*, **1,** 161
62. Einhorn, H. J. (1972). Expert measurement and mechanical combination. *Org. Behav. Hum. Perform.*, **7,** 86
63. Einhorn, H. J. and Hogarth, R. M. (1975). Unit weighting schemes for decision making. *Org. Behav. Hum. Perform.*, **13,** 171
64. Dawes, R. M. and Corrigan, B. (1974). Linear models in decision making. *Psychol. Bull.*, **81,** 95
65. Dawes, R. M. (1977). Predictive models as a guide to preference. *IEEE Trans. Sys. Man. Cyber.*, **SMC-7,** 355
66. Slovic, P. (1975). Choice between equally-valued alternatives. *J. Exp. Psychol. Hum. Percept. Perform.*, **1,** 280
67. Sjöberg, L. (1976). Self esteem and information processing. *Göteborg Psychol. Rep.*, **6,** No. 14
68. Sjöberg, L. (1977). Strength of belief and risk. *Göteborg Psychol. Rep.*, **7,** No. 2
69. Kunreuther, H. (1976). Limited knowledge and insurance protection. *Pub. Pol.*, **24,** 227
70. Swalm, R. O. (1966). Utility theory – insights into risk taking. *Harv. Bus. Rev.*, **44,** 123
71. Slovic, P., Fischhoff, B., Lichtenstein, S., Corrigan, B. and Combs, B. (1977). Preference for insuring against probable small losses: implications for the theory and practice of insurance. *J. Risk. Insur.*, **44,** 237
72. Langer, E. J. and Roth, J. (1975). Heads I win, tails it's chance: the illusion of control as a function of the sequence of outcomes in a purely chance task. *J. Pers. Soc. Psychol.*, **32,** 951
73. Lichtenstein, S., Fischhoff, B. and Phillips, L. D. (1977). Calibration of probabilities: the state of the art. In Jungermann, H. and de Zeeuw, G. (eds.) *Decision Making and Change in Human Affairs*, pp. 275–324. (Dordrecht-Holland: Reidel)
74. Lichtenstein, S. and Fischhoff, B. (1977). Do those who know more also know more about how much they know? *Org. Behav. Hum. Perform.*, **20,** 159
75. Fischhoff, B. (1975). Hindsight: thinking backward? *Psychol. Today* (April), 71
76. Fischhoff, B. and Beyth, R. (1975). 'I knew it would happen' – remembered probabilities of once-future things. *Org. Behav. Hum. Perform.*, **13,** 1
77. Fischhoff, B. (1975). Hindsight ≠ foresight. The effect of outcome knowledge on judgement under uncertainty. *J. Exp. Psychol.: Hum. Percept. Perform.*, **1,** 288
78. Fischhoff, B. (1977). Perceived informativeness of facts. *J. Exp. Psychol.: Hum. Percept. Perform.*, **3,** 349
79 Slovic, P. and Fischhoff, B. (1977). On the psychology of experimental surprises. *J. Exp. Psychol.: Hum. Percept. Perform.*, **3,** 544
80. Lusted, L. B. (1968). *Introduction to Medical Decision Making.* (Springfield, Ill.: Charles C. Thomas)

81. Kassirer, J. P. (1976). The principles of clinical decision making: an introduction to decision analysis. *Yale J. Bio. Med.*, **49,** 149
82. Raiffa, H. (1968). *Decision Analysis: Introductory Lectures on Choices under Uncertainty.* pp. 309 (Reading, Mass.: Addison-Wesley)
83. Pauker, S. G. (1976). Coronary artery surgery: the use of decision analysis. *Ann. Int. Med.*, **85,** 8
84. Aschenbrenner, K. M. and Kasubek, W. (1978). Challenging the Cushing syndrome: multiattribute evaluation of cortisone drugs. *Org. Behav. Hum. Perform.*, **22,** 216
85. Keeney, R. L. and Raiffa, H. (1976). *Decisions with Multiple Objectives: Preferences and Value Tradeoffs*, pp. 569 (New York: John Wiley & Sons)
86. von Winterfeldt, D. and Fischer, G. W. (1975). Multi-attribute utility theory: models and assessment procedures. In Wendt, D. and Vlek, C. (eds.) *Utility, Probability, and Human Decision Making*, pp. 47–86. (Dordrecht-Holland: Reidel)
87. Slovic, P., Rorer, L. G. and Hoffman, P. J. (1971). Analyzing use of diagnostic signs. *Invest. Radiol.*, **6,** 18
88. Bean, W. R. (ed.) (1950). *Sir William Osler: Aphorisms from his Bedside Teaching and Writings*, p. 125. (New York: Schuman) – cited in reference 2
89. de Finetti, B. (1937). La prévision: ses lois logiques, ses sources subjectives. *Annals de l'Institut Henri Poincaré*, **7,** 1
90. Moore, P. G. (1977). The manager struggles with uncertainty. *J. R. Stat. Soc. A.*, **140,** 129
91. Spetzler, C. S. and Staël von Holstein, C.-A.S. (1975). Probability encoding in decision analysis. *Manage. Sci.*, **22,** 340
92. Gini, C. (1952). The statistical bases of diagnosis and prognosis. *Acta Genet. Stat. Med.*, **3,** 280
93. Ledley, R. S. and Lusted, L. B. (1959). Reasoning foundations of medical diagnosis. *Science*, **130,** 9
94. Lusted, L. B., Bell, R. S., Edwards, W., Roberts, H. V. and Wallace, D. L. (1977). Evaluating the efficacy of radiologic procedures. In Snapper, K. (ed.) *Models in Metrics for Decision Makers* (Washington, D.C.: Information Resources Press)
95. Gustafson, D. H. (1969). Evaluation of probabilistic information processing in medical decision making. *Org. Behav. Hum. Perform.*, **4,** 20
96. Betaque, N. E. and Gorry, G. A. (1971). Automating judgmental decision making for a serious medical problem. *Manage. Sci.*, **17,** B-421–434
97. Gorry, G. A., Kassirer, J. P., Essig, A. and Schwartz, W. B. (1973). Decision analysis as the basis for computer-aided management of acute renal failure. *Am. J. Med.*, **55,** 473
98. Selvidge, J. (1975). A three-step procedure for assigning probabilities to rare events. In Wendt, D. and Vlek, C. (eds.) *Utility, Probability and Human Decision Making*, pp. 199–216. (Dordrecht-Holland: Reidel)
99. Humphreys, P. (1977). Application of multi-attribute utility theory. In Jungermann, H. and de Zeeuw, G. (eds.) *Decision Making and Change in Human Affairs*, pp. 165–207. (Dordrecht-Holland: Reidel)
100. Johnson, E. M. and Huber, G. P. (1977). The technology of utility assessment. *IEEE Trans. Sys. Man. Cyber.*, **SMC-7,** 311
101. Bell, D. E., Keeney, R. L. and Raiffa, H. (1977). *Conflicting Objectives in Decisions*, pp. 442. (Chichester, England: John Wiley & Sons)
102. Gustafson, D. H. and Holloway, D. C. (1975). A decision theory approach to measuring severity in illness. *Health Ser. Res.* (Spring), 97
103. Krischer, J. P. (1976). The mathematics of cleft lip and palate treatment evaluation: measuring the desirability of treatment outcomes. *Cleft Palate J.*, **13,** 165
104. McNeil, B. J., Keeler, E, and Adelstein, S. J. (1975). Primer on certain elements of medical decision making. *N. Engl. J. Med.*, **293,** 211
105. Pauker, S. G. and Kassirer, J. P. (1975). Therapeutic decision making: A cost-benefit analysis. *N. Engl. J. Med.*, **293,** 229

106. Thornbury, J. R. and Fryback, D. G. (1977). Cost-benefit analysis, medical decision making and the individual radiologist. *Curr. Probl. Diag. Radiol.*, **7** (Whole No. 2)
107. Lusted, L. B. (1971). Decision-making studies in patient management. *N. Engl. J. Med.*, **284,** 416
108. Lusted, L. B. (1971). Signal detectability and medical decision-making. *Science*, **171,** 1217
109. Neuhauser, D. and Lewicki, A. M. (1975). What do we gain from the sixth stool guaiac? *N. Engl. Med.*, **293,** 226
110. Fischhoff, B. (1980). Clinical decision analysis. *Operations Research*, **28,** 28
111. Brown, R. V. (1977). Modelling subsequent acts for decision analysis. In Aykac, A. and Brumat, C. (eds.) *New Developments in the Applications of Bayesian Methods*, pp. 313–336. (Amsterdam: North-Holland)
112. Fischhoff, B. (1977). Cost-benefit analysis and the art of motor-cycle maintenance. *Policy Sci.*, **8,** 177
113. Seaver, D. A. (1976). 'Assessment of group preferences and group uncertainty for decision making', pp. 56 (University of Southern California: SSRI Research Report 76–4)
114. Hammond, K. R. and Adelmann, L. (1976). Science, values and human judgment, *Science*, **194,** 389
115. Hammond, K. R. and Brehmer, B. (1973). Quasi-rationality, quarrels, and new conceptions of feedback. In Rappoport, L. and Summers, D. A. (eds.) *Human Judgement and Social Interaction*, pp. 338–391. (New York: Holt, Rinehart & Winston)
116. Price, P. B., Taylor, C. W., Nelson, D. E., Lewis, E. G., Laughmiller, G. C., Mathieson, R. Murray, S. L. and Maxwell, J. G. (1971). *Measurement and Predictors of Physician Performance: Two Decades of Intermittently Sustained Research.* (Salt Lake City: LLR Press). Cited in reference 3
117. Inman, W. H. W. (1977). Recorded release. In Gross, F. H. and Inman, W. H. W. (eds.) *Drug Monitoring*, pp. 65–78. (London: Academic Press)
118. Makridakis, S. and Wheelwright, S. C. (1978). *Interactive Forecasting: Univariate and Multivariate Methods*, 2nd Edn., pp. 650. (San Francisco): Holden-Day)
119. Peterson, C. R. (ed.) (1973). Special issue: cascaded inference, *Org. Behav. Hum. Perform.*, **10,** 315
120. Schum, D. A. (1975). On the weighing of testimony in judicial proceedings from sources having reduced credibility. *Hum. Fact.*, **17,** 172
121. Schum, D. A. (1977). Contrast effects in inference: on the conditioning of current evidence by prior evidence. *Org. Behav. Hum. Perform.*, **18,** 217
122. Koch-Weser, J. (1977). Validation of ADR's in Gross, F. H. and Inman, W. H. W. (eds.) *Drug Monitoring*, pp. 79–89. (London: Academic Press)

# 36
# Assessing cause and effect relationships of adverse drug reaction reports

J. VENULET

In monitoring suspected adverse drug reactions the assessment of whether the reaction is indeed causally related with drug treatment will come up at some stage in the analysis.

In epidemiological studies a higher incidence of an adverse event in the treated group will indicate the existence of causal relationship between the drug under study and the event. It will not, however, indicate whether a particular patient in the treated group developed the event *because* of taking the drug.

With spontaneous reporting of individual cases the statistical analysis is much more difficult, because at the initial stages the number of reports is small and there are problems in finding control groups suitable for testing hypotheses. Thus, the degree of causal relationship is assessed on the grounds of the strength of evidence provided by the details in the individual case report and interpreted by a knowledgeable evaluator, and is one of the factors which decides what steps should be taken. The other two factors are the severerity of the adverse event and the number of similar cases reported, even if poorly documented. Usually, this type of problem occurs before epidemiological studies are initiated since epidemiological studies may become necessary only after individual case reports have been received.[1] However, with the advent of such monitoring techniques as 'monitored release', it should be possible to monitor individual cases, and epidemiological studies could be conducted in parallel and within the framework of the same scheme. Unfortunately this is possible only for a limited number of drugs.

The causality factor is the most controversial of the three factors just mentioned, but at the same time the most crucial. Medical judgement is based on knowledge and experience which will vary from one doctor to another; but even different judgements by the same doctor are not uncommon in regard to causality. The level of disagreement among experts has been studied and demonstrated in several publications,[2–5] varying between 50 and 90% depending on the conditions of each study.

With such a high level of disagreement the practical informative value of a causality assessment may seem rather limited. Indeed, with data transferred from one monitoring system to another (e.g. from the pharmaceutical industry to drug regulatory agencies) and then pooled together with reports from other sources (e.g. in the WHO Collaborative Centre for International Drug Monitoring), the informative value of a subjective causality assessment becomes almost useless and potentially misleading. Yet even in cases where insufficient information is available, doctors, health authorities and manufacturers cannot always avoid making evaluations. This means that compromises have to be accepted, recognizing that the data available are poor but that their evaluation nevertheless has to be undertaken. In the absence of a scientific standard of reference, the evaluator's own experience, his subjective views and his tendency to keep on the safe side are factors which frequently influence the final assessment.

Not surprisingly, attempts have been made to remedy this situation. Various drug monitoring systems have selected lists of terms describing different levels of causal relationship (e.g. unlikely, possible, probable) and have indicated conditions which should be met in order to assign a case to a given causality level.[6–10] These provided a useful first step in the right direction, but for various reasons, mainly because of the limited number of variables considered and the vagueness of their description, they were not completely satisfactory.

In the last few years more formal approaches have been published, based on stricter criteria, and organized according to the principle of decision-making tables or other forms of algorithmic procedure. In these formal approaches items of information lead to the assessment in a predetetermined and standardized way, and with a logic which allows operational application largely (but not completely) independent of the subjectivity of the evaluation.[11–18]

The proliferation of methods of standardized assessment reflects the need for a more formal approach, and the hopes and expectations attached to this type of procedure. However, while each method may give reproducible results, differences between results obtained by different methods do occur, as has been demonstrated by Begaud *et al.*[19]

The purpose of all these efforts is not to replace human evaluators, but rather to find a practical standard presenting the most objective medical criteria with which an individual assessment can be compared. Nor is it the aim to force the evaluator to accept the verdict of the algorithm. Rather, any relevant discrepancy should lead to a 'dialogue' with the standardized procedure and to identification of reasons for the diverging judgement on a particular case; it should also bring about improvements in the method itself. In the case of disagreement, re-evaluation may result in a more accurate assessment. The role of the standardized assessment should be that of a 'supervisor' helping the evaluator to identify and avoid errors of judgement due to neglect of certain important information, and to reach the highest possible degree of consistency.

Any acceptable solution of the problem of standardized assessment of causality will require a thorough review of the particular needs of different users of such an approach, such as treating-physicians, drug regulatory agencies, pharmaceutical companies and other drug monitoring organizations. It will also require an analysis of the more immediate objectives set for particular monitoring systems; for example for early warning purposes the system should, in general, be more critical of the drug (to generate a signal) than in the case of regulatory decisions certainly requiring much more solid evidence.

It is also necessary to consider possible exceptions in the course of the assessment, because of specific pathognomonic patterns of the adverse reactions. And, last but not least, the legal consequences of causality assessments arrived at not by experts but by a standardized procedure should be considered.

Some of these aspects have been touched upon in different publications, but the whole matter of causality assessment of single cases was thoroughly reviewed at a workshop[20] held in Morges, Switzerland, in June 1981 – material from which was largely used in preparing this chapter. One consequence of this meeting was the organization of an informal group of those working in this field (Active Permanent Workshop of 'Imputologists' [APWI]).

The term standardized assessment implies that the same operational logic is always applied. This is achieved through strict adherence to an algorithmic design in which identical information always contributes to the final assessment in the same way. The presentation is usually either in the form of a classical algorithm,[18,21] or of decision tables,[12] or as a set of numerical values (weights) assigned to different items of information.[16] In this last approach the 'case value', which is the sum of weights of all questions, is calculated and, depending in what range it falls, is assigned a corresponding level of causality.

Various terms are used to express levels of causality. Five levels, (not drug related, unlikely, possible, probable and definite) are often used as this allows for a greater flexibility, but some systems do well with three levels. In any case, for all practical purposes the number of levels is more important than the names given to them: For example, is 'definite' a better term than 'very probable', or can one ever say that an event is not drug related unless it was already present before the drug was started? Practical implications of terms used may depend upon the method of assessment as explained later in this chapter. There is the feeling, particularly among the French authors,[11] that the individual case reports in most instances only allege causality, and that, therefore, the term imputability should be used instead.

If all evaluators interpreted each item in the standardized assessment in the same way, the resulting assessment of causality of cases with identical information would always be the same as long as the same algorithm is used. There is, however, a risk that while each method would give reproducible results differences between results obtained with different methods would still be possible. This, indeed was demonstrated by Begaud *et al.*[19] In only 27 of 100 cases were the results obtained with the four methods compared by him identical. The reason for this are the differences in the medical interpretations of the data in the case report, i.e. at the stage preceding the use of an algorithm.

Within a particular method, it is relatively easy to achieve a high degree of consistency of assessment, but the real goal is accuracy of assessment. Consistency both within the evaluator and between evaluators is a prerequisite of accuracy, and thus represents the first step of our efforts.

Achieving consistency should provide us with a point of reference, which would be very useful in this largely subjective domain, but accuracy of assessment is what we are really looking for. And it is here where the major difficulties begin. With largely observational type of data in case reports, and wide differences in experience between evaluators, disagreements occur quite often, and even an agreement does not necessarily prove that the assessment was correct. However, as long as there is no better way of proving accuracy than by the consensus of several evaluators, the quality of assessment with an alogorithmic approach will be judged by the level of its agreement with the opinions of experts. But even they rarely agree among themselves.

Standardization usually involves simplification and paying more attention to those items of information that are most relevant and readily available. For example, drug concentration in blood or the results of elaborate immunological tests may be conclusive, but are rarely available and, therefore, of less practical importance in standardized procedures.

The methods published so far have generally been intended for all drugs and all adverse reactions, which obviously increases the number of 'non-typical' cases which require special approaches. For example, depending on the type of reaction, any one item of information would carry a different strength of evidence. If the reported reaction was of a dose-related, pharmacological type, the lack of unwanted effect during previous administrations in the same patient would tend to militate against a causal relationship. With an allergic reaction, good tolerance in the past could not be interpreted in the same way. Such shortcomings could be remedied by enlarging the algorithm to include different types of reactions, such a dose-related and dose-unrelated, irreversible effects, application site reactions, etc. This would most likely increase the reliability of assessment and improve its accuracy.

There are no limitations to the development of special procedures for special situations. On the other hand, some drug/adverse reaction associations are so pathognomonic (for example bleeding with anticoagulants or bronchospasm after non-steroidal anti-inflammatory drug in patients allergic to acetyl-salicylic acid) that on the basis of such an association the existence of a definite relationship can be accepted. It would be too cumbersome and really unnecessary to develop special algorithms for such cases. The experienced doctor would do it faster and as well. In other words, standardized assessment is not necessary in obvious situations, but in those where differences could easily occur an objective yardstick (even one whose accuracy is unproven) provides a helpful point of reference.

Before even an algorithm is applied it is essential that the various items of information in the case report form are understood in a similar way by the medical evaluators. For example, rechallenge. It may mean only re-exposure for diagnostic purposes, or it may also include inadvertent taking of the drug by the patient. Or the important questions about whether similar symptoms may be caused by the disease or if the reported unwanted effect is known to occur with the suspected drug. What does 'known' mean?: one reported case of suspected adverse drug reaction, or five such cases, or only if causality was proven, etc.? Without clear guidance and definition inconsistency would be 'programmed in' even before the application of an algorithm, and independently from its quality.

In fact, most of the differences between the judgements of experts are probably caused by their different experience and interpretation of various data rather than by differences in the strength of evidence given to them. An important accomplishment of the Workshop in Morges[20] was to produce a list of definitions and clarifications regarding a number of items of information sought in most reporting systems or considered by evaluators.

Depending on the particular environment in which monitoring is conducted and its objectives, the type and amount of data collected may vary considerably. In a hospital where a decision has to be taken as to whether a potentially life-saving drug has to be discontinued because of a serious adverse event, the assessment of causality will have to be made without awaiting the results of dechallenge or rechallenge. In this situation the Bayesian approach, which takes into account past experience with the drug, will play a much more important role than when retrospectively assessing more complete case reports, as is the case with drug regulatory agencies or pharmaceutical companies. Dangoumau *et al.*[22] distinguish between initial assessment of causality (imputability) made at the time of occurrence of the adverse event and the final causality (imputability) made on the basis of additional information which may become subsequently available.

While no information can be discarded as useless, there is a certain amount of data which is usually easy to collect, and thus represents the basis for assessment of the majority of cases. In the method of standardized assessment proposed by us[16] the first and second part of the Check List and Assessment Form ('History of the present adverse reaction' and 'Patient's past adverse reaction history') are directly concerned with information asked for in the pharmaceutical company's adverse reaction reporting forms, and indeed by nearly all monitoring systems including WHO. The third part of the assessment form asks for the evaluating doctor's opinion on a set of questions represented in the reporting form. This opinion may vary from one evaluator to another according to their differing experience. Articles on adverse reactions, which contribute to the formation of this experience, are not always as informative as one would like them to be.[23] The questions considered in our standardized assessment method are listed below:

All questions refer to the Suspected Drug or in a case of interactions to both drugs:

I **History of present adverse reaction**

1. Dose or duration of treatment exceeded? *(as per 'Basis Text')*
2. Drug given prior to event? *(as per dates)*
3. Concomitant or preceding drug therapy?
4. Reaction at site of application? *(inj., supp., sublingual and topical)*
5. ADR immediately follows the drug? *(within approx. 1 hour)*
6. Dechallenge positive? *(if ADR reversible) (without treatment = W; with treatment = Y)*
7. Rechallenge positive?
8. Were concomitant drugs stopped at the same time? *(only if 3 = Y)*

II **Patient's past adverse reaction history**

9. Same ADR to this drug before?
10. Other ADR to this drug before?
11. Similar symptoms in the past? *(not related to drug treatment)*
12. Similar ADR with other drugs in the past?

III **Monitor's experience**

13. Drug/ADR interval compatible with the event? *(Typical = T; Compatible = Y; Incompatible = N)*
14. Adverse event of rare spontaneous occurrence? *(Y or N only)*
15. Similar events known to occur with the disease treated or with concomitant disease(s)?
16. ADR occurrence facilitated by the disease treated or by concomitant diseases?
17. Contributory role of non-drug therapies?
18. Other contributory factors (habits, environment etc.)?
19. ADR known with the suspected drug? *(K, Y or N only) (known = K; suspected = Y)*
20. ADR explainable by the biological properties of the suspected drug? *(only if 19 = N)*
21. ADR known with pharmacologically-related drugs? *(only if 19 = N)*
22. ADR known with concomitant or preceding drug therapy? *(only if 3 = Y; if well known = W)*
23. Drug interaction as a possible cause of ADR *(only if 3 = Y)*

Doctors are asked to answer each of the above questions by circling the appropriate letter Y (yes), N (no) or U (unknown) in the right hand column on the form. ADRs are categorized as follows:

A Dose-related
B Dose-unrelated
C Type I allergic
D At the site of application
E Interaction
F Drug dependence

G Irreversible
H Withdrawal symptoms
I Fetal malformation
Z Unclassified

A more detailed description of these categories is printed on the reverse side of the Check List and Assessment Form. Doctors are asked to tick at least one of the above categories.

The Check List is also intended to increase the likelihood that all relevant factors will be considered in a systematic way, and that no information will be left out. At the Workshop,[20] answers to the following questions were considered to be of 'greatest importance':

(1) Drug given prior to event?
(2) Reaction at site of application?
(3) Drug/ADR interval compatible with the event?
(4) ADR immediately follows the drug and of acute onset?
(5) Rechallenge positive?
(6) Dechallenge positive?
(7) Were concomitant drugs stopped at the same time?
(8) Same ADR to this drug before?
(9) ADR known with the suspected drug?

From these nine questions, seven directly refer to reported information, and only two (questions 3 and 9) reflect the opinions of the evaluator. Nevertheless, they influence the assessment considerably. The influence of items of information relative to knowledge and experience on the results obtained by employing different methods of assessment is greatest.

The shortest method[21] is based on seven questions, while the longest[15] lists 57 questions. The main reason for differences in the length of the algorithm are not only the very specific questions in the longer algorithms (e.g. drug levels in blood) but the more detailed way of enquiring about certain information (e.g. a question whether reported unwanted events are known to occur with the disease can be left as such or divided into two questions, one concerning the disease treated with the suspected drug and another concerning concomitant diseases). In shorter algorithms, many questions contain an assumption that related but unspecified details will be considered as well. But there must be a limit to adding more questions, if the algorithm is to remain useful. A simple but rigid algorithm might be easy to use, but would probably only have limited application. An 'all-encompassing' method would be unmanageable. The chances of obtaining a certain type of information must obviously play an important role in deciding whether to include a question about it or not.

The question of legal consequences of causality assessment is clearly an important one. Without at least assuming the existence of causal relationships the question of liability cannot be even asked; and much more would have to be known before it could be answered. This question of liability has been considered elsewhere in this book. It is, however, worth considering here the different possible outcomes of the same causality assessment of a particular case made by an expert as compared to the assessment with an algorithm. In the first situation it is an informed opinion based on whatever details are provided in the particular case report. In the latter it means only that certain criteria, clearly defined beforehand and applicable in the same way to all cases, were met allowing the case to be attributed to a certain level of causality; it does not imply that the assigned degree of causal relationship was proven beyond doubt.

In a diametrically different approach our group has tried to arrive at weights for the different questions, not empirically, but through mathematical analysis of a large series of cases already assessed by experts (method of correspondence analysis). The results were encouraging.[24]

A chapter devoted to causality assessment of single cases should end with a list of the main advantages of standardized assessment in general.

(1) *Communication between various users*: Standardized assessment improves communication, since the way the judgement was developed is clearly indicated; thus the information relative to causality becomes less equivocal.
(2) *Reproducibility of results*: Using standardized assessments, the same case report is more likely to be evaluated in the same way by different assessors.
(3) *Validity of results*: As with medical judgements in general the extent to which results obtained with standardized methods of assessment reflect the 'truth' needs to be evaluated. Different methods do not necessarily lead to the same conclusions; however, the results of a limited experiment with eight methods conducted at the Morges Workshop[20] were encouraging. One way of assessing validity is by comparing the results of an algorithmic method with experts' opinions. The concordance of the results obtained with all the published methods is encouraging, but falls short of definite proof.
(4) *Double-checking of case reports*: In several organizations, for example in Ciba–Geigy, our method of standardized assessment is used in parallel with expert evaluation to identify differences in opinion for the purposes of follow-up, re-evaluation, etc. Such comparisons could also lead to improvement in the method of assessment itself, and help to develop common understanding, acceptance of definitions, common standards for interpreting data, etc.

A discussion of the quality of case-reports to be assessed is not within the scope of this chapter, but it is clear that no system of assessment will give valid results if the information it uses is incomplete and of doubtful quality. Therefore, efforts towards improvement of adverse reaction reporting, both published and unpublished, should continue independently of whatever method of assessment is used. Better and more complete data would make the task of all of us much easier.

## References


1. Berneker, G.-C., and Venulet, J. (1982). About the problem. In Venulet, J., Berneker, G.-C. and Ciucci, A. G. (eds.) *Assessing Causes of Adverse Drug Reactions.* pp. 1–5. (London: Academic Press)
2. Karch, F. E., Smith, C. L., Kerzner, B., Mazzullo, J., Weintraub, M. and Lasagna, L. (1976). Adverse drug reactions – a matter of opinion. *Clin. Pharmacol. Ther.*, **19,** 489–92
3. Koch-Weser, J., Sellers, E. M. and Zacest, R. (1977). The ambiguity of adverse drug reactions. *Eur. J. Clin. Pharcacol.*, **11,** 75–8
4. James, D., Haller, E., Rosselet, G., Brooke, E. M. and Schelling, J. L. (1978). Fréquence des prescriptions de médicaments et de leurs effets indésirables dans un départment de médecine. *Schwiez. Med. Wschr.*, **108,** 1270–7
5. Joyce, C. R. B. (1982). Identifying causes of disagreement in assessment of causality. In Venulet, J., Berneker, G.-C. and Ciucci, A. G. (eds.) *Assessing causes of Adverse Drug Reactions.* pp. 95–103. (London: Academic Press)
6. Adverse Drug Reactions in the United States: Medicine in the Public Interest, Washington, DC
7. Meddelande fran Läkemeddsbiverknings Kommitten (1974): *Meddelande* No. 20 (in Swedish)
8. Australian Drug Evaluation Committee (1978). Report of Suspected Adverse Drug Reactions, No. 4, p.v. (Canberra: Australian Government Publishing)
9. Seidl, L. G. Thornton, G. F. and Cluff, L. E. (1965). Epidemiological studies of adverse drug reactions. *Am. J. Publ. Health*, **55,** 1170–5
10. Venulet, J. (1977). Methods of monitoring adverse reactions to drugs. In Jucker, E. (ed.) *Progress in Drug Research*, Vol. 21, pp. 233–92. (Basel: Birkhäuser Verlag)
11. Dangoumau, J., Evereux, J.-C. and Jouglard, J. (1978). Méthode d'imputabilité des effets indésirables des médicaments. *Thérapie*, **33,** 373–81
12. Karch, F. E. and Lasagna, L. (1977). Toward the operational identification of adverse drug reactions. *Clin. Pharmacol. Ther.*, **21,** 247–54
13. Irey, N. S. (1976). Tissue reactions to drugs. *Am. J. Pathol.*, **82,** 617–47
14. Blanc, S., Leuenberger, P., Berger, J. P., Brooke, E. M. and Schelling, J. L. (1979). Judgements of trained observers on adverse drug reactions. *Clin. Pharmacol. Ther.*, **25,** 493–8
15. Kramer, M. S., Leventhal, J. M., Hutchinson, T. A. and Feinstein, A. R. (1979). An algorithm for the operational assessment of adverse drug reactions. In Background, description and introduction for use. *J. Am. Med. Assoc.*, **242,** 623–32
16. Venulet, J., Ciucci, A. and Berneker, B.-C. (1980). Standardized assessment of drug-adverse reaction relationship. *Int. J. Clin. Pharmacol.*, **18,** 381–8
17. Emanueli, A. and Sacchetti, G. (1980). An algorithm for the classification of untoward events in large scale clinical trials. In *Agents and Actions*, Vol. 7, pp. 318–2. (Basel: Birkhäuser Verlag)
18. Jones, J. K. (1982). Adverse drug reactions in the community health setting: approaches to recognizing, counseling, and reporting. *Fam. Commun. Health*, **5,** 58–67
19. Begaud, B., Boisseau, A., Albin, H. and Dangoumau, J. (1981). Comparaison de quatre méthodes d'imputabilité des effets indésirables des médicaments. *Thérapie*, 36, **65–70**
20. Venulet, J., Berneker, G.-C., Ciucci, A. G. (eds.) (1982). *Assessing causes of adverse drug reactions.* (London: Academic Press)

21. Weber, J. C. P. (1982). Use of the computer to allocate a category of drug-culpability to adverse reactions. In Venulet, J., Berneker, G.-C. and Ciucci, A. G. (eds.) *Assessing Causes of Adverse Drug Reactions*. pp. 117–21. (London: Academic Press)
22. Dangoumau, J. Begaud, B., Père, J. C. and Albin, H. (1981). De l'imputabilité originelle a l'imputabilité terminale. *Thérapie*, **36,** 219–22
23. Venulet, J., Blattner, R., von Bülow, J., Berneker, G.-C. (1982). How good are articles on adverse drug reactions. *Br. Med. J.*, **284,** 252–4
24. Bastin, Ch., Wertheimer, P., Venulet, J. (1984). Adverse drug reactions – a computer assisted application of correspondence analysis for automatic causality assessment. *Meth. Inform. Med.*, **23,** 183–8

# Section 4:
# DRUG SAFETY AND THE LAW

# Editor's Introduction and Commentary

After reading the fourth section of this book which deals with the law in relation to drug effects, one might be forgiven for immediately seeking help from a psychiatrist. Words like 'nightmare', 'snakepit' or 'hallucination' spring to mind, but one thing is certain, only a tiny minority of the patients who are unfortunate enough to have become victims of drug accidents are likely to derive any benefit from the legal systems in the various countries.

In a civilized society, irrespective of the cause of an injury, it would be expected that victims should receive the highest possible standard of care that society can provide. Except where damage has been caused by negligence, there would seem to be no reason why an 'elite' of disabled people should be created simply because, as must inevitably happen on rare occasions, they have been disabled by an ADR rather than by slipping on a banana skin. There can be few greater tragedies, for example, than the permanent disablement of a child or young person, especially by brain damage. The great majority of such cases, however, are not due to drugs taken during pregnancy or to vaccination or to some form of treatment for a childhood complaint. Most patients and their families learn painfully to accept their misfortune with dignity and courage. Once a possible explanation for the damage has been suggested, however slender the evidence, the additional anguish associated with the search for compensation is often indescribable, and there is usually no way in which patients can be persuaded that a drug or doctor or manufacturer may not have been responsible. The search for compensation can become totally embittering, and it is infinitely preferable that relief for sufferers should be rapidly and generously provided by insurance, rather than by time-wasting and expensive law suits.

If he fears the legal consequences of ADRs and decides not to prescribe a drug and the patient dies, it is unlikely that a doctor would be pursued by lawyers with the same vigour afforded to those whose attempts to do good have resulted in harm. So far, there are no action groups for untreated patients whose quality of life might have been improved if a doctor had the courage to take a calculated risk. The present trend in litigation may seriously reduce the efficacy of medical care and the search for new treatment. Could new legislation reverse this trend?

The laws in various EEC countries are complex and, in striking contrast to the United States, there have been comparatively few cases of drug litigation in Europe. Mr Kurt Siehr tackles, in considerable depth, the complex legal systems on the continent of Europe, and predicts that insurance rather than law suits will eventually provide the best solution to problems faced by patients, doctors and manufacturers. Of particular interest among many strange and seemingly illogical concepts is that of *joint liability* which could lead to a manufacturer, a prescriber and a government drug regulatory agency all being sued, the latter because it failed to react appropriately to the ADRs reported to it. If one party was forced to pay the full compensation, he may then sue the others for a share of the settlement. Thus a manufacturer could sue the government for failing to warn about an ADR and also the doctor who prescribed the drug which caused it!

Howard Lester and Alan Fudim describe US society as 'litigious and consumer oriented', something of an understatement to those in other countries who fear that enormous US settlements will drive manufacturers out of business or encourage other countries to adopt similar legislation. Because most suits are against manufacturers, who are thought to be best able to bear the punitive costs of litigation (by increasing the price of their products), the cost of insurance is becoming prohibitive. Many products available in other countries are not sold in the USA, and the American public sooner or later will have to decide if the loss of a range of effective treatments for serious illnesses may not be too high a price to pay. But, as the authors explain, there is some hope that the trend may be reversed for, if drugs are adequately labelled with clear instructions for safe use, the manufacturer may be protected from all but accusations of negligence.

In the USA, the *Physicians' Desk Reference* provides the necessary instructions and warnings about proprietary drugs. The doctor who failed to read it before prescribing could be deemed to be negligent. The same could apply to the *Data Sheet* used in the United Kingdom. American law recognizes that the duty to warn the patient rests with the physician, or a pharmacist in the case of a non-prescribable medicine, rather than the manufacturer.

The contingency fee system in which an attorney advances and later, if he succeeds in the case, recovers all the expenses of litigation and retains perhaps as much as a third or more of the judgement, is unique to the USA, and it has the advantage that a patient of limited means may secure compensation where in other countries he might fail. At first sight this seems to be a considerable advance, but the risk of substantial loss to the attorney is great and he will often not accept a case unless there is a good chance of obtaining a settlement in excess of $100 000.

Although a number of drug tragedies such as thalidomide or practolol have been common to several countries, others such as cancer of the vagina caused by diethylstilboestrol (USA) and SMON (Japan) have been mainly restricted to a single country. SMON was unusual because it was not caused by a prescribed medicine (though it is now restricted to prescription in most countries), and because it affected a very large number of people.

Although somewhat confused, the development of relief systems for sufferers of ADRs may be more rapid in Japan than other countries, and it is encouraging to note that the Japanese Ministry of Health takes an active part in financing the relief fund. It is also interesting to note that at least the possibility exists for retrospective relief to the victims of past ADRs.

Mr Spink raises the question of who has the capacity to pay the huge sums involved in compensation for large-scale accidents, and he points to the complexity of scientific problems involved in proof of causation. In English law, an injured patient has to prove that the drug caused the injury, that it was manufactured by a particular company and that the product was defective through the manufacturer's negligence. Perhaps one of the strongest arguments against generic prescribing and any system which allows one manufacturer's product to be substituted for anothers' is that it virtually destroys the patient's chances of compensation should anything go wrong. The testing and quality control necessary to meet the requirements of the Medicines Act greatly reduces the chances that a manufacturer can be proved to have been negligent. With a new drug, the defendant company may have the scientific knowledge required to prove the plaintiff's case which the plaintiff's representatives do not have! The high cost of litigation may mean that justice may be available to the very rich who can afford it, or, paradoxically, to the very poor who receive legal aid, while it is denied to the great majority of middle-income groups.

The concept of strict liability, which removes the plaintiff's need to prove negligence, inevitably forces the manufacturers to insure against it, and this raises the question of whether the insurance market can provide the cover for such a high-risk industry.

By defining and enforcing the requirements for marketing a drug under the conditions of the Medicines Act, it would seem logical that the government should at least share, if not take over, the responsibility for compensating the victims of accidents which will inevitably happen from time to time through no fault of the manufacturer. However, this view was not accepted by the *Pearson Commission*, who excluded the defence of official certification (licencing) which would enable the manufacturer to avoid liability by showing that his product had been certificated by an official body such as the Committee on Safety of Medicine.

Clearly the greatest tragedy that can befall the community as a whole is that the cost of licencing, insurance and litigation, while securing compensation for a few individuals who may be the victims of accidents that were for the most part unpredictable and unavoidable, will result in the denial to millions of the undoubted benefits of drug innovation simply because the industry has been bankrupted.

# 37
# Drug reactions and the law in the European Economic Community

K. G. SIEHR

## LEGAL PROBLEMS: SURVEY AND LIMITATIONS

### Prevention and compensation

What is true of many other hazards of modern life applies also to drug reactions: prevention is better than compensation. Adverse drug reactions (ADRs) can be prevented or at least minimized by the licensing of drug manufacturers, pre-marketing testing, approval by a governmental drug regulatory agency (DRA), regulation of marketing, restriction to prescription-only dispensing, continuing medical education, post-marketing surveillance, and rapid withdrawal of dangerous drugs from the market. Most of these regulatory steps require statutory provisions because they considerably restrict the free enterprise of industry, pharmacists, hospitals and doctors. I need not emphasize how important these regulations are for the prevention of dangerous side-effects of drugs, but I do not want to elaborate on them. I would prefer to concentrate on compensatory remedies and on liabilities arising from monitoring of ADRs or from the omission of preventive measures.

### Compensation in mainland counties of West Europe

Although all mainland counties of West Europe have adopted the so-called civil law (in contrast to the common law of England, Commonwealth countries and the United States), their legal systems differ considerably. A comparison of all these legal systems would take too much space: therefore I intend to give a short account of the common principles of liability (p. 542) and to rely, with respect to special problems, mainly on West German law as a paradigm of West

European civil law. The laws of other West European countries will, however, be taken into consideration.

### Court practice on ADRs

ADRs are not an everyday subject of adjudication in law courts. World wide attention was drawn to deplorable catastrophes with thalidomide and some other drugs where ADRs affected large groups of people. Such spectacular trials should not lead us to believe that there is much court practice on ADRs. Very often painful or fatal calamities are either not attributed to ADRs, or their effect cannot be proved or no efforts are made to bring a suit against responsible persons. The last tendency arises in countries with comprehensive social insurance. In most cases the ADRs are covered by health insurance or other types of social security. In these circumstances it is up to the insurer to consider a law-suit against responsible persons. Because of the scarcity of court practice on ADRs, many questions of liability for ADRs are not yet settled.

## FOUNDATIONS OF LIABILITY

### Notion of liability

The term 'liability', when used by lawyers, has a specific meaning. They are not concerned merely with moral duties and liabilities which do not entail legal consequences. They have to deal with liabilities sanctioned by law in one way or another. These sanctions may consist of punishment pronounced by a court of law, of damages to be paid to the injured person or of both of these effects. A burglar, for example, will be sentenced to imprisonment by a criminal law court and, if sued, has to make good the loss suffered by the plaintiff. Hence, the burglar is liable in criminal law as well as in civil law. I shall not deal with criminal liability of persons dealing with drugs, only on their liability in civil law, which is their responsibility to compensate injured persons or their families and their duty to avoid injury to other persons. It should, however, be mentioned that criminal proceedings often precede an action for damages, so that the victim may make use of the evidence revealed during the criminal trial for his suit for compensation.

### General liability in tort

From time immemorial the main basis of civil liability is the law of torts or, as it is called in continental Europe, the law of delicts, civil responsibility or of prohibited acts. The gist of this liability is the same in all jurisdictions: in order to prevent a war of everyone against everyone, it is the general duty of everybody to abstain from doing harm to anybody. This duty, which has often been called the law of nature, has been reduced in the continental jurisdictions to a general statutory obligation to make compensation if damage has been caused by violation of this duty. As an example we may cite the provision of the French Civil Code (art. 1382) which has been copied by several countries:

> *Tout fait quelconque de l'homme, qui cause à autrui un dommage, oblige celui par la faute duquel il est arrivé, à le réparer.*

The general obligation to compensate an injured or wronged person seems to settle all questions about civil wrongs. This may be the case with *intentionally* committed torts such as murder or burglary. Problems, however, arise with actions which *unintentionally* cause injury. In such situations at least five questions have to be answered before the doer (e.g. the prescriber of a drug) can be held responsible:

(1) Is there a causal connection between the action and the injury suffered?
(2) Is it sufficient that the action is only a partial cause of the injury?
(3) Is it necessary that the doer knew or should have known that his action may cause damage?
(4) If lack of positive knowledge does not absolve the doer from liability, what efforts should have been made by him to obtain a better knowledge of the consequences of his actions or is he liable anyway, even if nobody could have foreseen the harmful consequences?
(5) Would the injured person's consent relieve the doer of any liability?

All continental European countries of the EEC agree on five propositions:

(6) There is no civil liability without a causal connection between the action and the ultimate damage.
(7) Contributory causes do not break such a causal connection.
(8) There is not tortious liability without fault. Nobody will be held liable in tort unless he can be blamed at least with negligence, i.e. with failure to take proper care under the given circumstances.
(9) Liability without fault is not covered by the general duty to do no wrong (see p. 542).
(10) Consent of the injured person is generally regarded as a defence in tort: *volenti non fit iniuria.*

All these principles also apply to the liability of doctors. Already the *corpus iuris* of Justinian mentions the tortious liability of a doctor for using bad drugs. Today damages for pain and suffering can be awarded only if a tort has been committed.

## Special liability in tort

Apart from the general liability in torts there may be liabilities in torts specially created by statute or regarded as special liabilities by common law. For doctors, however, there are no special provisions as to their liability in torts.

In various penal codes, however, there are codified special offences which relate to medical treatment with harmful substances (cf., e.g. Belgian Criminal Code art. 421). Such offences are to be distinguished from the provisions of codes of medical ethics which in many countries are the basis of disciplinary jurisdiction.

## Contractual liability

Liability in tort arises if the general duty to do no wrong is violated. By contract everybody may assume additional duties, and not only obligations to abstain from wrongful conduct. Such contractual duties may be assumed by a seller and a purchaser as well as by a doctor or a hospital if they are not obliged to render services even without any contract.

In such a contract the parties to it are generally free to stipulate everything on which they can come to an agreement. If something has not been expressly regulated by the terms of the contract, statutory provisions on contractual relations may help to fill this gap. Statutory provisions on standard forms of contract try to protect the weaker party against unfair conditions presented to him by the other party in small print as the general conditions of contracting.

The codified legal systems of continental Europe furnish statutory provisions for many types of contracts. They do not, however, contain provisions on a special contract about medical treatment. Hence, the parties and the law courts turn to provisions about contracts for services if individually stipulated terms are missing.

## Standards of care

Whether a doctor will be held responsible in tort or for breach of contract, one of the main issues is the question of careful treatment. Every doctor will ask about the standards of care to be pursued by him. There are three answers to this legitimate question – one rather cynical, one comforting, and one relieving. The cynical and somewhat exaggerated answer will be that subsequently the courts will finally decide whether, under the circumstances of the individual case and the knowledge of the profession at the time of treatment, the professional standards of care have been violated. It may be comforting that such an uncertainty is by no means restricted to physicians.

Everybody has to face the risk of being held responsible for injuries to others and of being told by the court the way he should have behaved to avoid the injury. Relief can only be given by liability or other insurance protecting the potential victims as well as the doctor himself. This answer conveys an idea of the importance of insurance law at present and in times to come (see p. 548 and p. 558).

## Strict liability

As outlined above, the general duty to do no wrong is incurred only if there had been at least a negligent violation of this duty, i.e. if a person did not act as he should have done according to the standards of care required under the given circumstances. Recently courts and legislatures of many countries have opted for another additional system of liability which is not based on failure to take care or blameworthy conduct. They thought it necessary that certain groups of people exposing their fellow citizens to a special risk should be held liable for any injury caused by their hazardous conduct or by their potentially dangerous products. The best-known illustration of this kind of strict, absolute or no-fault liability is the liability of car-owners for damage caused by their cars. Another hotly discussed example, which is pertinent to our problems, is the producers' strict liability for their products. In these examples of strict or absolute liability it is no defence for the defendant that he and his servants have observed the necessary standards of care. They will be held liable because they exposed the public to a certain risk. Mandatory or voluntary liability insurance may relieve the responsible persons of their risk of being exposed to unforeseeable claims for compensation for damage caused by them.

In the continental European countries of the EEC there does not exist a comprehensive provision which holds all producers strictly liable for all their products. In Germany, for example, a special provision has been introduced recently concerning the strict liability of drug manufacturers for damage caused by their drugs (Drug Act of 1976, art. 84). Two international pieces of legislation, however, have been prepared by the Council of Europe and the EEC Commission to deal with the problem of product liability more comprehensively. The United Nations Commission on International Trade Law is considering the harmonization of the liability for damage caused by products involved in international trade. None of these three international efforts has yet become effective in any national jurisdiction.

But the EEC Council Directive of 25 July 1985 on the approximation of the laws, regulations and administrative provisions of the Member States concerning liability for defective products (Off.J.EC 1985, No. L 210/29) obliges the Member States of the EEC to bring into force, not later than three years from the date of notification of the Directive, national legislative acts necessary to comply with this Directive.

## Vicarious liability

Of utmost importance in modern life is vicarious liability, which is the liability for other people's wrongful acts. The person who caused the injury to the victim may be a doctor in a public hospital, a drug company chemist or a pharmacologist employed by a DRA. If only one of these persons were reponsible for the injury they caused, the victim would have a very poor chance of recovering his damages. Therefore all legal systems defined the responsibility of that person, company or public body under the supervision, guidance or direction of which an individual person acts while causing an injury. Simply stated, the employer (whether he be a private person or a public body) may be held responsible for injuries caused by his employees while carrying out their duties. The vicarious liability of the employer may depend on his failure to supervise his employees or it may be independent of any fault on his part. In the first case the employer's liability is founded on his own failure to fulfil his supervisory duties. In the other case the employer is held responsible because he bears the risk for damage caused by his employees. Whether or not the employer is held responsible for his own failure to supervise, varies from one legal system to another, and even within one legal system it may vary according to the kind of liability. In all continental European legal systems the employer is responsible for any damage caused by his employees while fulfilling the employer's *contractual* duties towards third persons. The employer warrants the fulfilment of these duties. It does not matter whether he himself performs his contractual duties or whether they are performed by one of his agents or servants. In the law of *torts* most continental legal systems agree that the employer is also strictly liable for his servants' tortious conduct; in other words, he cannot escape liability by proving his own innocence and diligent supervision of, and instructions to, his employees. Even where, as for example under the German CC §831, such an exception would be possible, the standards of care are extremely high so that there are in practice no differences from the strict liability of the master for his servants' wrongful acts.

## Government liability

In all continental European countries the government is responsible for any wrong committed by governmental agencies and their officials. There is no principle that the government can do no wrong. There may be, however, a difference compared with the liability of private enterprises; the liability of the government may be only secondary, for example only if nobody else, other than the government and its employees is responsible for the damage caused by governmental activities.

Special rules in several countries provide that persons damaged by a compulsory programme of vaccination have to be compensated by the government irrespective of any fault (see p. 542).

## Joint liability

In very many instances of civil liability the injury is produced by several different causes. For an adverse reaction to drugs, for example, the manufacturer of the drug, the doctor prescribing the drug and the DRA which did not react properly to suspected ADRs reported to it, may be held responsible. All of them contributed to the injury and, in general, they are jointly liable for the damage. Each or all of them may be sued for the whole amount of damages. The victim need not be concerned about the percentage which each of them contributed to the injury. This problem is a matter to be decided between those jointly liable. If one of them completely compensates the victim he may sue the others for reimbursement up to their respective share.

## Relation between various causes of action

It may happen that a certain set of facts covers the prerequisites of more than one ground of civil liability. An injured passenger in a defective bus, for example, may base his claim against the bus-owner on the contract of transportation (p. 544), on the general duty to do no wrong (p. 542) or on the bus-owner's strict liability (p. 545). He may even sue the owner's insurer if the insurance contract provides for victims having a direct cause of action, he may sue the bus driver for negligent conduct and/or the maker of the bus because of his strict liability for damage caused by his products.

With respect to the relation between various causes of action there are three principles common to all continental European jurisdictions:

(1) The victim may sue any person who is responsible for the injury sustained.
(2) A responsible defendant is not allowed to deny his responsibility because another person may also have contributed to the injury.
(3) The injured person cannot recover more than once for his loss and injury.

There is no agreement on the answer to the following questions:

(4) Does a contractual claim – as in France – exclude any other claim against the same person based on statutory provisions such as tort or strict liability?
(5) According to which principles have several responsible persons contributed to the compensation either by direct payment to the victim or by reimbursement of the compensating debtor? It goes without saying that the public liability insurer has ultimately to bear the loss caused and made good by his insured client.

## Liability and civil procedure

Several differences between continental European law and especially American law can only be explained by differing court procedures. In the USA the trial by jury, contingent fees for attorneys, and insurance coverage seem to favour verdicts for huge amounts of damages for injuries caused by medical malpractice or defective products. In continental European countries, courts are reluctant to award general or punitive damages. They prefer to award pensions to be paid monthly and modified according to the cost of living. Damages awarded for pain and suffering are rather moderate in comparison with American standards.

Of utmost importance is the law of evidence. This is true of every system of individual liability, especially because the causes of ADRs are difficult to prove, and the outcome of an action for damages depends to a great extent on legal rules about the burden of proof. If the victim had to prove that beyond any reasonable doubt ADRs have been caused by a specific drug, he would succeed very rarely. This would, however, be different if the burden of proof is shifted to the defendant, as may happen when suspected ADRs are attributed to a certain drug, and it has been given to a patient without any therapeutic necessity.

## Intermediate summary

Eight preliminary conclusions can be drawn:

(1) Doctors cannot be held liable without fault, and strict liability cannot apply to them.

(2) The standard of care to be observed has to be determined according to the circumstances of the individual case and the knowledge of the medical profession at the time of treatment.

(3) In some countries manufacturers of drugs are strictly liable for injuries caused by their product.

(4) Companies, hospitals, DRAs and other institutions are vicariously responsible for injuries caused by their employees.

(5) There is no government immunity in respect of injury caused by government agencies or state institutions.

(6) All persons or institutions which contributed to the cause of injury are jointly liable to the victim.

(7) There is no agreement on the continent whether a contractual claim excludes any other claim against the same person based on statutory provisions about extra-contractual liabilities.

(8) Procedural questions, especially those about evidence and the burden of proof, may be more important than problems of substantive law.

## LIABILITY AND INSURANCE

### Social and private insurance

Social and private insurance play an important role in modern society. Their impact on liability for ADRs is also considerable, as has already been mentioned. The difference between social and private insurance need not be explained in detail because it is common knowledge. Suffice to say that in most legal systems social insurance does not yet cover all people and all hazards, whereas private insurance offers a broader coverage.

### Public liability insurance

Everybody knows of public liability insurance because everywhere in Europe there is a compulsory public liability insurance of motor-car owners. Four statements, however, are necessary:

(1) Public liability insurance is a branch of private insurance.
(2) Everybody may take out insurance, including doctors and hospitals. In West Germany, drug manufacturers only have to make sure that they can fulfil the obligations arising from their strict liability (p. 545 and p. 546). This may be done by insurance.
(3) Public liability insurance presupposes that the insured person is liable. If this is the case, the insurance company pays for the insured.
(4) Normally the victim has no direct action against the liability insurer.

### Health, accident and life insurance

If the victim is insured against illness, accidents or death, his social or private insurance has to pay as soon as the insured risk materializes. The victim's claims against persons responsible for the damage, at least up to the amount paid or to be paid by the insurer, are subrogated in favour of the insurer. Then the insurer may decide whether a lawsuit should be filed against the persons liable.

## LIABILITY OF THE DOCTOR

### Liability to the patient

There may be a contractual relationship between a doctor and a patient or not as, for example, in the case of medical treatment by a hospital and its doctors. Irrespective of this, most obligations towards the patient are the same or nearly the same.

*Prescribing new drugs*

Two problems arise with respect to new drugs: has the patient to be informed of his therapeutic treatment by new drugs and of the potential hazards, and has the patient's informed consent to be obtained? The Declaration of Helsinki, adopted in 1964 and revised by the 29th World Medical Assembly of 1975 in Tokyo, provides general affirmitive answers for cases of biomedical research involving human subjects (I, 9–11) and lays down exceptions for medical research combined with professional care (clinical research). These principles have been embodied in the German Drug Act of 1976 [cf. §§ 40(1) no. 2, (2), (4) no. 4; 41 no. 2]. It is unclear whether the same standards apply if no biomedical or clinical research is involved, that is, if a newly developed and officially approved drug is prescribed for a patient for purely therapeutic treatment. It may be expected that an exception to the general necessity for an informed consent will be more easily admitted than in cases of clinical research.

If the patient's informed consent had to be obtained, but was not obtained and ADRs materialize, the doctor may be held liable for the harm caused by the drugs. The same is true if the treatment with new drugs cannot be justified according to the standards of medical care and the circumstances of the individual case.

Of special interest are two lines of cases which deal with the general liability of doctors, but also shed some light on the doctors' liability for ADRs. In Italy it has been constantly held by courts that surgeons are not liable for damages unless they acted intentionally or grossly negligently. This preference is based on Italian Civil Code art. 2236 where 'independent intellectuals' are relieved from liability for simple negligence if they have to solve especially complicated technical problems for the execution of their obligation. This concession is unlikely to be applied to the doctor prescribing new drugs, although courts in many countries are inclined to hold a doctor responsible only if his treatment cannot be justified by any reasonable therapy.

German courts have decided that under certain circumstances the burden of proof should be shifted in favour of the victim. If his informed consent had to be obtained, but was not given and something went wrong, it is the doctor who has to convince the court that the patient would have consented to the treatment with its potential hazards. This case law is likely to be extended also to the treatment with new drugs.

*Prescribing drugs causing ADRs*

If ADRs are not yet known, no doctor will be held liable for prescribing drugs which cause them. Doctors are liable for fault only (p. 542), and ADRs not yet attributed to a specific drug with absolute certainty or reasonable suspicion do not justify blame for lack of medical care. Doctors need not fear that they will be held liable for ADRs in such areas.

Doctors may, however, be held responsible for ADRs which have already been attributed to a specific drug with absolute certainty or reasonable likelihood. There is not much case-law to specify the standard of care to be used by a doctor when prescribing and dispensing drugs with regard to his duty to give precise information about their use and possible dangers. This does not mean that there are no complaints about doctors and their prescribing practice. Floods of new drugs, drugs with new labels or labels which impart different instructions in different countries have threatened to submerge every doctor for many years. Newpapers quite often report ADRs with fatal outcome. In many cases the ADRs could have been avoided if contraindications, incompatibilities and directions given by the manufacturer had been taken seriously, if the prescribing doctor had asked his patient to disclose his use of other drugs, or if warnings issued by the DRA had been heeded. If an ADR could have been avoided by reasonable care, the prescribing doctor will be held liable.

ADRs are mentioned in the annual directory (*Rote Liste*) edited by the Federal Association of the Pharmaceutical Industry, which is distributed free of charge to every doctor practising in the Federal Republic of Germany. Medical and pharmaceutical periodicals report on proved or suspected ADRs. For several years the Federal Health Agency acting as the DRA, state health agencies, pharmacists, and special commissions set up by West German physicians and by drug manufacturers have gathered observations about ADRs. All observations are monitored by the Federal Health Agency and relayed to the WHO. Any doctor may ask the monitoring bodies for information about the ADRs that have been reported in connection with any drug.

It is possible that a doctor will be held liable if he ignores published notices and warnings by the manufacturer or the monitoring bodies in his country. There is no obligation, however, to refer to the monitoring bodies for information about suspected ADRs that have not yet been published. Unless there are published suspicions about potential ADRs he may rely on the manufacturers' literature or on warnings issued by the DRA or other monitoring body.

### *Breach of medical confidence*

For more than 2000 years the obligation to preserve professional confidence is part of every doctor's duty. Hippocrates included this in his famous oath, and nowadays a breach of medical confidence is a criminal offence (cf. French Criminal Code art. 378; West German Criminal Code § 203(1) no. 1). The patient may also bring a suit for damages for pain and suffering because a breach of medical confidence constitutes not only a violation of contractual duties, but also a tortious invasion of the right of privacy.

In West Germany no exception to the rule of medical confidence is made for purposes of drug monitoring. For this reason drug monitoring has to be conducted anonymously with respect to the patient unless he agrees to full disclosure of his name. The Drug Commission of the German Medical Association publishes report forms in the *Deutsches Aerzteblatt* and asks for information about ADRs. These forms do not provide a 'box' for the name of the patient. Only his initials, his date of birth, height, weight, and profession (not his address) can be given. Even these personal data may reveal too much. I do not know, however, of any case in which a patient objected to monitoring in general or to the use of the reporting form.

There is no legal requirement that a German doctor should report ADRs to the DRA, and he cannot, therefore, rely on such an obligation as an excuse for breaking medical confidence. Despite this, nearly 2000 reports about potential ADRs are voluntarily submitted by doctors to the Drug Commission of the German Medical Association each year.

### *Liability to a public hospital*

Doctors may become liable towards public hospitals if they are employed in them and are in breach of their duties towards them. This may be occasioned by treatment which is unjustified or for which consent has not been obtained. In these circumstances the patient may sue the government or other body running the public hospital (p. 545) separately or jointly with the doctor (p. 546). If the hospital or its organizing body has to pay damages because of the doctor's fault, it may recover them from the doctor. A doctor who is in breach of his duty to the patient is also in breach of his contractual duty to the hospital.

## Liability to drug manufacturers

### *Prescribing drugs causing ADRs*

Prescribing drugs which cause ADRs may cause the doctor to be held liable (p. 542 and p. 544). At the same time the drug manufacturer may become liable and have to pay damages to the injured patient. In such situations the manufacturer may try to recover the amount of these damages from the doctor (p. 547) who caused the ADRs, and who may have negligently disregarded the danger of ADRs. I do not know, however, whether this potential liability of a doctor towards a drug manufacturer is of great importance, and I have not found any examples of such a situation.

### *Monitoring of ADRs*

There is no doubt that ADRs cause considerable concern to the pharmaceutical industry. ADRs diminish the efficacy of a drug, they may provoke civil litigation and may lead to the withdrawal of the drug from the market. The suspicion that a certain drug may cause ADRs impairs its commercial future, and the need to monitor suspected ADRs may be unwelcome to the industry. Despite this, German manufacturers have encouraged drug monitoring following the thalidomide tragedy since the early 1960s. No legal proceedings have apparently been brought by them against monitoring doctors.

In the future it seems very unlikely that any monitoring doctor will run the risk of being sued by the manufacturer of the monitored drug. An action for damages would lie only if the doctor failed to monitor suspected ADRs, but maliciously invented them in order to do harm to the manufacturer's business.

### Liability to the DRA

A system of mandatory monitoring would be ideal, but it cannot be generally enforced. It is more realistic to limit compulsory monitoring to hospitals and to some professional bodies. In Sweden, hospitals have to report ADRs to the DRA. It is likely that this example will be followed in West Germany since the new Drug Act provides a national centre for observing, collecting and evaluating the hazards caused by drugs.

Whatever form of drug monitoring prevails in a country, the information must, of course, be given with due professional care. Violation of this duty, however, will not result in an action for damage since the DRA does not suffer damages.

As has already been mentioned, monitoring of drugs must respect the patient's right of privacy and the need for medical confidence (p. 551). So long as these rights are preserved, consent by the patient is not necessary for the monitoring of drugs.

## LIABILITY OF HOSPITALS

### To the patient

Hospitals have to make sure that the provisions regarding the treatment with new drugs are observed (p. 549), that no drug causing unacceptably frequent and serious ADRs is prescribed (p. 550), and that due regard is paid to medical confidence (p. 551). If one of these obligations is violated by doctors or other employees, the body running the hospital is vicariously and jointly liable for any damage suffered by the patient (p. 546).

### To doctors

Hospitals are obliged to furnish adequate facilities for medical treatment. Doctors must be in a position to fulfil their duties towards patients (p. 549). If the hospital fails to do this it is in breach of its legal obligations to the doctor.

## LIABILITY OF PHARMACISTS

### To the customer

The pharmacist selling drugs to his customers may become responsible for injuries caused by the drugs. This has been decided several times by the courts in cases where, by mistake, the wrong drug has been sold. A well-known example is the birth of a child when the wrong tablets have been sold to a woman who asked for an oral contraceptive.

Will a pharmacist also be held liable for ADRs caused by the drug? A seller usually warrants or guarantees that the goods sold have no latent defects which render them unfit for the purpose for which they are intended, but this contractual obligation does not necessarily entail liability for damages. The normal remedy for the buyer in a breach of warranty is the repayment of the price or part of it. In most jurisdictions the seller is liable for damages only if he was aware of the defects. Applying these principles and the general law of torts (p. 542) a pharmacist seems to be especially liable for damages in three situations:

(1) If he sells a drug which needs no medical prescription, knowing of well-founded suspicions that it can cause serious ADRs, and he does not reveal them to the customer.
(2) If he sells drugs already withdrawn from the market because of their ADRs.
(3) If he sells drugs which cause ADRs because they have been carelessly prepared by him (e.g. because they are old or have been stored improperly).

It is doubtful if a pharmacist has to pay regard to the customer's sensitivities to certain drugs.

### To the DRA

In most countries the marketing of drugs is regulated by statutory provisions. Breach of these provisions will be punishable by fines and administrative measures against the pharmacist.

## LIABILITY OF DRUG MANUFACTURERS

Sensational law-suits dealing with ADRs have been brought against drug manufacturers and, in many instances, jointly against the DRA.

This is not surprising because every seriously injured victim tries to sue wealthy defendants who can pay high damages or provide pensions for a long time.

## Liability to the patient

### *ADRs caused during clinical trials*

Clinical trials of drugs may be carried out with the patient's informed consent. If the hazards, which have been explained to the patient, materialize, the drug manufacturers will not be held responsible for ADRs. For this reason the new German Drug Act of 1976 provides that an insurance has to be taken out for the patient.

### *ADRs to drugs on the market*

As soon as a drug is marketed or used as an officially licensed drug, the manufacturers have to face the risk of being sued by people injured by ADRs.

The basis of responsibility differs in most countries. Up to now the liability of drug manufacturers has been mainly based on the law of tort (p. 542), that is on general principles about careful conduct and the avoidance of foreseeable injuries. In some jurisdictions, however, stricter standards apply to all producers in general, and drug manufacturers in particular. In France all producers may be held responsible for defective products because of the contractual warranty of quality (p. 544). They are liable to everybody who sustains damage as a final consumer in a chain of sales, even if there is no direct contractual relation (privity of contract) between the producer and the final consumer. This contractual remedy is not available to an injured party who does not himself form part of the chain of sales. In West Germany, on the other hand the new Drug Act has created a strict liability on drug manufacturers (p. 545); they have to make good, up to a certain fixed limit, all serious damage which has been caused by a proper use of the drug or which can be attributed to the development or production of the drug. The same responsibility applies if the harm could have been avoided by a careful description of the drug and adequate information as to its use. The strict liability of drug manufacturers does not exclude their unlimited liability in tort (p. 542) if negligence can be proved. This does not seem to be impossible to prove when ADRs have been attributed to the drug with a reasonable degree of certainty and the manufactuer does not react to well-founded grounds for suspicion by issuing warnings or by withdrawal of the drug from the market. Therefore, the manufacturers have to observe the need for drug monitoring in order to avoid unlimited liability.

Even if drug manufacturers are strictly liable for ADRs, it can be very difficult to prove that the ADRs have been caused by their drug, and that no other factors were decisive in causing the injury or contributing to it. These difficulties of evidence cause long court trials against drug manufacturers. Most jurisdictions have not yet found satisfactory solutions to shorten the law-finding process. Victims cannot afford to wait for compensation for years, and this may be prevented by insurance of all potential victims (p. 548).

### Liability to the DRA

#### *Information and Marketing*

Drugs should not be sold or advertised like apples. A free market for drugs would increase their hazards tremendously. Therefore, the industry is extensively regulated in many countries. The Council of the European Communities has issued several directives on the approximation of the laws of the member-states about the regulation of drugs and about the standards of applications for marketing authorization. The WHO has prepared requirements for Good Manufacturing Practices (GMP) which – although not binding – have been approved by pharmaceutical associations and published by national governments. Most important, however, is national legislation which has to bring into force provisions complying with the EEC directives, and which alone can create duties binding drug manufacturers. In many countries such legislation has already been promulgated. According to it, drugs have to be admitted by the DRA after they have been informed extensively about, *inter alia*, the component parts, the effects, the contra-indications, already known side-effects and incompatibilities. Further details need not be mentioned here except for a few words about the enforcement of all these duties. If drug manufacturers do not comply with their statutory obligations, they may be punished by fines, the DRA may order the withdrawal of a drug from the market, or the drug manufacturer may lose his licence for the production of drugs.

#### *Duty to monitor ADRs*

If drug manufacturers have not only to inform about known side-effects but also to monitor subsequently suspected ADRs, the same sanctions apply as described above (p. 552).

A voluntary monitoring system organized by the drug manufacturers themselves (p. 553) does not create obligations towards the DRA.

## LIABILITY OF THE DRA

### To the patient

Usually DRAs have comprehensive regulatory powers for the release of drugs and post-marketing surveillance of ADRs. The reverse side of these powers are respective duties towards the public, and these may be enforced by individuals injured by ADRs. Examples for such actions by victims have been reported from many countries. In other instances the government acknowledged its responsibility by substantial contributions to funds for the benefit of victims of ADRs.

Under which conditions will the DRA or the government be held liable towards patients? It is essential that the DRA can be blamed for the breach of a supervisory duty, and of utmost importance is post-marketing surveillance. It obliges the DRA to order the withdrawal of drugs from the market as soon as they know of any confirmed suspicion of ADRs which are considered to be unacceptable. If domestic law imposes such a duty and the DRA does not order the withdrawal of the dangerous drug, the DRA (the government) will be held liable for damages caused by ADRs.

### To drug manufacturers

The DRA may become liable in tort to a drug manufacturer if it bans a drug from the market without any reasonable suspicion that it causes ADRs. Apart from this rather theoretical case, the DRA does not run any risk of being held liable by drug manufacturers for the post-marketing surveillance. The measures to be taken by the DRA will be justified by its supervisory duties. Even the omission of appropriate measures will not create obligations towards the manufacturer, because they themselves have to withdraw their drugs as soon as ADRs are attributed to them.

## EVALUATION AND PROPOSALS

### Shortcomings of the present situation

The present shortcomings will not be discussed in detail. Briefly, they can be summarized under five headings:

(1) Today, *legal proceedings* are necessary to recover damages from liable persons, companies or governmental agencies. This raises problems of access to the courts and difficulties in finding a lawyer and paying him.

(2) The causation of ADRs has to be *proved*. This is difficult and in many cases may be impossible. Evidence has also to be produced of the defendant's responsibility, unless there is a strict liability even for development risks (i.e. risks which may develop in the future).

(3) These problems of evidence cause an enormous *delay* before the victims get a final judgement, whether in their favour or not. Up to this time the victims have to support themselves unless some emergency measures are taken.

(4) The *costs* of lengthy court proceedings with expert witnesses are extremely high. These costs are a burden for the plaintiff if he has to pay a deposit. But even if this is not the case and the plaintiff sues *in forma pauperis* the costs of the trial have to be paid by somebody. Whoever this may be, the money would have been better invested in compensating the victims.

(5) The present system tends to be *inequitable and unjust* for victims as well as for defendants. Compared with victims of isolated ADRs, the victims of sensational drug catstrophes are likely to find their way to court more easily, to hire better attorneys and to achieve more substantial judgements against their opponents. The responsible persons may be unable to meet their liabilities and to satisfy the substantial judgements. It also happens that damages awarded against powerful and well-insured defendants are computed more generously than those against financially weak adversaries. The result of these differences and anomalies is the danger of spiralling claims for compensation: substantial damages are awarded because the defendant is covered by a liability insurance; insurance premiums are raised because of the increased risk; even higher damages are awarded because they will finally be paid by the insurance company under the extended policy; and so on.

## Solutions to remove shortcomings

### *Voluntary insurance by victim and manufacturer*

A voluntary health, life, and liability insurance may meet some of the shortcomings mentioned above.

(1) A general health, accident, and life insurance policy taken out by the victim will cover him and his dependents against all or almost all risks. The insurer may have to suffer from the difficulties of enforcing the victim's subrogated cause of action against the manufacturer. All this presupposes that the victim has insured himself. What, however, happens when there is no insurance coverage as, for example, in at least some thalidomide cases?

(2) If the manufacturer has a product liability insurance, this may reduce the victim's risk of becoming a creditor or an insolvent debtor. In some jurisdictions, especially in the United States, it has become doubtful whether consumers should rely on such a product liability insurance. Because of the increased number of product liability claims and of the astronomical damages awarded and substantially raised insurance premiums, it has become difficult for smaller manufacturers to obtain product liability insurance.

*Elective no-fault insurance*

In the United States Jeffrey O'Connell, Professor of Law at the University of Illinois, advocated that tortious liability in general should be replaced by a voluntary elective no-fault insurance for many kinds of injuries, *inter alia*, for medical malpractice and product liability. His basic idea is a no-fault bargain; the victim will get quick compensation for out-of-pocket losses up to a certain amount irrespective of anybody's fault, in return for waiver of an uncertain cause of action in tort for a larger amount plus compensation for pain and suffering. I do not think that O'Connell's proposal can be transferred to non-American jurisdictions, because it is made to meet the special American need to reduce the excessive or punitive damages awarded by compassionate juries for pain and suffering. What is needed today is no cornucopia for a minority of victims, but equal and adequate compensation for all victims.

But even if non-American manufacturers who export to the USA are exposed to the American law of product liability, the elective no-fault insurance proposals share the shortcomings of every voluntary insurance.

*Strict liability and mandatory liability insurance*

In West Germany every drug manufacturer is strictly liable for injuries caused by his drugs (Drug Act § 84; p. 545). At the same time he has to make sure that he can meet his strict liability up to a certain limit. This may be done by buying a liability insurance or by furnishing a guarantee provided by a German bank (Drug Act § 94). The German solution may be a fair compromise between the needs of injured persons and the interests of drug manufacturers. It does not, however, cope with most of the above-mentioned shortcomings. A court procedure is still necessary, liability of the manufacturer has to be proved, and years may pass before the victim will be compensated.

*Mandatory drug insurance in favour of victims*

On July 1st, 1978, Sweden introduced an undertaking providing for a mandatory insurance of all citizens against ADRs. The insurance covers damages up to a certain amount, and the premiums are paid by drug manufacturers. This insurance supplements the Swedish insurance of patients against medical malpractice. Now Sweden has nearly accompished what has been urged for years in other countries, for example in the USA (Ehrenzweig), France (Tunc, Penneau), and recently West Germany (Weyers).

Whether this solution will work remains to be seen. There is at least one major advantage. The victim will be paid by the insurance without being obliged to bring a suit against somebody beforehand.

*Comprehensive accident insurance*

In New Zealand an Accident Compensation Act 1972 entered into force on April 1st, 1974. This statute was revolutionary and attracted world-wide attention. The New Zealand Act radically abolishes nearly all actions for damages, and fills the resulting gap by claims against certain compensation funds. Civil liability has been replaced by a comprehensive and compulsory insurance system for the 'compensation of persons who suffer personal injury by accident', and of 'certain dependants of those persons where death results from injury' (1§ 4(1)(c) of the Act).

With regard to our problem the effect of the Accident Compensation Act may be summarized as follows:

(1) All persons personally injured by any accident which happened in New Zealand, and their dependants, have cover in respect of the injury under one of the five schemes established by the Act. The injury may be caused, *inter alia*, by a defective or harmful product, or, as has been specifically emphasized in an amendment, by a 'medical, surgical, dental, or first-aid misadventure'. It is not clear whether pharmaceutical products are also included.

(2) The Accident Compensation Commission not only has to provide for the rehabilitation of the victim (§§ 48–53) but also to pay, out of the respective fund, for:
   (a) the medical treatment of the victims so far as he is not entitled to benefits under the Social Security Act (§ 111);
   (b) compensation for loss of earning capacity up to a certain maximum amount per week (§ 104; first schedule, part IV, new version):
   (c) compensation for pain and suffering up to a maximum lump sum payment (§ 120, new version);
   (d) compensation to the victim's dependants if the victim dies as a result of personal injury caused by an accident (§§ 122–125).

(3) The compensation to be awarded to the victim or his dependants is limited to a certain percentage of the victim's earnings up to a certain maximum amount. If somebody wants to recover the entire amount of his loss without any limitations, he has to take a private accident insurance.

(4) The five compensation funds (§ 31) are supplied with regular contributions by employers (§§ 77 ss.), by holders of drivers' licences (§ 97 ss.), and with money appropriated by Parliament (§§ 70, 102D). It is interesting to know that manufacturers of hazardous products do not contribute to the funds. They contribute only as employers and holders of drivers' licences.

(5) The victim of a personal injury accident does not have any cause of action independent of the Accident Compensation Act (§ 5). This means that he has claims against the Accident Compensation Commission only, and that he cannot take to court the person normally liable for the injury. The Commission cannot recover the payments awarded to the victim from those previously liable.

These persons may only be charged with penalty rates to be contributed to the fund (§§ 73(1)(a); 100(d)), and they can be prosecuted for criminal offences.

(6) The Act does not cover accidents which resulted in damage to property only. In such situations the common law remedies still prevail. Moreover, diseases caused independently of any accident are not included in this Act.

*Integrated full aid insurance of all citizens*

Even against the New Zealand Accident Act some objections may be raised. To a great extent they have already been formulated by Geoffrey W. R. Palmer, Professor of Law at the Victoria University of Wellington. First, it should be made clear that ADRs are covered by the insurance. The present uncertainty may be explained by the strange situation that producers in general do not have to contribute to the insurance funds, and would be relieved of any liability if damage caused by defective products were covered by the insurance. Another criticism relates to the separate administration of the accident insurance fund. It should be fused with the administration of the general social security funds. Such a fusion would *per se* create an integrated full aid insurance for nearly all citizens. If such an integration takes place the insured will be protected against all sorts of risks. Most of the shortcomings of the present situation will vanish.

Insurance may cause doctors, hospitals, pharmacists, drug manufacturers and the DRA to act with less diligence than before. This danger can be avoided to a large extent by pre-and post-marketing surveillance and other measures to prevent injuries; also differing premiums may have deterrent effects. The same is true of actions of the insurer to recover payments from persons or institutions acting recklessly. Finally it should not be forgotten that criminal procedures, medical ethics, and disciplinary measures are devices better suited as deterrents than insurable financial responsibilities.

## Conclusions

The civil liabilities of hospitals and doctors for prescribing and dispensing harmful drugs are based upon the law of contract and tort. It is very unlikely that they will be held strictly liable for defective or harmful drugs or drugs with serious side-effects. I venture to predict that, in the long run, insurance – whether social or private – will be the most convenient solution not only for product liability in general, but also for medical liability in drug prescribing and dispensing. This insurance may have to be bought by the drug manufacturer – at the consumer's expense, of course. It is, however, better to rely on a broad insurance coverage than to speculate in burdensome and uncertain civil law suits against the manufacturer of hazardous and harmful products.

Whether and to what extent the insurer may have a right of redress against a tortfeasor, is a collateral problem only. Such a right of redress may relieve the insurer of his expenses and may, perhaps, exert some deterrent effects. On the whole, damages caused by accidents should be settled by insurance. The law of torts, of product liability and medical responsibility cannot prevent serious injuries – which should be the ultimate goal of any manufacturer. Drug monitoring is of the utmost importance, a necessity, a need even more urgent than reform of the law of compensation for injuries which might have been avoided if monitoring was more efficient.

## Bibliography

Anrys, H. (1974). *La Responsabilité Civil Medicale*, 389 pp. (Brussels and Braine-L'Alleud: Larcier and Chambre Syndicale des Médecins)

Blair, A. P. (1978). *Accident compensation in New Zealand*. 195 pp. (Wellington: Butterworth)

Boyer Chammard, G. and Monzein, P. (1974). *La Responsabilité Médicale*. 281 pp. (Paris: Presses Universitaires de France)

Deutsch, E. (1978). *Medizin und Forschung vor Gericht*. 51 pp. (Heidelberg and Karlsruhe: C. F. Müller)

Ehrenzweig, A. A. (1951). Trends toward an enterprise liability for insurable loss. Negligence without fault. 95 pp. (Berkeley, Los Angeles: University of California)

Fleming, J. G. (1982). Drug injury compensation plans. *Am. J. Compar. Law*, **30**, 297

Gaskins, R. (1980). Tort Reform in the Welfare State: The New Zealand Accident Compensation Act. *Osgoode Hall Law J.*, **18**, 238

Gesetz zur Neuordnung des Arzneimittelrechts (German Drug Act) of August 24, 1976, (1976). *Bundesgesetzblatt*, **I**, 2445

Giesen, D. (1976). *Civil Liability of Physicians with Regard to New Methods of Treatment and Experiments*. 147 pp. (Bielefeld: Gieseking)

Giesen, D. (1978). Civil Liability of Physicians. In Max-Planck-Institut Für Ausländisches und Internationales Privatrecht Hamburg (ed.) *Deutsche zivil-, kollisions- und wirtschaftsrechtliche Beiträge zum X. Internationalen Kongreß für Rechtsvergleichung in Budapest 1978*. pp. 403–431 (Tübingen: Mohr)

Giesen, D. (1981). *Medical Malpractice Law*. 512 pp. (Bielefeld: Gieseking)

Gramberg-Danielsen, B. (1978). *Die Haftung des Arztes*. 52 pp. (Stuttgart: Enke)

Gross, F. H. and Inman, W. H. W. (eds.) (1977). *Drug Monitoring*. 311 pp. (London, New York, San Francisco: Academic Press)

Ison, T. G. (1980). *Accident Compensation. A Commentary on the New Zealand Scheme*. 201 pp. (London: Croom Helm)

Kornprost, L. and Dephin, S. (1960). *Le Contrat de Soins Médicaux*. 215 pp. (Paris: Sirey)

Kullmann, H. J. (1978). Haftung der pharmazeutischen Unternehmer nach dem Gesetz zur Neuordnung des Arzneimittelrechts. *Betriebs-Berater*, **33**, 175

Laufs, A. (1977). *Arztrecht*. 110 pp. (Munich: Beck)

Lawin, P. and Huth, H. (eds.) (1982). *Grenzen der Aerztlichen Aufklaerungs- und Behandlungspflicht*. 167 pp. (Stuttgart, New York: Thieme)

Lega, C. (1974). *Le Libere Professioni Intellettuali nelle Leggi e nella Giurisprudenza*. 1000 pp. (Milan: Giuffré)

Marinero, H. G. S. (1982). *Arzneimittelhaftung in den USA und in Deutschland*. 286 pp. (Frankfurt am Main, Bern: Lang)

Newdick, C. (1985). Strict liability for defective drugs in the pharmaceutical industry. *Law Quarterly Rev.*, **101**, 405

O'Connell, J. (1976). An alternative to abandoning tort liability: elective no fault

insurance for many kinds of injury. *Minn. Law. Rev.*, **60,** 501
Palmer, G. W. P. (1977). Accident compensation in New Zealand: the first two years. *Am. J. Compar. Law*, **25,** 1
Palmer, G. (1979). *Compensation for Incapacity. A Study of Law and Social Change in New Zealand and Australia.* 460 pp. (Wellington, Melbourne, Oxford: Oxford University Press)
Penneau, J. (1973). *Faute et Erreur en Matière de Responsabilité Médicale.* 409 pp. (Paris: Librairie Générale de droit et de jurisprudence)
Penneau, J. (1977). *La Responsabilité Médicale.* 331 pp. (Paris: Sirey)
Ryckmans, X. and Meert-van de Put, R. (1971–72). *Les Droits et les Obligations des Médecins.* 2nd Edn., 2 Vols., 487 and 487 pp. (Brussels: Larcier)
Savatier, R., Auby, J.-M., Savatier, J. and Péquignot, H. (1956). *Traité de Droit Médical.* 574 pp. (Paris: Librairies techniques)
Sjöström, H. and Nilsson, R. (1972). *Thalidomide and the Power of the Drug Companies.* 1st Edn., 281 pp. (Harmondsworth: Penguin Books)
Slyters, B. *et al.* (1974). *Medische aansprakelijkheid in Amerika en Nederland en De relatie ziekenfonds – arts – patient.* 130 pp. (Deventer: Kluwer)
Tunc, A. (1981). La responsibilité civile. 182 pp. (Paris: Economica)
Verberne, R., Rietveldt, M., van der Kolk, A., Geers, A., Gevers, S., Dassen, K., Witteveen, F., Verderne, R. and Pannenborg, Ch. O. (1976). Gezondheidsrecht – De rechten van de patiënt. *Ars Aequi*, **25,** 551
Weimar, W. (1976). *Arzt-Krankenhaus-Patient.* 2nd Edn., 172 pp. (Munich: Beck)
Weyers, H.-L. (1978). Empfiehlt es sich, im Interesse der Patienten und Ärzte ergänzende Regelungen für das ärztliche Vertrags- (Standes-) und Haftungsrecht einzuführen? *Verhandlungen des 52. Deutschen Juristentags*, **I.** (A). (Munich: Beck)
Wolter, U. (1976). Die Haftungsregelung des neuen Arzneimittelgesetzes. *Der Betrieb*, **29,** 2001

# 38
# Pharmaceutical law in the United States

H. LESTER and A. FUDIM

## INTRODUCTION

The United States is a litigious and consumer-oriented society. Recovery for pharmaceutical and medical device*-induced personal injury comes within the ambit of products liability litigation. As medical care has become more depersonalized, the incidence of use of the courts to address medically related injuries has accelerated. This expansion is likely to continue. Recoveries are now made in products cases which would have been previously dismissed.[1] The constant expansion of the basis of liability in the products field is consistent with the concept that the manufacturer is best able to bear the financial burden. Manufacturers of pharmaceutical and medical devices are now named as party defendants in cases which at one time would have been limited to medical malpractice issues. Manufacturers are now co-defendants with health care providers. Although certain products liability principles continue to invade medical device litigation, until recently the legal basis for recovery in drug products cases has been more restricted. If present trends persist, monetary exposure† and litigation expenses will continue to escalate.

* 'Device' is a term of art as defined by the Food and Drug Administration.
† 'Monetary exposure' is equivalent to the potential verdict.

1. *MacPherson* v. *Buick Motor Co.*, 217 N.Y.382 (1916), an early lead products case has today become an historical curiosity. Later cases typical of this expansion are *Henningsen* v. *Bloomfield Motors Inc.*, 32 N.J.358, 161A.2d 69 (1960); *Greenman* v. *Yuba Power Products Inc.*, 29 Cal.2d 57, Cal.Rptr. 697, 337 P.2d 897 (1963); *Goldberg* v. *Kollsman Instrument Corp.*, 12 N.Y.S. 2d 432, 240 N.Y.S.2d 592, 191 N.E.2d 81 (1963); *Vandermark* v. *Ford Motors Co.*, 61 Cal.2d 245, 37 Cal.Rptr. 896, 391 P.2d 168 (1964); *Rooney* v. *S.A. Healey Co.*, 20N.Y.2d 42, 228 N.Y.2d 383 (1967); *Larsen* v. *General Motors Corp.*, 391 F.2d 495 (8th Cir. 1968); *Codling* v. *Paglia*, 32 N.Y.2d 330, 298 N.E.2d 622, 345 N.Y.S.2d 461 (1973); *Bolm* v. *Triumph Corp.*, 33 N.Y.2d 151, 350 N.Y.S.2d 644 (1973).

## AMERICAN PRODUCTS LIABILITY DOCTRINE

To comprehend the American Law of Products Liability as it applies to pharmaceutical-induced injuries, one must first understand the general field of products liability. The development of the law on products is a result of a curious mixture of concepts of contract and tort law. Early products liability cases were founded on sales and contract law, but were subsequently modified, particularly during the last 20 years, by new developments in the law of negligence. The American Products Liability Doctrine is based upon three distinct theories of liability: that of strict liability in tort, negligence, or warranty (express or implied). The doctrine of strict products liability is a relatively new concept which has only been accepted in most American jurisdictions within the last 15 years. Under strict products liability the manufacturer, processor of material, maker of a component part, wholesaler, retailer or distributor of a product may be found liable provided that the injured party proves that:[2]

(a) a defect existed which rendered the product not reasonably safe at the time of the design, manufacture, assembly, installation or sale by the party against whom liability is sought;
(b) the defect was a substantial factor in bringing about the plaintiff's injury; and
(c) the product at the time of the occurrence was being used for the purpose and the manner normally intended.

American law is founded on the English common law principle of *stare decisis*. This doctrine mandates that courts should follow legal precedent in deciding similar cases. In the United States there are 50 State court systems, plus a Federal court system. While the Federal court system will look to the substantive law of the state having the most significant contact with the suit at issue, each of the states may develop its own law, as long as that law does not violate the Constitution or areas reserved to the Federal government. On a given set of facts, recovery may be available in one state, but not in another. The American Law Institute, a non-governmental advisory body has attempted through the 'Restatement of Torts' to codify prior legal decisions as a guideline for future judicial opinions. It should not be confused with statutes used in code countries[3], the legal system predominantly used in EEC countries. The Restatement of Torts is not a Statute, is not legally binding upon the court, but is favourably received and is utilized by the judiciary as a guideline in making legal determinations in particular cases.

2. *Codling* v. *Paglia*, 32 N.Y.2d 330 (1973); *Cascia* v. *Maze Wooden Ware Co.*, 29 A.D.2d 924 (1968), motion for leave to appeal denied and decision amended 30 A.D.2d 806, aff'd. 23 N.Y.2d 1000; *Rosenzweig* v. *Arista Truck Renting Corp.* 34 A.D.2d 542, (1970).
3. With the exception of the English-speaking countries, *stare decisis* is not followed and the courts are guided by statutes as codified law.

The American Law Institute in 1965 in Section 402(a) of the Restatement (2d) of Torts provided:

> 'Special Liability of Seller of Product for Physical Harm to User or Consumer:
> (1) One who sells any product in a defective condition or reasonably dangerous to the user or consumer or to his property is subject to liability for physical harm thereby caused to the ultimate user or consumer, or to his property if
> (a) the seller is engaged in the business of selling such a product; and
> (b) it is expected to, and does, reach the user and consumer without substantial change in the condition in which it is sold.
> (2) The rule stated in Subsection (1) applies although:
> (a) the seller has exercised all possible care in the preparation and sale of his product; and
> (b) the user or consumer has not bought the product from or entered into any contractual relationship with the seller.

In comments which follow this Section the American Law Institute explain that this special liability is justified on socio-economic considerations, based on the belief that the burden of loss caused by defective products should be borne by those responsible for the marketing of the product, and should be treated as a cost of production against which liability insurance can be obtained. Unfortunately the expansion of the legal basis for imposing liability and inflation in verdict value, has resulted in crisis in products liability in which insurance is no longer available or is available at a prohibitive cost.[4] Causality cost has increased product cost to the extent that its pricing has caused many worthwhile products to be withdrawn from the market. There are many worthwhile pharmaceutical products available in Europe which have either been withdrawn from the United States market or not introduced by reason of liability problems or licensing difficulties which prevent affirmative FDA action on a New Drug Application due to adverse reaction in a statistically insignificant percentage of users.[5]

The Commentators of the American Law Institute, in their comments under Section 402(a), recognized that the strict liability rule was intended to apply only where the defective condition of the product makes it unreasonably dangerous to the user or consumer, and that many products cannot possibly be made entirely safe for all consumption.

Any food or drug necessarily involves some risk or harm if only from over-consumption. The Commentators recognized that ordinary sugar

4. Proceedings of First World Congress on Product Liability, January 19–21, 1977.
5. Becotide by Glaxo is unlicensed in the US. This product is unavailable in the border areas of Mexico and Canada as many Americans on the recommendations of their physicians attempt to purchase the product in places like Tijuana and Vancouver and then bring it into the US. Marsalid by Hoffman-La Roche was withdrawn from the US market but is available in the rest of the world.

is a deadly poison to diabetics. Every pharmaceutical, in order to be effective, must be potent, and as potency is increased so too is risk of undesirable side-effects usually increased. It is also recognized that medication is used primarily by a diseased section of the population. Ingestion is dependent upon a prescription being issued by a doctor who exercises medical judgement by weighing benefit against risk. As a result the commentators have adopted comment K to 402 (a) which deals with unavoidably unsafe products, and applies primarily to pure prescription drugs and medical devices that can only be obtained or implanted through an intervening physician. Comment K excludes such products from the reach of strict liability by clearly stating that the whole question is whether reasonable care has been exercised in warning potential users. Comment K provides that:

> 'There are some products which, in the present state of human knowledge, are quite incapable of being made safe for their intended and ordinary use. These are especially common in the field of drugs. An outstanding example is the vaccine for the Pasteur treatment of rabies, which not uncommonly leads to very serious and damaging consequences when it is injected. Since the disease itself invariably leads to a dreadful death, both the marketing and the use of the vaccine are fully justified, notwithstanding the unavoidable high degree of risk which they involve. Such a product, properly prepared and accompanied by proper directions and warnings, is not defective, nor is it *unreasonably* dangerous. The same is true of many other *drugs, vaccines and the like* many of which for this very reason cannot legally be sold except to physicians or under the prescription of a physician. It is also true in particular of many new and experimental drugs as to which, because of lack of time and opportunity for sufficient medical experience, there can be no assurance of safety, or perhaps even of purity of ingredients, but such experience as there is justifies the marketing and use of the drug notwithstanding a medically recognizable risk. *The seller of such products, again with the qualification that they are properly prepared and marketed, and proper warning is given, or the situation calls for it, is not to be held to strict liability for unfortunate consequences attending their use, merely because he has undertaken to supply the public with an apparently useful and desirable product, attended with a known but apparently reasonable risk.' (All emphasis added by authors.)*

The legal distinction between pharmaceutical cases, and other product cases was recently eroded in New Jersey. In *Feldman* v. *Lederle Laboratories*, 97 N.J. 429, 479 A. 2d 374 (1984) the Supreme Court of that state held that 'we see no reason to hold as a matter of law and policy that all prescription drugs are unsafe and avoidably so, drugs, like any other products, may contain defects that could have been avoided by better manufacturing or design. Whether a drug is unavoidably unsafe should be decided on a case by case basis'.

## DUTY TO WARN: LABELLING

The legal obligation imposed upon pharmaceutical manufacturers is, therefore, primarily based upon the duty to warn. In the recent Fifth

Circuit decision in *Reyes* v. *Wyeth Laboratories*,[6] Judge Wisdom held:

> 'Prescription drugs are likely to be complex medicines, esoteric in formula and varied in effect. As a medical expert, the prescribing physician can take into account the propensities of the drug, as well as the susceptibilities of his patient. His is the task of weighing the benefits of any medication against its potential dangers. The choice he makes is an informed one, and individualized medical judgment bottomed on the knowledge of both patient and palliative. Pharmaceutical companies then, must warn ultimate purchasers of the dangers inherent in patent drugs, sold over the counter, and when selling prescription drugs are required to warn only the prescribing physician who acts as "learned intermediary" between manufacturer and consumer.'

Accordingly, the duty of the ethical drug manufacturer to warn is limited to those dangers which the manufacturer knows, or has reason to know, are inherent in the use of its drug.[7] The state of the art defines the duty owed. If the package insert succinctly and adequately sets the known contraindications and warnings, the manufacturer has effectively insulated itself from liability.[8]

An exception, however, exists in the case of pharmaceuticals, or biologicals, utilized in mass immunization programmes in which there is no intervening doctor–patient relationship. *Reyes* v. *Wyeth* held that where there was no individualized balancing of the benefits and risks by a doctor, the warning must be conveyed to the consumer. Under Reyes even a vaccination by a public health nurse does not insulate the manufacturer. The rationale is that a manufacturer is deemed to be familiar with the distribution/administration practices associated with its product. The absence of a physician/patient relationship is thus foreseeable. This exception has now been adopted in several states.

No discussion of negligence is warranted in this chapter. American Courts, as a practical matter, interchange the concept of negligence with that of strict liability in cases involving ethical pharmaceuticals. The negligence doctrine is guided by the same principles referable to the 'duty to warn' as are detailed in the comments concerning Comment K of 402(a) of the Restatement of Torts.

Causes of action for breach of implied warranty of merchantability have not passed from the general products liability field into drug products liability. While the general rule is to the effect that there is an implied warranty that goods are of fair and average quality and are fit

6. 498 F.2d 1264, 1276 (5th Cir. 1974).
7. *Sterling Drug, Inc.* v. *Cornish*, 370 F.2d 82 (8th Cir. 1966); *Parke-Davis & Co.* v. *Stromsodt*, 411 F.2d 1390 (8th Cir. 1969); *Love* v. *Wolf*, 226 Cal. App.2d 378 (1964).
8. *Magill* v. *G. D. Searle & Co.* U.S.D.C., East.Dis.Pa., Civ. Action No. 72-1118 (1975) unreported; *Vaughan* v. *G. D. Searle & Co.*, 536 P.2d 1247 (Ore. 1975); *Givens* v. *Gulf States Utilities Co.*, U.S.D.C. Mid.Dist.La. (1975) unreported; *Terhune* v. *A. H. Robins* 577 P.2d 975 (1978); *Chambers* v. *G. D. Searle & Co.*, 441 F.Supp. 377 (1975); *Dunkin* v. *Syntex*, 443 F.Supp. 121 (1977); *Wolfgruber* v. *Upjohn*, 72 A.D.2d 59, aff'd 52 N.Y.2d 768 (1979).

for the ordinary purposes for which such goods are used, this rule does not operate in drug cases.[9]

Where the manufacturer does not have knowledge or notice of a buyer's sensitivity or idiosyncrasy to the product, breach of implied warranty cannot attach.[10] The manufacturer is not an insurer of the public safety. The product need be no more than reasonably merchantable and reasonably fit for its intended use by normal individuals. The defence of an idiosyncratic reaction applies not only in the case of prescription products, but also in the case of cosmetics and over-the-counter products. The only instance in which the manufacturer will be held responsible is the case in which plaintiffs are able to prove an adulterated or impure product.[11]

The duty to warn as a general rule does not extend to the patient.[12] In *Fogo*, the court reiterated the general view that:

(1) The doctor is intended to be an intervening party in the full sense of the word. Medical ethics as well as medical practice dictate independent judgment, unaffected by the manufacturers control, on the part of the doctor.
(2) Were the patient to be given the complete and highly technical information on the adverse possibility associated with the use of the drug, he would have no way of evaluating it, and in his limited understanding he might actually object to the use of the drug, thereby jeopardizing his life.
(3) It would be virtually impossible for a manufacturer to comply with the duty of direct warning as there is no sure way to reach the patient.

There are, however, certain products in which warnings are given directly to the user. At the present time this class is small and is limited to birth control pills, IUDs and insulin. Legislative proposals have been advanced, however, to compel manufacturers to provide warnings to consumers for other pharmaceuticals. It is entirely likely that if patient package insert proposals are accepted a new duty to warn the patient may be created. At the present time, the warnings which accompany the 'pill' do not create liability, but ordinarily insulate the manufacturer from liability.[13] Should the regulatory authority mandate that the warning be given to the patient then one would expect the

9. *Dunkin* v. *Syntex, Supra.*
10. *Howard* v. *Avon Products*, 395 P.2d 1007 (1964).
11. 21 U.S.C.331. Present standards of quality control, government inspection make this class of case today almost unique. Obviously, if the product is adulterated and the adulteration is the cause of the injury, the manufacturer is liable.
12. *Stottlemire* v. *Cawood*, 213 F.Supp. 897 (1963). *Fogo* v. *Cutter Laboratories*, 68 Cal. App. 3d 744 (1977).
13. *Seley* v. *G. D. Searle & Co.*, 67 Ohio St.2d 192 (1981), held that an informational pamphlet provided by the physician for distribution to patients by the OC manufacturer did not extend the duty to warn, but the opposite view was expressed in Wisconsin in; *Lukaszewicz* v. *Ortho Pharmaceutical*, 510 F.Supp. 961 (1981).

Courts to rule that the warning must be understandable by an ordinary layman (the average patient) rather than the subjective standard of what the injured patient understood. This principle at present applies to the package insert and other material supplied to the medical profession.

It should be noted that, even in those cases in which it can be shown that there was a failure to adequately warn, the plaintiff must still prove that the alleged failure to warn was a causal factor in the physician's prescribing the drug, and in the patient's developing the alleged injury.[14] For example, when the patient fails to give the physician an adequate and accurate history it is the patient's negligence rather than the manufacturer's failure which is the cause of the injury. Another example is the case in which the patient begins to develop symptoms consistent with a known adverse reaction and the patient fails to notify the physician in spite of having previously been advised to report all unusual symptoms. Alternate causation can also defeat recovery on the part of the injured party. The plaintiff's injury may be the result of (a) genetic factors, (b) different dosages, (c) drug interactions, (d) intervening acts of malpractice on the part of the physician or (e) abuse of the product by the patient. Illustratively, cataracts can be caused by diabetes or by drug ingestion.

Where the prescribing physician has independent knowledge of reported side-effects or independent expertise, and testifies that he knew of the foreseeability of the adverse reaction, the manufacturer will be absolved of liability in spite of the failure to warn the physician.

Effective labelling can, therefore, create a defence that works. Ineffective labelling may, in itself, create liability. Labelling, to be effective, must be a joint effort of the manufacturer and its liability counsel.[15] More recent cases establish the principle that if this obligation is met and the prescribing physician accedes to the proposition that he understood the materials supplied by the manufacturer and made the requisite medical judgement with reference to the prescribing of the pharmaceutical product, then the action is dismissible against the manufacturer.[16]

Applicable statutes distinguish between over-the-counter drugs and prescription drugs. The basic provision is that a drug is misbranded if its labelling does not bear 'adequate directions for use'. 21 USC §352(f)(i). These directions are intended for the user, but the requirement only applies to non-prescription drugs. 21 USC §353(b)(c) provides that a prescription is necessary if a drug is (a) habit forming, (b) because of 'toxicity or other potentiality for harmful effect, or the method of its use, or the collateral measures necessary to its use, is not

14. The issue of causation is a question of fact for determination by the jury. PJI (N.Y.) 2:72; *Hoover* v. *Franklin Sewer Co.*, 444 S.W.2d 596 (1969); *Contra Evans* v. *U.S.* 319 F.2d 752 (1963).
15. Defences that work in Products Liability cases, 26 Fed. of Ins. Counsel Q 89 (1976).
16. *Terhune* v. *A. H. Robins*, *Chambers* v. *G. D. Searle & Co.*, *Dunkin* v. *Syntex*, supra.

safe for use except under the supervision of a practitioner licensed by law to administer such drugs', or (c) 'is limited by an effective application under §355 (new drugs) of this law to be used under the professional supervision of a practitioner licensed by law to administer such drug'.

Prescription drugs are exempt from the requirements for over-the-counter drugs, and they need not bear 'adequate directions for use' on the label going to the user 21 USC §353(b)(2). The label for the user is a simplified statement, which must bear the statement 'Caution: Federal law prohibits dispensing without a prescription 21 USC §353(b)(4). In addition the prescription drug label must contain the name and address of the dispenser; the serial number and the date of the prescription or its filling or refilling; the name of the prescriber; and, if stated in the prescription, the name of the patient and the directions for use and statements, if any contained in such prescription.

The directions for use of a drug which is sold by virtue of an approved NDA are provided to the physician in the form of prescribing information or package inserts; they are phrased in medical terms unintelligible to the consumer layman. The physician is obligated to educate himself fully about various drugs and devices from journals, articles, meetings, seminars and from his own past experiences. When taken in conjunction with an examination of the patient, their medical history, and other factors, and after considering all of the foregoing, the doctor exercises his own judgement and discretion in determining what treatment is indicated, and what information regarding the side-effects or risks inherent with that drug or device are to be passed on to the patient.

There is available, without cost, to every physician in the United States, the *Physician's Desk Reference*, colloquially known as the PDR. This volume is issued on an annual basis with twice-yearly supplements. Almost all ethical pharmaceuticals are listed. There is a generic index and a manufacturers index. There is also a section containing full-colour reproductions of selected products. A product information section, which makes up the mass of the volume, contains package inserts of almost every drug sold in the United States. The product identification section basically contains the word-for-word reproduction of the package insert as issued by the manufacturer. At least one court has held that the greater the potential hazard of a drug the more extensive must be the manufacturers efforts to make that hazard known to the medical profession. In *Baker* v. *St. Agnes Hospital*, 421 N.Y.S.2d 81 (1979) a New York State court found that Eli Lilly was negligent in failing to establish a Dicumarol warning in the PDR. A physician who concedes that he was unaware of the existence of the PDR, or failed to make himself fully familiar with the package insert as listed in the PDR prior to issuing a prescription could, by that act alone, cast himself in liability.

The doctor is, therefore, a learned intermediary between the patient and the manufacturer, and case law has consistently recognized and reaffirmed the proposition that a warning to the physician is the only effective way a warning can be given. Self-medication with these potent drugs is illegal. Prescribing information in the hands of a pharmacist is not to be displayed to purchasers 21 CFR §3.513.

Since May 28, 1976, the law, with respect to ethical pharmaceuticals and all new drug applications, has been made applicable to medical devices.[17] This makes eminently good sense, since items such as prostheses, diagnostic devices, pacemakers, IUDs and similar devices can only come into contact with a patient through the intervening acts of a physician.

If the action is dismissible against the manufacturer, it is dismissible against those parties whose liability derives from the manufacturer's obligation with reference to the duty to warn. Under American law on products liability, liability is imposed upon the seller of the product. Effectively this means, as far as ethical pharmaceuticals are concerned, the pharmacist who fills the prescription, the drug wholesaler who sold it to the pharmacist, any intervening vendors in the chain of distribution and ultimately the manufacturer.[18]

If the pharmacist has not adulterated the product or misfilled the prescription, the pharmacist's liability is a vicarious liability. He did not manufacture the product. He did not detail it to the medical profession. He had no involvement in the preparation of the package insert, made neither representations nor warranties with reference to the efficacy or safety of the product. The pharmacist merely follows the physician's instructions with reference to filling the prescription, and has sold a product which has been supplied to him by the drug wholesaler or distributor, who, in turn, was supplied the product by the manufacturer. Under these circumstances, in the event that the court holds that the plaintiff is entitled to recover, the pharmacist relies upon representations made by the person from whom he purchased the product, the drug distributor, and is entitled to be indemnified, not only for any adverse judgement, but also for the costs of defence against the person from whom he has purchased the product, the drug distributor. The legal rule applicable to the drug distributor is identical to that applicable to the pharmacist, and the distributor may in turn be indemnified not only for monetary damages arising from the sums he is legally obligated to pay to the injured party and to the pharmacist, but also the cost of his legal defence, and may recover the sum from the manufacturer. Basically, the legal system is such that the ultimate cost is borne by the manufacturer, who is once again best able to bear the financial loss.

Chief Judge Bailey Brown of the United States District Court for the Western District of Tennessee in *Dunkin* v. *Syntex Laboratories Inc.*,[19] held that:

17. 21 U.S.C.A. 360.
18. 402(a) Restatement of Torts.
19. Supra, n.8.

'This rule is based on the recognition that prescription drugs are sold on a prescription basis and not over the counter; because of the special expertise a trained physician is necessary for their use. Thus, an effective warning could only be to the medical profession, and not to an untrained patient. Moreover, concern has been expressed that attempts to give detailed warnings to patients could mislead patients and might also tend to interfere in the physician/patient relationship. On the other hand, it has been recognized that an effective warning regarding a prescription drug must go to the medical profession generally and not to the prescribing physician alone, since the patient may not return to the original prescribing physician when problems occur.

This is not to suggest that persons using prescription drugs should receive no warnings of the dangers involved in the use of those drugs. Rather, it is this court's determination that the duty to warn the patient, if one exists, lies with the physician and not with the drug manufacturer.'

## PHYSICIAN'S LIABILITY

The physician's liability arising from the administration of a drug can be the result of administration of too little, for instance antibiotics; too much, as in digitalis or a steroid product; too long, for instance in the case of 'Butazolidin' or 'Tanderil'; no indication for an administered variation,[20] for instance in an antibiotic not effective for the particular infection; or a misdiagnosis of the condition.[21] Administration of a drug in the presence of known contra-indication, as reported in the *PDR* or in the medical literature supplied by the manufacturer; administration without performing the required physical examination, as for instance in the case of oral contraceptives; administration without obtaining the informed consent from the patient as in chloramphenicol or streptomycin, can also create liability on the part of the physician.[22] Should the physician fail to keep abreast of current medical knowledge or of the latest data supplied by the manufacturer, he once again does so at his peril.

Since the pharmaceutical manufacturer does not practise medicine it is the responsibility of the physician to monitor the patient for side-effects, both those reported in the package insert and those which are basically allergic or idiosyncratic. The physician must be alert to the earliest manifestations of known and unknown side-effects.[23] The failure of a physician to determine a causal relationship between the ingestion of the drug and the side-effect and treat it, can cast him in liability.[24] His failure to stop the administration of the offending drug and the failure to obtain information from the manufacturer and the medical literature and to prepare to treat for known adverse reactions

20. *Koury* v. *Follo*, 272 N.C. 366 (1968).
21. *Rotan* v. *Greenbaum*, 273 F.2d 830 (1959).
22. *Mulder* v. *Parke Davis & Co.*, 181 N.W.2d 882 (1970). See D. H. Mills, 'Physician Responsibility for Drug Prescription', *J. Am. Med. Assoc.*, **192** (1956), 116.
23. Drug Product Liability, Marden G. Dixon, Sect. 7.16.
24. *Magee* v. *Wyeth Laboratories*, 20 Cal.Rptr. 322 (1963).

and side-effects can also cast him in liability.[25] A classic example is the failure of the physician to be prepared to administer epinephrine if the patient goes into anaphylactic shock on administration of penicillin.

The pharmaceutical manufacturer should be mindful that the prescribing physician is an ally in the defence of the case. His goodwill must be obtained, and should be maintained throughout the litigation. This is especially true since, in addition to the problems concerning the manufacturer in the individual law suit, the manufacturer, as always, must be aware that the viability of his product is dependent upon the physician's continuing acceptance of the product as relatively safe and efficacious. The manufacturer should under no circumstances do anything in the case which would alienate the physician.[26]

The gravamen of the duty imposed on a physician with reference to pharmaceuticals which are prescribed in accordance with the information provided in the package insert is twofold. There is first a duty to warn the patient of the hazards of the treatment prior to its administration.[27] The second duty is a separate and distinct duty to protect the patient from the dangers of an adverse drug reaction. This doctrine is called 'informed consent' and is in flux, but most commentators believe that the future will see an expansion of this doctrine. Commentators generally conceive that there is an obligation on the part of the physician to advise the patient of risks inherent in the medication and the alternatives available to the patient prior to the initiation of drug therapy. More recent cases indicate that the physician has a legal duty to assist the patient in selecting the proper course of treatment. This obligation cannot be met by having the patient sign a written consent form. The physician is under an obligation to inform the patient about the dangers of an adverse reaction attributable to the medication which may be more serious than, or as serious as, the disease.[28] Thus, prior to prescribing an oral contraceptive which is alleged to cause serious injury with a risk of morbidity, the physician must inform the patient of the risks of pregnancy, and let the patient join him in the election of a proper contraceptive method.

The emphasis under the informed consent doctrine is that the patient is legally entitled to, and must be afforded an opportunity by the physician to, participate in making the decision pertaining to the election of treatment. The only exception is emergency treatment. Even after the physician has met this legal obligation he also has a continuing obligation to monitor the patient, and to supply the patient with enough information so that the patient himself can recognize the onsets of a drug reaction and then might seek medical attention. The

25. *Fleischman* v. *Richardson-Merrell, Inc.*, 226 A.2d 843 (1967).
26. It should be noted, however, that if the physician fails to follow the package insert, it constitutes a break in causation which exonerates the manufacturer from liability. *Mulder* v. *Parke-Davis & Co.*, 181 N.W.2d 882 (1970).
27. *Natanson* v. *Kline*, 350 P.2d 1093 (1960), *Salgo* v. *Leland Stanford Univ.* 317 P.2d 170 (1957); *Canterbury* v. *Spence*, 464 F.2d 772 (1972).
28. *ZeBarth* v. *Swedish Hospital Medical Center*, 49 P.2d 1 (1972).

doctor must additionally be ever aware of the possibility of an anaphylactic reaction or an idiosyncratic reaction. Many package inserts bear admonitions to the physician that he be aware of the earliest signs of a drug-induced reaction. Unless the physician advises the patient in laymen's terms of the symptomatology that necessitates the patient securing medical treatment, the physician might well expose himself to liability.

## MANUFACTURER'S LIABILITY

The investigation, licensing, marketing, distribution, labelling and advertising of ethical pharmaceuticals comes within the jurisdiction of the Food & Drug Administration (FDA).

No drug can be marketed unless an NDA drug application has been approved. The drug application in reality, and in legal contemplation, is not an application as such. After the original chemistry, toxicology and clinical testing have been performed under an International New Drug (IND) a new drug application is made to the FDA. The NDA is in reality, and in legal contemplation, a continuing application. All changes in advertising and labelling must be submitted to the FDA prior to adaptation by the pharmaceutical manufacturer. There is a continuing obligation to monitor all medical literature, not only in the US but from sources all over the world which have any relevance or are applicable to the product as marketed. If a review of the medical literature, even in the first instance, indicates an adverse reaction causally related to the ingestion of the product which had not been recognized prior to that time, it must be immediately reported to the FDA. Immediate investigation of any claimed adverse reaction is obligatory on pharmaceutical manufacturers. All adverse reactions of serious consequence must be submitted to the FDA. A '1639' or 'Adverse Reaction Report' mandates the identity of the patient, the nature of the adverse reaction and the identity of the reporting doctor.

A manufacturer has three options available to him if he is to insulate himself from liability upon discovery of a new class of drug reaction. If the new class of reaction is one which bears the risk of immediate and dire consequences to the patient, the pharmaceutical manufacturer, after consulting with the FDA, should promptly send all registered physicians a so-called 'Dear Doctor' letter. This letter basically advises the physician that a recent medical development has established a new class of reactions involved in the ingestion of the drug. Basically, the 'Dear Doctor' letter provides immediate information referable to contraindications and warnings.

The 'Dear Doctor' letter has been traditionally followed at a later date by an appropriate package insert change. The second alternative is to submit a formal application to the FDA for an amendment to the package insert. The danger with this procedure is, of course, the delay inherent in dealing with bureaucracy. Substantial time is involved. There are wording changes and multiple meetings with the FDA. The hiatus between the initiation of the change, its approval by the FDA, its printing and its appearance on the pharmacist's shelves and in the *PDR*, may involve a period of 6 months or more. The third alternative is provided by Section 21 CFR 314.8(d) of the Food and Drug and Cosmetic Act which provide that in the event of a discovery of a serious adverse reaction the pharmaceutical company may immediately change its package insert without prior notification to the FDA. The nature of the adverse reaction usually dictates the method used. Details of the method adopted should be immediately disseminated to the detailing force.

The physician who reports a suspected adverse reaction either to the FDA or the pharmaceutical company has no liability exposure. On the contrary, most litigation involving the reporting of adverse reactions is almost exclusively directed to attempts by the injured party's attorney to secure copies of the adverse reaction reports (1639) either under the Freedom of Information Act directly from the FDA, or from the NDA which the pharmaceutical manufacturer is mandated by law to maintain on his premises. The discovery efforts by the injured party's attorney are directed to using this source to establish that the pharmaceutical manufacturer was under notice of a particular adverse reaction, but took no steps either to send out a 'Dear Doctor' Letter, a separate filing under provisions of 21 CFR 314.8(d) or make application to change the package insert.

Traditionally, the physician does not identify the individual patient but merely uses some appropriate initial or other designation. The physician by law is concerned primarily with his patient's treatment and secondly with maintaining the confidentiality of the doctor–patient privilege. The physician is morally obligated, where he suspects a drug-induced adverse reaction, to report it to the manufacturer. He often does so in order to secure from the manufacturer details that would help him in treating the suspected drug reaction. Physicians assume, and rightfully so, that the manufacturer can help them in exercising the proper medical judgement in the treatment of a drug reaction. Many adverse reactions reported to the manufacturer are of this category. Traditionally a flurry of reports of a specific adverse reaction occur during the period immediately after the reaction has been reported in the public press or medical literature. These reports must be analysed in detail.

## THE CONTINGENT FEE SYSTEM

To appreciate the exposure inherent in pharmaceutical litigation in the US one must understand the idiosyncrasies of the American legal system. The contingent fee system is unique to the United States.[29] Its rationale is that it provides a means by which an individual without

29. A study of contingent fees in the prosecution of personal injury claims. 33 *Ins. Counsel J.*, **197** (April 1966).

adequate funds can secure legal representation by highly skilled and competent trial counsel. The counsel who is retained advances all money required to prosecute the action. It is counsel, not the client, who in the first instance pays the cost of securing and reproducing hospital records, the retention of investigators, filing and court costs, the retention of experts, retention of other professionals to do medical and pharmaceutical research, pays court reporters as well as a plethora of other incidental costs. Prosecution of the action is, therefore, independent of the ability of the client to pay. These costs in the average pharmaceutical products liability or medical malpractice case can be staggering, and in many instances grossly exceed $30 000. The attorney, in turn, if he prevails, receives out of the recovery, reimbursement of all costs and disbursements advanced, and then after deducting these sums from the amount recovered, receives a fee of approximately one-third of the judgement. Depending on the jurisdiction and the nature of the cause of action, this fee may vary from 20% to 50%.

In many jurisdictions, the contingent fee is regulated by the court.[30] Unlike the United Kingdom and Canada, the losing party does not pay counsel fees. US legal costs are limited, as a general proposition, to filing costs and subpoena fees, all of which, even in an action in which the recovery exceeds a million dollars, are usually limited to a sum less than $1000. If plaintiff's counsel loses the case he receives no fee and absorbs the expenses advanced. Since the sum required to prosecute a pharmaceutical products liability case or a medical malpractice case is staggering, the well-trained, highly competent plaintiff's counsel will traditionally refuse to prosecute an action either for medical malpractice or pharmaceutical products case unless the injury is one in which he has first a reasonable expectation of recovery, and secondly, a reasonable expectation of securing a verdict in excess of $100 000.[31] If the injury is truly catastrophic, as in the case of a paraplegic or quadraplegic, or in the case of a catastrophic birth defect, the monetary incentive is so great that the case will be undertaken even in cases of questionable liability. The rationale is that since most negligence cases are reduced to a question of fact, they are determined by a jury. Experience teaches defence counsel, as well as pharmaceutical manufacturers and their insurers, that catastrophic injuries alone tend to create liability once they are submitted to a jury.

## ASSESSMENT OF DAMAGES

To appreciate the hazards presented in a drug case in the US some understanding must also be had of the legal basis on which damages

30. N. H. Rev. Stat. Ann. Sect. 507-C:8; N.Y. Jud. Law (McKinney) Sect. 474-a.
31. US Dept. of Commerce, Interagency Task Force in Products Liability (1977), suggests a figure of $25 000. The author's experience is such that they feel the higher figure of $100 000 is more appropriate.

are measured. The injured party, if he is entitled to recover at all, must recover all sums expended by the plaintiff for all medical services which are related to the injuries, including physician's services, X-rays and diagnostic procedures, hospital bills, costs of physiotherapy, medication and, if a basis can be established to show that it is causally connected to the injury, the costs of household help, etc. In addition, if the plaintiff were gainfully employed at the time of the injury, the wages lost by reason of the period of incapacity and the inability to return to work would be included. If proofs are adduced, during the course of the trial, that the injury has tendered the plaintiff unable to work in the future, or that the injured party requires future medical attention, plaintiff is entitled during the trial to introduce expert-opinion evidence as to the value of these prospective services. These proofs include, traditionally in a major negligence action, testimony from an economist as to the rate of inflation, the testimony of the former employer as to the prospects for advancement, and other emotional proofs to the effect that a most promising career was destroyed before it could mature. The inherent vice is that a paid expert is permitted to testify in an attempt to sway the jury. Prospective testimony is neither objective nor impartial. Typical testimony is to the effect that the injured party requires prospective medical care whose cost is ever increasing due to the inflationary spiral. As to loss of earnings, prospective testimony by plaintiff's economist may be to the effect that although at trial, plaintiff, a postal worker, is earning $20 000 a year, has a 20-year effective work-life expectancy, inflation and union contracts will mandate that at age 65, for the same job he will be earning $50 000 a year. This prospective testimony establishes the basis for multi-million dollar verdicts. Once again it is not the Court that determines the validity of these proofs, but the jury, which is oft-times swayed by consideration of sympathy and prejudice. In addition, under the American system, the plaintiff is entitled to receive as compensation a sum of money representing 'pain and suffering' that cannot be measured by any mathematical rule or scientific principle.[32] In actuality it is a sum of dollars which may be 'pulled out of a hat' by the jury. The type of instruction given to the jury by the Court prior to its deliberation in order to assist it in making a determination of what pain and suffering represents is called a part of the Charge. Under the Patent Jury Instruction, which might perhaps be termed the Judge's Bible, the instructions to the jury under Section PJI 2:280 are as follows:

> 'If you decide for the plaintiff on the question of liability, you may include in your verdict an award for the injury you find that he suffered and for conscious pain and suffering which you find to have been caused by the

32. *Interagency Task Force on Product Liability*, Vol. V at page 96 (1977) estimates that damages for 'pain and suffering' exceed pecuniary damages by a ratio of three to two.

negligence of defendant. The plaintiff is entitled to recover a sum of money which will justly and fairly compensate him for his injury and for his conscious pain and suffering to date.'

## THE AMERICAN JURY SYSTEM

The law mandates that all personal injury litigants are entitled to a 'jury of your peers'. Under the American jury system, six individuals, usually without university or scientific training, by occupation, retiree, postal worker, housewife, or taxi driver, will be asked to make a determination which will be legally binding on the physician or pharmaceutical manufacturer. Should a prospective juror have had formal training in toxicology, epidemiology or other scientific discipline which would be helpful in evaluating the issues in the case, he would be disqualified from sitting on the case. The US, unlike Europe, does not permit experts to sit on the jury, even in an advisory function. The jury will be presented evidence by way of oral testimony, documentation and expert-opinion evidence, during the trial presided over by the Court whose sole function is to moderate the trial, rule on objections and decide what is competent legal evidence, whether oral or documentary. At the close of the case the Court will instruct the jury as to what law to apply. The decision as to whether the plaintiff is entitled to recover, and how much, remains exclusively in the province of the jury. Should the Court invade that province, on appeal to a higher court, the verdict, whatever it may be, would be set aside and the case re-tried. It is not unrealistic to anticipate in an American jury trial to have a jury determine the cause of cancer, and whether or not the ingestion of an ethical pharmaceutical is involved in the causative process. Such determination, by other than an American jury sitting on a personal-injury drug case, would entitle one to a Nobel prize in medicine.

Catastrophic cases are also affected by monstrous jury awards in other categories of negligence trials involving automobile accident cases and other types of products cases. Awards which shock the conscience of the business community produce a plethora of human-interest newspaper stories which tend to emphasize the fact that multi-million-dollar verdicts are common occurrences in negligence cases. Newspaper articles, therefore, tend to affect jurors by creating a standard which pereptuates high verdicts. Many courts refuse to review jury verdicts on the grounds of excessiveness.[33]

In view of the high cost of processing multi-party, combined medical malpractice–products liability cases, the plaintiffs bar is continually

33. See, Report of California Citizen's Commission on Tort Reform, Righting the Liability Balance (1977). The Commission recommends the development of standards limiting awards for 'pain and suffering', the model statute of the Council of State Government proposes limiting damages for 'pain and suffering' to $25 000.

seeking to reduce the costs of discovery. Where many individuals claim injury from a single product the plaintiff's bar has attempted to join all of their cases together in a single class action.[34] The class action commonly seeks hundreds of millions of dollars. The key question is certification of the 'class'. If certification is granted, a determination in favour of the injured party is expanded to include all others similarly injured, even if their identity is unknown, and they themselves are unaware of the pendency of the suit. This type of litigation was previously restricted to mass disasters, such as aircraft accident cases. Recently a court in California, on its own motion, accepted a class certification in Dalkon shield litigation. That courts conditional order proposed a limited class on limited liability issues. The manufacturer, A. H. Robins, filed a motion for certification under the Federal Rules of Civil Procedure, Rule 23(b)(1) to combine all persons who had claims for punitive damages. The court found classification for that purpose particularly compelling where there was a finding that Robins had a limited fund of insurance and assets. Thus in the absence of a class there might be a rush to the courthouse so that the first plaintiffs to try their cases might leave later plaintiffs without a means of redress.[35] If present trends continue, it is likely that the courts will certify cases that have previously been rejected.

As distinguished from compensatory damages, punitive damages are awarded to punish and deter outrageous conduct. Punitive damages cannot be awarded unless the defendant's conduct contains elements of intentional wrongdoing or conscious disregard for the plaintiff's rights. The requisite misconduct must be chargeable either by participation or acquiescence by the corporate management. It is now quite common for plaintiffs to allege punitive damages. If the court does not order bifurcation and separate trial on this issue, a jury will hear proof on issues which would have otherwise been excluded from the trial, such as details of the corporation's fiscal structure. Since each plaintiff can seek punitive damages in their individual case, defendants are exposed to repeated punishment for the same wrong. In addition to seeking class certification on punitive damages issues, pharmaceutical manufacturers are also supporting a national product liability law to correct this situation and other inequities. Although insurance coverage is ordinarily available for compensatory damages it is seldom permitted in the event of an adverse verdict for punitive damages.

Another tactic employed by the plaintiff's bar, which is growing in acceptance, is the concept of collateral estoppel.* In the case of *Vincent*

*Estoppel, as used here, refers to a finding of fact by judicial determination so that a factual determination by one jury prevents that party from relitigating the same question in a subsequent case.

34. 14 C.J.S. 1193; C.P.L.R. (N.Y.) Art. 9.
35. In re Northern District of California Dalkon shield IUD Products Liability Litigation, 526 F. Supp. 887; *Payton* v. *Abbott Laboratories*, 83 FRD 382 (a DES class certification).

v. *Thompson*, 50 A.D.2d 211, 377 N.U.S.2d 118, the New York Courts considered the case of a child who had become ill following the administration of a vaccine known as Quadrigen. An earlier Federal decision had established that the Quadrigen vaccine was in fact defective, resulting in serious injuries to the plaintiff in that case. Plaintiff sought to invoke the doctrine of collateral estoppel to reduce the case to an issue of damages alone. The Court rejected this theory, noting that even assuming defective design the injuries to any one particular patient may have resulted from a variety of factors completely unrelated to the design defect, and there may in fact have been factors in the plaintiff's background which changed the risk. In *Ezagui* v. *Dow Chemical Corp.*, 598 F.2d 727 (1979), another Quadrigen case, the court ruled that plaintiff was not entitled to collateral estoppel as to chemical defect since new scientific evidence cast doubt upon the theory relied upon in prior cases, but collateral estoppel was available to prevent the manufacturer from denying the inadequacy of the warning contained in the Quadrigen package insert, since the manufacturer had been given an opportunity to litigate that issue in an earlier case. Collateral estoppel has since been applied in a DES case against Eli Lilly; *Kaufman* v. *Eli Lilly*, 65 N.Y.2d 449.

The diethylstilboestrol (DES) litigation presented a unique problem: product identification. This drug synthesized in England in 1937, received FDA approval in 1941 for many usages, including the maintenance of pregnancy. In 1971, Dr Herbst reported a statistical association between the use of DES by pregnant women and the development of clear cell adenocarcinoma in the vagina of the daughters many years later.

Most of the litigants could not establish whose product was ingested. In response to this predicament, the judiciary has created new legal theories to ease plaintiff's burden. In California the theory is called 'Market Share Liability'. *Sindell* v. *Abbott Laboratories*,[36] holds that once plaintiff joins manufacturers of a substantial share of the DES market and proves a *prima facie* case, except for identification of the tortfeasor, the burden of proof shifts to the defendants to prove that they did not cause plaintiff's injury. Another theory plaintiffs propose is called 'Concerted Action'. The underlying principle of this theory is that those who in pursuance of a common plan or design to commit a tort, actively take part in it or further it by co-operation or request, or who will lend aid or encouragement to the wrongdoer, or ratify and adopt his acts done for their benefits are equally liable. Express agreement is not necessary, and all that is required is that there be understanding between the companies. See *Bickler* v. *Eli Lilly*, 759 A.D.2d 317 aff'd 55 N.Y.2d 571 (1982). In Michigan the principle is called 'alternative liability'. Under this principle the plaintiff must prove that all of the defendants acted tortiously, that the plaintiff was

36. *Sindell* v. *Abbott Laboratories*, 85 Cal. App. 3d 1, 86 Cal. App. 416a.

harmed by the conduct of one of the defendants and that the plaintiffs, through no fault of their own, are unable to identify which act caused the injury. The court in Abel concluded that this remedy was available only where additional legal principles are unavailable to the plaintiff. Thus where the plaintiff knows who the manufacturer is they cannot sue all manufacturers and distributors.

In *Collins* v. *Eli Lilly*, 116 Wis. 2d 166 (1984) the Wisconsin Supreme Court allowed the plaintiff to sue only one of many DES manufacturers, even though the plaintiff could not prove that the manufacturer supplied the product ingested by her mother. The court in Collins stated:

> The plaintiff need commence suit against only one defendant and allege the following elements: that the plaintiff's mother took DES; that DES caused the plaintiff subsequent injury; that the defendant produced or marketed the type of DES taken by the plaintiff's mother; and that the defendant's conduct in producing or marketing the DES constituted a breach of a legally recognized duty to the plaintiff. In the situation where the plaintiff can not allege and prove what type of DES the mother took. As to the third element, the plaintiff need only allege and prove that the defendant drug company produced or marketed the drug DES for use in preventing miscarriages during pregnancy.

If more than one defendant is joined, the plaintiff can recover from each defendant damages proportionate to a jury assessment of liability pursuant to a comparative negligence scheme. Defendants may rebut the case by proving that they did not produce or market the DES during the period when ingestion was alleged, or that their distribution was not in the geographic area where the plaintiff's mother was located. The court explained: 'As between the plaintiff, who probably is not at fault, and the defendants, who may have provided the product which caused the injury, the interest of justice and fundamental fairness demand that the latter should bear the costs of injury."

Despite the hazards of the jury trial, there is still available to the defence, legal proceedings prior to trial which entitle the defence to a dismissal of the plaintiff's case as a matter of law. In essence this type of procedure is to the effect that even if the Court were to accept all the material allegations of the complaint as filed by or on behalf of the injured party, there is no legal basis on which the plaintiff may recover, thereby permitting the Court to grant judgement in favour of the pharmaceutical manufacturer. This doctrine affords a pharmaceutical company a dismissal of the action without trial, *Dunkin* v. *Syntex*, *Terhune* v. *A. H. Robins*.[37] The manufacturer's position is once again that the only legal theory on which the plaintiff can recover is for a breach of the duty to warn.

37. Report of the [HEW] Secretary's Commission on Medical Malpractice (1973).

## INSURANCE

Excessive verdicts, the expense of defending products cases, and the expansion of the legal basis of liability has created a crisis in products liability in the US, if not in the world.[38]

The insurance industry's experience with reference to such pharmaceutical products as thalidomide, diethylstilboestrol, MER-29, Dalkon Shield and, in the early days, the costs of defending oral contraceptive cases, has made that industry particularly sensitive to the liability exposure of the pharmaceutical manufacturer. The standard insurance contract today, by special endorsement, excludes coverages for injuries resulting on a products basis for injuries alleged to have been caused by diethylstilboestrol, IUDs and swine flu vaccine.[39] Insurance is no longer available on a primary basis. As a practical matter, if insurance coverage is available, it can only be purchased with a large SIR (self-insured retention). Today in the US most of the major pharmaceutical companies are self-insured and can only secure coverage in the London Excess and Surplus Market for so-called catastrophe insurance, and even then it is often unavailable. The lack of insurance mandates that the pharmaceutical company must train and organize its own legal staff to defend products cases.

## ORGANIZED PLAINTIFF GROUPS

The organized plaintiffs' bars in the US not infrequently, on a nationwide basis, have formed independent groups to exchange information to assist each other in the prosecution of personal injury actions against the pharmaceutical manufacturer, whose product has been indicted in the public press. Prime examples of a successful products group involve Richardson Merrill's MER-29 and the Dalkon Shield IUD group. In the 'IUD's Federal Loophole' in the November/December 1974 issue of *Trial*, the author states that a Dalkon Shield Group has been established which will,

> '. . . keep members informed of developments in the cases filed and in the medical administrative field. Copies of pleadings and various discovery will be exchanged. It is possible that friends of the group will be used to prepare expert witnesses for trial and to participate in joint discovery of the defendants . . .'

The pharmaceutical manufacturer, in order to protect the integrity of his product against this type of onslaught, usually co-ordinates

38. US Dept. of Commerce, Options Paper on Product Liability and Accident Compensation Issues (1978), indicated that increases in the number of claims from 1974 to 1976 averaged over 200% and that some industries with high-risk exposure faced premium increases of over 1000%, if insurance was available at all.
39. Universal in the Lloyds form.

products liability defence utilizing both house counsel and an independent expert retained for this specific purpose. Defence litigation is controlled from a central source and guarantees that local defence counsel in each of the 50 states will submit answers to interrogatories, which are not inadvertently contradictory. This prevents inconsistent statements in different cases in diverse states; it provides the pharmaceutical manufacturer with control and inspection of documentation. More importantly, legal input serves a prophylactic purpose in that all package inserts, advertisements, packaging and training aids for detailing personnel are reviewed, in order to prevent the inadvertent creation of liability. Legal review tends to guarantee that the package insert meets the mandate of the 'duty to warn', and prevents by inadvertent creation of a claim for fraudulent advertising, or excess puffing on the part of the detailing staff.[40]

Since primary insurance, as a practical basis, is no longer available, the issue becomes one of securing adequate catastrophe insurance in the excess and surplus market on a premium basis that is acceptable. Insurance placement is handled on a sophisticated basis by a knowledgeable broker and insurance manager. Premium rates are negotiated. One cannot trade dollars with insurance companies. This phrase in insurance circles signifies that the manufacturer cannot assume that the insurer will pay its casualty losses. In the event that losses exceed premiums paid, insurance is no longer available, or the premium is increased to reflect the losses incurred by the insurer in prior years, plus an additional premium for anticipated future losses. Insurance premiums always reflect prior experience. The problem is further complicated by the fact that the Statute of Limitations in so-called infants' actions is not time-barred until 3 years after the child reaches his majority. This is especially true in cases in which there is a teratogenic claim. Since the excess surplus market utilizes a 3-year accounting period, they may not be advised of a pendency of a claim until a decade after the insurer has closed its books on a particular pharmaceutical manufacturer. If a comprehensive loss control liability programme, under guidance of counsel by an outside expert, can be presented during the negotiating process, coverage can be secured, and at a premium that is livable. That is not to say that insurance will be inexpensive.

## 'NO FAULT' LEGISLATION

Commentators have suggested that no-fault insurance for pharmaceutically induced injuries is a solution to ever-spiralling casualty costs.[41] The US has adopted no-fault automobile laws on an almost universal basis. Under no-fault, if an individual is involved in an

40. Defenses that Work, supra.
41. Supra, n.31.

automobile accident, the common law tort principle no longer applies, and the insurer of the vehicle is legally responsible to compensate the injured party out-of-pocket losses incurred including his medical expenses, hospital bills and lost earnings. The right to additional compensation for payments for pain and suffering has theoretically been abolished. As a practical matter, if the injury is severe, in every no-fault law so far enacted in the US there is available to the plaintiff the right to bring a traditional negligence action, even though the injured party had previously received reimbursement from the insurance carrier for his so-called special damages. In many instances the no-fault benefits are utilized to prosecute a major casualty claim against the defendant who has paid no-fault benefits. Although the issue of pharmaceutical no-fault has been broached in the US it has been viewed with disfavour. First, it is a diseased section of the population who ingest ethical pharmaceutical products. Secondly, even the most liberal legal commentators have been unable to formulate no-fault legislation with a compensation system which would be economically feasible. Since morbidity is usually preceded by protracted illness, during which ingestion of medication is present, the pharmaceutical industry could be exposed to paying compensation in every drug case. No serious consideration has been given in the US, as far as the author knows, similar to the programmes which have been suggested in Sweden and Germany. The Swedish and German legislations basically provide no-fault benefits in instances where injuries have been caused by drug reactions which were unknown or unanticipated by the manufacturer. If the drug reaction is a known peril it is excluded from either the Swedish or German law. Under the German law insurance coverage is mandatory, and must be placed with a German insurer. The disparity in value of a personal injury case in the US, as opposed to Germany, makes the placement of this type of coverage in the US unavailable. Attempts at this type of legislation have to date received no serious consideration in the US.

Despite the idiosyncrasies of the American legal system, and what must seem to the rest of the world as absolutely shocking verdicts, there are defences which insulate the pharmaceutical manufacturer from liability or, at least reduce potential casualty losses to a workable level. These defences, however, require a substantial expenditure of time and expense by the manufacturer, its counsel and insurer. Substantial efforts must be invested in establishing the integrity of the product, the absence of any defect, and establishing that, if the accident occurred as described by the plaintiff, it was due to a misuse of the product. If, after the casualty occurs, it is determined that there is a basis for liability, in most instances the case should be disposed of by settlement with the least expense consistent with the value of the injuries.

# 39
# Relief system for sufferers of adverse drug reactions in Japan

N. IKEDA

## THALIDOMIDE AND SMON DISASTERS

It is not necessary to argue here that drugs are indispensable for health care. However, in spite of their obvious benefits, they often have harmful side effects. As a result, a balanced assessment of their efficacy and safety has been one of the principal aims of pharmaceutical jurisprudence.

In 1961, the year after an extensive revision of the *1948 Japanese Pharmaceutical Affairs Law*, a warning that congenitally malformed babies were being born to mothers who had taken thalidomide was made by Dr Lentz in West Germany.

As was happening elsewhere in the world, malformed children were born in Japan and the nationwide litigation for compensation from the pharmaceutical manufacturers responsible and the Ministry of Health and Welfare were made both on behalf of the suffering children and of their parents. Litigations began with a suit in the Nagoya district court in 1963. Later, the plaintiffs and defendants were conciliated, either in court or out of court, and the number of the victims rose to a final total of 309 including subsequent notifications.

As a result of this tragedy Japanese pharmaceutical regulators realized that attention should be paid to congenital abnormalities due to drug use when considering the policy of the toxicity-oriented drug approval review system. The thalidomide catastrophe has led to more stringent approval systems throughout the world.

In Japan, in 1967, Notification of the Director of the Pharmaceutical Affairs Bureau of the Ministry of Health and Welfare *Basic Policy Concerning Drug Manufacturing Approval* was issued, and the approval review procedure was made more rigorous, especially with regard to the safety of new drugs.

While thalidomide cases were still being discovered, early in 1965 cases of SMON (subacute myelo-optico-neuropathy) were reported. The first, mass outbreak of SMON occurred locally and was treated as a disease with unknown causes. A research team commissioned by the Health Ministry later discovered that the cause was quinoform, a drug used to treat gastrointestinal disorders, and an order was issued immediately for its production to be discontinued.

Drug manufacturers and the Ministry of Health and Welfare (MHW) were sued for compensation in courts throughout Japan. The first cases appeared before the Tokyo district court in 1971. To date, 11 district courts have reached the verdict that there is a definite relationship between SMON and quinoform.

The MHW, while admitting the legal liability of the state, tried to arrange out-of court settlements to provide early compensation for SMON sufferers. The first out-of-court settlement was achieved at the Tokyo district court in October, 1977, and subsequently, amicable settlements followed in many other districts. As of now, about 6300 of 6450 plaintiffs have settled out of court.

## DISCUSSION OF THE ESTABLISHMENT OF THE RELIEF SYSTEM

The tragic and widespread suffering resulting from adverse drug reactions (ADRs), such as occurred in the thalidomide and SMON disasters, prompted the MHW to set out relief measures for the sufferers, and a study group for a relief system was created in November, 1971. This study group made preliminary studies for detailed discussions of the relief system to be established in the future. The study group was dissolved when the new committee was formed.

The new committee, 'Committee for the Relief System for Sufferers from Adverse Drug Reactions', was created in June, 1973. This committee, which included experts on law, medicine, and pharmacology, submitted their reports in June, 1976 after investigating various aspects of relief system for three years.

An outline of their report included the following points:

– No-fault liability should not be introduced.
– Relief operations should be made through an independent body such as a foundation.
– Relief measures should be extended to sufferers of known ADRs as well as unknown ADRs.
– Resources for the benefit grants should, in principle, be supported by subscription charges from drug manufacturers.
– Certain relief measures should be extended to past victims such as SMON sufferers.

These fundamental points constitute the backbone of the present relief system.

The Ministry of Health and Welfare drafted a bill for the relief system based initially on the reports from the above committee, and in December, 1977, made public the *Draft of the Principle of Adverse Drug Reaction Sufferings Relief* (Bureau of Drug's Draft Bill).

The following comments on and criticisms of the Draft were expressed by various interested parties, and one year was spent reviewing and amending it.

(1) State subsidies for the Relief Fund should be introduced.
(2) Certification of relief grants should be decided by a third party organization independently from the Relief Fund.
(3) Limitations on the total benefits for any accident should be rescinded.
(4) The relief system should cover not only adverse drug reactions which occurred after the enactment of the relief system, but also ADRs that occurred before.
(5) The *Pharmaceutical Affairs Law* should be amended extensively in order to prevent further occurrences of adverse drug reactions.

Discussions on (1) were inconclusive, (2) was unadoptable because of practical restrictions, and (3) was not immediately acceptable because of the fundamental concepts of the relief system. However, (3) and (5) were acceptable and discussions continued to incorporate those opinions.

More importantly, amendments to the *Pharamceutical Affairs Law* were promptly initiated by the MHW, and resulted in the present Law for *Partial Amendment to the Pharmaceutical Affairs Law*, which has further tightened the approval review system of new drugs since the aforementioned MHW notification (Basic Policy Concerning Drug Manufacturing Approval) of 1967.

## Diet deliberations on the *Adverse Drug Reaction Sufferings Relief Fund Law (Relief Fund Law)*

The *Adverse Drug Reaction Sufferings Relief Fund Law* was introduced for discussion at the 87th National Diet session on February 28, 1979.

The *Partial Amendment to the Pharmaceutical Affairs Law* was introduced a little later, and both bills were deliberated simultaneously. The following amendments were unanimously proposed.

(1) Relief measures should be extended to previous ADR sufferers.
(2) Monetary relief grants as well as health and welfare relief should be extended to the sufferers.
(3) Judgment should always be placed before the Minister of Health and Welfare.

The above amendments were unanimously approved by the House of Representatives on June 5, 1979. However, during the subsequent deliberation in the House of Councillors, both bills failed to pass, because disorders in the Diet at that time resulted in that session closing.

The *Relief Fund Bill*, including all of the above amendments, was reintroduced at the 88th Extraordinary Diet Session on August 21, 1979, coupled with the *Partial Amendment to the Pharmaceutical Affairs Law*, and both bills were passed on September 7, 1979.

Then, on October 1, the Adverse Drug Reaction Sufferings Relief Fund Law (*Relief Fund Law*) was promulgated and became effective on the same day. The Relief Fund for Sufferers from Health Disorders Due to Adverse Drug Reactions (*Relief Fund*) was established on October 15, 1979 and the relief system came into operation.

## *THE RELIEF FUND LAW*

The *Adverse Drug Reaction Sufferings Relief Fund Law* is a public corporation statute which stipulates that the Adverse Drug Reaction Sufferings Relief Fund, will be organized for the rapid financial compensation of illness caused by ADRs.

This law is intended to ensure that financial aid is provided rapidly for individuals who have suffered ADRs, for medical expenses, personal pension, family pension, etc. In the case of serious diseases, disabilities and death due to ADRs aid shall be provided when compensation from a third party is impossible. The expenses incurred in operating this Relief Fund shall be financed by subscription charges from drug manufacturers and importers of drugs.

Although efforts are made to produce drugs which are safe as well as effective, serious adverse drug reactions do occur. Relief measures should therefore be extended. However, because it was felt that a no-fault liability system would be inappropriate, a system of granting benefits and fund contributions under the *Relief Fund Law* was stipulated.

This system may, therefore, be considered as a new social benefit relying on subscription charges from drug manufacturers. The manufacturers are willing to support this system in this way because it is their responsibility to provide effective and safe drugs.

The *Relief Fund Law* in its appendices also stipulates the compensation of victims of past ADRs.

Although there are, at present, relief systems operating in West Germany and Sweden, these are funded by private insurance companies. The Swedish system has no legal basis, the Japanese system is thus unique. The Japanese Relief Fund and its West German counterpart are compared below.

(1) The social responsibility of drug manufacturers is the fundamental basis of the system; thus a no-fault liability system which requires alterations in the present civil laws governing liability (liability arising from negligence) could be avoided.

– West Germany introduced the principle of no-fault liability.

(2) Establishment of an independent organization is stipulated as the principal relief operation body.

– West Germany legally mandated that drug manufacturers subscribe private insurance.

(3) Enactment of a special law for the establishment of the relief system.

– West Germany stipulated a relief system in its drug law.

(4) No limitation on the relief grants (limitation on the total relief benefit allowances for an accident) was set.

– West Germany restricted total relief benefits up to 200 million DM (about 20 000 Million yen). If the necessary funds exceed this amount, allowance grants to each sufferer are curtailed.

(5) The relief operation can receive state subsidies.

– The West German relief system has no provisions in this regard.

## Designated category of drugs in the *Relief Fund Law*

In this law, the drugs subject to subscription charges are the drugs defined in Article 2, Section 1 of the *Pharmaceutical Affairs Law*, and manufactured or imported after obtaining approval according to the procedures stipulated therein. Drugs manufactured or imported without valid licences and drugs prior to New Drug Application (NDA), i.e. investigational new drugs are excluded. In addition, the following categories of drugs are excluded even if they fall into the categories defined above:

(1) Drugs designated by the MHW, which are used for the treatment of diseases such as cancer. These drugs are considered indispensable, despite their high incidence of ADRs. 48 Drugs have been designated by government notices. Drugs for the treatment of malignant tumours (anti-cancer drugs), immunotherapeutic drugs and blood preparations are included in this category (MHW Notification No. 168, 1979 *Designated Drugs by the Minister of Health and Welfare*, in accordance with Article 2, Section 12, item 1 of the *Relief Fund Law for Sufferers from Health Disorders Due to Adverse Drug Reactions*).
(2) Drugs used only for the treatment of animals.
(3) Drugs used only for the manufacture of other drugs.
(4) Drugs manufactured for export only.
(5) Drugs not used directly on humans (insecticides, bactericides and disinfectants, non-internal diagnostic agents, etc.).
(6) Hygienic materials such as gauze, absorbent sanitary cotton and bandages, etc.

(7) 95 other items such as excipients, (designated in a separate table of the Ministerial Ordinance of MHW).

## Adverse drug reactions (ADRs)

The term 'adverse drug reaction' is defined as a harmful reaction occurring in spite of the proper use of the appropriate drugs in the treatment of a disease.

ADRs caused by improper use of medical negligence are excluded from benefits of the Relief Fund. Judgment in these matters are made by the Central Pharmaceutical Affairs Council which will be discussed in a subsequent section.

## The Adverse Drug Reaction Sufferings Relief Fund (Relief Fund)

### *Establishment and administration of the Relief Fund (Figure 1)*

The Relief Fund was established under the *Relief Fund Law*, as the sole authorized body under the auspices of non-government parties (i.e. the pharmaceutical companies) following approval by the Minister of Health and Welfare.

The existence of the Relief Fund as an authorized corporation, and not as a special corporation through legal procedures, indicates the social responsibility of the drug manufacturers in taking these steps voluntarily. The management of this Relief Fund includes one chief administrator, four or fewer directors and one auditor. All positions are currently filled.

The Relief Fund also has a board of trustees for the deliberation of important matters such as budget planning for its efficient operations. The board consists of ten members, comprising five persons belonging to associations and allied organizations, and five persons experienced in the operation of the Relief Fund. The board of trustees meetings discuss budget planning, relief grant ratios, revenues and financial statements.

### *Functions of the Relief Fund*

The Relief Fund performs the following functions.

(1) Granting of medical expenses, medical allowances, personal pensions, pensions for raising children, family pensions, lump sum benefits, and funeral expenses for diseases, disabilities, and deaths due to ADRs.
(2) Health and Welfare services with the approval of the Minister of Health and Welfare for sufferers receiving relief benefits.
(3) Collection of subscription charges.
(4) Jobs necessary for the operation of (1)–(3).

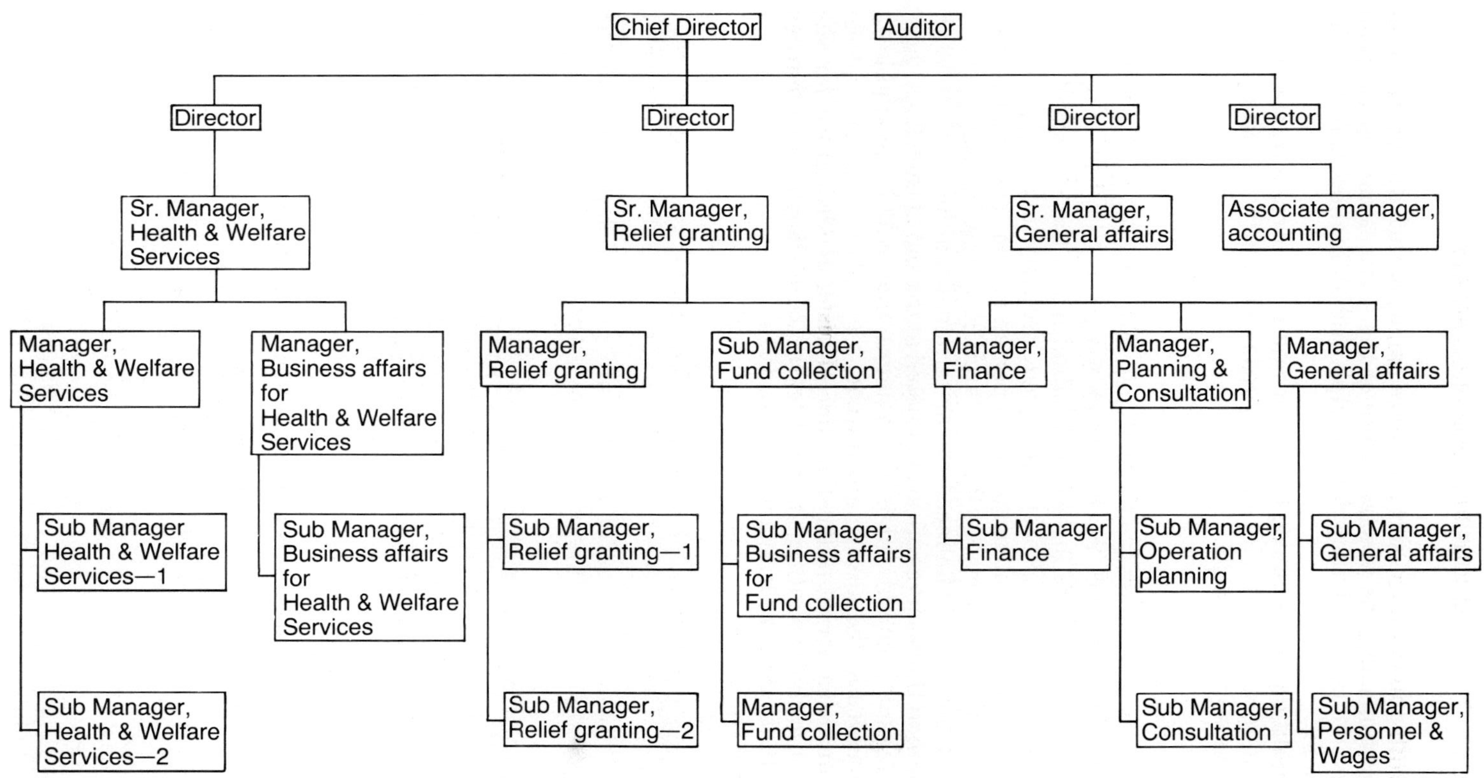


**Figure 1** Organization of the Adverse Drug Reaction Sufferings Relief Fund

Health and Welfare services were incorporated during the Diet deliberations, but the precise nature of the services has not yet been decided. It is hoped that, for example, rehabilitation care will be included.

In addition to the above, the Relief Fund has been entrusted with relevant operations and its monetary resources for the victims of past tragedies such as SMON.

*Finance and accounting*

Finance and accounting of the Relief Fund is supervised by the Minister of Health and Welfare. Each fiscal year, budget, operation, and revenue plans are formed and submitted to the Minister for his approval. At the end of each fiscal year, property inventory, balance sheet and financial statements are reported to him. The fiscal year of the Relief Fund is from April 1 to March 31 of the following year.

The Relief Fund is financed by the terminal-funding method. With this method the reserves are accumulated at the end of each fiscal year. The amount accumulated is the amount that will be available to beneficiaries in the next financial year.

Other rules are stipulated in the *Ministerial Ordinance for the Finance and Accounting of the Adverse Drug Reaction Sufferings Relief Fund* (MHW Ordinance No. 48, 1979).

## Relief benefits

The following seven relief benefits are granted depending on the degree and extent of illness caused by ADRs.

*Medical expenses* are granted towards the cost of medical care for the treatment of illness, resulting from ADRs, that requires hospital admission.

The need for hospitalization is judged from a medical stand point based on the ADRs suffered by the individual. Prior hospitalization in itself does not guarantee that this benefit will be awarded.

Request for this benefit must be made by the sufferer himself who received medical treatment and the application must be made within two years of the date the sufferer paid the hospital's fees.

*Medical allowance*: patients with diseases caused by ADRs that qualify for the Medical Expenses Benefit, receive a Medical Allowance on a monthly basis depending on the number of days of hospitalization and hospital visits as listed in Table 1.

Request of the benefit grant must be made by the sufferer himself who received medical treatment. A sufferer will be disqualified for this benefit if more than two years have passed from the first day of the month following his medical treatment.

**Table 1** Benefit Grant from the Relief Fund (June 1, 1984)

| | *Yen* | *US dollars* | *£* |
|---|---|---|---|
| *Medical allowance (per month)* | | | |
| hospitalization – less than 3 days | 25 600 | 107.78 | 71.05 |
| hospital visit – less than 8 days | | | |
| other cases | 27 600 | 116.20 | 76.60 |
| *Personal pension (per year)* | | | |
| Grade 1 | 2 013 600 | 8477.60 | 5588.37 |
| Grade 2 | 1 611 600 | 6785.11 | 4472.69 |
| *Pension for upbringing of ADR-damaged children* | | | |
| Grade 1 | 630 000 | 2652.41 | 1748.45 |
| Grade 2 | 504 000 | 2121.93 | 1398.76 |
| *Family pension (per year)* | 1 761 600 | 7416.64 | 4888.99 |
| *Lump sum benefit for bereaved families* | 5 284 800 | 22 249.92 | 14 666.96 |
| *Funeral expenses* | 105 000 | 442.07 | 291.41 |

(IMF International Financial Statistics, 1983)

*Personal Damage Pension*: The ADR sufferer whose illness is listed in Table 2 and who is 18 years old or older is eligible to receive this benefit, depending on the severity of illness (for allowances, see Table 1). The amount of this benefit may be changed if there are changes in, for example, the severity of the patient's disability. Requests for this pension should be made by the sufferer himself. No application period is set, and the personal damage pension will be granted from the month after the date of application.

*Pension for raising ADR damaged children*: This pension shall be granted to persons who are responsible for bringing up children below the age of 18 who are suffering from diseases caused by ADRs to the degree shown in Table 2 (for allowances, see Table 1). Eligibility for this benefit is limited to persons who are responsible for the child, and is awarded only after it has been verified that those who claim to be responsible for the child are in fact responsible. The amount of the pension is subject to change if there are changes from the initial designation, as in the case of changes in severity of disability.

Request for this pension should be made by the person who will raise the child. No application period is set, and the pension for raising children is granted from the month after the date of application.

*Bereaved Family Pension*: This benefit will be granted to the dependants of the person who died due to ADRs (for allowances, see Table 1). In order of eligibility, spouses, (including a person substan-

**Table 2**

| Grade | Disease conditions |
|---|---|
| *Grade I* | (1) Total visual power of 0.04 or less in both eyes<br>(2) Loss of hearing of 90 decibels or more in both ears<br>(3) Severe functional disorders in both upper limbs<br>(4) Severe functional disorders in both lower limbs<br>(5) Functional disorders of the body trunk to the degree that sitting or standing is impossible<br>(6) With the exception of the conditions in the previous items, cases where it is confirmed that there are functional disorders or disease conditions which require long periods of rest, which are of the same degree or more severe than those in the previous items and which make normal daily life impossible<br>(7) Psychiatric disorders found to be of the same degree or more serious than those in the previous items<br>(8) Cases of concomitant functional disorders, disease conditions or psychiatric disorders where the conditions are found to be of the same degree or more serious than those in the previous items |
| *Grade II* | (1) Total visual power of 0.08 or less in both eyes<br>(2) Loss of hearing of 80 decibels or more in both ears<br>(3) Severe disorders of the equilibrium function<br>(4) Loss of mastication function<br>(5) Severe disorders of the vocal or speech functions<br>(6) Severe functional disorders in one limb<br>(7) Severe functional disorders in one lower limb<br>(8) Functional disorders of the body trunk to the degree that walking is impossible<br>(9) With the exception of the conditions in the previous items, cases where it is confirmed that there are functional disorders or disease conditions which require long periods of rest, which are of the same degree or more serious than those in the previous items, and also which result in or require severe restriction on daily life<br>(10) Psychiatric disorders found to be of the same degree or more serious than those in the previous items<br>(11) Cases of concomitant functional disorders, disease conditions or psychiatric disorders where the conditions are found to be of the same degree or more serious than those in the previous items |

Note: Visual power will be measured by the International Eye Testing Table and cases of ametropia will be measured by means of corrected visual power

tially in the marital state), children, parents, grandchildren, grandparents, brothers and sisters and then closest blood relations can receive this benefit.

This pension is limited to a 10-year period. If the recipient of the benefit was receiving the Personal Damage Pension before his death, the terms of Family Pension will be for a maximum of 7 years.

If the primary pension recipient dies before the full term, the pension for the remaining term will be provided at his request to his next of kin. Application for this pension must be made within two years if the deceased has been receiving Medical Expenses, Medical Allowance, Personal Damage Pension or Pension for Raising ADR-Damaged Children before his death, and within five years in other cases.

*Lump sum benefit for bereaved families*: This benefit will be granted to families of persons who died due to ADRs, but were not dependent on him for their livelihood. If a family is already eligible for the Family Pension, then this benefit shall not be granted. If, however, the person who was receiving the Family Pension dies and the total sum of the pension has not reached the amount of the Lump Sum Benefit for Families, the balance will be granted as a lump sum. Relations who are eligible for the Lump Sum Benefit for Families are spouses, children, parents, grandparents, brothers and sisters, in that order. The primary recipient should be the closest relative in the above-mentioned order.

The application period for this pension is the same as Family Pension. However, if this lump sum benefit is granted as the difference of the Lump Sum Benefit for Bereaved Families and Family Pension, the application period is two years from the death of the recipient who was receiving the Family Pension.

*Funeral Expenses*: This benefit shall be granted for the funeral services of persons who died due to ADRs (for allowances, see Table 1).

Persons responsible for the payment of funeral services for persons who died due to ADRs are eligible for this benefit regardless of that person's relation to the person who died. The application period of this benefit is the same as the Family Pension.

*Granting of the remainder of benefits*: If a person who is eligible for any of the above benefits has died and there are allowances remaining, those benefits will be granted to his family at their request.

### *Refusal of benefits*

Benefits may be refused in the following cases even if the applications are made in accordance with the categories of diseases, disabilities and death due to ADRs mentioned earlier:

(1) The diseases, disabilities, or death following innoculation according to the *Preventative Vaccination Law* or *Tuberculosis Control Law*.

These exclusions exist because relief pensions provided by government and local government are available for people who have suffered diseases, disabilities, and deaths due to prophylactic innoculations.

(2) In cases where liability for compensation can be proved, for example, in the case of adulterated drugs, then compensation

should be received from the liable person rather than the Relief Fund. Civil liability is determined by the courts. In cases where liability is proven after benefits have been granted, the Relief Fund not only terminates the grant of benefits, but also is entitled to claim the amount the recipients have received in benefits.

(3) Diseases, disabilities, and/or death of the sufferer due to the large doses given to save his life.

This provision is included because there are often no alternatives for medical treatment in these cases even though the ADR effects are predictable, but must be accepted to save the sufferer's life.

*Judgement*

Provisions are made for medical and pharmaceutical judgements as to whether diseases, disabilities and deaths caused by ADRs qualify suffers to benefits from the Relief Fund. In this context, the most important consideration of the Relief Fund operation is how to make fair judgements; and hence judgements are not made by the Relief Fund, but by the Minister of Health and Welfare. The Minister makes his judgement after hearing the advice of the Central Pharmaceutical Affairs Council and notifies the Relief Fund of his decision. For this purpose the Subcommittee for the Judgement of ADRs Relief was incorporated in the Central Pharmaceutical Affairs Council on May 1, 1980.

*Other considerations*

The right of the relief grant shall not be transferred, mortgaged, seized, or be taxed or impose other taxations on the monetary benefits granted by the Relief Fund.

## Subscription charges

The costs of the operation of this Relief Fund are covered by subscription charges from drug manufacturers and importers.

Subscription charges are calculated using two formulae. One is imposed on drug manufacturers who manufacture or import the drug subject to this Relief Fund (*General Subscription Charges*), and the other is the compulsory additional subscription (*Special Subscription Charge*) for manufacturers who manufacture or import the drugs that cause ADRs subject to this Relief Fund.

*General subscription charge*

General subscription charges make up the principal part of this Relief Fund and are received from all drug manufacturers who manufacture and supply drug products.

The charges are calculated by multiplying the appropriate contribution coefficient (see below) by the basic transaction estimate (i.e. the total net sale or shipment value of the product).

The following four categories of drugs are given according to the likelihood of their causing an ADR. This enables a fair charge for drug manufacturers to be calculated.

(1) ***Prescription drug***

| | | |
|---|---|---|
| (a) | Newly developed drug (only for drugs prescribed or administered by physicians at medical institutions) | 2.0 |
| (b) | Injections, suppositories, inhalations, internal drugs and douches | 1.0 |
| (c) | Dosage forms other than (b) | 0.6 |

(2) ***Non-prescription drugs*** 0.1

(Drugs sold to the general public at drug stores)

Subscription charge ratios are arranged in order to acquire a long term balance for finances, because finances of the Relief Fund are not based on 'Pay-as-you-go system' for every fiscal year's budget, but on the 'Funded system' which allows the Relief Fund to accumulate liability reserve money. Financial checks are made at least every five years.

The ratios determined by the Relief Fund are authorized by the Minister of Health and Welfare. At present they do not exceed 2 yen per thousand.

For the fiscal year 1979, the ratio was only 0.02/1000 yen to cover office expenses since the benefits had not yet started. For the fiscal year 1980, 1/1000 yen was allocated and 0.3/1000 yen for the fiscal year 1981, since surpluses had developed because of the few cases of benefit applications during the previous year. The ratio was reduced to 0.1/1000 yen from fiscal year 1982.

*Special subscription charge*

Special subscription charges are the additional funds levied from manufacturers whose products cause ADRs. The intention is to encourage the prevention of further occurrences of ADRs. It is felt that it is unfair to impose the same burden on the manufacturers whose products do not cause ADRs as those companies whose products do.

This means that rough classifications are made according to the probability that ADRs will occur, and the fine-tuning is done on the basis of the past ADRs.

The annual amount of the special subscription charges is 1/4 of the corresponding amount of the nominal value of the allowances granted by the Relief Fund during the previous fiscal year (total estimation of the allowances with future grants, but without interim interests).

However, the amount does not exceed 1/100 of the monetary value of the drugs sold by manufacturers and importers in the previous year, because this Relief Fund is not based on the no-fault liability and because it is not appropriate to impose excessive burdens on the companies who manufacture or import the drugs which cause adverse reactions.

*Method of charges*

Drug manufacturers apply and pay both for general and special subscription charges by July 31 of every fiscal year. Deferred payments can be made in case of *force majeure* such as natural disasters.

The Relief Fund notifies manufacturers of its estimation of the special subscription charges based on calculations of corresonding monetary values from the previous year.

Manufacturers who do not apply and pay the above contributions are subject to coercive procurement under non-payment charges of the national taxation law's payment reminder and collection provisions according to the amount estimated by the Relief Fund.

## Other considerations of the Relief Fund

*State subsidies*

In special circumstances, the government may order the provision of subsidies to ensure the smooth administration of the Relief Fund. So far, however, this provision has not been called on.

At present, the total cost of the relief grant is covered by contributions from the drug manufacturers and importers. Government subsidies have, however, been allocated for part of the office expenses of the Relief Fund.

*Complaints procedure*

Those who have complaints regarding decisions concerning relief grants and estimations of contributions under the Relief Fund Law may ask the Minister of Health and Welfare to review their case. Those who have complaints on re-demand or non-payment charge of the contribution are able to appeal to the Minister of Health and Welfare under the Administrative Complaint Law.

This right to complain applies specifically to decisions made by the Relief Fund, which is an authorized corporation, and not provided for in the Administrative Complaint Law.

*Supervision by the Minister of Health and Welfare*

The Minister of Health and Welfare is able to authorize the establishment of the Relief Fund, its finance and the subscription charge ratios, as mentioned before, to order the reporting to the Relief Fund or those who are entrusted with collecting the contributions for the Relief Fund and further to make on-the-spot inspections of the offices.

### Relief procedure for ADRs that have already occurred

This Relief Fund is available not only for illnesses caused by ADRs after May 1, 1980, but also, for the time being, for illness caused by specific drugs before April 30, 1980. The following additional procedures may be performed after obtaining the approval of the Minister of Health and Welfare.

(1) Necessary procedures for the relief of illness.
(2) Necessary loans to those who grant relief benefits for drug-induced illness.

In addition the following procedures are being enacted for the SMON victims.

*Procedure (1):Trust proxy operation* of the payment of health care pensions and caring expenses agreed on between SMON sufferers and the drug manufacturers responsible, and,
*Procedure (2):*loans for conciliatory once-only payments agreed on between SMON sufferers and the drug manufacturers responsible.

As for the loan operation of (2), debts from city banks for this Relief Fund have the government guarantee, if the resource is for the joint relief of health disorders with the state. The government in this connection has already guaranteed debts for SMON compensation.

Those who grant benefits by obtaining loans of (2) are allowed to state the amount as assets of their financial statements, but depreciation should be allocated for each settlement within 15 years.

## PRESENT STATE OF THE RELIEF FUND OPERATION

Between the inauguration of the Relief Fund in May 1, 1980, and December 31st 1983, 191 applications were made for relief benefits (Table 3). Of these, the benefits were granted in 105 cases and 16 cases were rejected.

**Table 3** Granting of the Relief Benefits (to December 31, 1983)

| | | Relief Benefits | | | | | |
|---|---|---|---|---|---|---|---|
| | *No. of ADR cases* | *Medical expenses* | *Medical allowance* | *Personal damage pension* | *Family pension* | *Lump Sum benefit for bereaved family* | *Funeral expenses* |
| No. of requests | 191 | 86 | 150 | 27 | 27 | 19 | 44 |
| Granted | 105 | 45 | 86 | 9 | 17 | 10 | 26 |
| Rejected | 16 | 7 | 10 | 6 | 1 | 4 | 5 |

**Table 4** Subscription charges collected (1979–1983)

| *Fiscal year* | *Charge ratio* | *Charges (million yen)* |
|---|---|---|
| 1979 | 0.02/1000 | 92 |
| 1980 | 1/1000 | 3765 |
| 1981 | 0.3/1000 | 1291 |
| 1982 | 0.1/1000 | 484 |
| 1983 | 0.1/1000 | 581 |

The subscription charges collected from drug manufacturers by the Relief Fund for relief benefits and office expenses are shown in Table 4.

# 40
# Product liability in the UK

J. D. SPINK

## INTRODUCTION

Any statement at the present time on product liability as related to drugs can be no more than a snapshot of a slowly but inexorably moving scene. English law has a centuries old in-built capacity to adapt itself to changing social needs, but the mechanisms which bring about change tend to operate slowly. When the revolution in chemotherapy started in earnest in the 1930s and brought with it chemical entities which had both healing powers and a capacity for unforetold injury far greater than the natural substances to which medicine had hitherto been mainly confined, the advance of medical science rapidly outstripped the evolution of the law. Its inadequacy in dealing with the new life-saving but potentially maiming drugs crystallized with the failure of the system to cope with the thalidomide disaster in the 1960s. Although no real changes have yet been made in our civil law to cope with drug injury on a major scale, there have been *de facto* changes in its operation and minor statutory developments designed to rectify the most obvious deficiencies. Settlements have been arrived at under extra-legal pressures which do not stand up to close ethical examination. Thus, companies have felt obliged to meet claims which they might otherwise have been disposed to defend, because of pressure from the media. In the statutory context the *Congenital Disabilities (Civil Liability) Act 1976* did little more than establish, beyond previous possible doubt, that a child had a right of action in regard to injury sustained before it was born; and the *Vaccine Damage Payments Act 1979* provided limited assistance to children suffering serious disablement attributed, on a balance of probabilities, to the administration of a vaccine. Meanwhile, consideration of more radical changes of the law has been in progress over the last 12 years, but so far there has been no change, and there is little in close prospect. The fact that Britain is trying to bring about such fundamental changes in concert with nine other countries of the EEC, at least two of which already have strict liability in mutually inconsistent forms, and most of which follow a legal code of Roman origin with radical differences from ours, certainly does not aid the evolutionary process. Two major factors with which the present British system is unable to cope are, firstly, the possible scale of modern-day product-related disasters which brings in the question of who has the capacity to fund the necessary compensation; and secondly, the scientific complexity of the causative process which makes causation difficult, if not impossible, to prove. Both these factors apply particularly to latent drug injuries and aircraft accidents, in view of the number of persons who can be involved in one incident, and the seriousness of the injuries they can cause.

## THE PRESENT LEGAL POSITION

Under the present law a person who suffers damage or injury through a fault in a manufactured product has remedies, in the form of damages or compensation, in contract and in tort, the former of which is virtually irrelevant and the latter highly relevant to drug injury. In contract there is liability against the supplier of goods under the implied terms of the *Sale of Goods Act 1979*, which require that a product must be of merchantable quality and fit for the purpose for which it is sold, and clearly a product with a known and obvious defect will not be fit. This liability is strict, inasmuch as no amount of protestation that he had exercised every possible care to ensure that the goods were fit for their purpose will protect the supplier. However, one of the prerequisites of contract liability is that there must have been privity of contract between the buyer and the seller of the goods; that is to say that liability does not normally extend beyond the seller nor the availability of the remedy beyond the buyer. Thus, liability cannot be referred directly back to the manufacturer to whom the defect was probably attributable, and the remedy will not be available to the person injured if he was not the actual buyer, such as when a wife buys on behalf of her husband and he sustains the injury. The range of impact of contract liability is, therefore, too narrow to be of useful effect in dealing with drug injury as not only is the seller not responsible for an injurious defect in a manufactured product, except if it arises from a fault in his handling or storage of it, but he generally has neither the competence nor the facilities to assess the fitness of it. This is particularly the case with modern high technology products, and even more so with dispensed medicines which, when supplied in original unit packs, cannot even be seen by the supplier. Yet another factor which negates the effect of contract liability in the great majority of cases involving the supply of medicines on prescription is that it was established in the *Pfizer* v *Ministry of Health* patent case in 1963/5 (RPC 1963/173 and 1965/261) that there is no contract between the patient and the dispensing chemist when the product is prescribed and dispensed under the National Health Service. Contract liability can, therefore, be discounted as a remedy for drug injury for all practical purposes. This is probably just as well, as even if it had been established that there was a contract between the NHS patient and the dispensing chemist it is almost unthinkable from the moral viewpoint that the chemist, who only passes the product through his hands, should be held liable for a manufacturing defect which he has no capability to detect, or even less an intrinsic development defect which will have escaped detection by the developer of the product. Moreover, most dispensing chemists are private businesses which would be unlikely to have the means or the insurance cover needed to meet the level of damages awarded in present-day cases of liability for drug injury.

Product liability in tort, which is a much later and more sophisticated development in the history of English law, has two main differences from contract liability, and these are to some extent mutually opposed in their benefit to the injured party. On the one hand liability reaches out well beyond the contracting parties, in fact to the manufacturer of the product, but on the other hand it is weakened by the need for the plaintiff to prove that the manufacturer failed to take due care in the manufacture of the product, in other words that he was negligent, which is unnecessary in contract liability. Tort liability is, therefore, less discriminating but more difficult to prove. These two features derive from the legal concept of the duty of care one owes to one's neighbour. The extent of this duty and the limit of remoteness of one's neighbour to be owed the duty were established by Lord Atkin in the celebrated snail in the bottle case of *Donoghue* v *Stevenson* (1932) A.C.52. He defined 'neighbours' as 'persons who are so closely and directly affected by my act that I ought reasonably to have them in contemplation as being so affected when I am directing my mind to the acts or omissions which are called in question'. He went on to relate this to modern manufacture, thus:

> 'A manufacturer of products, which he sells in such a form as to show that he intends them to reach the ultimate consumer in the form in which they left him with no reasonable possibility of intermediate examination, and with the knowledge that the absence of reasonable care in the preparation or putting up of the products will result in an injury to the consumer's life or property, owes a duty to the consumer to take that reasonable care.'

Under the present law a person injured by a drug must prove the following in order to establish a successful claim against the manufacturer of the product:

(1) That the defendant company was the manufacturer of the product;
(2) That the defendant's product caused the injury;
(3) That the defendant's product was defective, and that the defect was due to the defendant's negligence.

At this point we should distinguish between two types of defect, namely manufacturing defects and development or design defects. The former occurs when a product is not manufactured in accordance with specification or falls short of the required official standard. Thus, for instance, a contaminated injection product or a product containing a wrong dose or a wrong active ingredient would amount to a manufacturing defect. For such obvious faults in manufacture, companies are generally prepared to accept liability as if it were already strict, and will want to settle claims brought against them as expeditiously as possible. Development defects on the other hand occur when a product is manufactured precisely in accordance with its officially approved specification, but the drug contained in it is subsequently found to have some intrinsic feature of its chemical structure which gives rise to serious adverse reactions.

## THE NEED FOR CHANGE

In some cases it will be quite clear that the manufacturer is liable, and this is particularly likely to be so in the case of a manufacturing defect. If there is *prima facie* evidence against him there is a presumption of negligence, and the burden of proof is placed upon him to show that he was not negligent. It is said that 'the thing speaks for itself' (*res ipsa loquitur*), and in most such cases the manufacturer will be advised to settle.

If on the other hand a development defect is involved the position is very different. Here the plaintiff carries the burden of proving identity (of the defendant), causation and negligence, and he is likely to find this a formidable task. Taking the three points in the same order:

(1) Establishing the identity of the manufacturer can itself be difficult, particularly when generic products are prescribed and, as is usually the case, no record is maintained of the manufacturer whose product was dispensed. Also, a pharmacy may dispense a different manufacturer's product on successive prescriptions, and a mobile patient taking prescriptions to different pharmacies may receive a different manufacturer's product on each occasion. This is a good reason for prescribing branded rather than generic products, also bearing in mind that there may be a long delay between treatment and detection of the injury over which memories would be assisted by a distinctive name and product dose-form, such as the colour and shape of a tablet.

(2) Establishing that the defendant's product caused the injury can put the plaintiff in real difficulty, as therapeutic activity in any drug is dependent upon an interaction between the drug and the patient, and in many cases it is not the drug itself but a metabolite of it which causes both the desired and any undesired effects. In many diseases, the patient's metabolism may be abnormal, and it may be further modified by other factors having an effect on the

metabolic chemistry of the drug. Secondary disease, whether detected or undetected, can also play a part in altering the effects of a drug, and some patients, by virtue of some peculiar abnormality in their genetic make-up, will also react differently. All these factors, together with the fact that a drug may produce a highly beneficial reaction in hundreds of thousands of patients and a serious adverse reaction in one individual makes one question whether the defect which caused the reaction is in the patient rather than the drug. Proof of causation against the defendant company's drug to the exclusion of other possible causes, in the absence of numerous cases following a common pattern in a catastrophe situation, can indeed be difficult.

(3) Proving negligence against the manufacturer is probably the most difficult hurdle of all. In the present situation, with the vast amount of testing over a period of several years in both animals and human volunteers needed to meet the licensing requirements of the Medicines Act, it becomes extremely unlikely that negligence could exist, let alone be proven, when it relates to a development defect.

In addition to these basic needs for a successful claim the injured plaintiff has to contend with other difficulties. He is faced with the need to initiate adversary proceedings in an unequal legal contest against a more powerful and financially interested party, bearing in mind that development defects tend to arise more in the early stages of marketing of the products of research-based companies which are usually the largest in the industry. The company will also be more knowledgeable in the highly scientific subject matter of the action than the plaintiff's representatives. Indeed, with a really novel drug the defendant company could be almost the only possessor of the advanced scientific knowledge needed to bring the plaintiff's action to a successful conclusion.

Finally, there is the enormous cost of a product liability action to be faced. The effect of this is to limit the availablity of justice to the very wealthy, who can afford the risk of an unsuccessful action out of their own pocket, and the less well-off who will be entitled to legal aid. This leaves a large gap of middle income earners who are effectively denied justice under the present system.

## THE PEARSON COMMISSION

It was against this background of inadequacy of the present law, and a rising public clamour for change stemming from the delays in providing support for the victims of the thalidomide disaster and injuries attributed to vaccination, that the Royal Commission on Civil Liability and Compensation for Personal Injury was appointed in March 1973 under the chairmanship of Lord Pearson. The Commission took written evidence from 766 organizations and individuals, oral evidence from 113 in the United Kingdom, and presented its Report to Parliament in 1978. Liability for drug injury was but a small section of the wide-ranging subject matter they had considered, and within the drug injury category they had been heavily pre-occupied with antenatal injury. Nonetheless, the Commission made some far reaching proposals, which can be broadly summed up as strict liability in tort for death or personal injury arising from the use of any manufactured product, including drugs.

They had, however, considered other alternatives. They rejected various forms of no-fault scheme, whereby injured parties would be compensated from a central fund regardless of whether the injury arose from fault or not, or whose fault it arose from, largely on the grounds of cost and the fact that for other reasons they did not recommend compulsory insurance. They also considered amending the law of contract to enable consumers to sue manufacturers and to enable parties other than the purchaser to bring an action against either the seller or the manufacturer, but they abandoned this in the light of unfavourable experience of such a system, known as 'enterprise liability', in the United States. Probably one of the most interesting alternatives they considered was a reversal of the burden of proof in an otherwise unchanged action for product liability in tort. This could appear at first sight to overcome the present problem created by the superior strength and knowledge of the defendant manufacturer in the subject matter of the case. In effect, however, there would be little difference in the plaintiff's favour, as he would still be obliged to overturn a strong defence put up by the defendant manufacturer which, in ultimate effect, would amount to a 're-reversal' of the burden of proof.

The Commission, therefore, settled on the recommendation of strict liability of manufacturers, that is to say liability without the need for the plaintiff to prove negligence against the manufacturer. The effect would be to create a hybrid between the strict liability of contract law with the farther reaching impact of tort extending not only to the manufacturer of the defective product but also to the manufacturers of its components. Culpability would no longer be an issue, and manufacturers would no longer be able to protect themselves completely by taking care since negligence would be eliminated from the issues to be considered in the case. Although the proposal is highly controversial and has been firmly opposed by manufacturing industry on which the burden of it almost entirely falls, the Pearson Commission were supported in it by the English and Scottish Law Commissions, who both reported before Pearson, the Council of Europe in its Strasbourg Convention and the European Economic Community in its draft Directives. While there are differences in detail and degree between the proposals of these five bodies, with the Strasbourg Convention being probably the most moderate, strict liability of manufacturers is common to them all. The unanimity of view between so many important law reforming bodies is not difficult to understand as the basic merit of strict liability is that it spreads the burden of compensation for product related injuries over all the people purchasing the products by forcing manufacturers to insure themselves against the liability and pass on the cost of the premiums in their prices. Whilst the increased cost of insurance for strict liability will be high with pharmaceuticals compared with the present cost of cover on less hazardous goods, the necessary increase in the prices of medicinal products would be relatively small. Against this, however, is the overriding question whether the level of cover needed by a company in a high-risk industry, such as pharmaceuticals, can be provided by the insurance market. Since we have to contend with latent defect, whereby a volume of virtually unlimited damage can be built up before one is even aware that one has a problem, the sums needed to cover catastrophe risk are greater than most insurers are prepared to underwrite; and no insurer is prepared to cover the unlimited liability that is really needed to make strict liability a secure proposition from the point of view of either the manufacturer or the public. It is a matter of fact that there are not more than five or six companies in the British pharmaceutical industry who could have borne the cost of the thalidomide settlement out of their own resources. Any one of the remainder would have been bankrupted which, apart from the elimination of the company, the resultant loss to its shareholders and the employment of all its staff, would have meant that those who suffered the injuries would have gone uncompensated. It is a matter of fortunate chance that the proprietors of the two drugs, thalidomide and practolol, which have given rise to accidents in catastrophic proportions in the United Kingdom, happen to be two of the largest companies in the whole of British industry. This is not to say that many of the highly reputable foreign-owned subsidiaries comprising a large part of the British pharmaceutical industry would have to rely only on their UK asset resources, but there is no legally enforceable requirement for a foreign parent company to finance the liabilities of a locally incorporated subsidiary.

Strict liability is, therefore, very much a two-edged sword, with the easing of the burden of establishing a successful claim counteracted by the difficulty in covering the level of compensation needed to meet multiple claims in a catastrophe situation. This difficulty could be overcome, but only by Government covering the top layer of risk above that which is reasonably insurable by the industry. Government catastrophe cover was one of the essential features of the scheme proposed by the Association of the British Pharmaceutical Industry to the Pearson Commission.

## PROPOSED ELEMENTS OF STRICT LIABILITY

Of the several bodies which have made proposals for reform based on strict liability the two most important we have to consider in the United Kingdom are the Pearson Commission and the EEC Commission, whose proposed Directive is now in its second full draft, though additional modifications are being considered. Common to both sets of proposals is the removal of the need to prove negligence against the manufacturer to establish a successful claim, which is the essence of strict liability. Beyond this there are both differences and agreement on the other elements of strict liability, and the most important of these are in the defences available to the manufacturer as these determine the measure of the strictness of liability.

## Defences available to the producer

Both sets of proposals allow the defence that the product causing the injury *was not defective when it was put into circulation.* This does not provide a defence for latent or unforeseen defect as this will have been present when the product was launched albeit that the manufacturer was unaware of it.

The defence of *prior notice* whereby the manufacturer escapes liability by giving due warning of the hazards of the product is implicit in the Pearson proposals by their adoption of Article 2 of the Strasbourg Convention as their definition of defect. This includes the proviso that a defective product 'does not provide the safety which a person is entitled to expect, *having regard to all the circumstances, including the presentation of the product*'. Thus, a warning printed on a label or package or on a leaflet provided with it would be a feature of its presentation and could be expected to protect the manufacturer. This defence was not included in the original EEC proposals, as the definition of defect in the draft Directive did not contain the proviso as to the circumstances of presentation. It has, however, been included in the second draft.

The Pearson Commission allows *contributory negligence* on the part of the user of the product as a partial or complete defence for the producer. While the first draft of the EEC Directive did not allow this defence the second draft does. It also allows *misuse of the product* for purposes other than those for which it is apparently intended, as a defence, but with an enigmatic qualification in an explanatory note that the word 'apparently' means that the use is determined by public opinion and not by the producer.

## Defences denied to the producer

The most controversial of the present defences which it is proposed by both Commissions to exclude is the one known as 'the state of the art'. This is the defence which allows a manufacturer to escape liability if the state of scientific knowledge at the time that the product was marketed was insufficiently advanced for the manufacturer to have been able to detect the defect. This exclusion makes the industry fully liable for development defects, including latent defects, whatever level of testing may have been carried out to avoid them. It is, therefore, seen as a serious inhibitor of innovation and a threat to research-based industry, to the extent that the British Government supports the industry's opposition to the exclusion of this defence. The exclusion was also voted against by the European Parliament, but the European Commission overturned the Parliament's decision. One does not need to look far for the reason why they did so as 'the state of the art' defence knocks the centre right out of strict liability. It would almost certainly be the defence of first choice in most cases of liability for development defects causing drug injury, and would probably have protected the producers of thalidomide and practolol if the cases had been brought to trial. Since thalidomide was one of the main reasons for setting up the Pearson Commission it is not difficult to see why all the reforming bodies were prepared to sacrifice the obvious equity of this defence.

The Pearson Commission also excluded the defence of *official certification* which, if allowed in respect of pharmaceuticals, could enable a manufacturer to escape liability by showing that his product's safety had been approved by an official body such as the Committee on the Safety of Medicines. The effect of allowing the defence would be virtually to remove liability from all lawfully marketed medicinal products, since the possession of a Product Licence issued on the advice of the CSM is a prerequisite for marketing. It is also worthy of note that the industry never sought this defence in its submission to the Pearson Commission, since it does not regard CSM approval as diminishing the company's own responsibility for its products. The EEC draft Directive is silent on official certification, but as it could possibly be used as a valid defence under present English law, it would probably be barred by statute in line with the Pearson Commission's recommendation.

*Contracting out of liability* for death or personal injury is already prohibited under the *Unfair Contract Terms Act 1977*, and the Pearson Commission endorsed the extension of the prohibition under a regime of strict liability. The EEC draft Directive also excludes contracting out, except in the one circumstance that a producer, who contemplates manufacturing a product to the specification of another party, warns that party that the specification is unsound. In this circumstance the producer is entitled to seek indemnity from the party for whom he is manufacturing the product.

The *withdrawal of a product* from the market or any attempts made by the manufacturer to effect a cessation of use will not serve as a defence under the Pearson proposals. This decision is a hard one for the industry to bear, as it is well known that doctors continued to prescribe practolol long after the manufacturers had withdrawn it, and after having received letters warning them of the drug's new-found hazards from both the manufacturers and the Department of Health. It therefore seems wrong that manufacturers should suffer from the perversity of others over whom they have no control. Again the EEC draft Directive is silent on this point, which means that although withdrawal would not be a positive statutory defence it might be pleaded by the manufactuer as part of his general defence, thus leaving the Court to decide how much attention to give to it.

## The bearers of strict liability

The EEC draft Directive makes strict liability fall primarily on the company which markets the product (described as 'putting the product into circulation'), but the Pearson Commission places it squarely on the producer. In most cases these will be one and the same company, but in many they will not. The Pearson proposals expressly exclude distributors from liability but, in the event of a claim being contemplated in relation to a product the distributor has sold, would require them to disclose their suppliers on pain of attracting liability to themselves if they do not. This requirement would apply to each link in a chain of suppliers so that liability would eventually reach the producer. The Strasbourg Convention made provision for relieving distributors of this requirement where they might be unable to identify a particular supplier, as possibly in the case of a product of mixed origin, but the Pearson Commission did not endorse this concession.

Both the EEC and Pearson Commissions make the producer of components (ingredients in the case of finished pharmaceutical products) liable in the event that the defect in the finished product is attributable to a defective component just as if he were the producer of the finished product. Exceptions are proposed where the design of the finished product makes the component unsuitable for incorporation in it or where the component is made to a faulty specification provided by the producer of the finished product.

In the case of so-called 'own brand' product, which are manufactured by one company and sold in the name of another to the exclusion of the name of the manufacturer, the Pearson proposals make both the manufacturer and the 'brander' equally liable. By making the person who put the products into circulation the target of liability, it would appear that the EEC proposals make the 'brander' solely liable; certainly so if the 'brander' represents himself as the producer by his presentation of the product.

The Pearson proposals make importers liable as if they were producers. This is clearly an expedient as most importers have no control over the quality of the products they import. It is, however, entirely reasonable since the foreign producer escapes liability by being outside the jurisdiction of British Courts, and it is open to importers to make their own arrangements for indemnification by their foreign suppliers. The EEC draft Directive makes similar proposals, but does not treat goods passing from one EEC state to another as imports; thus, liability will stretch across national borders within the Market.

As noted above under 'Defences Denied' contract manufacturers do not escape liability except when they warn the other contracting party that the specification is unsound and obtain an indemnity from him.

## LIMITATION OF LIABILITY

Both the Pearson Commission and the EEC Commission were agreed that there must be some cut-off point beyond which manufacturers would no longer be liable, both in time and quantum. The question of limitation was probably one of the most difficult problems they faced in relating it to strict liability, and in not making any attempt to distinguish between different types of goods there is an element of despair in some of the blunderbuss proposals they both made. This is even more evident with products other than pharmaceuticals, as for instance with hand tools there is no provision for the present freedom of choice to buy a cheaper product of lower quality and durability for light and infrequent use. Similarly, there is no discrimination in limits of liability in time between products such as fish paste, a ladder, or a piece of furniture which could be expected to remain safe for 100 years or more.

### Time limits

Both Commissions and the Strasbourg Convention propose that the manufacturer's liability should expire at 10 years from the date that the product was put into circulation, and both Pearson and Strasbourg make it clear that the limit relates to the particular article (e.g. a particular bottle of tablets) rather than the date on which the product was first marketed as a new line of merchandise. In the case of pharmaceuticals the limit is irrelevant, as most products are now expiry-dated up to a maximum life of 5 years (mandatory if it is 3 years or less) and there must surely be a presumption that anyone using a product after its openly indicated expiry date has passed does so at his own risk; in any event the fact that the product was not defective when it was put into circulation would also serve as a good defence. In the case of the draft EEC Directive it is not so clear that the limitation does not relate to the date that the product was first released on the market as a new line of merchandise. If this is intended, 10 years seems excessive, as even latent defects have generally manifested themselves within 5 years of first marketing the product. On the other hand, even a 10 year period would not be sufficient to cover long delayed adverse reactions, such as in the case of diethylstilboestrol, where a girl on reaching puberty can develop vaginal cancer which has been attributed to her mother having taken the drug during pregnancy.

Both Commissions and the Strasbourg Convention were agreed that the maximum lapse of time in which a claimant could start proceedings against a manufacturer should be 3 years from the date that the claimant became aware, or should reasonably have become aware, of the damage, the defect and the identity of the defendant, not the date when the damage occurred. This is also in accordance with the present English law.

## Financial limits

In attempting to find, in strict liability, a solution which would provide support for the largest number of people injured by manufactured products, all the reforming bodies ran into the problem of where the funds would be found to compensate all those injured in a catastrophe resulting in a total of damage beyond the limits of insurability. This was also one of the reasons why compulsory product liability insurance was not proposed, as insurers cannot provide cover for the unlimited liability that would be needed to cater for a catastrophe. Against this insuperable problem it is perhaps not surprising that the three reforming bodies came up with three different proposals. The Pearson Commission, although recognizing that the absence of a limit would mean that compensation beyond insured limits would be dependent on the financial strength of the manufacturer and that bankruptcy could result in no compensation being paid to those injured, proposed that there should be no limit of the manufacturer's liability. The EEC draft Directive proposes a limit of 25 million units of account, equivalent to about £15 million, for all injuries arising from a single cause throughout the Common Market. The Strasbourg Convention leaves the matter optional for the decision of national governments.

Whilst the EEC proposal is more pragmatic and constructive than that of the Pearson Commission it does give rise to questions which have yet to be answered in relation to catastrophe where the sum involved exceeds the limit. Is the limit to operate on the first-come-first-served principle, so that any claims decided after the limit has been reached go uncompensated? If it is, we would very soon be back into the situation of 'trial by newspaper' in which manufacturers are forced by emotively stimulated public opinion to pay in excess of the limit. Alternatively, if the sum is to be evenly distributed over all those injured in proportion to the extent of their injuries this would mean waiting until all claims had been heard before any could be compensated. In the case of latent or delayed injury this would be even more intolerable. Aggregate claims in excess of the £15 million limit are surely a case in which governments must step in with their support to ensure that justice is done to all alike and within a reasonable time.

## Non-pecuniary losses

The EEC draft Directive eschews the award of damages for non-pecuniary losses such as pain and suffering in a strict liability situation. The Pearson Commission, whilst making provision to prevent minor claims, does not propose to exclude claims of substance; and the Strasbourg Convention leaves the matter open to national governments to decide.

## THE PHARMACEUTICAL INDUSTRY'S VIEW

While prepared to accept strict liability for manufacturing defects the pharmaceutical industry is firmly resistant to it for development or design defects, though its attitude is somewhat mitigated by HM Government's support for the preservation of the 'state of the art' defence. The industry's resistance is partly due to the natural concern of companies for their own survival, and the welfare of those injured in a catastrophe causing damage beyond the company's means or insurance cover to provide, but also because of the inhibiting effect that strict liability would have on innovation.

Medical research is organized to detect development defects, firstly by extensive experiments on animals and subsequently by clinical trials in man – and, of course, it usually does detect them. But sometimes a defect will escape detection by animal experiments because man is the only species susceptible to the particular adverse reaction, or it may occur so rarely that it does not manifest itself in the clinical trials. With most modern new drugs the clinical trials will involve several thousand patients, but if the incidence of an adverse reaction is one in tens of thousands, it is unlikely to be revealed until after the drug has been launched on the market and its use expands into hundreds of thousands of cases. Even then it may be a considerable time before an adverse reaction is recognized as such. There is nothing which shows up a drug injury for what it is, and nothing which points directly to any particular cause. They are usually no different from adverse effects, which could result from any one of a large number of causes. It is only when an increase in the incidence of a particular effect in patients who have received the same medicine, is noticed by an unusually observant physician, that a cause and effect relationship is even suspected. This may take several years, as it did in the case of thalidomide. This particular instance is noteworthy, as the deformity of phocomelia caused by thalidomide is rare in comparison with other congenital deformities such as cleft-palate and hare-lip. If it had caused one of these more common deformities, it is possible that the hazard would have remained undetected for much longer than it did. It is thus that a company can, without warning, build up a pile of damage amounting to many millions of pounds.

The pharmaceutical industry, in keeping with other high technology industries producing high-risk products, regards strict liability for development defects with very real concern as a threat to future advances in drug therapy. It would only need one small or medium-sized research-based public company to be bankrupted through strict liability arising from a multiple-case adverse reaction for public investment in the whole industry to be seriously affected. However, it would not even need a disaster like this for the threat of strict liability to result in a severe and progressive braking effect on the industry's capacity to invent and develop new products. This would begin with companies finding it more difficult to cover the costs of increased testing needed to maintain innovation at its present level.

Research and development in the pharmaceutical industry is a higher risk investment than in most other industries, and statistics show that the profit returned from it is at about half the level of the average return on industrial research generally. Not only does the industry face the risk of not finding new products which every research-based company faces in any industry, but it also faces the risk arising from adverse reactions. In purely financial terms, this itself is a twofold risk, firstly from the liability to compensate for the injuries caused; and secondly, from the fact that, at a stroke, the company has lost an important profit-earning product, which could otherwise have been expected to make a substantial contribution to future research and development costs for several years to come.

It is the research-based companies which would be hit hardest by the advent of unlimited strict liability, as latent development defects tend to occur more in new drugs. One of the most important factors tending to slow down innovation will almost certainly be a further escalation in the mandatory testing of new drugs, in both animals and man, demanded by regulatory authorities. Because of the extent to which Government participates in the control of safety and the fact that they have to approve new products before they can be marketed, regulatory authorities become very embarrassed when unpredicted adverse reactions occur in substantial numbers. Therefore, as the number of claims would undoubtedly rise under a situation of strict liability, Government will want to show that they are doing something about it, and they will quickly turn to a further increase in safety-testing standards to demonstrate their concern. There is a natural tendency with Government authorities throughout the world, to believe, or perhaps to be persuaded, that the degree of safety achieved is in proportion to the volume of animal experiments and clinical trials carried out. In point of fact, additional safety is achieved only on a rapidly diminishing return. The adverse effects of this on research and development investment will come, first, from the non-productive depletion of research and development funds, but secondly, and even more important, the additional time it will take. The average time taken to develop a new product from the time that the compound is invented to the time that it reaches the market and begins to show a return, is now about 10 years, which is exactly half of the life of a patent, and is still increasing. This will mean that the time during which the product enjoys monopoly protection will be further curtailed, and the capacity to earn the level of profits needed to finance the company's future research will be correspondingly reduced. There is clearly a critical point at which the extension of development time makes it no longer possible for pharmaceutical research to be self-financing.

Another effect of the extension of development time will be that new products will arrive on the market and become available to the patients needing them, considerably later than is now the case. This is exactly what has happened in the United States, where strict liability has existed for many years. In the case of the anti-asthmatic drug 'Intal' there was a 6-year delay between its release in the UK and the USA. This so called 'drug lag' has produced controversial discussion on the opposing merits of releasing a drug on the market as completely safe as it could possibly be, against the lost benefits to sick patients who could have had the drug several years earlier and accepted a marginally greater risk. When the drug is intended for the treatment of mortal disease, and patients actually die waiting for the release of a drug already available in other countries, the controversy surrounding 'drug lag' is indeed acute.

There is a peculiar irony in the inhibition of development which unlimited strict liability will bring, inasmuch as the industry is at present not only striving to find more effective drugs, but also safer drugs. There have been several instances in which a new product has been well received by the market and has rapidly outstripped its competitors, not because it is any more effective, but because it is safer. Under strict liability in a situation in which a company has had a successful product for the treatment of a certain disease on the market for several years, and then discovers another product for the same disease which is equally effective, but apparently safer, it will be very wary of marketing it, in the knowledge that it could later exhibit a latent hazard. Most companies, if they cannot get some kind of protection against the catastrophe risk involved in such a hazard would probably prefer to go on living with a profitable product which, although less safe, has shown up all its hazards, of which the company has given notice in its literature and thereby protected itself against strict liability.

Another likely effect of strict liability without Government support is that in the early years of a new product's life, when unpredictable adverse reactions are most likely to appear, the product will be first marketed in countries outside the United Kingdom, where the arrangements for dealing with product liability are less adversely disposed against the innovating manufacturer. There would also be effects on the practice of medicine generally, insofar as it involves the use of drug therapy. With the defences that it is proposed to deny to producers, the manufacturer will be forced to rely more heavily on the defence of prior notification of all possible hazards, and as it is the doctor who selects the medicine it will be his responsibility to pass on information provided to him by the manufacturer. Not only will this be an additional burden on the already overworked general practitioner, but it will encourage the development of a form of defensive medicine in which, for fear of not giving notice of all the possible hazards of their medicine to all his patients, the doctor will be encouraged to prescribe safer, but less effective medicines, to the detriment of both the patient and the innovating manufacturer's sales and profits, and thus his potential for innovation.

One could have gone some way towards accepting the adverse effects that unlimited strict liability would have on research and on the practice of medicine generally if one could have seen compensating advantages in it. But it is the industry's firm view that it would not achieve its intended object of ensuring that persons injured by drugs are provided with the support they need to sustain them, possibly for the rest of their lives. Elimination of the need to prove negligence against the manufacturer overcomes only one of the problems now facing the injured party. He will still have to prove a cause and effect relationship between the drug and the injury, which can present real difficulties.

## THE SPECIAL CASE OF CLINICAL TRIAL PRODUCTS

For some years the pharmaceutical industry has been under growing pressure from hospital ethical committees to accept strict liability voluntarily for injuries suffered by patients involved in clinical trials when the injury is attributable to a drug under trial before being placed on the market. There is also an increasing willingness of companies to accept a degree of liability well in excess of their legal liability under the present law, first because they have a vested interest in having the trials carried out; and, secondly, because the unlimited liability, which is the main reason for the industry's resistance against strict liability for marketed products, does not apply in a clinical trial situation.

Under the present law the position of the company, in the absence of some specially agreed indemnity, is exactly the same as if the injury was caused by a marked product, that is to say, liability for negligence in tort; again, contract liability is irrelevant as it is very rare for a pre-marketing clinical trial product to be the subject of a sale. Negligence on the part of the company would have to be proved in circumstances in which this would be virtually impossible. In the event of the injury being caused by a development defect the 'state of the art' defence would in most cases protect the company, bearing in mind that clinical trials are usually carried out on the borderline of new scientific knowledge. This situation is accepted by all, including the industry, as wholly unsatisfactory from the patient's point of view.

There are a number of reasons why the industry can look upon a clinical trial product differently from a marketed product in regard to the level of liability it should reasonably accept, without prejudice to its resistance against strict liability for marketed products:

(1) The number of patients involved is not only very much smaller, but is also known in advance which enables the risk faced by the manufacturer to be both limited and quantified.
(2) There is a consciousness that one is operating in the area of the unknown at the borderline of new scientific knowledge. The clinical trialist, therefore, proceeds with extreme caution, starting with fractional dosage and only raising this as safety is assured.
(3) There is a close monitoring of patients in a hospital trial, where trained nursing and medical staff are in a position to observe the slightest untoward effect which could well pass unnoticed in a general practice situation with a marketed product.
(4) In the event that any sign of a reaction occurs, remedial measures in the form of staff, equipment and antidotal drugs are immediately available.
(5) With the trial drug being administered by nurses, there will be a much higher level of patient conformity to the protocol dosage than could be expected with a marketed product in general practice.
(6) As clinical trials are carried out under the direction of consultants, there will be a better selection of patients appropriate to the intended treatment, and patients at special risk can be selected out.

The overall effect of these factors is that the aggregate sum of maximum liability will not only be but a small fraction of what it could be with a marketed product, but it will be determinable in advance. Moreover the level of risk to any individual patient is generally lower in a clinical trial than it is with a newly marketed product used in general practice. This also means that the risk may be insurable. It certainly should be insurable, but unfortunately it is often difficult to persuade lay insurers how safe a clinical trial really is.

If the industry could agree to accepting something more favourable in the patients' interest than the present negligence liability, then a number of factors would need to be taken into account in assessing a just and proper level of compensation in each case:

(1) In the case of a disease without a satisfactory treatment and where the clinical trial drug shows promise of being the first useful remedy, it may well be the best, or in some cases, the only option that the patient has.
(2) In the case of a patient suffering mortal disease, the effect of a serious adverse reaction could be no more than to further shorten an already much shortened life expectancy.
(3) The disease itself may in many cases give rise to injuries which must be measured against any caused by the drug.
(4) There may be an interaction between concomitant treatments, or an adverse reaction may arise which could be attributable to either of two or more drugs.
(5) When there is associated secondary disease, it may be impossible

to determine whether an injury is associated with the trial drug or the secondary disease, or a combination of both.

(6) It is difficult to see how it is reasonable that liability could attach to a manufacturer when the drug is given to a patient who reacts to it idiosyncratically or there is some other hypersensitivity perhaps associated with a genetic factor.

(7) Probably one of the most important factors determining the level of compensation must be the relative prospective efficacy of the trial drug and that of existing treatments. In cases where the advantage of the trial drug is speculative or marginal, the patient is undertaking a relatively greater risk in volunteering for the trial and, in the event of an accident, should be compensated more generously.

(8) There is also an important difference in the level of the company's responsibility to patients involved in trials on drugs intended for treatment of serious or mortal disease on the one hand and relatively trivial complaints on the other. For instance, the level of acceptable risk will be much higher with a drug for the treatment of cancer than if one is conducting a comparative trial on drugs for the treatment of cough. Thus, whereas in the former case the justification for compensation is relatively minor, if in fact it is justified at all, compensation in the latter case would need to be much more generous. In drawing comparisons of this kind, it is entirely reasonable to take into account the prospective benefit that the patient can derive from the trial. Generally, drugs under clinical investigation start with a good prospect of being an advance on existing therapies, so in many cases the patient can look forward to receiving a more effective treatment than any other available. This point is often overlooked by those demanding unqualified strict liability for manufacturers of clinical trial products.

(9) In a number of disease states, particularly in most of the neoplastic diseases, it is necessary to use the drug, whether it is on trial or an established drug, at the maximum tolerated dosage. In these cases it is well understood in advance that the drug will almost certainly cause side-effects and that the risk of serious adverse reaction is much greater. Provided that this is explained to the patient at the time of seeking his consent for the trial this recognition of risk must be taken into account.

(10) It must also be taken into account, that most anti-cancer drugs have a predisposition to cause damage to other organs than the one treated.

(11) The problems covered in the last four points are particularly relevant in the case of a drug for the treatment of serious disease where there is a high prospect of success but this is associated with a high and already known level of risk of serious adverse reaction. Assuming, for example, one has a drug under investigation for the treatment of a neoplastic disease with a virtual 100% mortality, and in previous trials it has shown a 75% success rate

but 20% of all cases receiving the drug have been struck blind; this means that 15% of the patients involved in the trials will come out of it cured but blind. Although this presents a cruel choice, the risk/benefit ratio is one which it could be expected most such patients would accept. In such a case, it would be unthinkable that the company whose drug is on trial should be asked to bear strict liability. This hypothetical case is perhaps extreme, but the principle is highly relevant in varying degrees to many cases.

(12) One of the most difficult problems to evaluate in this assessment is whether it is reasonable to compensate injuries arising only from hitherto unknown hazards or whether those which are known in advance, particularly if they are extremely rare, should also be covered. The Swedish compensation scheme compensates for known adverse reactions, and women suffering thrombotic episodes while taking oral contraceptives have already been compensated. It is morally difficult to justify a distinction to the extent that one patient is compensated simply because the hazard which caused his injury was unknown at the time he took the drug whereas another patient goes uncompensated simply because the risk, albeit a very rare one, was known in advance. The patient facing a known hazard needs more courage to volunteer for the trial and would seem to be even more deserving of compensation. One also has to bear in mind that both patients equally need the support that compensation would provide to sustain them, possibly for the rest of their lives.

If it could be agreed that compensation, calculated in gross by the established rules for assessing damages for personal injury, should be abated by any of the foregoing factors which were relevant to the case, there would also need to be agreement on the procedure for deciding in which cases the manufacturer should be liable. Under the present law, even if one eliminates the need to prove negligence it will still be necessary for the plaintiff patient to prove causation. The kind of indemnity which most manufacturers are already prepared to give effectively relieves the hospital authority and the physician in charge of the trial of liability which is taken instead on to the shoulders of the manufacturer. This still leaves the plaintiff needing to prove his case against a more powerful opponent, so the aim should be to find a non-adversarial solution. The industry has considered the possibility of agreeing with the medical authorities some kind of standard form of indemnity which is more directly to the benefit of the patient and accepts a degree of liability well in excess of the present legal liability. However, it is difficult to devise any such indemnity which justly covers the wide variety of circumstances which can prevail in all or even a majority of clinical trials.

Generally in such circumstances, solutions are to be found in a fairly loose framework of principles which can be applied to most, if not all, the relevant cases, rather than a rigid set of rules of which one or several will be found unacceptable and can become sources of disagreement or even legal dispute. It has, therefore, been suggested that a non-legal and voluntary Convention of Principles, or Guidelines, could form the basis of indemnities which could in turn be adapted to the particular circumstances of any given clinical trial. Within such a Convention it could be agreed, for instance, on the form that a patient's consent to participate in a trial should take and that signing it would in no way prejudice his rights under the Convention. This would in effect nullify any possible defence that he had voluntarily assumed any risk involved (*volenti non fit injuria*), subject to the exceptions and causes for abatement of compensation previously referred to, as listed (1)–(12) above. Manufacturers would also need to agree not to rely on the 'state of the art' defence, and that causation would be established either on the balance of probabilities, as in cases covered by the *Vaccine Damage Payments Act*, or by a presumption that the drug was defective if there was no good reason to attribute the injury to another cause. Manufacturers should also be prepared to accept unlimited liability, since the potential for liability is already limited by the number of patients involved and is probably insurable.

In summary, what is suggested here is a qualified form of strict liability for injuries from clinical trial products subject to a graded defence of *volenti*, with damages determined insofar as possible by an agreed set of principles. It is emphasized that these suggestions are related exclusively to clinical trial products, as the very factors which make it possible to treat these products differently from marketed products are precisely those factors which call for Government to bear the risk of catastrophe with a marketed product.

## The ABPI guidlines

Proposals along the lines of the above were first presented by the author at the *Fourth Annual Symposium of the British Institute of Regulatory Affairs* held in June–July, 1982. After discussion by appropriate committees within the Association of the British Pharmaceutical Industry (ABPI) and with leading representatives of the medical and legal professions, 'Guidelines' based in large measure on the proposals were commended by the Board of Management of the ABPI to its membership in the following statement issued on 12th August, 1983, and reproduced here by kind permission of the Association:

## GUIDELINES

*Clinical Trials – Compensation for Medicine-Induced Injury*

It is becoming common practice for ethical committees to expect assurance that patients participating in clinical trials will be appropriately compensated, by a simple procedure, should they be adversely affected by reason of their involvement in the trial. While such adverse effects are very uncommon, the Association of the British Pharmaceutical Industry (ABPI) accepts this as a guiding principle and has noted that quite different considerations apply to medicines undergoing clinical trial compared to medicines generally available on prescription. Consequently, in cases where injury is attributable to a medicine in clinical trial, the ABPI recommends to its member companies that the following guidelines should be accepted without legal commitment on the part of the member companies:

(a) The company should favourably consider the provision of compensation for personal injury, including death, in accordance with these guidelines but without the requirement for negligence to be proved against the company.

(b) Compensation should only be paid when there is a balance of probabilities that the injury (including exacerbation of an existing condition) was attributable to the company's medicine under trial.

(c) Compensation should only be paid for the more serious injury of an enduring and disabling character, and not for temporary pain or discomfort or less serious or curable complaints such as skin rashes.

(d) These guidelines only apply to injuries to patients involved in clinical trials, conventionally known as Phase II or Phase III trials, that is to say, patients under treatment and surveillance (usually in hospital) and suffering from the ailment which the medicine under trial is intended to treat. These guidelines do not apply to injuries arising from studies on healthy volunteers (Phase I), whether or not they are in hospital, for which separate guidelines for compensation already exist. These guidelines also do not apply to injuries arising from clinical trials on marketed products, except when the trial is on a marketed medicinal product being tested for a prospective indication not yet authorised by inclusion in a product licence.

(e) These guidelines apply to an injury whether or not the adverse reaction causing the injury was foreseeable or predictable although compensation may be abated or excluded in the light of the factors mentioned in paragraph (j) below.

(f) Compensation should not be payable (or should be abated, as the case may be) (i) when there has been a significant departure from the agreed protocol, (ii) where the injury was attributable to the wrongful act or default of a third party, including a doctor's failure to deal adequately with an adverse reaction, or (iii) when there has been contributory negligence by a patient.

(g) Compensation should only be payable to patients receiving the medicine under trial and, therefore, not to control patients not receiving the trial medicine nor to patients receiving placebos, nor to patients receiving other non-trial drugs or medicines for the purpose of comparison with the medicine under trial.

(h) The giving of consents to participate in a clinical trial, whether in writing or otherwise, should not exclude a patient from the benefits of compensation or in any way prejudice his position under the guidelines, although compensation may be abated or excluded in the light of the factors mentioned in paragraph (j) below.

(i) No compensation should be paid for the failure of a medicine to have its intended effect or to provide any other benefit to the patient. This includes the failure of any vaccine or other preparation to provide the preventive or prophylactic effect for which it is under trial, and the failure of any contraceptive preparation or device to prevent pregnancy.

(j) The amount of any compensation paid by the company should be appropriate to the nature, severity and persistence of the injury. However such compensation may be abated, or in certain circumstances excluded, in the light of the following factors (on which will depend the kind of risk the patient should be expected to accept):
   (i) the seriousness of the disease being treated, the degree of probability that adverse reactions will occur and any warnings given;
   (ii) the hazards of established treatments relative to those known or suspected of the trial medicine, and
   (iii) the availability and relative efficacy of alternative treatments that the patient could have had if he had not volunteered for the trial.

   *Note:* This guideline assumes that the level of any compensation paid will depend upon the circumstances in the light of the factors mentioned above. As an extreme example, there may be a patient suffering from serious or mortal disease such as cancer who is warned of a certain defined risk of adverse reaction. Participation in the trial is then based on an expectation that the benefit/risk ratio associated with participation is better than that associated with alternative treatment. It is, therefore, reasonable that the patient accepts the high risk and should not expect compensation for the occurrence of the adverse reaction of which he or she was told.

---

## RECENT DEVELOPMENTS

Since the first draft of this chapter was written in 1983 there has been a great deal of discussion between the representatives of the Member States of the EEC on the type and form that the Directive on Product Liability should take. At the time of going to press in the Spring of 1985 no agreement had been reached on a number of the most controversial problems relating to liability for injury caused by defective products on the market. It had not even been decided whether the Directive should require a minimum of legislation to which member states could add their own national requirements, or the more inflexible type which lays down in fairly precise form the requirements to be enacted by the Member States without allowing these to be exceeded or mitigated. Since the original objective of the Directive was to harmonize legislation in order to avoid unfair competition it is clear that the latter more rigid type of Directive is needed, but with such fundamental differences of view on some of the important issues still unresolved it appears that a Directive based on an expedient of minimum requirements will be the only possible outcome. This inevitably raises the question whether there is any real justification for a Directive, as the effect of a minimum Directive could well be to highlight the differences in the ensuing national legislation and result in the exploitation of these differences to the disadvantage of free trade within the EEC, thus doing more harm than good in the context of the original objective.

Whilst all the Member States are agreed that manufacturers should bear strict liability for injuries caused by their defective products, the main stumbling blocks as to the form liability should take are:

(1) *Development Risks* – Whether the manufacturer should be liable for development risks and in this connection, whether the 'state of the art' defence should be allowed. The delegations of four Member States are in favour of manufacturers bearing such liability without recourse to the 'state of the art' defence and six Member States, including the United Kingdom, are against.
(2) *Limitation of Liability* – Three member states, led by Germany, are in favour of limiting the producers' overall liability, and seven member states, including the United Kingdom, are against.
(3) *Property Damage* – Eight member states are in favour of the Directive covering property damage as well as personal injury, whereas the United Kingdom and Italy are against such an inclusion, on the grounds that existing laws on compensation for property damage are adequate and reasonably consistent between Member States.

In an attempt to bridge these wide divergences of view various compromise solutions have been proposed based on a linkage between the principles of the acceptance or exclusion of liability for development risk and the limitation of overall liability. Thus, if liability for development risks were excluded it has been suggested that there need be no limitation of liability, presumably because the catastrophes that have occurred have with one exception arisen from development defects, but if it were included limits of overall liability would be a set at variously suggested levels of 50 or 75 million EEC units of account (currently equivalent to roughly M£30 or M£45). Sweden and Germany are often cited as examples of countries which are successfully operating drug injury compensation schemes in which there is a limitation of liability. However, neither of these countries' schemes has yet been tested by a catastrophe of the order of thalidomide, possibly because their longer than average licensing procedures have delayed marketing until after a development defect has been revealed in another country.

Another suggestion has been that liability for development risks and the limitation of that liability should apply only to the pharmaceutical and chemical industries, where the chance of encountering a substantial disaster is greater, and the risk is augmented by the possibility of latent or deferred injury. This takes account of the enormous sums that can be involved in a drug catastrophe, and the fact that neither the manufacturer nor his insurers can be expected to carry risks above a substantial but reasonably limited level. What is much more important, however, is that it fails to take account of the problem of administering a limitation in a situation of catastrophe in which the total damage exceeds the limitation, possibly by several-fold; that is to say, whether to settle claims on a first-come-first-served basis until the limit has been reached, leaving the rest to go uncompensated, or to wait possibly for years until all the claims have been made and then meet all of them probably inadequately, which is almost equally unacceptable. Most of the discussions on these difficult issues have led up to and then foundered on the question of who pays for catastrophe, and it appears that an increasing volume of authoritative opinion is coming to realize that whilst the industry can be expected to cover itself for business risks up to a considerable maximum, subject to insurability, it is only Government that has the capacity to cover the top layer of liability that can arise from the use of modern medicines. Once this is accepted by the Governments of the EEC Member States it would be reasonable to expect that agreement on the other outstanding issues would follow.

# Section 5: COMMUNICATIONS

# Editor's Introduction and Commentary

The success or failure of all the activities so far described in this book depend on whether or not all the groups of people involved communicate with each other. While planning the final section, the editor drew a flow-chart resembling a wheel. The patient was placed at the centre. Close to the hub of the wheel were his most immediate sources of information, his general practitioner, his TV set and his newspaper. At the rim of the wheel were other bodies such as pharmacists, consumer organizations, pharmacologists, the drug industry, the regulatory authorities and the scientific press. Representatives of each of these bodies were then asked to describe how they believed they interacted with each of the others, how they communicated, directly or indirectly, with a patient at the centre of the wheel, and how these communications might be improved. No attempt was subsequently made to edit out repetitions of central themes because this helped to emphasize the more important ones.

Professor Gavin Kellaway sets the scene by reminding us of the wide spectrum of attitudes adopted by patients, ranging from that of well-informed super-critic to unquestioning stoic. Although a minority of patients may be discouraged by knowledge of the possible side-effects of drugs they are about to swallow, Doctor Kellaway feels that a simple explanation of the nature of their illness, how a drug might help, how to take it and what side-effects might be anticipated, is the key to compliance and effective therapy. How much better than overdramatized warnings in the Press about serious and rare ADRs, if patients could learn from their doctor in unemotional terms how a small incidence of ADRs should be viewed in the light of symptomatic or possibly life-prolonging effects of treatment. However, even assuming that the doctor takes the trouble to explain the risks and benefits, only part of his advice will be understood or remembered.

Since the first edition of this book some progress has been made towards the acceptance of *patient package inserts*. Obviously no single set of instructions is appropriate or even understood by all patients, and the prescribing doctor is still the most important target for information relevant to drug safety and efficacy. Only the doctor is adequately equipped to digest the information and appropriately interpret it for each of his individual patients in the light of their ability to comprehend and comply with his advice.

The thrust of consumer interest has changed over the years. What was originally intended as a means of ensuring that scientific jargon was translated into meaningful instructions has become confused with 'action groups' and anti-drug or anti-doctor propaganda. In many diseases, the risks of non-compliance far outweigh those of rare side-effects. If, for example, we consider the non-steroidal anti-inflammatory drugs, the risks of failing to comply with treatment, in terms of the lethal consequences of immobility, pain and loss of enjoyment in life, far exceed the very small risks that the drugs themselves will have lethal side-effects. Kellaway points to the cards which warn patients about the risks associated with monoamine oxidase inhibitors, corticosteroids and anticoagulants, all of which carry significant risks if the patient fails to avoid certain food or drugs. Such advice is essential in the interests of safety. It is questionable, however, whether it is desirable or appropriate to warn patients of risks such as those of aplastic anaemia, which are so small as to be almost beyond comprehension, but which, if attention is drawn to them, will seriously affect compliance.

In Chapter 42, Professor Michael Drury, speaking for the general practitioner, estimates that the average patient spends about 22 hours during his lifetime in the company of his general practitioner. Most doctors regularly prescribe between 400 and 500 products, and about half of the average of six prescriptions received by each patient annually are issued in the form of 'repeat prescriptions', usually without a consultation between doctor and patient. Many factors may influence the choice of treatment but consultants' letters are seen to be the most important. Although the length of a consultation is short, a great deal is said. Damage to confidence in treatment by fortuitous advice from people outside the surgery is likely to do more harm than ADRs.

Good doctors tend to use a small list of drugs well, but this does not mean that the list should be predetermined for them. What is most important is the ability to prescribe appropriately for the individual patient, and this requires a wide choice of treatment. Drury suggests the communications from regulatory authorities are sometimes the most important and best-informed. This view is difficult to reconcile with the fact that, while no fewer than eight drugs were removed from the market by the Committee on Safety of Medicines between 1982 and 1984, not one paper was published either by the CSM or its secretariat which provided a scientific basis for this action. This is in striking contrast to the regular flow of scientific communications during the 1960s and 1970s. Perhaps Drury's most telling statement is that society must be taught that risk-taking is part of normal living, and that risks must be measured before they are taken. We have seen elsewhere (e.g.

Chapter 15) that drugs have to be used on a large scale before risks can be measured, because risks are so small.

Professor Charles Fletcher (Chapter 44) became very familiar to television viewers in the 'black and white days' through the programme '*Your life in their hands*', and probably made a greater contribution than any other single person to breaking down the prejudice against attempts to popularize and encourage a healthy interest in medicine. Members of the medical profession are no longer shunned by their colleagues if they appear on television or radio broadcasts. Patients are more knowledgeable about medicines and more wary of their harmful effects. In the 1970s, the tendency was to sensationalize rare complications, e.g. with contraception or vaccination, and halfway through the 80s, there is little sign that this has diminished. Reporters work under the pressure of 'deadlines', and this rubs off on those whom they interview. Sub-editors tend to select the bad news, such as mortality from drugs, and edit out any statement which might suggest that the case against drugs is unproven. Fletcher's chapter gives much useful advice on how to handle press enquiries, and emphasizes the need to use clearly understandable lay phraseology and to avoid medical jargon.

At this point in the commentary it might be appropriate to remind readers of the statement made by Lord Rothschild in his Richard Dimbleby Lecture of 1978 that 'comparisons, far from being odious, are the best antidote to panic'. Risks must be explained to people in simple numerical terms (e.g. 1 in 1000) and referred to as a period of time (per week, per year etc) and then compared with familiar risks such as those associated with travelling or being bitten by a snake (a very significant risk in some countries, but negligible in others).

In Chapter 45, Doctor Oliver Gillie, an experienced journalist, gives us considerable insight into press methods for capturing and processing the 'news'. He uses the word 'story' candidly, and admits that the need to dramatize the facts can lead to prejudice, and that the news value of a story may not be related to the medical importance of the issue under discussion.

Newspapers have successfully campaigned for compensation for thalidomide victims and children damaged by vaccines. In the case of whooping cough vaccine they have uncovered disagreement between experts and differing governmental advice in various countries. In drawing attention to the plight of victims they may well have done some good. In the long run, some public exposure probably does no harm; for example, too many women take unnecessary drugs during pregnancy. On the other hand to create alarm about rare side-effects of important drugs is to shoulder a great burden of responsibility because of the effect it may have on compliance with essential treatment.

It may be helpful to give a hypothetical example of what could happen if some serious, but uncommon, side-effect of a life-prolonging drug were given wide publicity. Let us suppose that the drug was being used to treat a chronic disease which had an anticipated annual mortality of 10%. Let us further suppose that the drug produced a fatal side-effect in one in every 10 000 patients treated. If 100 000 patients were complying with treatment with the drug and if it was effective in 80% of them, instead of the anticipated 10 000 deaths each year there would only be 2000 plus a further 10 deaths from the adverse reaction. If a news article had the effect of reducing compliance by 20%, so that 20 000 patients stopped taking it, the expected mortality among those who continued to comply with treatment may be calculated as 1608. Among the non-compliers, there would be no adverse reaction deaths, but 2000 would have died from the disease after a year. The overall annual mortality would thus be 3608, or 1598 more than would have occurred without the publicity. It could, of course, be argued that the drug might not be unique and that patients could be switched to an equally effective and possibly safer treatment if such a treatment existed. Unfortunately, so little information is available about the true risks and benefits of drugs that nobody is able to report authoritatively on the relative risks and benefits, and in practice publicity almost invariably does harm. The adverse effects of publicity on compliance with the whooping cough vaccination programme has almost certainly been harmful to some children living in high risk communities.

The work of Doctor Andrew Herxheimer, Editor of *Drug and Therapeutics Bulletin*, published by the Consumers Association is concerned with objective comparisons of the risks and benefits of treatment and in the need to communicate this information. It should be clearly distinguished from the activities of 'consumerist' groups who see the pharmaceutical industry and the medical profession as soft targets for their political attacks. The tobacco industry, whose product is three or four orders of magnitude more lethal than drugs, retains its immunity because smoking is still very much a 'class' activity, promoted by many of our most successful young sportsmen.

Herxheimer reviews the various attempts which are being made to encourage patients to ask questions and to understand the medicines they take, and there is much emphasis on written information for patients. The most important message must surely be – 'talk with your doctor', who in turn should have read and comprehended the contents of *Drug and Therapeutics Bulletin*.

The sudden death on the 26th March, 1984 of Franz Gross, removed one of the most effective contributors to drug safety. His chapter from the first edition is published posthumously (Chapter 47). The Editor would like to pay tribute to the memory of a personal friend who did more than most to 'internationalize' work in this field, and who was certainly the best conference chairman he has ever been privileged to work with. Gross suggested four principles for prescribing. First, doctors should be taught to prescribe only where treatment is essential and to avoid polypharmacy. Secondly, they should, where possible, prescribe the least toxic and most effective drug available. Thirdly, they should reserve new treatments for patients who do not respond to well-tried remedies. Fourthly, they should learn the elements of pharmacokinetics in order to understand therapeutic responses and side-effects and the rather small number of drug interactions that are of practical importance. If they followed these simple rules, most 'ADRs', which are the result of overdosage or otherwise inappropriate treatment, would be avoided, as would the need for drug withdrawals and much of the adverse publicity that is so harmful to patients.

Writing about the relationships between the pharmaceutical industry and the drug regulatory authorities, Drs Cromie and Slater (Chapter 48) draw attention to diseases for which new drugs are needed as urgently as ever, and to the continuing need to improve the therapeutic ratio of older remedies. Dramatic advances such as cimetidine and cromoglycate are rare and many of the improvements in therapeutic ratio are marginal, though worthwhile.

The authors question whether the demand for certain types of clinical trials is realistic. Drugs are still tested against placebos rather than active medications, and clinical testing is often restricted to studies by experts conducted in highly selected groups of patients who are less likely to develop adverse effects than the target population. Although the authors do not name it, the benoxaprofen incident could have resulted from a regulatory climate in which drugs aimed at the elderly were prevented from being tested in the elderly. The authors stress the need to replace the ritual of randomized, double-blind, controlled trials with active 'real-life' carefully supervized Phase IV studies.

Compliance can be improved by apparently minor formulation modifications which would be lost completely if generic prescribing or substitution was the rule. The authors also draw attention to the importance of identification of medicines. This can only be ensured by *original-pack dispensing*, where the pack shows the batch number and, of course, the manufacturer, so that a defective batch may be withdrawn. Generic prescribing or substitution leaves the patient unprotected. The authors finish on a hopeful note in recalling the objectives of the *US Drug Regulation Reform Act of 1978*, and they stress that the DRAs must try and live up to a tradition in which they conduct their activities 'unmoved by political considerations or media campaigns', and to continually evaluate regulatory requirements and discard those of unproven value.

Next (Chapter 43) we consider the responsibility of pharmacists who can bridge a number of communication gaps between the patient, the doctor and the pharmaceutical industry. Since a patient may visit any one of several different pharmacies in his area, it is likely that only regular patients will be well known to their local pharmacists. Not content with their existing role, however, many pharmacists are seeking additional responsibilities, not the least of which is to fill the information gap created by doctors. Pharmacists are responsible for the handling and advice about 'over-the-counter' medicines. The influence of pharmacists is likely to increase as more products become freed from the prescription-only lists.

The authors touch on the possibility of inequivalence of generic formulations, but not on the legal consequences of generic prescribing. As we mentioned earlier, pharmacists may become prime targets for litigation when something goes wrong and the manufacturer cannot be traced.

The authors state in unequivocal terms that pharmacists lack the knowledge of clinical medicine necessary to recognize adverse drug reactions. This runs contrary to the idea that pharmacists should take an active part in reporting ADRs to prescribed medicines. If patients complain of side-effects to over-the-counter medicines it must clearly be the duty of the pharmacist to discuss the problem with the patient's doctor since he, rather than the pharmacist, is ultimately responsible for the care of the patient.

In Chapter 49 Doctor Edmund Harris, outlines the structure and workings of the UK Drug Regulatory Authority and its relationship with other divisions of the health departments and outside bodies. He points to the dilemma of communications with the profession. Perhaps the most important example arose in 1969 when an analysis of the ADR reports suggested that the risks of oral contraceptives were larger when higher doses of oestrogen were used (this is also discussed in Chapter 1). On that occasion the Committee's attempts to minimize the risk of alarm misfired when the press got hold of the story prematurely. On a similar occasion in 1982 when the decision was reached to withdraw benoxaprofen from the market, a statement was issued to the media in the knowledge that doctors would be aggrieved because patients would be first to hear about the withdrawal. In practice, whatever action is taken by a health department or an advisory committee it is likely to be seen to be wrong by somebody. The DRA is either accused of delay in conveying early warnings or is seen to be scare-mongering.

In chapter 50, Doctor John Marks enumerates the responsibilities of the pharmaceutical medical director. The industry, he feels, should be responsible for the distribution of detailed information rather than the Drug Regulatory Authority, while the latter should ensure that acceptable general guidelines are followed. The responsibility for individual communications should lie squarely on the shoulders of the company director who is in a position to influence its marketing policy. On the other hand, when an urgent warning about toxicity becomes necessary, he must collaborate closely with the Drug Regulatory Authority because both must tell the same story. If the DRA insists on a withdrawal, the medical director must ensure that the mechanism for recall of material already distributed to pharmacists or dispensed to patients is rapidly mobilized.

Commenting on the reasons why recommendations may vary from one country to another, he sees no reasons why the therapeutic indications or warnings should differ. However, while agreeing in principle one would question, whether this need always be true. For example, there seems little point in alarming Asiatic women using oral contraceptives by warning that Western women may develop thrombosis as an occasional complication, when the former are at little or no risk. The risk-benefit analysis may be quite different in countries in which maternal or infant mortality vary by one or more orders of magnitude.

Referring to communication between companies, Marks points to the conflict of commercial interests and the fact that people are suspicious about cartels and restrictive practices. These inhibit discussions with other companies, regulatory authorities and private research organizations. This is one of the main reasons why company sponsored post-marketing surveillance usually fails. No company is prepared to volunteer one of its products as a 'control' for comparative purposes.

Finally, Doctor Stephen Lock (Chapter 51) Editor of the *British Medical Journal* describes how articles are selected for publication. Eighty per cent have to be rejected either because they are unsuitable or because of lack of space. He does not believe that the correspondence columns are the correct place for large numbers of anecdotal accounts of side-effects. Rather they should be sent to the appropriate national monitoring centre. In contrast with the popular press, where scientific truth may not always be the prime consideration, medical journals have a complex system for assessing the quality of work sent to them, including the use of independent referees. Nevertheless, many of the principles of good journalism apply. The medical editor, who is usually a doctor, has to capture and maintain the interest of subscribers and to ensure that important reviews and original research articles are fairly represented in the limited space available. An important new role has been the decision to send referees' opinions to young authors if their articles are rejected. Another important innovation is the decision that most editorials should be signed. Since public policy is often influenced by them it is vital that the person with the power to influence opinion should be identifiable.

The medical journals exert a profound influence on the media, and very frequently provide the original material for the 'stories' described by Gillie. In a sense the medical journalist, unlike almost anyone else in the editor's 'wheel', is in the best position to influence all the people concerned with health care, including the patient.

# 41
# The patient

G. KELLAWAY

The express purpose of monitoring for drug safety is to protect patients against unnecessary risks of drug misadventure. The fact that this book is written at all and the wide diversity of backgrounds seen in its contributors amply reflects the genuine concern felt for the safety of those who have problems necessitating drug therapy. It is also entirely appropriate that in this era of widening patient interests and involvement in their own treatment, their particular role in drug safety monitoring should be clearly established. Although there are still many patients who would prefer to leave the choice of drug and the responsibility of what is best prescribed for their particular ailment to their medical advisor, there are a growing number of people who wish to know more about what advantages, potential hazards, side-effects and any other features which might result from even short-term drugs use. With long-term therapy this interest is often even greater.

This is especially the case in the more developed countries where, even if the prescribing clinician fails in his educative role to the patient, the news media, and indeed many other agencies, will arouse a laudible demand for information. Most patients are now aware that adept drug selection enhances the chance of a successful outcome with a minimal risk of untoward drug reaction. As consumers, patients who make their own choice of over-the-counter drugs, expect to have sufficient information to be able to make a reasonable choice for a particular problem. In an era when advertising has reached intense heights, aimed particularly at the consumer, it is perhaps an anomaly that prescribed drugs, those which are most likely to be potent and have the greatest risks of producing side-effects, are little known by the lay public; since information sources have been somewhat difficult to find, education is seldom forthcoming from prescribing clinicians, and lay advertising is considered unethical. How then does the patient become better informed, and how does he look upon the endeavours of others towards making his drugs safe?

## THE PATIENT

Quite obviously there is no such thing as a 'standard patient', and it is probably an oversimplification to equate the 'patient' with the 'public'. The background each person exhibits in terms of experience and education makes it extremely difficult to obtain statistically sound information about the attitudes of patients to drug monitoring, safety, and even their own medical practitioners. There are studies which purport to show that even though doctors feel that patient acceptance of therapy and consequent well-being are excellent and patients feel that the results are quite good their relatives are often disappointed with the outcome of treatment. Beauty perhaps does indeed lie in the eye of the beholder.

Patients vary in intellect, education, enquiry of mind, specific desire to be involved with drugs or drug treatment (especially where this is long-term), their aptitude to become involved, interest, economic means, personality and numerous other characteristics. Again, racial and national traits often modify the experience, and studies comparing one country with another demonstrate both regional and international differences in drug choice and patient involvement. Probably the greatest attribute any patient can have in relationship to drugs is commonsense. From a very wide background then of preparedness to take an interest in drugs and their use one can delineate the ends of the patient spectrum. One extreme is the 'on the ball' consumer who demands:

(1) All of the most up-to-date and effective drugs that anyone else in the world has, available for his own use as needed;
(2) A guarantee in the safety of these drugs if taken as prescribed;
(3) Assurance that the local medical practitioner knows exactly how the preparation can be used to best effect and with most safety; and
(4) Knowledge that those responsible for drug regulations in any country ensure that only the finest quality preparations are available as cheaply as possible.

As in fields outside medicine he is a hard man to satisfy, is critical of drug wastage, unnecessary prescribing and inadequate patient education; expects to know what each drug is meant to do, how effectiveness can be judged and what to do if he has doubts about this; demands to know if everything is being done to ensure quality control, correct use, safety and effective surveillance of the overall scene.

At the other end of the spectrum is the patient who accepts his medication from the doctor without demur. He is ignorant of drug preparation names, has no idea how they act, does not question their need and may even accept unpleasant side-effects without query. In between, every variation can be expected from full involvement to complete disregard. That so few patients' views have been analysed in the literature perhaps reflects that those interested in the field of monitoring and drug safety have themselves been recipients of prescribed or over-the-counter drugs. Perhaps subconsciously they expect patients to share a similar philosophy to their own about drug use; a premise which in many instances, is probably false.

## ADVERSE DRUG REACTIONS

It is sometimes difficult for patients to differentiate between drug toxicity and unpleasant side-effects. Adverse reactions are basically either 'harmful' (reactions of sufficient magnitude to result in time off work, or, at worst, death) or a 'nuisance' (where there is no serious interruption to daily living.) Patients often ask for help in recognizing adverse drug reactions. The following classification is largely self-explanatory and easily understood:

(1) Excessive therapeutic effect (e.g. digoxin intoxication, anticoagulant bleeds, hypoglycaemic coma),
(2) Unwanted pharmacological effect (e.g. postural hypotension, constipation, diarrhoea, blurring of vision, impotence, urinary obstruction),
(3) Pathological reaction
    (a) allergic (e.g. penicillin hypersensitivity, hepatitis, thrombocytopenia)
    (b) non-allergic (including mutagenic, teratogenic and carcinogenic),
(4) Super-infection, and
(5) Drug interaction.

Life-threatening drug effects probably occur as commonly with excessive therapeutic endeavour as with pathological and pharmacological reactions. Super-infections with antibiotics may impose a serious threat to life, and are sometimes devious in presentation; as with pseudomembranous colitis.[1] Drug interactions probably account for no more than 1% of total reactions, but again can threaten safety. Expert knowledge is required by prescribers and drug counsellors alike if problems are to be avoided.

For safety then, attention is focussed on the drug itself and its ability to produce unwanted reactions in the human body. In addition, particularly for drugs with a narrow therapeutic/toxic ratio, safety depends upon both prescriber and patient recognition of the potential dangers with potent drugs, and being prepared to cope with adverse reactions when they occur.

## INFORMATION SOURCES FOR THE PATIENT

If drug reactions or misuse can be hazardous or even life-threatening it seems obvious that successful treatment needs patient co-operation.

The barest informational requirements[2] include dose, dose frequency and proposed length of therapy, particular instructions about dose-times in relationship to meals, what risk situations (e.g. driving a car or operating machinery) accompany treatment, whether alcohol may potentiate drug effects, and whether there are any adverse effects which may necessitate prompt attention. The labels pasted by pharmacists on medication containers usually contain lamentably inadequate drug information by modern day standards.

Since the last edition of this book there has been an encouraging upsurge of interesting patient drug education. In the United Kingdom the methods of doing this include preparation of patient education drug leaflets,[3] patient and community group participation in general practice,[4,5] patient committees[6] and more extensive women's journal columns answering increasing numbers of patient write-in questions.[7] Greater emphasis has been placed on encouraging doctors to consider patients in their prescribing,[8] and Drury rightly points out[9] in a recent leading article on patient information leaflets that whatever the advantages or disadvantages of these leaflets are, patients have the right to this type of information.

In the United States there is much more emphasis on booklets, brochures and textbooks for patients. In 1982 the National Council on Patient Information and Education (NCPIE) was established as a non-profit making organization concerned with patient education issues. Strongly supported by the FDA the NCPIE has promoted an active campaign of 'Get the Answers' in an attempt to improve dialogue between health care professionals and patients about prescription drugs. Apart from producing their own quite clear and decisive advertising material they have published lists of patient leaflets, patient consumer education programmes, relevant textbooks, books, booklets, magazines and journal articles, news letters, instructional material, surveys and information about patient education resource centres. The list includes some 17 books, seven booklets and of course much other informative data. This major attempt to promote patient education concerns aspects other than adverse drug reactions (ADRs). Nevertheless, as most regulatory agencies discover sooner or later, their main concern with drugs is to establish efficacy, maintain quality control and ensure a high degree of safety. The occurrence and recognition of ADRs is therefore, of extreme importance to them.

In the past most drug safety information has been aimed at the prescribing doctor and perhaps to a lesser extent, the dispensing pharmacist. Patients were largely left to discover what information they could about drugs from reference sources such as dictionaries, home compendiums and encyclopaedias (e.g. Pears, Britannica). The numbers who have used such sources for drug information is quite unknown, but it is likely that a desire for broader information about drugs has always existed. Acceptance that successful drug treatment often needs patient co-operation has re-directed attention to the value of patient education, and in the past decade many clinicians have developed enthusiasm for involving patients in at least some of their own drug treatment. Recognition of substantial compliance-failure with many forms of drug therapy demonstrates convincingly that the patient is often determined to play a part in his own self-medication. Examples of counselling and the use of drug cards leading to improved compliance in adults[10] and children[11] support those who believe patient education about drugs is worthwhile. Even with the best of drug counselling, however, a hard core of patients continue to exhibit independence by making personal decisions and failing in compliance. Is it not better to offer them better educational opportunities about prescribed drugs so their decisions can be made on a more rational basis? It would seem that in the past 4 years there is a large body of opinion which has come to accept this philosophy.

A number of countries prepare warning cards for certain drugs with particular characteristics which may lead to safety risks. In Britain such cards are produced for patients taking monoamine oxidase inhibitors, systemic corticosteroids and anticoagulants. Special bodies such as the British Diabetic and Epileptic Associations also produce their own information cards. Again, many drug manufacturers produce patient information leaflets for their particular products. In the United States the FDA requires patient package inserts (PPIs) to be provided for patients[12] using certain devices and drugs. Five years ago there appeared to be pressure to extend PPIs to include the most prescribed drugs. The concept of simplified patient drug education cards appears now to be gradually superseding the PPI concept. This would seem to be much more appealing to patients themselves, since instructions are usually simply stated and information made clearly obvious even to the most casual of observers. Even some monthly publications have entered the act (*Current Prescribing*, 1977, 1978; *New Ethicals*, 1983). In this modern era, however, there always seems to be something more that can be done to improve on the previous 'best'. The next step beyond excellent drug reference material is the talk-back programme on drug use and ADRs (a telephone service has already been functional in Uppsala, Sweden for some 4 years), while the obviously potent appeal of the home video market must make it only a matter of time before home video drug education (including ADRs) will be available for considered use.

Naturally the whole topic of educating the patient about drug use has engendered some opposition. To the busy practitioner pressure of work and patient numbers, it is contended, leave insufficient time to discuss the principal qualities of drugs prescribed and the reasons for these. The hoped-for advantages, potential drug effects, interactions and education about drugs in general may have to be reinforced on several occasions for adequate educational results. Critics have suggested that drug information, apart from that offered by the prescribing clinician, might interfere with doctor/patient relationships, increase the tendency towards malpractice suits, and pose problems of non-compliance by making patients afraid to take medications for fear of listed ADRs.[13] There is perhaps a hint, in the insistance by government sources that PPI material be given to patients by pharmacists, that this type of information is unlikely to emanate from the prescribing doctors themselves. Some might consider this a method of circumventing doctors while establishing drug use criteria that may provide rigid legal standards. There is also a possibility, with PPIs for example, that without some additional counselling explanation or tuition the data presented may be misconstrued. Despite these possible disadvantages, in reviewing modern published literature there appears to be an increasing acceptance that used as a back-up to practitioner/patient drug education, prescriber leaflets, doctor/patient drug participation groups, textbooks, pamphlets and even well informed replies to women's journal questions, all help in providing useful information sources for the patient about drugs and the adverse effects of these.

## CAN THE PATIENT BE INVOLVED IN MONITORING FOR DRUG SAFETY?

In developed countries all but the very simple are capable of understanding at least something concerning their medication. Younger patients in particular[14] often wish to know how their drugs act, the manner in which they can be expected to help their disease, why there is a need to take them, what adverse reaction might occur with their use and what should be done if these do occur. With this degree of involvement the patient is in a strong position to contribute to drug safety monitoring. Even those with a lesser educational background can usually recognize adverse effects when provided with a suitable check list.

Many physicians bemoan the fact that offering patients lists of possible adverse effects increases the apparent incidence of ADRs.[15] In reality this is probably of little importance, since a falsely high incidence of adverse reactions involves mainly nuisance symptoms rather than dangerous or life-threatening reactions. As it is only critically important to recognize the latter early, it can be argued that encouraging prompt recognition of serious reactions is worth the excessive yield of trivial nuisance reports. In fact, there is some recent evidence, in a general practice pilot study of prescription information leaflets,[16] to suggest that improved patient knowledge does not increase the incidence of adverse effects, but enhances patient recognition of reactions which they then discuss with their prescribing doctors.

There are those who are concerned that greater patient education about potential ADRs may encourage an increase in therapeutic liability actions. When a litigation-minded population has the 'bit between the teeth' such an attribute must naturally interfere with the educational process. There is a strong risk, however, that in time such patients will prove to be greatly disadvantaged compared to those who live in environments with a less avid eye to lucrative opportunity, but with better knowledge about the drugs they use.

As the consumer in whom adverse drug reactions might occur, basic recognition of their appearance lies with the patient. It is interesting to see how frequently studies on occurrence and incidence of adverse effects concentrate attention on the doctor and his reporting of such reactions[17,18] without reference to methods of data collection. It is this concentration on data collection which has made the Boston Collaborative Drug Surveillance Program most authentic in establishing the relative incidence of adverse drug effects. Only daily interview is likely to establish 24 hour occurrence of untoward reactions. Second best in accuracy of recording adverse effects is the use of a check list, completed as a daily task. The records can then be discussed at visits with the interviewing doctor, resulting in information that is more likely to be accurate than that obtained from computerized programs depending on memory to periodically fill in answers. It seems extraordinary how few people in this field recall the simple dictum that transferred information from one person to another is often associated with distortion of the original content. Basically, therefore, the patient taking medication in surveillance monitoring for ADRs has to be the prime recorder of untoward events; not the second string doctor, or the third string statistician.

It would seem to me, therefore, that for a more complete and accurate data collection the patient should not only be intensively involved in monitoring for drug safety, but in most instances ought to be better prepared to play an accurate role with daily check list recording of adverse events as well as reactions.

## WHO EDUCATES THE PATIENT? : DOCTOR TO PATIENT

Traditionally the responsibility for telling patients about their drugs has rested primarily with the prescribing doctor. Apart from the shortage of time to properly discuss treatment with patients during busy practice times, it is tempting to wonder whether inadequate prescriber knowledge of basic pharmacology may not sometimes be a bar to good tuition. To some it will appear that the introduction of greater information for patients to assimilate themselves may supplant inadequate prescriber attention to the important task of doctor/patient drug-education, while perhaps blunting the omnipotent image of those doctors who expect patients to accept prescribed drugs without question.

The responsibility for patient education then should really lie firmly with the prescribing clinician. If he chooses to delegate this task to trained paramedical staff, the overall responsibility is still his. It is probable that much of what is being offered from government sources, the pharmaceutical industry, the news media and independent information publications will provide a splendid back-up to prescriber–patient drug intercourse. If this responsibility is neglected by the doctor there is a clear implication that other sources will take over his educative role by default, and an important aspect of the doctor/patient relationship will be undermined.

Good patient compliance with prescribed drug treatment necessitates good prescribing. Examples abound where compliance-failure on the patients' behalf have been life-saving. The patient then who takes potent drugs with potentially serious adverse reactions should be adequately informed about these preparations if the drugs are to be used as effectively and safely as possible.

Only 14 years ago one reads that 'as control of administration passes from the doctor to the patient, drug efficacy tends to diminish, beneficial effects produced by the drug in the defined clinical situation becomes less, and adverse effects occur more often and may be more serious'.[19] Despite this harbinger of gloom the trend appears to have been quite steadily in the opposite direction. It is not quite standard practice for diabetics and asthmatics to manipulate their own therapy, based on objective measurements of satisfactory response (namely blood sugar estimations and PEFR recordings), but almost. Many clinicians would also rate a number of the drugs used in coronary artery disease, chronic rheumatic disorders, certain skin conditions, many gastrointestinal complaints, anxiety, tension problems, haemophilia, migraine, essential hypertension and a number of other medical conditions, as equally requiring patient recognition of what can be expected from the self-manipulation drugs used in their treatment.

This can be combined with education about necessary changes in drug dose, unwanted drug effects which might ensue and the actual manipulation of different drug dosages as appropriately indicated. My own practice of giving hypertensive patients their own sphygomanometer with permission to manipulate their drugs to maintain minimally effective dosage almost completely overcomes any problem of non-compliance. Economically this has been an outstanding success in that the patients, almost invariably, find that they can reduce dosage while still maintaining good blood pressure control; and in doing so have taught me that good blood pressure control can be maintained with a single daily dosage, no matter what the β-blocker, once good control has been achieved.

A word of warning about patient freedom in self-management with chronic illnesses in relationship to drugs. Relying only on a feeling of well-being for dose changes[20] can result in a less than satisfactory response (e.g. with essential hypertension, diabetes mellitis and many other conditions), and it is essential under such circumstances for patients to have a simple method of obectively assessing progress. It is also important I believe, for them to have an adverse drug reaction check list in which they can record suspected drug-related events as well as adverse reactions, so that at doctor/patient interview these can be carefully discussed; rather than leaving specific event recall to hopeful memory or even clinician inspiration to ask the appropriate question.

Opposition to closer involvement of patients in their own therapy arises largely from the medical profession itself, and particularly from those in whom recognition of non-compliance as a problem is probably least. A search of the literature has failed to unearth any patient-orientated studies of how deeply patients might wish to be concerned in their own drug treatment; although it is likely that doctor/patient committees as they become more involved in the process of doctor/patient relationship, will find that this question demands their early consideration. Some scepticism has been expressed about patient textbooks with a viewpoint that only the intensely introverted will be tempted to obtain and read such material. How do you yourself use a textbook of internal medicine and drug treatment? Do you read the publication from cover to cover or simply peruse the chapter or chapters to which you specifically wish to refer? There seems to be a worldwide trend of favourably publicizing minority groups. Materials and facilities for the man in the street are sometimes curtailed for fear that a small minority of cranks may abuse these privileges. It is unlikely that Mr Average will use a patient medical textbook for anything other than the specific information he requires. In the same way studies in compliance are often aimed at detecting the patients who wish to deceive rather than concentrating on those who would wish to comply if they were only better informed. A guide to prescription drugs including their uses, actions and potential adverse effects would clearly be valuable for those who wish to know more about their drug treatment, but are less than adequately informed by their medical advisors.

There is a possible alternative which may find increasing popularity in the future. The drug counsellor, particularly with the help of take-home information videos, attached to a group practice or clinical pharmacology department, trained to discuss drug therapy with patients and be available to answer questions about problems which arise, may fill an increasingly important role. As more information directly aimed at educating the patient becomes available, group patient tuition could well reinforce or even replace the immediate needs of the prescribing clinician to spend time with patients discussing their therapeutic drugs. Group education for patients already flourishes in diabetic, asthmatic, psychiatric and neurological centres as well as cardiac rehabilitation, etc. Such an approach appears practical to assist even those patients who are not prepared to accept a large measure of responsibility for their own drug treatment.

## WHO EDUCATES THE PATIENT? : PATIENT TO DOCTOR

Having prescribed what one believes is the most suitable drug for a particular medical problem, even the most sanguine of doctors is inclined to feel a twinge of annoyance when the patient describes a new complaint and asks: 'Could it be due to the drug, doctor?'. If a 'nuisance' type of unwanted effect, the immediate reaction is often to dismiss the complaint. Its persistence, however, necessitates careful evaluation because, even if not a genuine drug side-effect, it is likely to result in therapeutic default.

The experienced clinician takes patient complaints of adverse drug reactions as probably true until proven otherwise. Even so, where a particular reaction has not previously been reported, it is often hard to accept a relationship. Thalidomide produced many congenital abnormalities before the connection was established. Even recognition of practolol complications occurred only after many examples had occurred.

With recognized but uncommon reactions it is quite often the patient who alerts the doctor to the existence of a problem. Two brief case history examples follow:

*Mr J. McC.*, aged 40, architect. Previous myocardial infarct, at 32; hyperlipoproteinaemia (Fredricksen, type 2a), treatment with clofibrate and cholestyramine. Coronary arteriography aged 38. Triple vein graft operation followed by treatment with warfarin. Difficulty experienced by GP in controlling anticoagulant dosage. Patient experimented and found that with warfarin taken $1\frac{1}{2}$ hours before cholestyramine the dose was stable. Cholestyramine taken before warfarin led to fluctuations in warfarin dose with inadequate anticoagulant control. Patient presented at hospital clinic stating 'there must be a reaction between cholestyramine and warfarin; the cholestyramine appears to prevent satisfactory warfarin action'. This observation was made without reference to textbooks, news media or PPIs; simply an ability to observe, consider and deduct.

*Mr W. D. D.*, aged 66, motor engineer. Treatment in 1966 for paroxysmal supraventricular tachycardia with procainamide. In March 1967, polyarthritis treated with aspirin then indomethacin. Pains became generalized. He suspected procainamide, discontinued treatment and later returned to GP with relief of painful symptoms, but complaining of palpitations. Procainamide was recommenced and joint symptoms returned. Reference by general practitioner to textbooks revealed no reported evidence of procainamide causing such symptoms. Patient insisted syndrome was due to drug. Referred for consultation in June 1967; positive LE phenomena discovered at a time when textbooks made no mention of the complication. By manipulating his medication, the patient was convinced the drug was responsible and, persisting with his viewpoint, he was ultimately vindicated.

There is no documented evidence of how often patients are correct in recognizing harmful adverse drug reactions. Elucidation of this might provide evidence on whether patients are capable of accepting a responsible role in drug treatment. There would be some older patients who would not wish to have the present status quo altered, being prepared to leave all matters relating to drug therapy to their medical practitioners. It is likely, however, that amongst the younger brigade there will be some who are not only willing to participate actively in drug selection, dose manipulation and changes in therapy, but in the future may even come to demand such recognition as of right.

## PATIENTS WITH ESTABLISHED DRUG HYPERSENSITIVITIES

Certain patients are particularly likely to suffer with serious ADRs. Some have allergic diatheses (asthma, eczema, hay fever, hives), while others seem particularly prone and give histories of established reactions to several drugs. Often such patients seem either too shy to relate this information in the circumstances of a hurried consultation or, with the passage of time, appear to forget that they ever occurred. Once a serious drug reaction has been exhibited, steps should be taken to ensure the patient will be spared any recurrence with the same drug in the future.

Various forms of medical warning procedures have been introduced to cope with this situation. Warning discs worn around the neck or on the wrist (MEDIC-ALERT), with instructions to telephone a 24-hour information reference source, are a popular precautionary measure in many developed countries. Such reference agencies perform an extremely useful function but there are still patients who, after suffering a serious ADR, leave the hospital or doctor's office without any clear idea of the drug responsible, and what advice they should carry forward with them to any future consultations. This deficiency is possibly in part due to the well-recognized tendency for patients to forget the spoken word within a few minutes of leaving the consulting room. It is important, then, not to rely on verbal communication with patients about adverse reactions, but to provide them with written information in some suitable form. This is an important doctor responsibility.

An interesting method of helping protect such patients is being established in New Zealand. A nationwide computerized admission/discharge system is being introduced, initially in the major cities. A medical alert section, concerned with reactions which are acute and potentially life-threatening, is included in the computer input. The list of severe reactions recorded is approved by the National Committee on Adverse Drug Reactions. Two types of reactions are recognized – Medicine Danger (reactions which are acute and potentially life-threatening) and Medicine Warning (reactions of a lesser immediate risk). The former require verification by the Committee on Adverse Drug Reactions. The latter can be verified by a clinician or submitted by other hospital staff such as a nurse or admitting clerk as an unverified warning. Where there has been a previous hospital admission anywhere in the country, this computerized information is available at readmission. It is expected that information will gradually accumulate about most patients in New Zealand with established serious reactions; thereafter available for nationwide use in the hospital service.

## CONCLUSIONS

Some important conclusions arise.

(1) Drug information material for patients is escalating. The interested patient has an increasing number of sources from which he can obtain information, including newspapers, television, drug calendar cards, pharmaceutical handout leaflets, patient medication instruction notes produced in medical publications and by independent sources, patient package inserts, patient textbooks and patient/doctor community groups.

(2) The primary health clinician is still responsible for prescribing drugs for patients, and is the most likely person to receive queries about drugs, drug treatment and adverse drug effects, whether the patient has recourse to drug education or information material, or not.

(3) There is little statistically established information as to whether patients wish to know more about drugs prescribed for them, their actions, reasons for use, unwanted effects and what to do if they feel the treatment is unsatisfactory or inappropriate.

(4) Greater drug education does not result in a falsely high incidence of adverse reaction reports, but enhances more sensible and compliant drug use.

(5) With greater drug education, some patients may wish to share responsibility in drug selection. There is a need to know more about the desires of the public regarding active participation in drug treatment including manipulation of therapy and selection of drugs.

(6) Patient rights as regards their own drug therapy may well arise as an important issue in the foreseeable future.

(7) As a source of information and even doctor education the patient appears to be generally somewhat under-rated. Patient attitudes to drug safety remain largely unknown.

## References


1. Check, W. (1978). Colitis following antibiotic therapy due to *Clostridium difficile*. *J. Am. Med. Assoc.*, **239,** 2101
2. Hermann, F., Herxheimer, A. and Lional, N. D. W. (1978). Package inserts for prescribed medicines: What minimum does the patient need? *Br. Med. J.*, **2,** 1132
3. Gray, J. A. M. (1982). Preparing a Leaflet for patient education. *Br. Med. J.*, **284,** 1171
4. Pritchard, P. (ed.) (1981). Patient participation in general practice. (London: Royal College of General Practitioners)
5. Bergen, J. (1981). Berinsfield Community Participation Group. *Br. Med. J.*, **282,** 1593
6. Thomas, D. J. (1981). Abadare Patients Committee. *Br. Med. J.*, **282,** 1761
7. Smith, R. (1983). Part time agony aunt in trousers. *Br. Med. J.*, **287,** 1029
8. Drury, M. and Sabbagh, K. (1982). Think more about prescribing. *Br. Med. J.*, **284,** 313
9. Drury, V. W. M. (1984). Patient information leaflets. *Br. Med. J.*, **288,** 427
10. Kellaway, G. S. M. (1980). Facing up to compliance failure with prescribed drug therapy. Methods and Findings in Experiment 1. *Clin. Pharmacol.*, **2,** 205

11. Kellaway, G. S. M. and Brown, S. A. (1983). Compliance failure and counselling in paediatric drug therapy. *N.Z. Med. J.*, **96,** 207
12. Ryan, K. J. (1977). The FDA and the practice of medicine. *N. Engl. J. Med.*, **297,** 1287
13. Dorsey, R. (1977). The patient package insert. Is it safe and effective? *J. Am. Med. Assoc.*, **238,** 1936
14. Patient package inserts (1978). *Br. Med. J.*, **2,** 586
15. Rickels, K. and Downing, R. W. (1970). Can patients judge which symptoms are caused by their medications? *Clin. Pharmacol.*, **10,** 298
16. George, C. E., Waters, W. E. and Nicholes, J. A. (1983). Prescription information leaflets: a pilot study in general practice. *Br. Med. J.*, **287,** 1193
17. Drury, M. and Hull, F. M. (1981). Prospective monitoring for adverse reactions to drugs in general practice. *Br. Med. J.*, **283,** 1305
18. Rawlins, M. D. (1984). Postmarketing surveillance of adverse reactions to drugs. *Br. Med. J.*, **288,** 879
19. Wilson, C. W. M. (1969). The social implications of drug use. *J. Irish. Med. Assoc.*, **62,** 1
20. Learning from our prescribing: a conference. (1978). *Drug Ther. Bull.*, **16,** 57

# 42
# The doctor

V. W. M. DRURY

## INTRODUCTION

An inhabitant of Britain will, during his lifetime, consult a general practitioner on about 260 occasions.[1] The frequency is greatest at the extremes of age, and each consultation will last for an average of 5 min, though this average conceals great variation. At the current rate of prescribing 65–70% of these consultations will include the prescribing of a drug. Each year the doctor will see about 65% of the population for whom he is responsible, and over a period of 3 years this figure will rise to 90%. Thus it is that the general practitioner sees more of, and prescribes more for, each person in Britain than any other type of doctor.

The number of prescriptions issued annually has risen steadily since 1948. It is currently about six items per person on the doctor's list per year.[2] Despite this the cost of general practitioner prescribing has not increased as much as the total cost of the National Health Service, and thus constitutes a progressively smaller fraction of NHS costs as each year goes by. As the national average of consultations is just over three per person per year, that is half the number of prescriptions, it is apparent that a considerable part of prescribing, up to 50%, takes place without a direct consultation at that time. Nearly all of this is repeat prescribing of medications initially issued during a consultation usually by a general practitioner, but occasionally by a hospital doctor. The sophistication of this medicine has increased greatly since 1948, increasing both the benefits and the risks.

The experience that an individual doctor has of each drug is more limited than that of the specialist. He is prescribing a wider range covering disorders of every system of the body. Although there are great individual variations it has been shown that most doctors have an armamentarium of between 400 and 500 preparations that they use in a year, but around 70% of the prescribing is accounted for by 25% of this list so that the doctor becomes really familiar with about 80 drugs.[3–5] Some of the less frequently used drugs are prescribed for uncommon conditions, but in most cases it is the influence of other doctors that cause it, letters from consultants or drugs prescribed by the patient's previous general practitioner.

All these factors will influence how well the doctor knows his patient and how well he knows the drugs that he uses. There are two others that are important in this respect: the advent of group practice and the mobility of the population; 83% of all doctors now work in conjunction with other general practitioners, sharing accommodation, staff and expenses. In many cases patients are shared as well, so that the patient may, during the course of 2 or 3 years, see each doctor in the group even, occasionally, during the course of one illness. In rural and small-town practice the population is relatively static, but in some city practices up to one in four patients may move each year, and the difficulty in providing continuity of care and keeping continuous records for this population is great. It follows that the drug armamentarium of a group practice is at least as important as that of the individual practitioner.

This is the background against which communication about adverse reaction between doctor and patient takes place and it is, clearly, a very varied background. The central event is the consultation, and it is the impact upon this consultation and the two people involved that we have to look at.

## THE CONSULTATION

There is an important principle that the doctor and his patient will want to see observed in any communication about ADRs impinging upon them and this is that nothing shall be said or done to lessen the strength of the doctor–patient relationship. This implies that the patient's confidence in the doctor's skills shall not be undermined, that the patient's confidence that the doctor's actions will be motivated only by the desire to do the best for him individually shall not be undermined, and that the confidentiality of the consultation shall be sacrosanct.

In any consultation, however short, a lot takes place. Patient and doctor have a great deal to communicate with each other by word and deed. The communication patterns are extremely complex, going far beyond the simple procedure of transmitting necessary information to and fro. Much is ritualistic and concerned with establishing or maintaining the individual's position *vis à vis* the other. Much is concerned with transmitting the perceived problem of the patient, which may be different from the real problem; or the perceived needs, which may be different from the real needs. False assumptions are frequently made by both parties about what the other wants to hear, and will affect what is reported by one to the other. Even if information is communicated it has to be both understood and capable of being recalled, and the selection of this information from other information is subject to equally complex filtering processes.

For example, a patient will select out from information that which he perceives to be important. This will depend on how it is said, where it is said, whether it is repeated, what previous information he possesses and so on. A patient will select out from information he gives to the doctor things that he thinks will please the doctor, or anger the doctor or confuse him according to his, the patient's, wishes at that time. All this shows that even in the consultation, facts about ADRs for drugs that have been prescribed, or are to be prescribed, will not pass backwards and forwards in a straight line but will be obscured, or exaggerated, or affected in other ways by either party. There are patients who blame everything they are given. There are patients who delight in reporting the bizarre. There are patients who 'never complain'. There are doctors who will not accept that any action they have initiated could harm the patient. So whatever care the lines of communication from ouside the consultation are given the consultation itself is so infinitely varied that the results of communication may not be what is desired. Nevertheless, with care they are more likely to be so.

We have already seen that in 70% of consultations in general practice a prescription is given to the patient, and there can be little doubt that this represents considerable over-prescribing. The reasons for this are complex and have been discussed elsewhere,[6,7] but in the same way that 'the doctor' is undervalued by the prescriber as part of the therapy so is the 'drug' overvalued by him. It is the most tangible weapon the general practitioner has. He cannot usually admit patients to hospital, perform complex investigations and so on, but he can easily prescribe. In his prescribing he is 'doing' something for the patient that is visible and satisfying, and the intrusion of a risk into that act is an unwelcome complication. It is also complicated by the lack of facts on which an assessment of that risk can be based. The doctor should be able to balance the benefit to the patient of his prescribing against the cost to the patient, and unfortunately the numerators and denominators on both sides of this balance are usually uncertain. Risk, therefore, is presented to the doctor as a largely unquantifiable danger. For example, the risk of causing haemorrhage by the administration of a drug should be measured by the frequency and severity of haemorrhage among all patients and sub-groups of those patients, and set against, say, the relief of pain in all patients and sub-groups of patients compared to no drugs, or other drugs. The doctor is rarely in possession of data at this level.

Furthermore the doctor is only one of the parties in this transaction. The patient is in possession of other facts, and also has a developed pattern of behaviour in response to medicine, prescribing, doctors, risks and so on.[8] The doctor will attempt to assess this in his communication to the patient about risk. He will try to use language and metaphor that is understandable to the patient. He will try to determine whether the patient is likely to be worried less by being given information than by having it withheld, and so to assess whether compliance will be helped or hindered by his communication. Clearly this will be different in an articulate, middle-class patient with a scientific background who is an enthusiastic supporter of the local parent/teacher association and a working-class wife with a full-time job in a shop and a young family in the care of a child-minder. But in either case if asked to quantify the level of risk he is usually unable to do so.

## THE MEDIA

Patients are more informed today about medical matters in general, and drugs in particular, than in the past. There can be little doubt about the effect of publicity about ADRs on patients. It is becoming increasingly common to hear patients expressing a dislike of taking tablets, and probably most doctors welcome this as a healthy trend. It is more doubtful whether they welcome the impact of specific publicity leading to a mass assault on the waiting room. During the past few years publicity given to vaccines, oral contraceptives, antihypertensive drugs, antidepressants and others have been followed by immediate increases in patient attendance. Occasionally the doctor is embarrassed by the fact that patients have acquired the information before he has, and at other times by the effect of headlines and dogmatic statements. Most 'news' is condensed to make a generalization based on scientific evidence, and this then has to be adapted to the individual.[9] Doctors tend to become less dogmatic, the older they get, and words like 'never' and 'always' are less frequently used. It is a pity that the discipline of journalists and programme producers does not always lead them to change in the same way. The criticism is usually of the manner in which information is presented to patients by the media, and if the public and the media would regard the personal doctor as the appropriate interpreter for the individual all would usually be well.

There are a number of special interest groups whose impact upon the patient is often out of all proportion to the scientific evidence upon which their message is based; anti-vaccination, anti-fluoridation and anti-medication groups exist, gaining support frequently from the isolated adverse event or the misquoted expert comment. It is unusual to be able to discuss matters with the members of such groups, but the case for the protagonists of vaccination, fluoridation and so on is helped by their being able to provide factual information in an easily digestible form.

## SOURCES OF INFORMATION FOR THE DOCTOR

Most doctors, and their patients, would be best served by confining prescribing to the smallest possible range of drugs available. In that way their experience of an individual drug and its potential for good or harm would be greatest. In fact, as we have already noted, the general practitioner prescribes between 300 and 400 drugs in a year very infrequently indeed. Many of these are prescribed at the behest of a consultant or a previous doctor of the patient, and many of them are variants of drugs he is already familiar with. In this case there is much to be said for changing the medication to one from his own preferred list. By keeping this list as small as possible the doctor becomes aware of important drug interactions and common side-effects, and becomes alerted to information reaching him about known or suspected ADRs on his 'list'.

Many hospitals now have their own 'formulary' with a limited range of drugs to be used on both in-patients and out-patients. These are chosen with an eye on both efficacy and cost. Many practices have developed their own formularies on the same basis. There is much to be said for a district attempting to define, with the practices who use that hospital, a joint formulary which would serve the needs of most patients.

General practitioners receive information from many sources about drugs. A major problem is the tidal wave of papers, journals, advertising material and information letters that flood in with every post. The volume poses a threat in itself because it dilutes important messages which may become lost. Amongst the most widely read are two weekly papers, *Pulse* and *General Practitioner;* a monthly journal, *The Practitioner;* and a journal confined to short articles on therapy, *Prescribers Journal.* If a company had an important product to promote it would advertise in the papers with the largest readership. In medicine it seems that the smaller the readership the more 'respectable' is the journal thought to be. Perhaps it would be appropriate for those responsible for the dissemination of important information about ADRs to look at circulation figures and take space appropriately that would ensure that it had the smallest chance of being thrown away unopened.

Consultants, when writing letters to general practitioners, are usually writing from a base of familiarity with the therapy they are advising. They may assume, quite wrongly, a similar base of familiarity in the recipient of the letter. It must be unusual for such letters to draw the attention of the general practitioner to reports of adverse events. For example, it might be that in advising drug X in his letter the specialist might add 'You will be aware that some cases of jaundice have recently been reported in association with this drug'. In this way an alert may be given without either party taking offence. Consultants should also recognize the need for keeping the general practitioner's range of drugs small, and where possible advise the prescription of a drug selected from a group, writing, for example, 'I suggest you put him on the tricyclic antidepressant you favour', unless there is a specific reason for one drug to be chosen.

Communications from drug regulatory authorities are sometimes the most important and best-informed advice arriving upon the doctor's desk about the dangers of a particular drug. It is important to retain their scarcity value. This helps to avoid the message being diluted. The envelope should be clearly identified on the outside to avoid loss. The message should be as clear and unambiguous as possible and presented in a standard format so that it is easily recognizable.

Advertising literature is an unrealiable source of information. *MIMS* (*Monthly Index of Medical Specialities*) provides a useful guide to products available and costs, but as a source of information on adverse effects is virtually useless. The *Data Sheet Compendium* is much more helpful, but the information is grouped illogically and it is difficult to read. *The British National Formulary* is a pocket sized volume, published twice yearly and contains useful and comprehensive advice on drugs available, preparations and cost and some guidance on usage. *Treatment*[10] is a larger, loose-leaved production which is updated every 3 months, and contains extended guidance on ADR risks as well as guidance on use, cost, preparations available and so on.

There are now available, or in the course of preparation, at least two drug data bases held on computer. It will shortly be possible to gain access to a drug data base via a 'viewdata' system using the telephone system. Whilst still in an experimental format in which the content and mode of access is being tested it should be possible in a year or two for a prescriber, using a video terminal which is either free standing or part of a microcomputer, to obtain much more detailed and up-to-date information. This will be particularly important in the field of new drugs and in the interaction and reactions reported that occur with more well established drugs. It should be possible to combine this with a message passing system giving the possiblity of obtaining faster information from the CSM and of notifying suspected ADRs to the CSM. Other possibilities that need exploring in relation to this include the storage of the data base on a 'laser disc' thus obviating reliance on outside telephone lines.

A second exciting step will take place when the drug data base begins to interact with electronic prescribing within the doctor's surgery; giving, for example, the opportunity to automatically flag potential interactions between two drugs on the same prescription, or printing out cautions that the doctor might observe or even hand to a patient. It will be important that the information contained within such a data base covers proprietary and generic preparations and has an independent provenance.

The hospital based pharmacist, and particularly the information pharmacist who is often based in the region, can provide extremely helpful advice and they should be used much more actively.

## COMMUNICATION FROM DOCTOR AND PATIENT

So far I have considered information about adverse events arriving and impinging upon the consultation. The source of most of this information should, however, be the doctor and the patient, and as most prescribing takes place in general practice it should be from the general practitioner.

I have already referred to the complexity of the transaction occurring in the consultation. Doctors are now being trained in the skills of interviewing and most are taught the importance of the 'open' question. It is well known that this is capable of acquiring a wider range of data than the 'closed' question. Greater adoption of these techniques must mean that a wider range of symptoms is reported to the doctor when patients are on drug therapy. If the doctor is also taught to think of drugs as a possible cause of any adverse event occurring to the patient, there is a chance that the general practitioner will receive early information about any possible ADRs occurring in his patients. This would facilitate the first step in the gathering of information.

The second step, the assessment of such information and its transmission to a drug monitoring service, is even more difficult. The dilemma faced by the general practitioner is whether to report all events or only those which are likely and serious. He is never, and I suspect can never be, given guidance on this, for it is at least as likely that the unexpected will be important as the expected. There are a few doctors who report regularly; there are many who never do. It might be more effective and cheaper to take advantage of those regular reporters than to attempt to convert the unconvertible. However easy you make the system there will be a sizeable number who do not make use of it. For this reason I suspect that a sampling technique providing a statistically sufficient number of patients would give a more complete and quicker line of communication from general practice to the drug monitoring system than any other. It might require 500 or 1000 doctors to be involved. This would mean that in the United Kingdom 1 250 000–2 500 000 patients would be recruited and arguably careful monitoring by this group would result in a much greater input of information from general practice than is achieved by the present system.

The reasons for non-reporting by general practitioners have been discussed elsewhere.[11] They include lack of time, lack of knowledge and guilt. A sampling technique might help with time constraint by putting the responsibility upon one group of doctors who then make time to do it. Better information methods would help with the problem of ignorance, and methods I have suggested may improve this. Guilt as an attitude can only be changed by education. Until society and doctors can be taught that taking risks is a part of normal living and that what is important is that the risk is measured before it is taken, we shall not overcome this. As far as doctors are concerned the educational change needs to start in the undergraduate period and be built into both vocational and continuing education. If this is allied to better communication with the patient the most important steps will have been taken.

## References


1. *Morbidity Statistics from General Practice. Second National Study.* 1970–1971. (London: HMSO)
2. *DHSS Annual Report of Chief Medical Officer* (1976). (London: HMSO)
3. Berkeley, J. S. and Richardson, I. M. (1973). Drug usage in general practice. *J. R. Coll. Gen. Pract.*, **23,** 155
4. Bain, J. G. and Hains, A. J. (1975). A year's study of drug prescribing in general practice. *J. R. Coll. Gen. Pract*, **25,** 41
5. Harris, C. M. *et al.* (1984). Prescribing – a suitable case for treatment. *J. R. Coll. Gen. Pract.*, Occasional Paper 24
6. Balint, M. *et al.* (1970). *The Treatment or Diagnosis; a Study of Repeat Prescriptions in General Practice.* (London: Tavistock)
7. Howie, J. (1977). Patterns of work. In Fry, J. (ed.). *Trends in General Practice.* (British Medical Journal)
8. Stimson, G. and Webb, B. (1975). *Going to See the Doctor; The Consultation Process in General Practice.* (London: Routledge & Kegan Paul)
9. Sabbagh, K. (1977). ECT and the media. *Br. Med. J.*, **2** (6096), 1215; **2** (6103), 1669
10. Drury, V. W. M., Wade, O. L., Beeley, L. and Aylesbury, P. (1978). *Treatment – a handbook of Drug Therapy.* (London: Kluwer Publishing)
11. Drury, M. (1977). Monitoring ADRs in General Practice. In Gross, F. H. and Inman, W. H. W. (eds.) *Drug Monitoring*, pp. 119–121. (London: Academic Press)

# 43
# The pharmacist

J. POSTON and P. PARISH

## INTRODUCTION

Traditionally, the responsibility of pharmacists for patient safety has focused on events prior to the act of drug use, that is manufacture, compounding and dispensing. These activities lacked contact with patients and have not required the pharmacist to have knowledge of diseases and therapeutics. Recently, however, pharmacists are becoming increasingly involved with patient care. They are acting as advisers to physicians and counsellors to patients, and their education is changing in order to meet these roles. To consider such activities in terms of the contribution which pharmacists could make to drug safety, it is necessary to consider historical events which have lead to the present developments and to discuss relationships between pharmacists, physicians and other health professionals, and to examine the influence of government and other agencies in defining the responsibilities and boundaries of pharmacy practice.

## HISTORICAL PERSPECTIVE

Pharmacy became established as a profession on the basis that the knowledge and skill of its members contributed to the welfare of society by providing patients and physicians with accurate and stable medicines of quality.[1] Economies of scale initiated the industrialization of pharmaceutical manufacture, and this was accelerated by the advent of pharmaceutical technology, notably tablet production, and the development of specific therapeutic agents.[2,3] This resulted in the transfer of responsibility for the accurate compounding of pure and stable medicines from the individual pharmacist to the pharmaceutical industry. This transfer and subsequent reduction in the need for the traditional knowledge and skill of dispensing pharmacists contributed to dissatisfaction among pharmacists. This was exacerbated in community pharmacy by systems of remuneration for dispensing which were based on the provision of the product rather than the provision of a service, this has resulted in the classic profession versus trade dilemma of community pharmacists.

Dissatisfaction within pharmacy, together with a desire to contribute to rational drug use produced a concept for the future practice of pharmacy clinical pharmacy. There are several definitions of clinical pharmacy, each emphasizes a role for pharmacists in ensuring the safe and effective use of medicines.[4–6] However, this concept is not new. For decades pharmacists have aspired to an advisory role to physicians on the basis of their superior knowledge of pharmacology.[7] Impetus to develop a clinical role was provided by the recognition of problems associated with inappropriate and unsafe drug use,[8–11] and subsequent government reports.[12]

New service roles have been developed, for example, monitoring drug therapy in individual patients by participation in ward visits and doctors' ward rounds,[13,14] monitoring and interpreting drug concentrations in body fluids,[15] drug history taking,[16] patient counselling,[17,18] drug information services[19] and services to patients requiring total parenteral nutrition, both in the home[20] and in hospital.[21]

Evaluation of these new services provided by pharmacists have been limited. Most studies have been descriptions of problems solved by pharmacists, rather than evaluations of benefits conveyed to patients.[14,22] However, studies have demonstrated how pharmacists can improve documentation of and compliance with drug therapy,[23] improve cost effectiveness[24] and reduce drug use and costs in long-term care.[25]

New educational programmes have been developed to produce pharmacists more able to provide these services,[26–28] and new organizations to foster the development of clinical pharmacy services have been founded.[29–31]

## PHARMACISTS IN HEALTH CARE

Three models of drug use may be identified; self-treatment by the lay person, counter-prescribing by pharmacists, and drug prescribing by the physician. The latter may be further differentiated because in the community the patient self-administers medicine, whereas in hospital this is the responsibility of the nurse.

### Self-treatment and counter prescribing

The accessibility of the community pharmacy to members of the public has often been cited as a rationale for the pharmacist to play a greater role in primary care.[32] This role would be concerned with health education,[33] advice on self-treatment and the diagnosis and treatment of minor ailments[34] and advising other health care professionals.

Research on the potential role of the community pharmacist has indicated that pharmacists are discontented with their existing role, are willing to develop a greater involvement with patients but see inadequate facilities, lack of remuneration and legal restrictions on the products available for counter-prescribing as important constraints.[35]

Studies of the advice given by community pharmacists in Australia[36] and in Northern Ireland,[37] endorse previous studies in the United Kingdom, which have shown that despite some deficiencies, the advice given by pharmacists is generally useful and appropriate.[38,39] However, studies have also indicated a need to provide pharmacists with appropriate interviewing skills and greater knowledge of clinical medicine and therapeutics in order for them to provide a more competent service. These points were also emphasized in the report on *Response to Symptoms* by a working party established by the Council of the Pharmaceutical Society of Great Britain.[40]

## Drug prescribing

The process of safe and effective drug use by an individual physician comprises several stages – a correct assessment of initial and changing needs; selection of the most appropriate drug; selection of an appropriate formulation, dose, route and dosage regimen; supply of appropriate information to the patient; and the surveillance of outcome of therapy. These processes demand decisions based upon the physician's knowledge of medicine, pathology, pharmacology and therapeutics. Such decisions also require a skill in the evaluation of reports of clinical trials. However, this routine approach to drug prescribing often ignores the social context in which drugs are prescribed, dispensed and consumed, which may influence important determinants of safety.[41]

It has been shown that drug selection by physicians in practice is influenced principally by information supplied by the pharmaceutical industry.[41,42] Reliance on the latter is often criticized because of the association between information necessary to ensure optimum use of a product and the information which is used to promote that product. To rectify this situation it has been suggested that the pharmacist should act as an independent source of information, acting as an unbiased mediator between the manufacturer and the physician. This goal is being met in the United Kingdom where a study of the national drug information network indicated that hospital pharmacists are becoming increasingly involved in the provision of information to hospital doctors on drugs and drug use. However, use of the service by general medical practitioners and community pharmacists appears to be limited.[19] In addition, local policies to rationalize drug use both in the hospital and community have resulted from pharmacists providing drug information to Pharmacy and Therapeutics Committees, developing and implementing hospital formularies and reviewing patterns of drug usage.[43]

Much contemporary debate on the use of medicines has focused upon the extent to which patients should be self-determinant in their own care. Evidence from patient compliance studies[44] and drug collections[45] indicate that a significant number of patients either knowingly or unknowingly fail to take prescribed medicines as directed by the physician and or pharmacist. Identification of this so called non-compliance has been used to promote a new service role for pharmacists – counselling patients to take medicines as directed. However, pharmacists have often lacked the time, skill and often the facilities in their pharmacies to effectively develop patient counselling. Instead there has been the development of alternative methods of supplying information to the patient. Notably additional labelling[46] and patient information leaflets.[47] Often these are poor substitutes for a failure of the doctor and the pharmacist to spend time talking to patients. A need exists for better education of the patient with respect to the use of medicines, and attempts have been made to clarify what the patient should be told, how he should be told and by whom.[48]

While pharmacists have been involved in developments to promote rational and effective drug use, their role in controlling costs, at least in the community, has been small. This is despite recommendations in early government reports that they could make an important contribution.[49]

Schemes to limit the range of medicines (limited lists) available under government health programmes, and thereby reduce costs, have recently been introduced in a number of countries.[50] Whether or not such schemes are successful at making drug use more rational or economic remains to be seen. Critics see them having little effect on overall costs.[50] However, such lists, together with increased prescription fees may lead to an increase in the number of patients seeking advice and treatment with non-prescription medicines from pharmacists. Such changes will emphasize the need for community pharmacists to be adequately trained in order to perform these functions.

## THE PHARMACIST AND ORGANIZATIONS

The service role of the pharmacist is determined by economic, legal, administrative and professional controls. Each of these may act as a constraint to the development of new service roles, and often only limited changes may be possible within these existing controls. In particular, controls specific to pharmacy act as strong shackles on any change in the role of the community pharmacist.

### Governments, professional associations and health care systems

Legal limitations of products available off prescription and the medico-legal constraints on community pharmacists restrict their responsibility and potential contribution to the community. Relaxation of controls in the United Kingdom over products such as ibuprofen and loperamide is potentially a valuable development in that a more useful selection of drugs becomes available for the pharmacist to counter prescribe.

### The pharmaceutical industry

Several aspects of the professional relationships between pharmacists and the pharmaceutical industry have important consequences for the safe and economic use of drugs. These include brand versus generic formulations, procedures for product re-call, the promotion and availablity of non-prescription medicines and the role of the pharmacist as an independent disseminator of drug information.

Economics and safety are key issues in the brand versus generic formulation controversy. Although the dangers associated with the inequivalency of generic formulations have been exaggerated.[51] Pharmacists, particularly in hospitals, have to balance economic benefits against any risks associated with product inequivalency.

Economic pressures also create problems in respect to the sale of non-prescription medicines. Pharmacists have argued strongly for restricting the sale of non-prescription medicines, to pharmacies.[52] But a more critical issue is the relationship between the appropriateness of a medicine for an individual and the profit on its sale. Clearly conflict can arise between the economic pressures created by sales promotion and the pharmacists need to trade on the one hand and the desire to provide a safe, effective remedy for patients on the other.

## THE PHARMACIST AND ADVERSE REACTION MONITORING

Pharmacists lack the knowledge of clinical medicine necessary to recognize adverse drug reactions. However, their knowledge of pharmacology and toxicology should ensure a role for them in the prediction and prevention of adverse drug reactions.

Where non-pathological indices of adverse effects are used, pharmacists have played an important role in the prospective surveillance of adverse reactions. Such studies have principally been confined to general or specialist hospital in-patients.[53–57] Some studies have involved pharmacists participating in regional schemes to improve spontaneous reporting of adverse drug reactions.[58] Together with nurses, physicians and clinical pharmacologists, hospital pharmacists have contributed to the epidemiology and evaluation of adverse drug reactions. Community pharmacists could also play a significant role in the detection of adverse reactions. In recent years representatives of the pharmacy profession have requested the involvement of the community pharmacist in direct voluntary reporting systems based upon the pharmacists accessibility to the patient, his knowledge of drugs, and his knowledge of any non-prescription medicines the patient may be taking.[58,59] Post-marketing surveillance of new products[60–62] and the advocacy of 'event' monitoring[63] should provide an opportunity for community pharmacists to play a greater role in adverse drug reaction monitoring in the future. Furthermore, there are several examples of serious adverse drug reactions in the past which have been associated with non-prescription medicines.[64–66]

An important development supporting the role of the community pharmacist in monitoring drug therapy is the maintenance of patient medication records in pharmacies.[67] Such schemes would ensure that pharmacists keep records of patients' drug histories with additional information from patients' medical histories relevant to drug use. The application of computer technology to pharmacy practice should make the maintenance of these records simpler in the future.[68] Furthermore the application of similar technology in general medical practice could allow for record linkage between general medical practitioners and pharmacists in the community. Subsequent improvement in communication could result in improved monitoring of drug therapy in the individual patient, but could also provide a method of studying many aspects of drug use in the community, including adverse reactions and prescribing costs.

## IN CONCLUSION

Pharmacists are capable of making a greater contribution to the safe and appropriate use of drugs. Changes in pharmacy education, health care policies and pharmacy practices should further these developments. However, critical management of resources, particularly in hospitals, will make it necessary for the benefits of the expansion the pharmacists role to be clearly demonstrated. In the community, much will depend on the effects of new information technology and even more sophisticated methods of drug packaging and distribution. However, society will always be concerned about the costs and safety of drugs and the pharmacists' knowledge and skill equip them to make a useful contribution to safe, effective and economic drug use. It is to be hoped that protection of professional territories will not prejudice such a contribution.

## References

1. Bell, J. (1841). On the constitution of the Pharmaceutical Society of Great Britain. *Pharm. J.*, **1**, 4
2. Bull, B. A. (1947). The changing face of pharmacy. *Pharm. J.*, **159**, 199
3. Dale, H. (1932). Some therapeutic problems of the future. *Pharm. J.*, **129**, 515
4. Parker, P. F. (1967). The hospital pharmacist in the clinical setting I. The Hospital Pharmacist's viewpoint. Presented at the *Second Annual Mid-Year Meeting of the American Society of Hospital Pharmacists.*

5. Sperandio, G. J. (1965). *Hospital Pharmacy Notes*. No. 1 (Jan–April) (USA: Eli Lilly and Co)
6. Brodie, D. C. and Benson, R. (1976). Evolution of the Clinical Pharmacy Concept. *Drug Intell. Clin. Pharm.*, **10,** 506
7. Burn, J. H. (1933). The Outlook for Pharmaceutical Students. *Pharm. J.*, **131,** 238
8. Jick, H. (1970). Comprehensive Drug Surveillance. *J. Am. Med. Assoc.*, **213,** 1455
9. Gardner, P. and Cluff, L. E. (1970). The epidemiology of adverse drug reactions. A review and perspective. *Johns Hopkins Med. J.*, **126,** 77.
10. Crooks, J. (1965). Prescribing and administration of drugs in Hospital. *Lancet*, **1,** 373
11. Vere, D. W. (1965). Errors of complex prescribing. *Lancet*, **1,** 370
12. Department of Health and Social Security (1970). *Report of the Working Party on the Hospital Pharmaceutical Service.* (London: HMSO)
13. Fitzpatrick, R. W. (1981). The pharmacist in a clinical area: a practical account. *Br. J. Pharm. Pract.*, 3, **18**
14. Shaw, P., Hollebon, C. E., Mason, S. K. (1980). An investigation into the role of pharmacists on consultant ward rounds. *Br. J. Pharm. Pract.*, **2,** 13
15. Maddox, R. R., Vanderveen, T. W., Jones, E. M. *et al.* (1981). Collaborative clinical pharmacokinetic services. *Am. J. Hosp. Pharm.*, **38,** 524
16. Dodds, L. J. (1982). An objective assessment of the role of the pharmacist in medication and compliance history taking. *Br. J. Pharm. Pract.*, **4,** 12
17. MacDonald, E. and MacDonald, J. B. (1977). Improving compliance after hospital discharge. *Br. Med. J.*, **2,** 618
18. Rehder, T. L., McCoy, L. K., Blackwell, B. *et al.* (1980). Improving medication compliance by counselling and special prescription container. *Am. J. Hosp. Pharm.*, **37,** 379
19. Smith, J. C. and McNulty, H. (1982). The national drug information network. *Pharm. J.*, **228,** 67
20. Dzierba, S. H., Mirtallo, J. M., Grauer, D. W. *et al.* (1984). Fiscal and clinical evaluation of home parenteral nutrition. *Am J. Hosp. Pharm.*, **41,** 285
21. Hoxey, E. and Athey, S. (1981). Patient specific parenteral nutrition based on a standard regimen. *Br. J. Pharm. Pract.*, **2,** 5
22. Fink, A., Kosecoff, J., Oppenheimer, P. R. *et al.* (1982). Assessing whether a clinical pharmacy program is meeting its goals. *Am. J. Hosp. Pharm.*, **39,** 806
23. Moson, R., Bond, C. A. and Schuna, A. (1981). Role of the clinical pharmacist in improving drug therapy. *Arch. Intern. Med.*, **141,** 1441
24. Suzuki, N. T. and Pelham, L. D. (1983). Cost–benefit of pharmacist concurrent monitoring of cefazolin prescribing. *Am. J. Hosp. Pharm.*, **40,** 1187
25. Strandberg, L. R., Dawson, G. W., Mathieson, D. *et al.* (1980). Effect of comprehensive pharmaceutical services on drug use in long-term facilities. *Am. J. Hosp. Pharm.*, **37,** 92
26. Francke, D. E. and Whitney, H. A. K. (1976). Patterns of clinical pharmacy education & practice in the USA. *Drug Intell. Clin. Pharm.*, **10,** 511
27. Poston, J. W. and Parish, P. A. (1981). Developing an undergraduate course in clinical and social pharmacy. *Pharm. J.*, **226,** 439
28. Anon. (1976). Guidelines for Pharm. D. programs. *Drug Intell. Clin. Pharm.*, **10,** 409
29. Anon. (1980). Clinical Pharmacy group formally established. *Pharm. J.*, **225,** 702
30. Barrett, C. W. (1980). The European Society of Clinical Pharmacy. *Br. J. Pharm. Pract.*, **1,** 29
31. Anon. (1979). American College of Clinical Pharmacy. *Drug. Intell. Clin. Pharm.*, **13,** 564
32. Dunnell, K. and Cartwright, A. (1972). *Medicine Takers, Prescribers and Hoarders.* p. 96, (London: Routledge and Kegan Paul)
33. Harris, J. W., (1983). Health education and preventive medicine in community pharmacy. *Pharm. J.*, **231,** 381
34. Whitfield, M. (1968). The pharmacists' contribution to medical care. *The Practitioner*, **200,** 434
35. Edwards, C. and Newcombe, C. (1980). Clinical pharmacy in community practice. *Br. J. Pharm. Pract.*, **2,** 11

36. Feehan, H. V. (1980). Study of pharmacists counselling competency. *Pharm. J.*, **225,** 172
37. D'Arcy, P. F., Irwin, W. G. and Clarke, D. (1980). Role of the general practice pharmacist in primary health care. *Pharm. J.*, **225,** 539
38. Elliot-Binns, C. P. (1973). An analysis of lay medicine. *J. R. Coll. Gen. Pract.*, **23,** 255
39. Edwards, J. and Attan, J. (1975). General practice pharmacists: How good is the advice they give patients? *Pharm. J.*, **214,** 568
40. Anon. (1981). Response to symptoms in general practice pharmacy. *Pharm. J.*, **226,** 14
41. Hemminki, E. (1975). Review of literature on the factors affecting drug prescribing. *Soc. Sci. Med.*, **9,** 111
42. Smith, M. C. (1977). Drug product advertising and prescribing: A review of the evidence. *Amer. J. Hosp. Pharm.*, **34,** 1208
43. Kleijn, E. and Jonkers, J. R. (eds.). (1977). *Clinical Pharmacy.* (Amsterdam: Elsevier/North-Holland Biomedical Press)
44. Sackett, D. L. and Haynes, R. B. (1976). *Compliance with Therapeutic Regimens* (Baltimore: Johns Hopkins University Press)
45. Nicholson, W. A. (1967). Collection of unwanted drugs from private homes. B. Med. J., 3, **730**
46. Anon. (1985). *British National Formulary Number 9. Appendix 4, Cautionary and Advisory Labels for Dispensed Medicines.* pp. 439–42
47. Griffith, H. W. (1978). Drug Information for patients. (Philadelphia: W. B. Saunders)
48. Herxheimer, A. and Davies, C. (1982). Drug information for patients: bringing together the messages from prescriber, pharmacist and manufacturer. *J. R. Coll. Gen. Pract.*, **32,** 93
49. Anon. (1959). Final Report of the Committee on the Cost of Prescribing. The Hinchcliffe Report. (London: HMSO)
50. Taylor, D. and Griffin, J. (1985). Does Britain spend too much on pharmaceuticals? *Pharm. J.*, 234, **228**
51. US Department of Health, Education and Welfare (1969). *Task Force on Prescription Drugs, Final Report.* pp. 31–35. (Washington DC: Department of Health, Education and Welfare)
52. Statement by Council of Pharmaceutical Society of Great Britain. (1974). *Pharm. J.*, 212, **216**
53. Gardner, P. and Watson, J. L. (1970). Adverse drug reactions: A pharmacist-based monitoring system. *Clin. Pharm. Ther.*, **11,** 802
54. Miller, R. R. (1973). Drug surveillance utilizing epidemiologic methods. *Am. J. Hosp. Pharm.*, 30, **584**
55. McKenzie, M. W. (1973). A pharmacist-based study of the epidemiology of adverse drug reactions in pediatric medicine patients. *Am. J. Hosp. Pharm.*, **30,** 898
56. Bergman, H. D. (1971). A new role for the pharmacist in the detection and evaluation of adverse drug reactions. *Am. J. Hosp.*, **28,** 343
57. Collins, G. E. and Clay, M. M. (1974). A prospective study of the epidemiology of adverse drug reactions in pediatric hematology and oncology patients. *Am. J. Hosp. Pharm.*, **31,** 968
58. Veitch, G .B. A. and Talbot, J. C. C. (1985). The pharmacist and adverse drug reaction reporting. *Pharm. J.*, **234,** 107
59. Anon. (1977). Report of the Council of the Pharmaceutical Society of Great Britain. *Pharm. J.*, **218,** 501
60. Wilson, A. B. (1977). Post-marketing surveillance of adverse reactions to new medicines. *Br. Med. J.*, **2,** 1001
61. Lawson, D. H. and Henry, D. A. (1977). Monitoring adverse reactions to new drugs 'restricted release' or 'monitored release'? *Br. Med. J.*, **1,** 691
62. Dollery, C. T. and Rawlins, M. D. (1977). Monitoring adverse reactions to drugs. *Br. Med. J.*, **1,** 96
63. Finney, D. J. (1971). Statistical aspects of monitoring for dangers in drug therapy. *Methods. Inf. Med.*, **10,** 1

64. Inman, W. H. W., and Adelstein, A. M. (1969). Rise and fall of asthma mortality in England and Wales in relation to use of pressurised aerosols. *Lancet*, **2,** 279
65. Reynolds, J.E. F. (1982). Clioquinol. In *Martindale, The Extra Pharmacopoeia, 28th Edn. p. 975. (London: The Pharmaceutical Press)*
66. Reynolds, J. E. F. (1982). Analgesic Abuse. In *Martindale, The Extra Pharmacopoeia, 28th Edn.* p. 234. (London: The Pharmaceutical Press)
67. Poston, J. W. and Shulman, S. (1985). Patient medication records in community pharmacy. *Pharm. J.*, **234,** 442
68. Winters, J. (1980). Computers within pharmacy practice. *Pharm. J.*, **225,** 384

# 44
# The media

C. M. FLETCHER

## INTRODUCTION

Since general practitioners write nearly 400 million prescriptions every year (an average of eight per patient) it is safe to say that more than half the population in the United Kingdom are prescribed some sort of medication (drug, inoculation, or a dietary component) every year, and, if we include those who buy non-prescribed drugs, the proportion must be over 75%. Many of these drugs have no significant pharmaceutical action and are taken solely for their placebo effect. Many are never taken. Most of those that are potentially beneficial are useful or at least harmless. But some of them – it is impossible to give a precise figure – cause undesirable side-effects. In a minute proportion of these the harm is serious or even fatal. Although the proportion is low the total number of serious reactions to drugs is large. In one recent study of old people who were on diuretics, which can have serious side-effects, it was found that only one in three needed them and one in eight had potentially dangerous hypokalaemia.[1]

Doctors clearly have a heavy responsibility to ensure that the drugs they prescribe for their patients do prevent or cure illness, and do not themselves cause or worsen illness. Doctors also have to face the problem of how and what they should tell their patients about the benefits and risks of medication. Their prescriptions are beneficial or harmless to nearly all patients but a few will be harmed; this is a difficult point to get across to ignorant and often anxious patients. The essence of it is that patients must somehow be warned to look out for any new symptoms they develop while taking drugs and to report them to the doctor so that he can judge whether or not they are due to, or independent of, the medication.

I shall consider first what doctors themselves can do about this problem and then look at the contributions, positive and negative, that the mass media (press and broadcasting) make or could make towards educating people about this problem.

## DOCTOR AND PATIENT

A doctor's prescription is usually the culmination of a consultation. He has, or should have, discovered, by skilful interviewing, what his patient's problem is and should, by any necessary physical examination and technical investigation, have reached a diagnosis. Many patients need only to be given reassurance or counsel, but more often than not they need, or are thought to need, a prescription. This is not so simple a matter as many doctors, who take out and complete a prescription sheet, believe it to be. Stewart and Cluff in their article on medication errors and non-compliance[2] point out that: 'People get much clearer instructions when they buy a camera or a transistor radio than they do when they are given a life-saving antibiotic or cardiac drug'. One consequence of this clinical casualness (apart from high rates of non-compliance) is that many patients ask their pharmacists what their prescriptions are for, how important it is that they should take them, and what harm they may do.

It is clear in Byrne and Long's report[3] on nearly 2500 recordings of general practitioner consultations that doctors seldom refer to side-effects of drugs when they prescribe. Indeed since few GPs can give more than an average of 6 min to each patient they have little time to enter into any worthwhile discussion of possible side-effects of any drugs. Nor, in my experience, do consultants regularly give much more information. It was certainly my practice, and I am sure this was true of most of my consultant colleagues, to warn patients of common or potentially serious side-effects such as nausea from aminophylline preparations, diarrhoea or pruritus from antibiotics or visual disturbances from drugs such as chloroquine, but not to give a detailed account of all the possible harmful effects of every drug prescribed.

What then should a doctor do in this regard? If doctors were to read out the full accounts of all recorded side-effects of drugs listed in the 'contraindications and warnings' of the comprehensive data sheets supplied by the pharmaceutical companies for their products, few patients would understand them. If they did they would be unlikely to take any medication without full discussion of the statistical balance between benefit and risk for which there is no time in most consultations.

The first step, of course, which all doctors could and should take is to ask any patient who is put onto or maintained on medication to report any unusual or new symptoms, however mild, which he develops. They should tell patients, except in rare circumstances where it could be dangerous to discontinue the drug, to stop taking a new drug temporarily to see if any symptoms improve and then to see whether they recur if the drug is started again.

But this would also be time-consuming. Somehow we have to develop better techniques of communication between doctors and patients. The second part of the consultation is in effect a short lecture. No medical teacher would expect his students to remember all that he had said in a lecture without either encouraging them to take notes or giving them a summary of his lecture's content. Yet few, if any, doctors use such techniques to help their patients remember what they have or should have been told about their medication.[4]

Studies abroad[5–7] have shown that brief, simply written pamphlets about the prescribed drugs leads to an increased knowledge, satisfaction and consequently compliance amongst patients. These pamphlets, known as Patient Package Inserts or, preferably, Prescription Information Leaflets, describe the purpose of prescribed drugs, how they should be taken, what to do about omitted doses, what side effects are harmless and which ones should lead to stopping the drug and reporting to the doctor. It has been found that such leaflets increase the number of side effects reported to doctors without increasing their frequency.

A small pilot trial in general practice in the UK[8] showed that such pamphlets do increase patients' satisfaction and knowledge, both of which should improve compliance and reduce serious side effects. This year (1985) the pilot study has been extended in the form of a controlled trial to examine the effectiveness of these pamphlets and to look at their use and issue by doctors or by pharmacists. Considerable difficulty was found in obtaining finance for this simple but important study which shows how uninterested most doctors and medical agencies in the UK still are about the clinical importance of better communication between doctors and their patients, even in relation to better use of the drugs that they prescribe.

## THE MEDIA AND THE PUBLIC

Until the middle of the last century doctors seem to have had little objection to popular interest in the treatment of illnesses. Buchan's book *Domestic Medicine: or The Family Physician*, first published in 1769, ran through many editions over 100 years and met with no professional disapproval. Medicine was regarded as a topic of which any educated man should have some knowledge. But at some time in the nineteenth century a strong prejudice developed against lay interest in clinical matters. The origins of this change of attitude are not easy to trace. Victorian prudery about the naked body, and still more about internal organs, may have played a part. Perhaps the Medical Qualifications Act of 1858 gave qualified doctors a feeling of having the unique privilege of knowing about and advising on the treatment of illness. They were also rightly concerned about the harmful effects of unbridled commercialism in advertisements of patent medicines. Respectable 'home-doctor' books continued to appear, but their use was frowned upon by the profession. Preventive medicine was quite a different matter. The great nineteenth century sanitary movement began, through Acts of Parliament, to provide conditions of housing, sanitation and occupation which transformed the lives of the disease-ridden poor. In the early years of the present century health education began to be developed to help the public protect themselves from disease. Doctors considered it entirely respectable to encourage attendance at ante-natal and infant-welfare clinics.

But the predjudice against giving public information about medical practice continued. In 1906 William Osler warned an audience of nurses and medical students:

> 'In the life of every successful physician, there comes the temptation to toy with the Delilah of the Press – daily and otherwise. There are times when she may be courted with satisfaction but beware: sooner or later, she is sure to play the harlot and has left many a man shorn of his strength, viz. the confidence of his professional brethren.'[9]

In 1950, the British Medical Association, which had been very active in the health education movement, proposed to start a popular health journal. It was first published in 1951 as *The Family Doctor*. But an eminent physician wrote to the *British Medical Journal* suggesting that it should have been called *The Hypochondriac*.[10] This suggestion reflected a common medical fear that public information on the nature and treatment of illnesses would encourage morbid anxiety. There was no logic in this attitude for people who were not worried about illnesses would presumably not bother to take the preventive measures that were encouraged by doctors.

Many doctors continued to take this narrow-minded view, but advances in general education led to a widespread, and entirely natural, increase of public interest both in the science and practice of medicine and in its social consequences. This interest was inevitably noticed and increasingly satisfied both by the press and by broadcasting. In particular, as the National Health Service developed, the consumer movement led to an increasing demand that patients should have a larger say in the way they were treated. They realized that they must have more knowledge if they were to play an effective part in ensuring that the Health Service was as effective, efficient and convenient as possible, and they wanted to have a readier means of voicing dissatisfaction. This pressure led eventually to the establishment of Community Health Councils, and more recently to a 'College of Health' to represent consumer interest in medicine.[11]

The first major break in professional reticence about public discussion of disease was made by Dr Charles Hill (now Lord Hill of Luton) in 1943 when he was Secretary of the British Medical Association and Chairman of the Central Council for Health Education. He was asked by the British Broadcasting Corporation (BBC) to broadcast a series of radio programmes under the title 'The Radio Doctor'. In these he described in gruff and picturesque, but simple, terms, a large variety of common illnesses; and indicated what ordinary people could do about them. It is strange to look back to the shock which, for instance, his public mention of constipation caused. There were murmurs of disapproval among doctors which became more pronounced as medical programmes began to appear on television. When in 1958, the BBC started a series of television programmes from hospitals, including films of surgical operations, under the title 'Your Life in Their Hands' (which I was invited to introduce), a storm of protest broke out in the columns of the *British Medical Journal*. For four consecutive weeks leading articles were published under the title 'Disease Education by the BBC' voicing the traditional view that while prevention should be discussed in public, 'dramatizing' the treatment of disease would frighten and bemuse people. In fact, public reaction to these programmes was increasingly favourable. In defence of the doctors who objected, it can be said that they then had little realization of how many people resented doctors' unwillingness to provide, and incompetence at providing, them with information about their illnesses. Ann Cartwright's study of a sample of patients discharged from hosptial, 70% of whom wished to have full information, was not published till 1965.[12] A few quotations from what some of these patients told her illustrate this feeling.

> 'They leave you in the dark too much. If only they treated you as though you could understand something. The doctors especially were very superior: they didn't tell you anything.'

> 'They would give you pills and if you asked what they were for you were told to take it and never mind. You were treated like a child, as if it were nothing to do with you if the medicine were changed. There was no reason given.'

> 'When I am confronted with something I don't understand I like to know as much about it as possible – the danger of complications, the possibility of survival – what it is all leading up to – an overall prospect.'

Another objection raised by doctors was that it is futile to try to teach people about disease in short television programmes. 'A little learning,' they quoted, 'is a dangerous thing.' This showed how irrational they were. If incomplete knowledge were more dangerous than no knowledge, doctors themselves should have stopped practising for they then knew nothing about what we have since learnt. The fact is that some knowledge is always better than total ignorance. One of the patients Ann Cartwright interviewed was dissatisfied about what she had been told in hospital after an operation. She said:

> 'I would like to have known all that they had to do inside me. They did not give me any details. While I was at my brother's I saw the operation on telly and that told me more about it than they did.'

But doctors were also worried that medical broadcasts might interfere with their relationship with their patients. They expected that patients might come and ask them for treatment which had been shown on television, but about which they themselves knew nothing. But why shouldn't patients know about treatment which could help them? In the event such fears were not fulfilled. A few years later the BBC started a series of educational programmes for doctors, called 'Medicine Today'. There was an eavesdropping audience for these programmes of about 500 000 lay people, but no complaint of this kind was ever received from a GP. Richard Asher summarized the doctors' illogical concern about this aspect of medical broadcasts in his usual succinct style:

> 'A little knowledge of medicine in the hands of our patients may benefit doctors. It is hard for the salesman to remain honest if his customers have no idea whether his goods are satisfactory or not. Blind ignorant faith in doctors is not always to their benefit, although we appreciate it highly on the rare occasions we obtain it.'[13]

Medical feature programmes on BBC radio and television and on Independent Television during the 1950s and 1960s presented medicine and surgery in a way which one BBC executive described as 'doing a public relations job for medicine'. They skilfully presented in visual form many of the new treatments, both medical and surgical, which doctors then had to offer their patients. Relatively little was ever said about the negative side of the story. Operations were always successful. Post-operative pain and the side-effects of drugs, whether mild or serious, were hardly ever referred to. This may have been why the storm of medical protest was stilled.

Doctors, however, continued to complain, justifiably, about misleading reports on news and current-affairs programmes. In some of these prominence was, and still is, given to useless quack remedies and mistaken criticisms made of orthodox medical opinions. In some current-affairs programmes doctors were, as it were, put in the witness box with the interviewer acting as prosecutor and judge, particularly in relation to occasions where it appeared that a doctor had made a mistake. Such programmes are still broadcast from time to time, but much less frequently.

A new development in the 1970s was that feature programmes began to appear on television which gave prominence to medical and surgical procedures about which medical opinion was divided. These tended to over-emphasize the dangers of one form of treatment so that a one-sided view was given and doctors who were on the other side were made to look complacent about any risks to their patients. Examples were programmes on children reputedly damaged by pertussis vaccination in which the connection between vaccination and damage was assumed without full discussion of the difficulty of establishing cause and effect, and the advantages were not presented; programmes on ECT, in which psychiatrists whose patients had not responded well to it were presented almost as sadists and little mention was made of the thousands of patients who had greatly benefited from it; and on induction of labour whose risks were emphasized with no emphasis on the very low risk of labour whether induced or spontaneous.

This change of approach in broadcasts reflected a growing reaction from many intelligent patients, and particularly from social scientists[14] against the dominant role assumed by many doctors in handling their patients. Such doctors tend to ignore their patients' desire for full information about their illnesses and to deny them any right to exert choice about their treatment, for they felt that they, the doctors, were the best judges of what should be done. They gave 'doctor's orders', which patients should obey. Patients who did not comply with treatment were described in derogatory terms as 'liars, uncooperative, negligent, deviant, or disobedient'. Above all such doctors felt it to be unwise and harmful to therapeutic efficiency to admit to patients any possibility of failure or risk of treatment, whether pharmacological, physical or surgical.

It was not surprising that television producers tended to cater for the new critical attitude of many of their viewers towards authoritarian doctors. It was also inevitable that doctors should begin to protest at the harm such programmes could do to their own patients, and at the anxiety and loss of confidence they caused. This view was expressed in a review article in the *British Medical Journal*.[15] In the correspondence which followed a further leading article,[16] the broadcasters tried to justify any harm that their programmes might do on the grounds of freedom of speech. One television executive asked 'Should television in its institutional role as "honest reporter" be allowed the same freedom to deal with a medical topic as it has to deal with, say, politics, gardening, civil engineering, physics, sport or foreign affairs?' He continued: 'If you answer "No" to this question then you are on the side of a type of censorship that operates nowhere else in the press today.'[17] He appeared quite unconcerned that patients, most of them justifiably confident in the safety of their treatment, might be unduly and harmfully alarmed if television programmes disclosed with dramatic emphasis that it carried risks of which they were unaware. He did not seem to realize that plants, buildings, athletes and foreign secretaries do not suffer from anxiety of this kind, but patients often do. To give one example: in 1969 the BBC described the epidemic of increased asthma deaths between 1964 and 1967 attributed to overuse of isoprenaline sprays. In the next 2 weeks patients came to their asthma clinics having stopped all aerosol treatment – including beclomethasone – with serious relapse of their asthma.

Fortunately this period of discord between broadcasters and doctors was short.[17] In a review prepared for their General Advisory Council[19] the BBC concluded: 'The essential ingredient is trust, between the medical world and the world of broadcasting, and without this there can be no satisfactory way of serving the lay audience or of meeting the public need for understanding about the scope and application of medical knowledge'. They did not discuss the means by which such trust should be engendered and maintained. I believe that constant, regular meetings between senior programme producers and doctors could do much to achieve this. Although I first suggested this in 1973[20] no steps have yet been taken to arrange such meetings except in Scotland.[21] Perhaps the rest of the United Kingdom will one day come to follow the Scottish example in this as they have in previous years followed them in other matters of medical education.

But what useful contribution can broadcasting make towards telling patients about the harmful effects of drugs that they take, while getting them to appreciate fully the benefits they can receive from their treatment? Recently the BBC broadcast a feature programme which had nearly 6 000 000 viewers, 'The poisons that heal'. At the end of this Caroline Medawar, who linked the programme, said:

> 'How could we improve things? Well, it's possible that doctors could prescribe less and listen more and certainly patients might then stop thinking of drugs as the first or only method of treatment. We've almost come to believe that whatever there is wrong with us there'll be a medicine to make it better. A pill for every ill. And also it's as though we believe that medicines are somehow magical, that they can only do us good and our doctors can help us. Now here's some practical advice. Next time you collect a prescription ask your doctor these questions:
>
> What kind of drug is it and how will it help me?
>
> How important is it for me to take it; what would happen if I didn't?
>
> Does this drug have any other effects?
>
> Can I drink or drive or take other medicines at the same time?
>
> How long do I take it for? And do I need another appointment?
>
> Now some of this may seem obvious, but a lot of doctors don't offer this information, or give it only reluctantly, and it's important that they do give it, for in the end, knowing about what we take when we're ill, like what we eat when we're hungry, is not only our responsibility but it's also just plain common sense.'

This is good advice, but how many patients followed it? They could not possibly have had time during the programme to write down all the questions they should ask their doctors. I asked several GPs about this, some of whom saw the programme and expected to receive questions from their patients. Not one of them had a single patient who appeared to have taken any notice of the BBC's advice. This does not mean that all viewers of this programme rejected the advice they were given; many may subsequently have been more cautious and critical of their doctor's advice. But BBC audience research has often shown that viewers remember the visual content of television programmes better than anything that is said to them, which they usually forget. We need to learn more about how best to use television for giving people practical advice about precautions in taking drugs.

What about the press? Doctors, on the whole, make as many complaints about the handling of medical matters by the press as they do about broadcasts on medicine. This is probably because most coverage of medical matters is written by non-medical reporters who have little understanding of the subject. Only one or two of the major national dailies have medical correspondents who have any real knowledge the subject. Their reports are therefore often written more with regard to their news value than to their truth, relevance or their effects upon patients. But when articles are written by people with medical experience who are skilled at presenting complicated issues, their articles can be of great value and, unlike broadcasts, they can be cut out and kept for further reference. Although in many respects the same criticisms can and have been made of press, as of broadcast reporting on therapeutic matters, on the whole, the press could fulfil a useful role. The impact of the written word is less dramatic than television and the readership of any one newspaper is usually small in comparison with television audiences. The important thing about such articles and programmes is that they should not be over-dramatized.

In summary: so many people are taking medicines of one kind or another today that large viewing or reading audiences could be obtained for articles or programmes on commonly used drugs. These should consist of simple expositions of the nature and use of drugs and of any possible risks. They should reassure patients about the rarity of nearly all the side-effects, but give them some indication of the sort of side-effects that are most important for them to report to their doctors. Programmes of this kind need not be broadcast at peak viewing or listening times, nor need they appear on the main feature page of newspapers. People taking drugs will notice any one which concerns the particular drug they are taking and will take the trouble to read, listen to, or view them. This is the sort of public service with which the media express their concern to carry out, but they do not do very much about it. Such articles and broadcasts could also help doctors, many of whom are aware of their relative ignorance of the pharmaceutical complexities of many of the drugs they prescribe.

## THE MEDIA AND DOCTORS

Newsmen and broadcasters are always on the lookout for interesting news about medical affairs of all kinds. For this reason doctors may find themselves approached by radio or television producers or by news-reporters about their experience with particular drugs or forms of treatment. Doctors not infrequently complain that when they have given interviews to reporters, or have recorded interviews for broadcasting, the eventual article or broadcast seriously misrepresents their stated views by subtle omissions or juxtapositions. This has not, however, been the experience of doctors who have had extensive experience of medical journalism or broadcasting. They find that misrepresentation and misreporting may be avoided by reaching a clear agreement with the writer of the article or the producer of the programme about the content or purpose of the article or programme and how it is proposed that this purpose should be attained. It may emerge in discussion that the purpose is quite contrary to what the doctor had supposed, in which case he may not wish to contribute. The reporter may, on the other hand, have had mistaken views which can be corrected.

This sort of complaint may arise because doctors, particularly research workers, do not always appreciate the sort of abbreviation and simplification of their views which are inevitably needed in presenting them to the public. In some instances of complaint, it has appeared that the doctor was chiefly concerned about criticisms which his specialist colleagues might make of the simplified version of his views or research findings which had been presented, and that he had not recognized the essential differences between a broadcast or newspaper article and a scientific paper.

It may be possible to arrange for a doctor to see and correct the draft of an article (but there is little safeguard against misleading headlines for which the reporter is usually not responsible). Broadcasting authorities insist on editorial control. It is difficult to arrange to see edited programmes before transmission because the final version is usually ready only shortly before transmission, when it may be too late to make alterations. Moreover, if there are several contributors, each of whom wishes to adapt his contribution, chaos would result. There is really no alternative to establishing mutual confidence between doctor and producer or refusing to contribute.

When asked by a press reporter for an interview on the telephone, it is wise to discover where and in what form the reported interview is to appear, and also whether the enquirer's experience in medical reporting, and understanding of technical matters, are sufficient for him to be able to produce an accurate report. If this is not the case, special care will be necessary to ensure that there has been no misunderstanding: the doctor should insist on being given an opportunity to correct any errors in the report. If time is short the reporter should be asked to read back his report over the telephone.

Occasionally, a misleading report may result from a doctor allowing a reporter to put words into his mouth: 'You have said, Doctor, that . . .' and subtle misrepresentations of what has been said may follow which the doctor may not refute, but just suggest a more accurate account of his point of view. The report may then appear as 'Dr X agreed that he had said . . .' without the correction. Any suggestion by a reporter that a doctor has said what he has not said should be firmly met by stating 'No, you have got that wrong. My opinion is . . .'.

In relation to broadcasts, any doctor approached to participate in a programme should find out:

(1) Who else is to participate. This is essential in order to avoid being faced, without preparation, by people with whose views the doctor may strongly disagree.
(2) What points are to be discussed and for what purpose. The

producer of the programme may wish to raise issues which the doctor feels are inappropriate for him to discuss in public. In this case, a firm assurance must be obtained that such issues will not be raised. On the other hand, the producer may persuade the doctor that it is desirable to raise these issues; agreement may then be reached on how they should be handled.

(3) Who is conducting the interview. This is often not the same person as the one who has invited participation. In this case, it must be established that the interviewer has also agreed not to raise issues which the doctor has refused to discuss.

(4) Whether the programme is to be live or recorded. In general, recorded interviews or discussions are easier to manage, because if the doctor has a slip of memory or expresses his point of view inappropriately, this part of the interview can be re-recorded. If the interviewer revokes his prior agreement and asks a question which he has agreed not to ask or asks a question of the 'have you stopped beating your wife?' type or makes an offensive or damaging statement, a forcible objection should ensure that the recording is stopped and is not broadcast. Such situations have indeed occurred, and are much harder to handle in a live transmission. When this happens it is probably best to use the politician's technique of blithely answering a question other than that which has been asked. If the interviewer persists with his question, it may be necessary to remind him of his undertaking and ask him to proceed with the interview along the agreed lines.

Doctors are occasionally concerned about anonymity and advertising. The 'rule' of anonymity is in effect only a tradition derived from the profession's rejection, as unethical, of advertising personal skill in order to attract patients. There is no firm rule about what constitutes such advertising except that doctors should not do anything that is, or appears to be, intended to attract patients. For this reason, accusations of advertising are likely to arise only in regard to public presentation of methods of diagnosis or treatment of patients. To state in public: 'Since I have used this new technique, my results have been far better than those of doctors who use the old technique', might well be regarded as advertising. Whereas to say 'this new technique has enabled doctors to obtain far better results than they used to obtain with former techniques' would not. Even so, the mere fact that an identified doctor has made it clear that he uses improved methods could encourage readers, listeners or viewers to consult him, and might lead his colleagues to feel that he had used his article or broadcast to his own advantage. This risk can be avoided if public statements by individual doctors about clinical methods are given anonymously. Reporters and broadcasters are becoming less willing than formerly to accept the need for anonymity. They will agree to it if it is insisted on, but prefer to use a doctor who agrees to be named.

One reason for this is the relatively small number of doctors in private practice today so that there is less competition for patients. There may also be difficulties in radio or TV discussions between several anonymous doctors, which would be much easier to follow if the participants were named. References to what 'the last doctor but one' has said are clumsy and confusing. Christian names can now often be used to preserve anonymity. Surnames may be used in introducing speakers, but are better not shown on the television screen in writing nor given in the *Radio Times* or *TV Times* in presentations or discussions concerned with clinical practice.

There is one particular situation in which anonymity must be carefully guarded. This is when a reporter telephones an enthusiastic practitioner of some particular clinical method. The doctor may feel flattered and give details of what he does and his reasons for believing that it is effective. When the report appears, perhaps under a headline 'Doctor X can Cure Aches and Pains', an accusation of advertising may well follow, whereas if the heading had just been 'New Cure for Aches and Pains' without any mention of the doctor's name or locality, no accusation would lie.

The patients' point of view has to be considered with special care when a doctor is asked his opinion on some relatively new method of treatment, the advantages and disadvantages of which are still uncertain. The doctor may have strong feelings on such a question and may forcibly express his views on the hazards or benefits of one or other method of management. In doing so, he should be particularly careful not to cause unnecessary alarm to patients who are on one or other method of treatment or are likely to need it. It may be helpful if he finds out which doctors are being asked to present the opposing point of view and to discuss with them ways in which the issue can best be presented without causing distress.

All these precautions sound as if talking to reporters or agreeing to broadcast is hazardous. While there are some risks, these are not difficult to overcome by taking the precautions suggested. It is important today that our profession should regard informing the public about what we do to prevent and treat disease as a necessary responsibility. It would be helpful if more doctors were trained in the special skills that are required so that they could themselves tell the public what they want to, and need to, know rather than having to leave it to professional reporters and broadcasters to do this for them. If they were trained in these skills their own patients too would probably find it easier to understand what they tell them. Doctors need to be better taught how to communicate both with the public and with their patients.[20]

Doctors are so used to talking about their work using the convenient 'shorthand' of technical jargon that they often find it difficult to write or talk about it in simple terms which will enable lay people to understand them. They forget that simple anatomical or diagnostic terms may have meanings to laymen which are different from those that they have for doctors. Some doctors even feel it beneath them to use simple lay English to describe technical matters, although they are often grateful to those in other specialities who avoid their own specialized jargon and talk simply about their work at medical meetings.

It is usually the role of the reporter in newspaper articles and of the 'anchor-man' in broadcasting to interpret jargon to the laity, but it is much better if the doctor himself can write or speak simply. This requires practice. A good way of preparing for a broadcast is for the doctor to try out what he proposes to say on a layman of the same educational level as that of the audience to which the programme is directed. It is helpful to make a tape recording of what has been said and to assess what the 'audience' would and would not be likely to follow, and then to try out a simplified version if necessary.

In the case of an article for the press a draft should be given to a layman of the kind for whom it is written, to see if he or she finds it interesting and easy to understand.

The simplified version will inevitably be much longer than the jargon version because words like 'mortality', 'epithelium' or metabolism' may require one or more sentences to explain. Even the verb 'to diagnose' may need expanding into a phrase such as 'to find out just what is wrong'. If doctors practise this sort of simple speaking and writing about medical matters they will be fully rewarded by the better understanding their patients will have about the value of the drugs they prescribe for them and the precautions they must take to avoid serious side-effects.

## References


1. Burr, M. L., King, S., Davies, H. E. F. and Pathy, M. S. (1977). The long term effect of discontinuing long-term diuretic therapy in the elderly. *Age and Ageing*, **6,** 38
2. Stewart, R. B. and Cluff, L. E. (1972). A review of medication errors and compliance in ambulant patients. *Clin. Pharmacol. Ther.*, **13,** 463
3. Byrne, P. S. and Long, E. L. (1976). *Doctors Talking to Patients. A Study of the Verbal Behaviour of General Practitioners Consulting in their Surgeries.* (London: HMSO)
4. Ley, P. (1979). Memory for clinical information. *Br. J. Soc. Clin. Psych.*, **18,** 245–55
5. Morris, L. A. and Halpern, J. A. (1979). Effects of written drug information on patient knowledge and compliance: a literature review. *Am. J. Pub. Health.*, **69,** 47–52
6. Eklund, L. H. and Wessling, A. (1976). Evaluation of package enclosures for drug packages. *Lakartidningen*, **73,** 2319–20
7. Institute of Medicine (1979). *Evaluating patient package inserts.* (Washington: National Academy of Sciences).
8. George, C. F., Waters, W. E. and Nicholas, J. A. (1983). Prescription Information Leaflets: a pilot study in general practice. *Br. Med. J.*, **287,** 1193–6
9. Osler, W. (1906). Internal medicine as a vocation. In *Aequanimitas, with other Addresses to Medical Students, Nurses and Practitioners of Medicine.* (London: H. K. Lewis)
10. Hutchinson, R. (1950). Popular health journal. *Br. Med. J.*, **1,** 1942 (Correspondence)
11. Young, M. (1983). The College of Health. *Self Health*, **1,** 3

12. Cartwright, A. (1964). *Human Relations and Hospital Care.* (London: Routledge & Kegan Paul)
13. Asher, R. (1959). The medical education of the patient and the public. In Jones, F. A. (ed.) *Richard Asher Talking Sense*, p. 102. (London: Pitman Medical)
14. Davis, H. and Horobin, G. (1977). *Medical Encounters.* (London: Croom Helm Ltd)
15. Leading Article. (1978). Doctors and television. *Br. Med. J.*, **1,** 348
16. Leading Article. (1978). Television medicine again. *Br. Med. J.*, **1,** 667
17. Sabagh, K. (1978). Television medicine (letter). *Br. Med. J.*, **1,** 713
18. Swann, M. (1978). Television medicine (letter). *Br. Med. J.*, **1,** 1274
19. British Broadcasting Corporation (1976). *The BBC's Medical Programmes and their effects on lay audiences.* (London: BBC Publications, 35, Marylebone High Street)
20. Fletcher, C. M. (1973). *Communication in Medicine.* (Rock Carling Monograph). (London: Nuffield Provincial Hospitals Trust)
21. Oliver, M. F. (1978). Television medicine (letter). *Br. Med. J.*, **1,** 917

# 45
# The journalist

O. GILLIE

## INTRODUCTION

Journalists and doctors have one special thing in common: they are both trained to able to diagnose what is happening in what may be a rapidly changing situation. They both know how to work against the clock in an emergency, and they both work backwards from symptoms to find out what is happening underneath. However the doctor has a great advantage in the battery of scientific tests he can bring to bear on the patient whose co-operation he can generally take for granted.

The journalist cannot assume that the person he must deal with, the 'contact', will be co-operative, and if the contact appears to be co-operative the journalist still has no simple test to tell whether he is telling lies, or, even more difficult to detect, half-truths. If a journalist is able to capture 75% of the truth then he reckons he has done well. If the public relations man manages to conceal 50% of the truth then he feels he has done well. This is far from the 100% truth aimed at by the scientist, albeit in a narrow area.

The journalist, particularly on a national newspaper, has to describe unique and often bizarre events which are likely to be extremely rare, occurring only once in perhaps thousands or millions. It may be a political scandal, murder, drug overdose or the story of one drug in thousands which has some unwanted effect. Here again he has the same problem as the doctor dealing with rare disease. However the journalist has no textbooks to guide him in diagnosing the situation, and must rely on experience built up during his apprenticeship.

## THE ESSENTIAL QUALITIES OF A JOURNALIST

What are the qualities a journalist must acquire to deal with these problems?

Nicholas Tomalin, who worked for *The (London) Sunday Times* before he tragically lost his life in the Yom Kippur war of 1973, has left us an entertaining definition:

> 'The only qualities essential for real success in journalism are rat-like cunning, a plausible manner, and a little literary ability. . . . Other qualities are helpful, but not diagnostic. These include a knack with telephones, trains and petty officials; a good digestion and a steady head; total recall; enough idealism to inspire indignant prose (but not enough to inhibit detached professionalism); a paranoid temperament; an ability to believe passionately in second-rate projects; well-placed relatives; good luck; the willingness to betray, if not friends, acquaintances; a reluctance to understand too much too well (because *tout comprendre c'est tout pardonner* and *tout pardonner* makes dull copy).'

Tomalin captures the essential schizophrenia of journalists who daily face people who may have no wish that the truth be known. Rat-like cunning, a phrase Tomalin admits 'stealing' from another *Sunday Times* journalist Murray Sayle, is necessary in confrontations with uncooperative contacts. The contact may have to be pushed, but not too far, or he may cease to provide any information at all.

People reveal confidential information for all sorts of reasons. They may be angry with a colleague or an institution and want revenge. They may be public-spirited, they may be motivated by moral indignation, or vanity may lead them to wish to influence events. The reporter must attempt to recognize these human characteristics and use them to help him obtain what information he can.

All the common features of human intercourse: politeness, humour, friendship and flattery, are part of the reporter's stock in trade. Ceremony in the form of food and drink may help. And if other methods fail a stern lecture on the citizen's duty to let the truth be known, or the civil servant's responsibility to the taxpayer sometimes, amazingly, helps to obtain information. The cunning reporter uses these instruments, as a surgeon might, in carefully chosen order so that application of one will not interfere with the application of the next.

Tomalin's definition sets out to be entertaining and in so doing, at least in this brief quotation, perhaps distorts the truth. The qualities used by the journalist are no different from those used by everyone every day in their personal lives. The journalist is acutely aware of them because he is using these personal qualities for professional ends. The results of his labour are published and he has to live with his story – it usually becomes evident, days or years later, how much of the truth he managed to obtain.

However, it is misleading to respresent the journalist's occupation simply as that of cynical sleuth. He usually maintains relationships with trusted contacts who he does not betray. He must also be familiar with all the technical resources for obtaining information from libraries, government and commercial resources. The reporter has to know how to get such information quickly. In reporting about drugs for example, he may have to obtain sales figures, demographic data on illness, clinical information about effects of drugs, and advertising material. He has to know how to get all these and also know how to interview patients who have experienced benefits or side-effects. He must then present the facts as a coherent story.

The reporter must also have sufficient background knowledge of a subject so that he can rapidly become familiar with a new technical area and talk to experts with some basic understanding. An increasing proportion of medical journalists now have science degrees, and a few have medical degrees. Some first-rate medical reporters have no university degree at all and have gained their knowledge of the subject through reporting it. This is, of course, an excellent way to learn about a subject and provided the reporter can recognize when he gets out of his depth is not a hazard to the reader. Most medical subjects have sufficient 'human interest' attached to them for a reporter to be able to choose a way of handling a story which is well within his competence.

Formal qualifications in medicine can be a disadvantage, and lead the writer to give too much weight to received medical opinion at the expense of the consumer viewpoint. Familiarity with medical problems may also stifle the apparently naive – but nevertheless important – questions which a journalist must often consider in writing for the general public. For example when oxytocic drugs began to be used on a massive scale to induce childbirth some women began to ask simple but awkward questions. In an epidemic of medical enthusiasm more than 60% of women in some British hospitals were being induced before term during the early 1970s. The risks of this procedure used on so large a scale have only been understood in detail and accepted by many obstetricians following the public outcry which began after articles written in *The Sunday Times* (October 13th and 20th, 1974) by my wife (Louise Panton) and myself. Although the risk of uterine rupture has been known for 20 or more years, the risks of unnecesary premature delivery, of jaundice to the baby and the increase in Caesarian delivery with attendant risks and major discomfort were not appreciated or acknowledged by many obstetricians. Such a procedure may be relatively safe in the hands of a senior man, but have a much higher risk factor if left to juniors, as it must often be in hospitals where 30–60% of all labours are induced.

## THE DISCIPLINES OF JOURNALISM

Like the doctor the journalist is always working under pressure, because it is always possible to spend more time to get a better picture of the situation before committing words to paper. The journalist sometimes follows particular stories for months or years, keeping extensive files, but more often he must finish his story by the end of the day or the end of the week. The journalist needs certain diciplines and ethical guidelines to enable him to work under such pressure.

Reporting ideally entails and enforces disciplines which have been developed to provide the reader with what might be called the best estimate of the facts together with some measure of reliability. These diciplines are evident in the way information is collected and in the way the story is written. One rule is that information should be attributed to its source. The reader can then judge the reliability of the information from his own knowledge or subjective feelings about the source.

This is why it is important wherever possible to publish a doctor's name. If the doctor is misquoted he will complain, the journalist will be castigated by the editor, and the newspaper will be forced to publish a letter.

It is another principle that any error of substance should be corrected at the earliest possible moment. In cases of disagreement readers in Britain may refer to the Press Council whose rulings are published in the newspaper concerned, whether favourable or not. The pressure is thus on the reporter to be accurate. If a source is quoted anonymously then there is no pressure, either on the journalist or the source, to be accurate or cogent. Many people will say things anonymously which they would not say with attribution, not least because they may not be absolutely sure of the facts.

Another basic rule is that anyone who is accused of something should be given the opportunity to reply to the accusation whenever possible before a story is published. The reporter must make every effort to approach the accused party and be sure to publish whatever cogent points are made. Quite often of course a party confronted in this way will admit the facts and as often will supply new information. This may change the whole story or sometimes 'knock it down' as journalists say in office jargon. Interestingly *The Lancet* deliberately does not pursue this policy over reports of drug side-effects. This was discussed in its columns in several letters during 1978 and the editor ruled that drug companies must wait until after publication to reply.

When the reporter has written his story it is examined by a series of editorial executives. The exact procedure varies on different newspapers and in different sections of newspapers, but the basic process involves checks for internal consistency and fairness to all parties referred to in the story as well as legal checks for libel. *The Sunday Times* employs two permanent lawyers and extra part-time lawyers on Friday evenings and Saturdays.

On *The Sunday Times* the procedure for editing news is as follows. The news editor reads the story to check that all the necessary information is there and that all parties have been approached and that the information is presented in a lively and engaging way. Stories are frequently rewritten several times – even by the most senior reporters – before everyone is satisfied. If the news editor is satisfied the story will then be passed on to the manager of home news who makes the final decision whether to put it into the newspaper and if so at what length and with what headline. He will already be expecting the story, which will usually have been discussed at the editorial conference, but only makes his decision about what to put in the paper as the copy becomes available. The editorial conference decides the general policy about what stories should be tackled and what approach should be taken.

The news manager then passes the story on to the chief sub-editor who together with the news manager decides how the story might be cut in length, 'tightened' by elimination of redundant words or paragraphs, or projected in a more lively way. Having decided what to do he may then do it himself or delegate the job to a sub-editor. If the reporter is available the sub-editor will usually check detailed points with him. When the sub-editor has done the job the work is checked by the revise sub-editor before it is sent to be set in type.

The reporter will then check galley proofs for accuracy if he is available, or sometimes check them by having them read over the telephone. Usually this elaborate process has the effect of clarifying awkward points and making the story easier for the reader to understand. Occasionally it can result in the introduction of errors when the reporter is not able to make the final check.

On *The Sunday Times* the reporter is also personally responsible for showing his story to one of the newspaper's lawyers whose job it is to protect the newspaper against libel claims. Stories involving drugs which allege that a company has been slow to act on scientific information, and in effect negligent, are of course potentially libellous and are checked particularly carefully by lawyers. The lawyer is mainly concerned that any statement which might be considered to be libellous can be, if necessary, proved in a court of law. This means that only provable facts may be stated, hearsay evidence is inadvisable, and any implications of corruption or cover-up must be left for the reader to make for himself.

British libel law is much stricter than American Law, and has the effect of making newspapers reluctant to assert foul play unless they are very certain of their facts and are able to prove them. Whether this is good or bad is, of course, arguable. Our libel laws have sometimes had the effect of making a newspaper refrain from publishing an important story because the newspaper was financially in too poor a state to defend itself against a major libel suit.

When it comes to ethics as opposed to law the reporter may also be faced with difficult decisions. Is the reporter ever justified in acting as an *agent provocateur*? To what lengths is it justifiable to tell lies or to adopt some false name or disguise in order to obtain information? It is impossible to answer these questions sensibly without reference to concrete cases because circumstances change judgements. There is, however, an important control on how far a reporter can go in using deception. The reporter should ultimately be able to justify any deception he may use in getting his story, and obtain the sympathy and moral sanction of the reader.

At its best reporting is a tight discipline which presents facts accurately. The reporter's task is comparable with that of the scientist. Both are endeavouring to find a kind of truth and present it clearly. A newspaper story, like a scientific paper, is replete with data; and in its editorial columns a newspaper discusses the data. Scientists exchange other more diffuse types of information at conferences. A newspaper does the same in its gossip columns.

The scientist is usually working on some theory or hunch which may or may not be explicitly stated. Built into the theory are assumptions which may be entirely wrong. At another level the scientist makes value-judgements or tacit assumptions about the sort of problems which are worth tackling, and which small part of the universe he should attempt to explain. Beyond these assumptions are the scientist's motives for his choice which may be deeply personal or simply conditioned by the types of questions which have been asked by his teachers or generations of scientists before him.

A newspaper is committed to exposing certain issues to the public eye – yet it must not degenerate into crude propaganda. It wishes to entertain – yet it must avoid distorting issues or events in doing so. It wishes to inform, but it can never have enough space to give all information – so it must select without misleading. The judgement a journalist brings to these problems is rather like that of the scientist in working out new hypotheses and subject to the same sort of bias.

How, for example, should a newspaper tell its readers of the major dangers to health? How can the public be warned about the dangers of smoking without the newspaper becoming boring by repeating the same old story? A news editor on *The Sunday Times* will almost certainly jump at the opportunity to print a genuinely new story about smoking, but may say that a story about hazards of smoking is familiar, boring health propaganda. He is right because it is much less effective to repeat the old story than to look for new ways to dramatize it.

However, there is an obvious danger that in dramatizing a story the journalist will lose objectivity; but this need not be the case. For example, I wrote a story about Liverpool having the world record for lung cancer as listed in WHO statistics. I wrote this story in *The Sunday Times* the week that Liverpool won the Football League Cup in 1977 (May 31st, 1977) and included a quotation from the captain to the effect that none of the team smoked. All the facts were true and they illustrated a larger truth in a dramatic way.

Some people might criticize this approach because it can be seen as a type of propaganda. However, newspapers make it a point to campaign for causes they believe in and to bring home to the public the facts. In so doing they look for objective data which illustrate the issues for which they are campaigning. Sometimes the basic understanding of the facts which led to the campaign may be mistaken. Journalist may then compound the erroneous diagnosis by selecting facts to support a mistaken campaign, and in so doing spread misunderstanding. Hopefully if this happens readers or other newspapers will take issue and the truth eventually emerge. Exactly the same process occurs in the medical literature when one school of opinion disputes with another.

Nevertheless selection of facts and the dramatization of facts in order to engage the attention of readers is an important source of prejudice in newspapers. One British national newspaper, for example, has published stories about the benefits of smoking because the proprietor, a smoker, believes that smoking is beneficial.

The journalist is afflicted with the same dangers as the scientist in pursuing his own or his editor's prejudices and assumptions and neglecting genuine and important issues. If these are sometimes difficult to spot in the newspaper stories they are more evident in the choice of story.

What, then, are the curious values which make a story news? As Bill Inman, editor of this book, asked me: 'Why do people get excited if one or two of every 100 000 women using the pill die as a result, and not by the incidence of deaths following operations which is often whole numbers per cent? Why have newspapers given so much adverse publicity to pertussis vaccination with the effect that the public may forget the benefits of other vaccinations?'

## THE JUDGEMENT OF NEWS VALUE

Murray Sayle, for some years a feature writer on *The Sunday Times*, is quoted by colleagues as having once said that there are only two kinds of stories. The first he called: 'arrow points to the defective part'; for example, the classic story of how the back door fell off the aeroplane. The second type was: 'we name the guilty men'; for example, the classic story of how the company director took bribes or the doctor prescribed drugs illegally. These may be two principal ingredients of the most sensational newspaper stories, but they are not the mainstay of the news.

The main content of newspaper and TV news is reports of meetings, movements of public figures, announcements by commercial firms, rows over political policy, or other policies from education to medicine, and then there is always the 'human interest story'. It is, of course, impossible to report news straight and unedited. It is usually too long, too complicated, badly written or perhaps wrong.

What is the basis for editorial decisions about which stories are published and which are not; and how do editors decide how much space is given to a subject and the way in which it is presented? These decisions are taken by editorial executives who, unlike reporters, may have little or no direct contact with the source of the story. The reporter is usually concerned about pressing for more space for the stories which he thinks are interesting, whereas editorial executives are concerned about keeping a balance of different types of stories each day or each week. In this they are guided by the discussions they have in daily conference. If an editor has two interesting medical stories then he will not be specially interested in a third. And in any case he may not have a spare reporter with sufficient background knowledge to handle a third. For this reason important stories are sometimes neglected.

The suggestion for a story may come from an editor or from a reporter. Specialist reporters such as medical correspondents are expected to find and develop most of their stories themselves. The specialist usually suggests a story to one of the editorial executives to gauge his interest. In deciding whether a story is interesting an editor wants to know how many people will feel directly involved in the subject matter. The newspaper has a constituency of readers whose votes are expressed in newspaper sales – these votes are never far from an editor's mind, although he may deliberately decide to ignore them and make a big issue of a minority problem. *The Sunday Times* campaign for the thalidomide children was a remarkable example of this (June 27th, 1976). In the early stages of the campaign when the Distillers Company, distributors of thalidomide in Britain, took legal action to prevent publication of the article, *The Sunday Times* kept the issue alive by publishing stories about the children on its front page.

If a story concerns a particular disease the editor will want to know how many people it affects. Cancer and heart disease, because they are the commonest killers, are immediate candidates for a story, provided the story is new. Anything about which it can be said: 'One of the commonest causes of . . . e.g. death in childhood' is a possible story.

Journalists talk about the news value of a story, but this is difficult to define and even more difficult to quantify. Violent death is always considered to be of potential interest to readers especially if it occurs in some sort of situation where the reader may be able to say to himself: 'there but for the grace of God go I'. Rail and air crashes, floods and storms, which insurance contracts call 'Acts of God', are all considered to be prime news material. However an, interesting inverse square law applies to such catastrophes. The farther away a disaster is the more people must be killed for it to be news. One person shot in London is national news. Perhaps ten must be shot in Chicago to have the same impact in London. News editors and the public expect people to be shot in Chicago, and anyway it is statistically more common. And in Chicago itself an ordinary gunshot killing is minor downpage news. A major flood in Britain is national news whether or not anyone has been killed. A flood in India must kill hundreds, possibly thousands, before it is news in London. As everyone knows people die from floods every year in India. We expect it to happen and so its newsworthiness is diminished.

Rare diseases have to be specially interesting to break through the threshold of interest which will get them into newsprint; but certain diseases such as haemophilia, or Huntington's chorea have nevertheless caught the public interest and been the subject of newspaper stories recently. There has been an important change in the way

British newspapers have covered medical stories in the last ten years or so. It used to be thought that the public did not want to know about certain 'unmentionable' diseases such as cancer and multiple sclerosis.

The old *Daily Express* did not carry any stories about cancer although their medical correspondent at the time, James Wilkinson, was specially interested in the subject and wrote a book on it. I was told by another ex-*Daily Express* journalist that his old newspaper would not use the word 'periods' in the weather report because of its taboo meaning and so a sub-editor was especially instructed to change 'sunny periods' into 'sunny spells'. I have not asked *Daily Express* executives if this anecdote is true, as the old newspaper adage goes: the story is too good to check.

*The Sunday Times* has pioneered popular writing about disease in its coverage of multiple sclerosis. I wrote about the controversial treatment with sunflower oil added to the diet (July 1st, 1973), but much more important was an article we published written by Jeremy Saise, an advertising executive, who discovered that he had the disease and wrote movingly about what this meant to him and his family (April 28th, 1974). This succeeded in sparking articles in magazines and items on radio and TV which have made the public much more aware of one of our commonest diseases. It is no longer unmentionable. But now more importantly the publicity has stimulated the Department of Health and Medical Research Council to look for better ways of supporting research in this field.

## The contraceptive Pill

Anything new about the contraceptive Pill is news simply because so many women take it. There are nagging doubts compounded with moralistic worries lying at the back of most people's minds about the sense of taking a pill which alters body chemistry. The one or two deaths reported in newspapers from Coroners' Courts in the early days have proved to be the tip of the iceberg, and in retrospect editors were not wrong to dramatize these reports. Even now we are learning that the Pill was never thoroughly monitored in epidemiological surveys for effect on the fetus, and there is still an important question mark over minor illness such as headaches and allergies caused by the Pill. Editors judged, and I am sure they were right, that the public were just as interested as doctors in details of the first-ever mass medication.

It is impossible to discuss here how individual newspapers have handled particular stories on the Pill. Obviously scare stories which persuade women to give up the Pill suddenly and risk pregnancy cannot be justified. But stories emphasizing the risks of the Pill do not seem so unwarranted now that we learn that a woman aged 35 who took the Pill until she was 45 may have a risk of death of 1 in 1000, over this 10-year period. Many women who started taking the Pill when they were younger are now moving up into this danger age. If I understand the research correctly we still know relatively little about the effects of taking the Pill for periods of 5–10 years or more, and whether certain side-effects may be cumulative. Editors, like scientists, often have to work on hunch, and in this case hunches were not so far wrong.

**Pertussis vaccination**

Why have newspapers given such adverse publicity to pertussis vaccination? The newspaper stories on this subject all originated in a campaign led by Mrs Rosemary Fox who founded the Association of Parents of Vaccine-Damaged Children. Her own daughter was damaged by polio vaccine. She approached newspapers and other media and made out a reasoned case for compensation for children who were damaged as a result of government policy on vaccination. Her case appealed to the press because she had social justice on her side.

*The Sunday Times*, together with other newspapers, particularly the *Daily Mail*, took up her campaign during 1976 and 1977. The *Daily Mail* concentrated largely on presenting heartrending cases of different children damaged by vaccine. I found very little interest in this approach at *The Sunday Times* (*ST*) because we had printed so many similar stories about thalidomide children, and news editors were worried about boring or alienating readers with a never-ending series of such stories.

Instead I decided to look into the evidence for the safety of whooping-cough vaccine which was the vaccine implicated most frequently among the parents in Mrs Fox's Association before publicity may have influenced her membership. I found that the Medical Research Council had no satisfactory data to show safety. In fact their data on safety, such as they were, were widely misquoted in the medical literature. Only a proportion of vaccinees in their trials during the 1950s have been properly followed up to record any subsequent illness, and vaccinees who dropped out before the course was finished were often excluded from the follow-up. There were scant satisfactory data on the incidence of brain damage in the sample investigated in the MRC trials. However it was widely claimed by experts that the MRC trial showed the vaccine to be safe because the trial found no cases of brain damage. Mrs Fox had one case on her books of a boy who was vaccinated during one of these MRC trials and subsequently suffered from brain damage. I wrote about this case to illustrate the defects in the MRC trial (*ST*, May 30th, 1976).

This story showed that the government, through the MRC, had a direct responsibility for children who had been damaged by the vaccine. Regrettably the Department of Health were slow to recognize the justice to the claim for compensation for these children. David Ennals, Secretary of State for Health, defended his policy in the House of Commons on February 8th, 1977, but his briefing was inept, and he made some important errors which aroused further suspicions that the advice given to govenment may not have been thought out with sufficient care. I exposed these errors in *The Sunday Times* (March 6th, 1977).

Vaccination with pertussis fell by about half over the next 2 or 3 years and in the summer of 1978 we had an epidemic with a roughly two-fold increase in the number of cases of pertussis as compared with the last epidemic 4 years before. However, the number of deaths seems to have been reduced as compared with the last epidemic year when there was full uptake of vaccine. It seems as if improved treatment of the disease may have reduced deaths. Alternatively earlier vaccination at 3 instead of 6 months (which was brought in through a rethinking of policy resulting from the campaign) may have provided better protection.

In addition clinics are now being more selective and not vaccinating children with certain histories such as birth trauma, possible brain damage, or severe reaction to the first vaccination. Manufacturers have also altered their vaccine, presumably in order to reduce risks. None of these improvement, would have occurred without newspapers taking up the story. However, it is still not clear whether the benefits of pertussis vaccination justify the risks of damage – research to provide evidence pertinent to this issue is now in progress, but it would never have been undertaken without the publicity. Furthermore the justice of the claims made by vaccine-damaged children against the government has been conceded in principle, and each child will get a minimum of £10 000 compensation. The children have yet to take their claims to the courts.

The whooping cough compensation campaign has caused considerable acrimony among doctors and expert government advisers who understandably resent having their policies publicly challenged. They blame newspapers for scaring the public. However, it would be impossible for a newspaper to take up an issue of this kind if there were not a division of opinion within the profession. Newspapers cannot conjure such issues out of thin air. Here it should be borne in mind that experts advising another government, West Germany, have come to conclusions diametrically opposite to those of our own advisers and recommended abandoning pertussis vaccine for routine use and recommended it only for children living in crowded conditions.

There is a more cogent criticism: why choose one set of handicapped children and campaign for compensation for them while ignoring children who have been handicapped in other ways? There are several reasons. One important one is that damage by vaccines was being minimized by government, the social and financial cost of it was being borne entirely by a few unlucky individuals. If government is forced to accept full responsibility including the cost then it is more likely to be careful about its policy in administering the vaccine. A cynical view, some will say, but it is all too easy to underestimate the human and financial costs of caring for a brain-damaged child when risks and benefits are compared. However, the fundamental reason for giving these children compensation is that they suffered so that all might benefit. The medical maxim: 'First of all do no harm' has been violated in their case, and the public as well as doctors must accept responsibility. Finally, by improving the standard of life of one set of handicapped children a new higher standard is set for all; eventually we may be shamed into giving better provision to all.

## Other stories about drugs

I have written in *The Sunday Times* about dozens of drugs, for a variety of reasons. Most, not all, have been cautionary tales which warn about side-effects. Why, it might be asked, do journalists not write more about the major new developments in therapeutics. The answer is that there have been relatively few in the last decade. During the same period there has, however, been an increasing awareness of the risks of even ordinary drugs such as tranquillizers and aspirin.

Drug companies understandably believe in their products and want to obtain as wide a sale as possible for them. Doctors often complain that the public tries to pressure them into prescribing when it is not necessary. The media have a role here in educating the public about drugs so that patients are able to have a more sensible dialogue with their doctors. To this end organizations such as CURB have been sponsored by the BMA to enlist the help of the press to reduce the use of barbiturates

The press also has an important role in exposing the worst sorts of malpractice perpetrated by drug companies. Here I will only briefly mention the important contribution of Milton Silverman, ex-science editor and writer for the *San Francisco Chronicle*, *Saturday Evening Post*, *Collier's* and *Reader's Digest*, who has shown how international drug companies exaggerate claims for effectiveness of their drugs and gloss over side-effects in order to sell their drugs to the widest possible market in Latin American countries. He does this by comparing claims made for drugs on package inserts distributed with drugs in various parts of South America. His book *The Drugging of the Americas* (Milton Silverman, University of California Press, 1976), shows that the probity of these international drug companies cannot be taken for granted.

Another important role for the press is the monitoring of national drug-regulating agencies. Decisions about whether or not to permit the sale of a particular drug, and under what conditions to permit the sale, are not simply medical decisions. They involve political and commonsense considerations which may be ignored by an agency which takes a narrow scientific approach.

Clioquinol (the best-known brand names being Ciba-Geigy's Enterovioform and Mexaform) has been implicated in Japan as the cause of SMON, a crippling and blinding disease. In Britain sale of the drug continued to be permitted for treatment of diarrhoea after the connection between clioquinol and SMON was discovered in Japan. In the United States the sale of the drug has never been permitted for this purpose because FDA officials questioned its efficacy at an early stage. Despite the appearance of side-effects in animals, reported first in 1929 and later in Japanese people, the official view of the Committee of Safety of Medicines was apparently that no cases of SMON were known in Britain and, therefore, British people were not susceptible to the drug at the recommended dose. No good evidence existed for the efficacy of the drug as a diarrhoea treatment, and there was published evidence of short-term neurological damage in British people and other Europeans who took the drug. However, the CSM argued that even if it was not effective clioquinol was a popularly accepted treatment for diarrhoea and took the view that it should not prevent the public from using such a popular remedy. This ignored the disturbing, but apparently transient neurological, effects of the drug reported in Britain which may have been a more widespread sequel of the drug, usually overlooked because they are attributed to the original illness. *The Sunday Times* supported critics such as Dr Olle Hansson of Gothenberg, Sweden, who argued against the continued sale of such a potentially toxic drug (*ST* May 22nd, July 17th, 1977). The CSM finally acted and put the drug on prescription.

Another case in which *The Sunday Times* took issue with the CSM was over hormone pregnancy tests (May 25th, 1975; April 23rd, 1978). In a front page article in 1975 we pointed out that the sale of these drugs continued to be permitted by the Committee after evidence had been published by Committee experts which showed that they suspected that the drugs might be the cause of birth defects. The Committee's reason for not acting on the report of their own experts was that their scientific evidence concerning the drugs was not complete. Although the risk of damage to the fetus from these drugs is not accepted by many experts today, the risk of abortion as a result of taking these drugs was known in 1975 and has inceasingly been accepted. These drugs were being abused as abortifacients but still many women using HPTs wanted their babies, and nothing was done to warn them of this risk. The Committee's initial decision to do nothing ignored the fact that these drugs were no longer necessary to test for pregnancy since the more reliable slide tests had been introduced several years before. The benefits from such drugs therefore approached zero while there was a strong suspicion of risks. The logic of this was apparently appreciated by the CSM and a decision to withdraw the drugs was taken the following week.

## RELATIONSHIPS WITH EXPERTS

The medical journalist usually obtains his information in the first instance from doctors, scientists or pressure groups. He will often have to obtain more information from companies or from patients in order to complete his story. Often a journalist will approach an expert for information, perhaps because he has read an article by him in a learned journal. Almost always I have found the greatest co-operation under these circumstances.

In other cases an expert or a concerned member of the public may approach a newspaper or an individual journalist with a dossier of information on some matter which he thinks is of public importance. In newspaper slang such a person with inside knowledge is called a 'fink'. The fink is seldom interested in money but rather in exposing an injustice or a public menace. They sometimes supply the kind of information which could never be obtained by an outsider. Others bring information which may be publicly available, but which can only be brought together by years of study devoted to one theme.

Difficulties generally only arise for the journalist in relationships with government officials or commercial companies who naturally want to protect commercial interests, and also to project their view, sometimes regardless of the truth. In the UK there is no Freedom of Information Act and so all sorts of background information which would be available to journalists in the USA or Sweden remains an official secret. Civil servants who reveal such information can in theory be prosecuted and so they are fearful of talking. On one occasion Department of Health officials refused to tell me even in the most general terms what types of food contained the British food colour, brown FK, which had been shown to be mutagenic in the Ames test. They said that this was a commercial secret entrusted to them even though it was potentially available from other sources (*ST*, June 6th, 1976, with Louise Panton).

In the USA government experts and high officials can be directly contacted on the telephone and are usually most friendly and helpful. As a foreign journalist I have arranged to see officials privately without any trouble and have telephoned them from London without problems. Once I tried all morning to get the information I wanted from the UK Department of Health and three UK commercial firms about the cause of a botulism outbreak known to have originated from a tin of infected salmon. This was the first case of botulism in Britain for 20 years and the first caused by tinned food, two of four people affected have died at the time of writing. All UK sources refused to release information which they had, and furthermore denied that they had any fresh information. Rat-like cunning was of no help. However one phone call to the Food and Drug Administration in Washington obtained the information in 20 minutes. The senior medical officer responsible at the Department of Health refused to see me or to talk on the telephone. The refusal of the commercial firms to talk was more understandable since they had to defend their legal position, but they could have provided factual information and need not have refused to admit that any fresh information was available (*ST*, November 20th, 1977).

Major improvements could be made in the UK by making public officials more accessible to the media, and by providing journalists with more detailed background documents. Government Departments also should be much more conservative in agreeing with commercial firms to preserve commercial secrets. Agreement to maintain secrecy should only be conceded to a commercial firm by government departments where its interests in competition with other firms might be damaged. Commercial secrecy should not be used as an excuse for depriving the consumer of relevant information.

Civil servants in government departments regularly meet the representatives of commercial firms to discuss their problems and to ensure that statutory regulations are met. Inevitably these civil servants are exposed to the arguments and the philosophy of these companies. The companies devote a great deal of time and money considering how they can quite properly best influence public officials to their own ends. The professions are also given a full hearing by the same officials who are well versed in their special interests. The experts develop their consensus, whether it be about the labelling of food or the uses of drugs, without knowing what weight to attach to any consumer view which comes their way, if any does. The decisions made behind these closed doors, and the arguments and assumptions which are used, cannot easily be questioned by the public because the background papers are not available to anyone outside government departments.

Yet amid this myriad of technical matters there are issues where public opinion is relevant. For example, everyone is entitled to his or her own opinion on whether he or she would prefer to take a chance of having a baby die of whooping cough or a baby permanently damaged by vaccine. To raise that question does not mean that other more sophisticated statistical questions can be ignored. Everyone is entitled to comment on whether he would like to be able to go on spending money on a medicine which is useless apart from any placebo value and could be positively harmful. Everyone is entitled to an opinion on whether it is a good idea to allow pregnancy tests to be sold when they carry a risk of causing abortion and possibly abnormalities. It is the job of newspapers to put such difficult questions to the public.

Full disclosure of technical information and decision-making is important so that it can be monitored and discussed by non-government technical experts in, for example, universities. These experts would be the first-line monitors who would be able to raise an issue in the media if it became contentious. Only a tiny proportion of the many technical issues considered by government committees could ever be taken up by newspapers. But newspapers are likely to choose those issues which involve points of principle. If a public consensus then develops it may influence future decisions made by technical committees.

In the last 20 years popular writing in science and medicine has changed dramatically. It has moved away from the simple popularization of expert knowledge towards analysis and criticism. Science writing in the spirit of the Huxleys or H. G. Wells was didactic and tended to assume that science was an unqualified force for good. The benefits of science were perhaps more evident then while the dangers of uncurbed pollution, uncontrolled use of drugs were appreciated, if at all, by a tiny minority. Since these dangers are now known, reporting of science cannot be so unqualified and the reporter must also act as the reasoning critic.

# 46
# Consumer organizations

A. HERXHEIMER

---

## INTRODUCTION

If we want to benefit from medicine, we must accept some risks. We first need to consider the risks when deciding whether or not to use the medicine. When we have decided to take the medicine, because the likely benefit sufficiently outweighs the risks, we have to understand how to minimize these risks. The user thus needs two quite separate kinds of information about possible harm: first, a realistic assessment of benefits and risks when the drug is properly used; second, what precautions and circumspections 'proper use' requires. For the first kind of information the user depends entirely on the prescriber, except in the case of self-prescribed drugs for which the pharmacist and the package insert can provide it. Information on dosage, precautions, on what effects to look out for and what to do if unwanted effects occur, should be provided by the prescriber and the pharmacist. Unfortunately, the information given is often insufficient, and what is given is frequently not properly understood and used. So much communication about medicines between professionals and patients is ineffective because many give it a low priority. For example, if writing a prescription is used and accepted as a device for ending a consultation, there will be no time for discussing that medicine with the patient. But the problem does not only lie with the prescriber and the pharmacist. Many patients lack basic notions about how to use medicines sensibly, and need education which cannot be provided in a busy surgery or pharmacy. The ultimate aim must be to have health professionals and patients understand each other's responsibilities in relation to the problems they have to deal with. To achieve that, they must learn to speak a common language, and get used to two-way conversations. Both doctor and patient should be aware of what it is that the patient needs to know about the drug. If the doctor forgets to mention something that is important to the patient, then the patient should know enough to ask him about it.

## THE ROLE OF CONSUMER ORGANIZATIONS

Consumer organizations have an interest in improving communications between health professionals and patients in all possible ways. This includes making doctors,[1] pharmacists and manufacturers more aware of what patients need to know about their medication, as well as teaching patients what important information they need.

A list of questions which patients may wish to ask the doctor about their medicines offers an approach that deserves wide trial.[2] The list has been reproduced in various forms, some simplified and illustrated, in magazines, pamphlets and books,[3] but in Britain no systematic attempt has been made to encourage or evaluate their use. Similar questions were very widely distributed in the USA in 1983: as a part of an 'Ask the Doctor' campaign the Department of Health and Human Services enclosed a leaflet with social security cheques sent to 36 million recipients. An assessment of the effect has not yet been published.

Health professionals have done nothing to encourage the use of such questions. Doctors do not welcome questions which they are not used to answering, and which they may not be able to answer. Pharmacists do want to give patients more advice and information than they have done in the past, but some questions from patients can be answered only by the prescriber, for example: 'Do I really have to take these tablets? What is likely to happen if I don't?' 'Are there any undesirable effects that I should look out for?' Even where the pharmacist could give a helpful answer, he will hesitate to do so for fear of contradicting what the doctor may have said or intended, and so upsetting the doctor-patient relationship. These obstacles need to be overcome by bringing together and harmonizing the information which the patient may get from the doctor, the pharmacist and the manufacturer. Detailed proposals for doing this have been published.[4] The central idea is that for each drug every doctor and pharmacist should have a summary of those points that patients need to know. This could be printed next to or as part of the data sheet for that drug.

Recently consumer organizations have begun to be more active. In September 1984, two 'Know your Medicines' campaigns were launched in South East Asia: in Singapore jointly by the Consumer Association of Singapore (CASE) and the Pharmaceutical Society of Singapore, and in Malaysia by the Federation of Malaysian Consumer Associations (FOMCA). Both are aimed at the community at large, including schoolchildren, and use material in Chinese or Malay as well as English. In the UK the National Consumer Council published useful advice in a book on 'The Patient's Rights in the National Health Service', and consumer magazines and TV programmes have to some extent increased public awareness of the need for more information.

Consumer organizations are also concerned that schoolchildren should learn about the use of medicines in general, and material for this purpose has been developed.[5] In most schools, however, children learn nothing about the subject.

## WRITTEN INFORMATION FOR THE PATIENT

Because patients need much more information than they can reliably remember, written information must be provided about particular treatment problems and about individual drugs. Articles, pamphlets and books on self-care and self-medication have been published by consumer organizations in various countries, but these publications reach only a very small proportion of medicine-users. It would be much better if the necessary information were distributed together with the medicine – then every user would be in a position to use it. The traditional method of doing this is to put as much information as possible on the container, and in some instances to provide a package leaflet. It is now widely accepted that labels can rarely carry sufficient information, and that leaflets are desirable, but there is no general agreement about what kinds of information they should contain, nor how they should be prepared.[6]

Proposals for the minimum information that should be provided about self-prescribed medicines have been made by an international *ad hoc* Working Group of clinical pharmacologists and clinicians,[7] and have been actively supported by the International Organization of Consumer Unions (IOCU). In the USA, the Food and Drug Administration did a great deal of work to produce model package inserts for patients for a wide range of products, and was preparing regulations to make their use mandatory. This programme was stopped by the Reagan administration. The American Medical Association and the US Pharmacopeia have now each published extensive sets of patient medication information (PMI) leaflets for issue to patients, but they are not yet widely used, and their usefulness has not so far been formally assessed. Some pharmaceutical companies are also developing information for patients on their products.

The US National Association of Retired Persons is interested in this area and its participation will be important. Consumer organizations have been little involved, apart from some background work sponsored by IOCU on the information that a leaflet should provide. This proposed that the information content should be determined by the responsibilities that the patient has to assume when he is handed a medicine by the pharmacist.[8] Essentially he or she becomes responsible for taking the medicine correctly, for storing it correctly, for understanding what it is intended to do, and for recognizing problems that it may cause. Items of information that do not help the patient with one of these responsibilities should be excluded from the PMI. Examples were prepared giving information on three different drugs. Various ways of presenting the information need to be tested, to find the format which best enables the patient to understand and act upon the advice given. At that stage health educationists and consumers, as well as pharmacists, can make important contributions; if they are fully involved in working out and testing information packages, then they are likely to encourage their wide use by patients.

Two specific initiatives have been taken. A major campaign about the use and dangers of benzodiazepine tranquillizers and hypnotics was run in 1984 by MIND, the National Association for Mental Health. The campaign was associated with the BBC TV programme 'That's Life', and included the distribution of over 40 000 leaflets with detailed information to people who requested it. The programme also invited viewers to complete a questionnaire about their experience of their own benzodiazepine use, and 2150 of 3000 who asked for a questionnaire did so. An analysis of those questionnnaires has been published by BBC Publications. The Crosby Women's Action Group in Liverpool has been concerned with the use of drugs in pregnancy. Since February 1983 it has campaigned (1) to have warning labels on all medicines which could harm the unborn child; (2) to educate women about potential dangers when they are taking any kind of medicines; and (3) to make doctors more circumspect when prescribing for women of childbearing age.

## INVOLVING PATIENTS IN ADVERSE REACTION REPORTING

The yellow card system has in its first 20 years yielded far fewer reports than might have been hoped. Over 80% of doctors have not contributed a single report.[9] If patients were encouraged to play a part in the reporting of adverse drug reactions (ADRs), the efficiency of the system might be improved. This is especially worth considering for two categories of drugs: those recently introduced, for which the CSM wants reports of *all* suspected reactions; these drugs are identified by a black triangle symbol (▼) in the BNF, MIMS and on data sheets. The second category are products which do not require a prescription and are, therefore, often bought over the counter. The direct reporting of suspected ADRs to the CSM by patients would probably be counterproductive, because such reports would be very difficult to assess and many would be unreliable. However, patients could, and in my view should, be encouraged to consult their doctor or pharmacist if they notice any new symptom or any unexpected effects that develop while they are taking the drug. The *Drug and Therapeutics Bulletin* has produced a card for patients prescribed a 'black-triangle' drug, to encourage them to do this.[10] It seems especially important to give such a card to patients buying terfenadine, the first black-triangle drug available without prescription.[11]

## ADVICE FOR INDIVIDUALS

Many people wonder whether they should really be taking the medicines that have been prescribed for them, for example because they may be against drugs in general, or they do not trust their doctor sufficiently, or because they think the drug may be harming them in some particular way. It often seems difficult to discuss such problems with the doctor, or the nurse or pharmacist who works with the doctor, and people may find it easier to talk about them with someone less involved in their treatment.

In Britain the Community Health Councils (CHCs), the Patients Association and most recently the College of Health are specialized consumer bodies which are presented with such questions. In the Netherlands experimental 'Health' and 'Medicine Shops' were set up in the 1970s to try and answer peoples' questions about health or medicines in an informal way. Although they took great care to co-operate with the patient's own doctor, some doctors nevertheless feared that they would sow discord.[12] It is clear that if doctors, nurses and pharmacists were better at discussing medicines with their patients, the need for alternative discussion partners would disappear; and this would be best in the end.

Some consumer organizations are also, in principle, concerned with cases in which individuals appear to have been harmed by drugs. It is highly desirable that there should be straightforward methods for investigating such cases, and for ensuring that patients who suffer are properly looked after, and if necessary compensated. Beyond that, each case should lead to public discussion of how similar harm can be prevented in the future. The investigation and follow-up of individual cases requires special skills and experience, and is not normally undertaken by national consumer organizations. Some CHCs, the Patients Association and the College of Health in the UK have begun this type of work, but little has been published about it. Many CHCs gave publicity to the practolol syndrome to try to ensure that the patients who had suffered damage from the drug were aware of the compensation offered by ICI and could make claims. The campaign brought to light a significant number of previously unrecognized cases. In this context one should also mention the special associations formed by people who have suffered damage – the parents of children damaged by thalidomide, or by whooping-cough vaccine, the large associations of victims of SMON (subacute myelo-optic neuropathy) in Japan and recently the Opren Action Committee in Britain. Perhaps a national organization with a wider view and greater ability to influence national policies on drugs could usefully take over some of the functions of such narrowly based pressure groups.

## References

1. Anon. Helping the patient to remember what the doctor tells him. *Drug and Therapeutics Bulletin* (1973), **11,** 81
2. Herxheimer, A. (1976). Sharing the responsibilities for treatment. *Lancet*, **2,** 1094
3. In (1980) Leach R. Coping with the system. London: National Extension College and Interaction Inprint; in Shenton, J., Adams, J. A. D., Eds. Drug Injury. (1983). London: Channel 4.
4. Herxheimer, A., Davies, C. (1983). Drug information for patients: bringing together

the messages from prescriber, pharmacist and manufacturer. *J. R. Coll Gen. Practit*, **32,** 93–7

5. Whichcraft (1978). *No.17: Doctor In The Home.* (London: Consumers' Association)
6. *Joint Symposium on Drug Information for Patients* (1977). *Drug Inf. J.*, 11, **(Suppl.)**
7. *Ad. hoc* Working-Group (1977). Minimum information for sensible use of self-prescribed medicines. *Lancet*, **2,** 1027
8. Hermann, F., Herxheimer, A. and Lionel, N. D. W. (1978). Package inserts for prescribed medicines: What minimum information do patients need? *Br. Med. J.*, **2,** 1132

8a. Lacey, R. and Woodward, A. (1985). *The 'That's Life' Survey on Tranquillisers.* (London: BBC)

9. Speirs, C. J., Griffin, J. P., Weber, J. C. P., Glen-Bott, M. and Twomey, C. (1984). *Health Trends*, **16,** 49–52
10. *Drug Ther. Bull.*, (1983), **21,** 93–4
11. *Drug Ther. Bull.*, (1984), **22,** 21–3
12. *Lancet* (1978). **1,** 654

# 47
# The clinical pharmacologist

**F. H. GROSS***

## INTRODUCTION

When in 1970, a WHO Study Group prepared the Technical Report on 'Clinical Pharmacology', the chosen subtitle was 'Scope, Organization, Training', and the functions of the clinical pharmacologist were defined as:

> (1) to improve patient care by promoting the safer and more effective use of drugs; (2) to increase knowledge through research; (3) to pass on knowledge through teaching; and (4) to provide services, e.g. analysis, drug information, and advice on the design of experiments.[1]

At that time, drug monitoring was considered to be one of the services under the heading 'Monitoring of drug usage', where:

> Clinical pharmacologists can fulfil an important service by surveying prescribing patterns and the incidence of adverse reactions. Collaboration between local and international centres may help to minimize delays in recognizing drug toxicity. Clinical pharmacology units also provide trained personnel who can quickly begin an investigation of a suspected adverse reaction.[1]

Such a description of the role that the clinical pharmacologist may play in the process of drug monitoring, although appropriate at the time it was written, meets only in part the major function of clinical pharmacology in the various procedures to be applied to drug monitoring for safety. There are several reasons for this situation, the main ones being the still limited number of well-trained clinical pharmacologists and the relatively few specialized centres which have been established during the past decades.[2] Clinical pharmacologists see only a small number of patients; in addition, they work in a hospital environment, and usually do not monitor drugs under 'natural' conditions.[3]

*Deceased 26th March 1984.

As has been stated recently, serious ADRs or uncommon adverse events, which may occur during a well-accepted therapy, applied already for many years, have been related to drugs not by the toxicologist or the pathologist, nor by the clinical pharmacologist, but by the epidemiologist, who has been called 'the new bearer of bad news'.[14] This does not, of course, exclude the clinical pharmacologist from the group of specialists closely involved in the drug-monitoring process, but his part differs somehow from what has originally been thought to be his major service contribution. With respect to drug safety, the clinical pharmacologist has the most important function: (1) by promoting the safer and more effective use of drugs, by teaching medical students, hospital staff, and practising physicians; (2) by providing all available information about drugs; (3) by surveying drug consumption; and (4) by giving advice to drug control agencies as well as to drug manufacturers.[1] All these activities are related to teaching and to the educational role of the clinical pharmacologist in the evaluation of drugs and their proper use.

## CLINICAL TRIALS

The first administration of a new drug in man and the planning of the various phases of clinical trials, especially phase I and phase II studies (the latter in the form of controlled clinical trials), should always involve the clinical pharmacologist. During these periods, he is the link between the experimental pharmacologist and toxicologist, who have both studied the new drug in various animal species, and the clinical scientist, who is responsible for the first use of a drug in man and later on for the controlled clinical studies. It is important that, during the early studies of a new drug in man, close co-operation is maintained between the clinical pharmacologist and the scientists in the laboratory, since observations in man may necessitate further work in animals, especially pharmacokinetic studies. If the clinical pharmacologist cannot undertake the early human studies himself, he should at least act as adviser to the responsible clinician. It is regrettable that clinical pharmacologists are quite often not consulted during the planning of early human studies, or that they participate only intermittently. This results in errors and omissions, which, in later phases, may be difficult to correct. On the other hand, clinical pharmacologists may not be very interested in doing or planning early studies, because the new drugs are not sufficiently attractive and lack innovation.[5] Most major drug companies have among their staff-members capable clinical pharmacologists, but not infrequently they are too far from medical practice; therefore the plans drawn up by them may be fine in theory, but do not come up to the difficulties of the local conditions in a hospital.

Several drug companies have their own clinical research facilities for early studies in human volunteers, and in most cases these units are run by a clinical pharmacologist. This is an efficient way of getting information about dose-tolerability relationships and pharmacokinetic data, and of comparing the results obtained in animal pharmacology with those observed in human beings. On the other hand, one has to be careful that such a procedure does not lead to the creation of professional drug testers with all its unwanted consequences.[6]

It has been suggested that, in view of the methodological progress made in early drug-evaluation in man, instead of one representative of a new series of drugs, two or three derivatives which have similar pharmacological and toxicological profiles, should be submitted to human studies; these may differ with respect to their therapeutic efficacy in man.[7] Such a comparison of closely related new compounds offers better prospects for the selection of the substance with the best therapeutic potential. However, studies of this kind have to be restricted to a few centres where the necessary know-how is available. Such trials may also be carried out – at least to a certain degree – in a human pharmacology unit within a drug company, but of course no information on the possible therapeutic efficacy can be obtained there.

One of the teaching responsibilities of the clinical pharmacologist is that he informs clinicians and doctors in the pharmaceutical industry – pharmaceutical physicians as they are called today – of the feasibilities of clinical trials: what has to be done, and what can be done for a certain drug under the existing conditions. One of the important pieces of advice to be given relates to the selection of the first dose and the dose increments. Various suggestions have been made for these procedures, but no strict rules can be set in view of the wide variety of drugs, their possible indications, and their use. It is obvious that drugs which are given only once, e.g. as a diagnostic agent or an anaesthetic; those which are administered for a limited period of 1 or 2 weeks, such as antibacterials for acute infections; or those to be used for months or years, such as antidiabetic or antihypertensive drugs, have to be investigated in quite different ways, with respect not only to establishing their efficacy, but also to monitoring their safety.

During the various phases of clinical trials before the marketing of a drug, monitoring for side-effects and for ADRs, done by the clinical pharmacologist himself, under his supervision, or with his advice to the clinicians directly responsible for the patients, is relatively easy because of the limited number and size of the studies. It will, however, not infrequently be hard to decide whether a recorded event is causally related to the administration of the new drug or purely coincidental. The limited number of patients who receive a drug before its marketing, as well as the restricted period of administration, are all inhibiting factors, which are not compensated by the possibilities of a more careful observation and follow-up of the patients. An ADR occurring in 1% of the cases may be a severe health problem if 10 000 people receive the drug, but may pass unobserved if only a few hundred patients are treated with it by different investigators, of whom some may have seen less than, say, 20 patients.

Despite the awareness that ADRs may happen, despite the experiences of the past, when severe side-effects were not discovered during the clinical trials – because they had either been overlooked or had not occurred at all – the possibility that severe adversities may still escape the watching eye of the clinical pharmacologist cannot be excluded. All he can do is to train himself to observe attentively the course of the disease when a new drug is applied, and to teach medical students, hospital physicians, and practising doctors to scrutinize every event during or after the administration of the drug most carefully.

## THE CLINICAL PHARMACOLOGIST AS A TEACHER

The promotion of the safer and more effective use of drugs is the main task that the clinical pharmacologist has to fulfil in relation to drug monitoring. This should begin with the teaching of medical students, but it is a deplorable fact that in most European countries not enough time is available in the curriculum. Furthermore, there are quite often discrepancies between the 'usual' therapy, taught in medicine, and the requirements of the effective and safe use of drugs within the whole treatment plan. Since drugs are easy to prescribe, since patients expect to receive drugs for the cure of their diseases or the relief of symptoms, and since numerous active drugs are available, the closest attention must be paid to them. This is certainly justified in the case of diseases in which a specific drug treatment is possible or where a substitution therapy is indicated, and it may also be valid in chronic diseases, for which there is an effective symptomatic therapy, e.g. in high blood pressure, coronary heart disease, or cardiac failure. There is, however, no doubt that polypharmacy is applied in hospitals and in general practice, and that non-pharmacological treatment is definitely neglected today. The first and most important piece of advice that the clinical pharmacologist has to give in order to improve drug safety therefore is:

(1) To prescribe only the drug(s) really necessary for the treatment of the disease, to keep strictly to the indication, and to avoid, if possible, additional drugs, given mainly to increase comfort; to stay away from polypharmacy and to ask oneself whether giving a second, third, or fourth drug is really indicated.

The opportunity for the clinical pharmacologist to teach and to train depends on the available facilities and the position given to the discipline in medical schools and in continuing education. In most European countries, except Great Britain and Sweden, clinical pharmacology is not included in the curricula of medical students. Despite the fact that the importance of the discipline is continuously emphasized, little is done in practice, and neither the responsible ministerial or university authorities nor the medical faculties have done much to improve this situation. In continuing education programmes, clinical pharmacology is nowadays included, but it is obvious that the majority of practising doctors are scared of being reminded of pharmacology, which they generally remember as one of the least liked disciplines during their studies.

The fact that basic pharmacology is taught in most European countries as a *preclinical* science has the great disadvantage that attempts to emphasize therapeutic aspects face insufficient pathophysiological understanding and clinical experience on the side of the students. Instead of clinical pharmacology being included in the clinical part of the curriculum, therapeutics are left to the clinicians, who of course are competent in practical matters, but cannot provide the theoretical background and the general information that are necessary for the assessment and correct use of new drugs. On the other hand, if clinical pharmacology is taught in the frame of continuing education programmes, the basic knowledge is hard to mediate, since most of the participants left medical school long ago.

## THERAPEUTIC SAFETY

In principle, monitoring for therapeutic safety has to distinguish between predictable and unpredictable events. Predictable consequences of the administration of inappropriate doses include those which are absolutely or relatively too high or too low; neglect of complications, such as impaired renal or liver function, or of the presence of a complicating disease, such as a peptic ulcer in a patient who needs anticoagulants, and the rare cases of increased sensitivity caused by genetic deficiencies, such as the lack of plasma-pseudocholinesterase. Side-effects may be expected according to their known frequency, such as allergic reactions to the pencillins, exanthema caused by sulphonamides or by some anticonvulsants, but here difficulties already exist, when it comes to the more rare granulocytopenic response caused by pyrazolone derivatives.[8] Unwanted reactions may also be part of the pharmaco-dynamic profile of the prescribed drug, but in such cases the association can easily be established and mostly avoided by adjusting the dosage. The difficulty arises with the unpredictable or hardly predictable events, where the frequency is unknown, which may differ in the data available from the literature, or may vary from one country to the other. These differences may be real and the consequence of racial, genetic, or environmental influences, but they may also be caused by various methodological approaches or simply by more careful attention at one centre or in one given country than in some others, or by more shrewd inferences by one observer than by others. Hence, it may be difficult to draw cogent conclusions and make generalized statements. I may recall the agranulocytosis caused by clozapine, seen more frequently in some countries than in others.[9a,b]; the aplastic anaemia caused by chloramphenicol, for which a different incidence has been reported; the occurrence of neurological disorders during prolonged treatment with clioquinol, which, in Japan, has been associated with the syndrome of

SMON (subacute myelo-optic neuropathy); the unexplained higher death rate in a group of subjects with high normal plasma concentration of cholesterol, when treated with clofibrate,[10] many more examples could be quoted. The practical consequence that the clinical pharmacologist has to draw from these observations for his teaching is the following advice:

(2) If in doubt about the tolerability of a drug and the possible occurrence of ADRs, one should not prescribe it, unless it is for vital reasons. If possible, some other drug should be chosen, which causes fewer or less severe ADRs.

In view of the continuous innovation of drugs, the literature which usually accompanies them has to be carefully assessed. This applies not only to the pamphlets written by the manufacturer, but also the papers published in the medical press, which in quite a few instances are not subjected to peer-review. To give the practising physician or the doctor in the hospital some guidance as to how to deal with the pile of printed material, he should be taught how to interpret data put before him and how to apply them to his therapeutic decisions. On the basis of his training in basic pharmacology, he should be able to assess the pharmacodynamic profile and to compare it with those of related drugs. This may not be easy, especially if marginal advantages are over-emphasized or if the presentation tries to hide the similarities.

The clinical pharmacologist may have to decide whether the claimed advantages, with respect either to efficacy, to differences in the pharmacodynamic profile, or to tolerability, are such that the use of the new product should be recommended, or whether it is better to 'wait and see'. Quite recently, it has been suggested that new medicines which do not represent any significant therapeutic advance over available drugs should not be accepted by drug regulatory agencies.[11] Such a requirement may be extremely difficult to comply with and may put expert committees in quite tricky situations, because only in very rare cases do two drugs differ – even if chemically closely related – other than quantitatively from each other; they will do so also in qualitative respects. Furthermore, a 'weak companion' may be preferable to a more powerful drug, especially in symptomatic treatment. Despite the fact that marginal advantages may be of little practical significance for the majority of patients, they may have benefits in selected cases, especially as regards tolerability. For this reason the clinical pharmacologist, besides recommending reservation in prescribing new drugs, should also warn against oversimplifying drug assessment. Exposing patients to unnecessary drugs is as unsuitable as depriving them of medicaments which might be useful to them.

If a drug is of an entirely new type – as at one time were propranolol as a $\beta$-adrenoceptor blocker, sodium cromoglycate as an anti-asthmatic, cimetidine, as an $H_2$-receptor-blocking drug, or allopurinol as a uricostatic – then the clinical pharmacologist has to explain where the drug fits in the armamentarium and what its possible advantages and limitations may be. He must warn of unjustified enthusiasm, recommend reserved use, and avoid an uncritical trial-and-error attitude. The general rule may be the following:

(3) To be conservative and have reservations *vis-à-vis* new drugs which offer only marginal advantages or are nothing but analogues of drugs already available and of satisfactory activity. If a new type of drug treatment becomes available for a so-far well-controllable disease, it is advisable to make use of it only when the established method fails. If, however, a so-far uncovered field may be opened by a new drug, cautious and vigilant application will be the best way to avoid possible harm. The more conservative the attitude towards new drugs, the smaller the risk of provoking severe ADRs.

## DRUG CONSUMPTION

Recently, clinical pharmacologists have become involved in the analysis of drug consumption. The fact that there are national preferences for certain types of treatment and, consequently, for certain drugs has been described by various groups of authors, but little is known of the reasons for such differences, which may be quite remarkable and often lack a scientific basis. Why is digitoxin the preferred digitalis drug in Norway, whereas, in Sweden, it is digoxin,[12] what is the reason for the preference of reserpine-diuretic combinations in the treatment of high blood pressure in Germany and Finland whereas in Great Britain, methyldopa is still one of the leading drugs; why is the consumption of antibiotics lower in Germany than in Great Britain, where also tricyclic antidepressants are prescribed more widely than in Germany? This list of national or even local preferences could easily be extended, but what is completely unknown is how these different types of drug treatment affect the course and the outcome of the disease.

Here the clinical pharmacologist should try to prepare a more solid basis for the use of certain drugs and to find out the reasons that have resulted in favouring or neglecting a medicine. He should also make use of such examples in teaching therapeutics; should point out to advanced medical students, as well as in continuing education, the numerous facets that drug therapy has; and should make clear that it may be dangerous to make absolute claims for one or the other drug or mode of treatment. At first sight, such complexity may confuse the student; a skilful teacher will demonstrate these differences in a way which helps clarify the principles of drug treatment instead of obscuring them.

## THE TEACHING OF PHARMACOKINETICS

Medical students and doctors in hospitals, and in practice, have problems in understanding pharmacokinetics. The student, when he receives his training in this field, has not yet had sufficient contact with clinical problems to appreciate the importance of the topic. He has not seen a case of digitalis overdosage or the appearance of toxic reactions with apparently correct doses of an aminoglycoside antibiotic in a patient with renal failure, and he has not seen bleeding induced by drug interaction with an anticoagulant. He hears of bioavailability studies and the use of plasma concentrations for measuring the degree of absorption, but he does not fully realize their practical significance, for example when a less expensive generic product may be ineffective, and ultimately more costly, because of poor bioavailability. Medical students have difficulty in applying the general principles of pharmacokinetics to individual drugs. This is even more so with practising physicians, who, despite the best intentions, lack insight into the various ways in which the human organism may handle a drug. Terms such as 'biological half-life', 'drug distribution', 'distribution volume', or the various possibilities of metabolizing and excreting a drug are ill understood.

One example of providing too detailed information of little practical importance is the extensive listing of possible drug interactions. Only a few of them are of clinical relevance, such as the competition for plasma protein-binding between oral anticoagulants and sulphonylureas with antidiabetic activity or phenylbutazone. Drug interactions have attracted too much interest, and too much has been published about data which are of theoretical, but not of practical significance. It may be stated that:

(4) Pharmacokinetic data are of substantial practical importance for effective and safe use of drugs. They are, however, nothing but aids in the assessment of correct dosage and treatment. Of the numerous possible drug interactions, only a few are of practical significance and will affect prescribing. Such data should be provided by drug manufacturers for new, as well as established drugs.

## TEACHING IN DRUG MONITORING

Although the clinical pharmacologist can play an active part in the process of drug monitoring, this will be an exception. In most cases he will play an auxiliary role, mainly in the assessment of a possible association between the administration of a drug and the occurrence of an adverse event. However, in his function as a teacher, he should instruct doctors to watch the course of a disease carefully and to consider every possible association between an unexpected event and the use of a drug. He should also warn against unjustified drug hysteria and of being overcautious and suspicious of drugs.

Modern methods of data processing are of great significance in monitoring for safety, and the clinical pharmacologist has to know how to make the best use of them.

He has to work closely with others, especially epidemiologists, who, today, make even more important contributions to drug monitoring and post-marketing surveillance of drugs. Drug epidemiology is a rapidly developing branch of monitoring for safety and efficacy of drugs, particularly postmarketing surveillance.

## THE INFORMATION OF DRUG CONTROL AGENCIES

The process of drug regulation varies from country to country. The larger organizations have clinical pharmacologists among their staff or at least doctors who had some training in this discipline, and they will also profit from the knowledge of expert advisers. Governments should make sure that clinical pharmacology is established as a discipline in their countries.

In the WHO Report on Clinical Pharmacology[1] it was stated that 'when difficult decisions have to be made, it is desirable that responsibility be shared with independent advisers rather than being borne by one or two government officials'. It would be profitable if regulatory agencies, especially if they have no trained clinical pharmacologists among their staff, invited them as consultants.

## CONCLUSIONS

In conclusion, then, the clinical pharmacologist, besides being a specialist in certain areas of drug research, has to fulfil a most important task by teaching and training medical students in basic principles of therapeutics; he has to provide information on new drugs and on those already available; and he has to draw attention to the principles of drug monitoring. In the course of continuing education programmes, practical advice for the monitoring of therapeutic efficacy and safety will be the most important contribution that he can make. If the clinical pharmacologist also succeeds in curbing the number of prescribed drugs and in eliminating polypharmacy, he will contribute much to a better and safer drug treatment. He should act as a consultant and adviser to the DRAs and try to complement regulatory decisions regarding the release, surveillance, or withdrawal of drugs.

### References

1. *Clinical Pharmacology; Scope, Organization, Training*. Report of a WHO Study Group. WHO Technical Report Series No. 446, Geneva, 1970

2. Gross, F. (1978). The thorny path of clinical pharmacology. *Clin. Pharmacol. Ther.*, **24,** 383
3. Lasagna, L. (1974). A plea for the 'naturalistic' study of medicines. *Eur. J. Clin. Pharmacol.*, **7,** 153
4. Crout, J. R. (1978). *The Nature of Regulatory Choices.* The Center for the Study of Drug Development, University of Rochester Medical Center, Rochester, NY. Publication Series No. 7812
5. Dollery, C. T. and Bennett, P. N. (1975). Clinical trials. *Br. J. Clin. Pharmacol.*, **2,** 479
6. Hassar, M., Pocelinko, R., Weintraub, M., Nelson, D., Thomas, G. and Lasagna, L. (1977). Free-living volunteer's motivations and attitudes toward pharmacologic studies in man. *Clin. Pharmacol. Ther.*, **21,** 515
7. Dollery, C. (1978). Problems of clinical assessment of new therapeutic agents. In *Triangle for Progress in Therapy* pp. 63–68. Plenary Meeting, Merck, Sharp & Dohme International, Medical Advisory Council, Paris, May 1977. (Rahway, NJ: Merck & Co., Inc.)
8. Dausset, J. and Barge, A. (1967). Anaemia, leucopenia, and thrombocytopenia due to drug allergy: The importance of cross-reactions. In Wolstenholme, G. and Porter, R. (eds.) *Drug Responses in Man.* pp. 91–105. (A Ciba Foundation Volume), (London: Churchill Ltd)

9a. Idänpään-Heikkilä, J., Alhava, E., Olkinuora, M. and Palva, I. P. (1977). Agranulocytosis during treatment with clozapine. *Eur. J. Clin. Pharmacol.*, **11,** 193

9b. Anderman, B. and Griffith, R. W. (1977). Clozapine-induced agranulocytosis: a situation report up to August 1976. *Eur. J. Clin. Pharmacol.*, **11,** 199

10. Report from the Committee of Principal Investigators (1978). A co-operative trial in the primary prevention of ischaemic heart disease using clofibrate. *Br. Heart J.*, **40,** 1069
11. Clarke, Sir Cyril (1979). Can medical practice be free of risk? *J. R. Soc. Med.*, **72,** 35
12. Lunde, P. K. M. (1976). Differences in national drug-prescribing patterns. In *Clinical Pharmacological Evaluation in Drug Control.* Report on a Symposium. Deidesheim, November 11th–14th, 1975 (Regional Office for Europe, WHO, Copenhagen), pp. 19–47 (IC/SQP 004)

# 48
# The pharmaceutical industry and the drug regulatory authorities

B. W. CROMIE and M. SLATER

---

## INTRODUCTION

The safety of medicines cannot be considered in isolation, as there is no such thing as absolute safety in an effective medicine. Safety can only be assessed in relation to efficacy. Every effective medicine has a balance of benefit to risk and anybody taking or prescribing a medicine, to obtain the anticipated benefit, must recognize and accept the concomitant risk of an adverse effect.

While accepting that this balance holds true for both new and established medicines, research for new drugs must continue. For diseases with existing treatments, new medicines will be needed to improve the therapeutic ratio or to overcome bacterial resistance that has developed. In addition, the Workshop of European Clinical Pharmacologists has stressed that: 'There remains a large number of diseases for which new drugs are needed as urgently as ever and advances will be achieved only if research and development are actively encouraged.[1]

It is against this background of a need for new medicines and the balance of benefit to risk for every medicine, that the responsibilities of the pharmaceutical industry and the regulatory authorities must be surveyed.

## PHARMACEUTICAL INDUSTRY

The pharmaceutical industry exists to invent, manufacture and make available medicines, and to have a profitable business with a return on the investment of its shareholders. The industry has to bear responsibility for the safety of its products. However, many of its attitudes and actions, in relation to drug safety, are influenced by drug regulatory authorities (DRAs) and by other government activities, such as the black-listing of certain prescription medicines so that they can no longer be prescribed in the UK.

It is difficult to study any aspect in isolation, but each function of the industry will be considered in turn.

## Innovation

The most striking advances in drug therapy come from breakthroughs, e.g. sodium cromoglycate and cimetidine, which completely replace previous therapies, but these are rare occurrences. The steady improvement comes from the introduction of new medicines which have a better therapeutic ratio (greater effectiveness/lesser risk of adverse reaction) than existing remedies. Although medicines tend to be compared for their average effect in test populations, it is not necessary for the new medicine to have a better average effect for it to be an advance in therapy; if it provides a more effective or safer alternative for individual patients this can be a major contribution.

Virtually all medicinal therapeutic advances in recent years have come from innovative research by the world's pharmaceutical industry. Unfortunately, this source of improved new medicines is now at risk.[2]

Due to increased regulatory requirements, the percentage of the pharmaceutical industry's research and development budget devoted to innovation is decreasing,[3] and the analysis for one major company demonstrated a trend that, if continued as a straight line, would bring all innovative research to an end by 1990.[4]

Apart from the burden of regulatory requirements, the total environment is no longer conducive to innovative research. The cumulative effects of price controls, WHO 'lists', no-fault liability, discriminatory post-marketing surveillance, low returns on high-risk research investment,[3,5] public antagonism and the threat of nationalization[4] and compulsory generic substitution has tended to push the pharmaceutical industry away from innovative research into safer, less risky areas, such as drug reformulation, licensing and diversification.

In addition to these general pressures against research, there are now deterrents in selected therapeutic areas. The UK government has introduced generic substitution and limited lists of prescribable medicines in certain therapeutic categories, including analgesics and anti-anxiety agents. It is to be expected that this will dissuade companies, for which the UK is an important market, from conducting research in those therapeutic areas.

A further problem is that of patent-life erosion. Walker and Prentis[6] have shown (Figure 1) that the average effective patent life for newly introduced New Chemical Entities (NCEs) in the UK is under 9 years

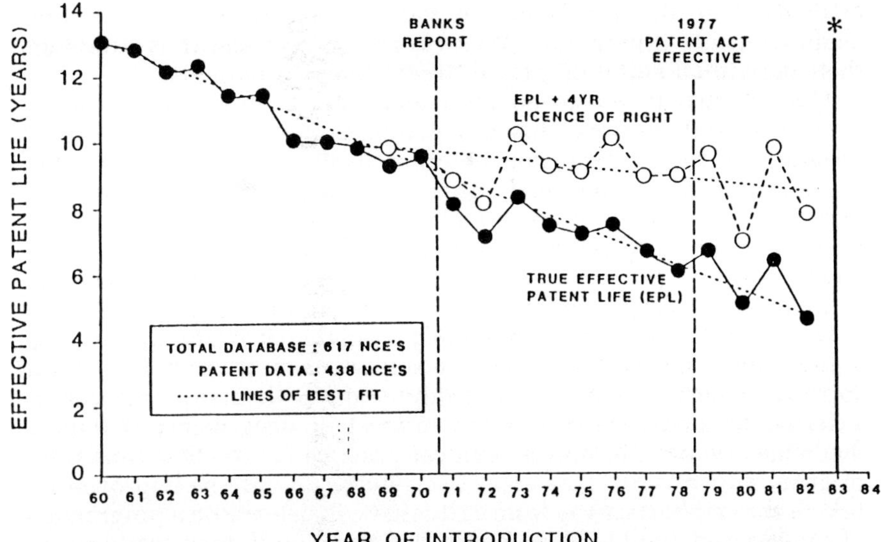


**Figure 1:** The erosion of effective patent life (1960–1982),* From this point the new chemical entities marketed with the full 20-year patent term will influence the slope of the true effective patent life line

Reproduced from Walker, S. R. and Prentis, R. A. Reference 6 with permission from the Pharmaceutical Journal vol 234, p. 12

and decreasing. With the general extension of generic prescribing in some form, the duration of patent life is increasingly important and the industry should oppose any measures which reduce residual patent life even further. It is inconceivable that safety testing should be conducted under pressure, and yet the longer the safety or surveillance before full marketing the shorter the residual patent life. The only way of ensuring that all safety and surveillance studies are carried out in an unhurried way for full patent protection is to have a reasonable period of patent protection starting with licensing approval or for a similar period of 'exclusivity', as has been suggested in EEC draft directives,[7] and as has been implemented in the USA by the Drug Price Competition and Patent Term Restoration Act of 1984.

## Realistic trials

It is the responsibility of the pharmaceutical industry to test its new medicines and assess their safety and efficacy under realistic conditions of clinical practice. Unfortunately, many DRA pressures tend to push clinical trials in the opposite direction.

Some authorities, though not all, automatically demand trials against placebos, which may be useful to test the sensitivity of trial methods, but do not have the value of comparisons of active medications, to differentiate their characteristics and thus establish their individual suitability for different types of patients.

There is also an overwhelming demand for so much double-blind, controlled trial data that this may dominate the clinical development programme, to the exclusion of other useful clinical testing. This inevitably leads to the main pre-marketing usage being limited to experimental studies by expert physicians on homogenous populations, with informed consent, careful supervision, a constant environment and exclusion of other common external factors such as medicines that might complicate the 'pure' results of therapy.[8]

Once a medicine is made generally available, it is administered to sub-groups that may not have been exposed to it before, with capricious compliance and in conjunction with many and varied external factors. It is not in the interest of drug safety that new medicines be used in normal clinical practice for the first time with minimal supervision. This aspect of safety can only be improved by taking the emphasis away from a ritualistic insistence on a programme of randomized, double-blind, controlled trials (with their well-known shortcomings)[9] or by shortening the whole regulatory procedure and substituting a period of Phase IV 'real-life' supervized usage.

However, to add any form of post-marketing surveillance as an extra phase, without other changes, would only increase the drug-lag, with disastrous consequences.[10] Therefore, it becomes crucial to restructure the entire approach to drug evaluation, so as to provide the really important information without excessively time-consuming and burdensome requirements.

## Improved therapy

The pharmaceutical industry can also contribute to safety by aiding compliance and by providing optimum formulations.

Compliance can be improved by modifying the size, shape or coating of the medication or by altering the flavour or concentration of liquids. It can also be improved by special calendar-type or blister packs, which are easy to carry and which make it easy to see if a tablet has been forgotten. Of course, such advantages are only obtained if the tablets are dispensed in their original packs which have also been tested for stability, and allow instructions and basic information to be seen whenever the medicine is taken, and not transferred from bulk containers into a pharmacist's bottle.

Compliance can also be improved by combination tablets, which reduce the number of medicaments that have to be remembered, although the official view of combinations is rather less pragmatic.[11]

Drug safety may also be improved by modifying the formulation, to decrease gut irritation, to aid absorption or to alter the bioavailability in order to produce more consistent or more appropriate blood levels.

The work undertaken to obtain such improvements tends to be dismissed as 'mere reformulation' work, and can be lost completely if generic prescribing or substitution takes place.[12] Advances in formulation should not be minimized; they can be significant contributions to overall drug safety. Another way of improving therapy is to search for formulations or congeners whose pharmacokinetic profile favours increased compliance, e.g. once daily rather than more frequent medication.

## Surveillance

The pharmaceutical industry has an obligation to report world-wide information which it receives on adverse reactions, but must do so accurately, so that it differentiates between confirmed, substantiated reports and those which are not substantiated.

The industry must also be prepared to follow up all reports of adverse reactions, and to encourage prescribing doctors to report any new or significant side-effects they might observe.

There is a danger, however, that an unwitting stress upon side-effects will discourage the necessary use of medicaments, so it is important that side-effects be put always in the context of the disease being treated and the benefit obtained. It is also important to separate side-effects related to the therapeutic action of the drug, and which may have arisen from inaccurate dosing or undue patient sensitivity, from unrelated reactions or from variations in the pattern of the disease being treated. Finally, the number of reported side-effects must be considered in the light of overall usage to get some idea of the percentage incidence.

These aspects must be considered in any Phase IV studies or post-marketing surveillance (PMS) systems that are undertaken.[5,13] The industry has a duty to co-operate with schemes which are practical and realistic, but to resist any ideas that will not contribute to safety but merely increase drug-lag and create further barriers against innovation.

## Identification and withdrawal

Medicines that cannot be identified are dangerous. Patients must know what medicines they are taking, so that they can report benefit or side-effects. Medicines must also be identifiable in cases of overdosage or when patients move from one medical attendant to another.[14]

This can best be achieved by ensuring that medicines are always dispensed in their original packs, with the name clearly shown. This original pack will also have a batch number and the date marked, so that it is possible to withdraw a defective batch or even total supplies of a medicine from the market right down to the level of the final consumer.

Experience has shown[15] that adverse reactions can occur from excipients and apparently inactive ingredients such as fillers, colouring agents and the like. These agents will vary between different manufacturers of medicines available from different sources, so it is imperative that sources are known when reporting adverse reactions. With generic prescribing and substitution this becomes almost impossible, unless original pack dispensing is mandatory with all details of the ingredients and source on the pack.

## Education

Current trends show that innovative research to find improved medicines is steadily decreasing,[4] and that patients are being deprived of the useful medicines already discovered.[10]

This danger to the development of further safe and effective medicines is clear for all to see, but it is most obvious to the pharmaceutical industry, which is at the heart of the matter.

The industry has a responsibility to improve drug safety. If it accepts this responsibility, it will not quietly abandon innovative research and move into generic sales or non-pharmaceutical diversification, but will fight against counter-productive legislation and against unreasonable regulatory demands and requests. In order to achieve this, the industry must try to educate DRAs, politicians and the public.

DRA requirements continue to increase and few older tests have been removed, however invalid they may now appear. All such tests of doubtful relevance should be challenged to slow down the exponential growth of regulatory requirements.[4]

Apart from formal requirements there are increasing requests for additional data. These include efficacy studies on indications for which approval has not been requested, informal systems of PMS or extra toxicological studies, carcinogenicity tests or similar work. It often appears easier to comply with the informal request from a DRA member handling a submission than to risk an adverse recommendation. By quietly accepting an extra load, the industry encourages the move away from innovation and, thus, the patient is deprived. The industry must, therefore, educate DRAs by challenging requests for unreasonable extra work and by explaining the challenge at appeals or hearings.

The industry must also educate the public and politicians about the fact that increasing drug-lag may allow large numbers of people to suffer unnecessarily.[4,10] As the European Clinical Pharmacologists' Group has noted, 'a balance must be found between the benefits of prolonged studies of safety and the possible deprivation of patients'.[1] The public must realize that deprivation of new medicines will increase as innovative research is blocked; and the public must finally recognize that all medicines have risks, which must be accepted if patients want the benefits. The educative role could be accomplished if everybody understood the slogan on a popular paperback about medicines: 'To get relief, you must take some risk'.[14]

## DRUG REGULATORY AUTHORITIES

DRAs have an overall responsibility to do more good than harm. Their goal should be to maximize the public good, and not simply to pursue politically expedient courses to cope with pressures from emotive but often uninformed pressure groups, whether from the public, from minority interests, from politicians, from the pharmaceutical industry or from the medical profession.

The recognition of the DRAs responsibility has been apparent in one DRAs defence of its performance relating to drug-lag,[16] its articles on 'Why our drug laws need to be changed,[17] and the US Drug Regulation Reform Act of 1978.[18]

It is worth listing the main points of this Act as stated by the then Health, Education and Welfare Secretary:

*To* get valuable new drugs on the market as rapidly as possible without compromizing safety requirements.
*To* permit more rapid removal from the market of drugs posing unacceptably high risks.
*To* make publicly available the experimental data on which drug approvals are based, thus ending the secrecy that has surrounded the approvals of new drugs.
*To* require monitoring and reporting of dangerous side-effects of drugs after they are on the market and to expand the powers of the Food and Drug Administration to deal with other problems that arise after drugs are on the market.
*To* provide patients with more information about the drugs that are prescribed for them.
*To* make drug regulation more rational and understandable by setting forth the clear standard that safety is always a relative matter – that using any drug always presents some risks that have to be weighed in the light of benefits.
*To* stimulate drug innovation and research.
*To* foster competition in the drug industry.
*To* create new jobs for American workers and markets for American drug producers by relaxing the rules for overseas sales of drugs.
*To* expand the FDAs enforcement powers but, at the same time, impose fairer standards of compliance on the drug industry.
*To* end abuses in the promotion and advertizing of drugs.
*To* focus attention and resources on the drug sciences through the creation of a National Center for Clinical Pharmacology.
*To* make drug regulation more uniform by ending arbitrary regulatory distinctions based on type of drug or date of development.

Since this was formulated, there have been changes in the US health administration, and major changes have been ordered to the FDAs management and administration of new drug application review by the new Secretary of Health and Human Services.[19] At the same time, the US Commission on the Federal Drug Approval Process issued a report which recommended: 'clearance of Investigational New Drug (IND) clinical studies by non-FDA Outside Review Boards, more use of external advisers, simplification and clarification of IND and New Drug Approval (NDA) requirements, improved relationships with the industry, revision of the review process and other measures designed to streamline and shorten the approval process'. These FDA recommendations, which have now been implemented as the February 22, 1985 revision of the New Drug and Antibiotic Regulations, should also facilitate drug approval solely on the basis of foreign data.[20]

It has been estimated by the FDA that the more efficient review procedure which reduces the approval time by 2 months for 15 therapeutically significant applications each year, could result in about 500 000 additional prescriptions in their first year of marketing.

## Patient deprivation

The time between the first publication about a drug and its marketing is now about 10 years in the UK, with a trend towards a steadily increasing time requirement.[4,6]

In the USA the period was greater,[10,16] and the President's Biomedical Research Panel[21] concluded that the delays and costs of the FDAs protective systems constituted a hazard to public health. The number of people that may have died unnecessarily because of the drug-lag varies according to different authorities, from a quarter of a million[22] to 10 000 a year[10] for the delays in beta-blockers alone in the USA.

Whatever country is involved, DRAs have a responsibility to balance benefit to risk, and not to delay drug introduction because of bureacratic, political or other reasons unconnected with proven safety tests or clinical experience.

In order to live up to these responsibilities, DRAs must try to achieve two main objectives:

(1) The first is to conduct their activities under impartial medical and scientific disciplines and remain unmoved by political considerations or media campaigns.

In the UK this is largely achieved by ensuring that decisions are taken by part-time expert committees of clinicians and academics who are not exposed to political, public or commercial pressure. There is a risk that any increase in the volume of data will make the part-time members more dependent on summaries by the licensing authority secretariat, but the basic protection from external influences remains.

In the USA there is no such protection. The FDA is regularly and frequently exposed to public and political examination. This occurs, in part, because there is no divided responsibility between external assessors and government implementation, and the officials have to fulfil both functions.[23] In keeping with this omnipotent role, it is important to have personnel of the highest calibre, and this is probably easier with part-time committees than with full-time government employees, where budgetary restraints may make it difficult to retain the services of the most able personnel.

(2) The second objective is to evaluate all regulatory requirements and discard those of unproven validity.

The UK now asks for tests which, *in toto*, take over 20 years to perform; the curve of increase in the test load is exponential so that, at the present rate, the total duration will approach infinity within 10 years.[4] Despite the fact that these tests have 'developed arbitrarily and by casual accretion,[1] and authoritative doubts on their value have been expressed,[22] no single significant reduction has been made in the total test requirements for new product approval and the growth continues. Even a leading member of the UK advisory committee to the DRA has gone on record as saying: 'What the authority must attempt is to prevent the uncontrolled growth of bureaucracy, the demands for endless dotting of i's and crossing of t's in toxicology . . .'.[24]

In the UK, however, there have been advances in recent years as the DRA recognized the shift by multinational companies towards performing early clinical studies abroad as a consequence of the inordinate requirement for pre-clinical data.[25] The requirements had previously been allowed to grow to the stage where the preclinical data needed in the UK, before the first administration of a new drug to the first patient, were sufficient in some other advanced countries for the full marketing approval application to be granted. Recognition of this fact led to the introduction of a new clinical trial exemption procedure (the CTX procedure).[26] This scheme enables pre-clinical data to be generated and submitted, in summary form, as clinical trials proceed and expand. It thereby allows an early assessment of a drug's potential in man, before the expensive and time-consuming full set of pre-clinical data has been produced. The new procedure was greeted with great enthusiasm by the industry and also seems popular with the DRA.[27] To date, there appear to have been no problems of unacceptable toxicity in man, and it is to be hoped that this pragmatic trend will be adopted by other DRAs.

## Innovation

Some DRAs have, directly or indirectly, accepted a responsibility to encourage innovation and to encourage the availability of new agents with an acceptable benefit to risk ratio, good examples being the US Orphan Drug Act of 1982 and the Drug Price Competition and Patent Term Restoration Act of 1984.

Despite this responsibility, DRAs (and other official organizations) suggest and implement many changes which might appear sensible in isolation but which, taken together, alter the environment for innovation so that commercial pharmaceutical companies are less likely to invest capital and effort in new drug discovery and development. Included in these measures are Good Laboratory Practice (GLP), Standards for Institutional Review Boards, Obligations for Clinical Investigators, requests for clinical trials in conditions where companies are not seeking approval and discriminatory systems of partial release or PMS.

When these are added to the limited list of allowed medicines in some categories, the regulatory workload already described and the additional requirements which are informally suggested as being necessary, innovation is no longer encouraged, but stifled.[28]

## Sensible response

For every medicine under investigation or in general use, there will be a mass of reports from research workers or clinicians. DRAs have a duty to respond sensibly to these various reports and to evaluate each in the context of the probable balance of benefit to risk in man.

Nevertheless, there is a tendency to accept toxicological findings in species that handle the drug differently from man and where the doses used probably overload the detoxifying mechanisms, even though such results can have little or no validity for routine clinical use. As stated by the Royal Society study group:

> 'Great efforts are made in 'toxicity testing' of new chemicals and drugs, with expenditure in the region of £50 million per annum in the UK alone. This activity tends, however, to be diverted into a sterile routine exposure of many animals, without attention to mechanisms. Only if mechanisms are understood is it possible to extrapolate toxicity measurements across species and from the larger doses used in experimental animals to the exposures experienced by man, commonly a thousand-fold smaller.'[24]

Despite this, cyclamates were banned and chloroform restricted in many countries and saccharin held in disrepute, on just such evidence, even though this last had been widely used in diabetics for decades, and any tendency towards the bladder cancers seen in animals would undoubtedly have been detected in such a closely supervized group of patients.

## Scope of involvement

DRAs have an accepted responsibility to consider the evidence on new medicines submitted to them and to make a judgement on the balance of benefit to risk which they feel is in the public interest. They come to this decision by their own expertise and that of external experts whose opinions they request.

However, there is now a tendency for some DRAs to seek wider involvement in drug research and in therapeutics. It is questionable whether such increased participation in non-regulatory aspects of science and medicine is socially wise.

It is also desirable that DRAs limit their involvement to a scientific study of the issues raised. On many occasions, minority groups raise issues which highlight an isolated aspect of toxicity or hazard, which are magnified by the media to the extent that public pressure eventually interferes with normal clinical practice and the good use of medicines.[29] When such things happen, the DRA should come out into the open and publicly put the issue into a realistic context. In this way, there should be a gradual education of the public, to the eventual benefit of all.

## References

1. Weatherall, M. *et al.* (1977). Towards a more rational regulation of the development of new medicines. *Eur. J. Clin. Pharmacol.*, **11,** 233
2. Steward, F. and Wibberley, G. (1980). Drug innovation – what's slowing it down? *Nature*, **284,** 118
3. Thesing, J. (1977). *Drug Research in the Pharmaceutical Industry.* (Frankfurt: MPS)
4. Cromie, B. W. (1978). *Medicines for the Year 2000.* (London: OHE Symposium)
5. Schwartzman, D. (1975). *American Enterprise.* (Washington DC: Institute of Public Policy Research)
6. Walker, S. R. and Prentis, R. A. (1985). Drug Research and Pharmaceutical Patents. *Pharm. J.*, (5th Jan.) 11
7. Council of the European Communities. (1984). Proposal for a Council Directive Amending Directive 65/65/EEC – Relating to Proprietary Medicinal Products COM (84) 437. *Official Journal*, **27,** (C293), 43
8. Lasagna, L. (1978). *Why Study Drug Usage in Medical Practice?* (Paris: Masson)
9. Cromie, B. W. (1963). The feet of clay of the double-blind trial. *Lancet*, **2,** 994
10. Wardell, W. M. (1978). A close inspection of the 'calm look'. *J. Am. Med. Assoc.*, **239,** 2004
11. WHO. (1977). The Selection of Essential Drugs. *Report of WHO Expert Committee. Technical Report Series, 615* (Geneva: World Health Organization).
12. Editorial. (1981). First substitution-linked death raises major issues. *Pharm. J.*, **227,** 482
13. Remington, R. D. (1978). *Post-Marketing Surveillance. A Comparison of Methods PS 7811.* (Rochester NY: The Centre for the Study of Drug Development)
14. Laurence, D. R. and Black, J. W. (1978). *The Medicines You Take.* (London: Fontana Books)
15. Napke, E. and Stevens, D. G. H. (1984). Excipients and additives: Hidden hazards in drug products and in product substitution. *Can. Med. Assoc. J.*, **131,** 1449
16. Kennedy, D. (1978). A calm look at drug-lag. *J. Am. Med. Assoc.*, **239,** 423
17. Kennedy, D. (1978). Why our drug laws need to be changed. *Science*, **18,** 11
18. Califano, J. (1978). Drug Regulations Reform Act of 1978. *H.E.W. News*, 16th March (Washington)
19. Editorial. (1982). NDA changes ordered and proposed. *Scrip. Nos.* 690 and 691, 13
20. Budiansky, S. (1982). FDA regulations. Saving time, but carefully. *Nature*, **298,** 598
21. President's Biomedical Research Panel (1976). The place of biochemical science in medicine and the state of science. Appendix A. *US Department of H.E.W. Publication No.* (OS) 76–50, 19, 21 and 236

22. James, B. G. (1977). *The Future of the Multinational Pharmaceutical Industry to 1990.* (London: ABPI 102, 103 and 148)
23. Long-Term Toxic Effects. *Final Report of a Royal Society Study Group.* July, 1978. (London: The Royal Society)
24. Grahame-Smith, D. G. (1981). Problems facing a regulatory authority. In Cavalla, J. F. (ed.) *Risk-Benefit Analysis in Drug Research.* pp. 51–61. (Lancaster: MTP Press.
25. Cromie, B. W. (1980). Testing new medicines in the U.K. *J. R. Soc. Med.*, **73,** 379–80
26. Griffin, J. P. and Long, J. R. (1981). New procedures affecting the conduct of clinical trials in the United Kingdom. *Br. Med. J.*, **283,** 477–9
27. Griffin, J. P. and Stewart, A. G. (1982). Six months' experience of new procedures affecting the conduct of clinical trials in the United Kingdom. *Br. J. Clin. Pharmacol.*, **13,** 253–5
28. May, M. S., Wardell, W. M. and Lasagna, L. (1983). New drug development during and after a period of regulatory change. Clinical research activity and major United States pharmaceutical firms, 1958 to 1979. *Clin. Pharmacol. Ther.*, **33,** 691
29. Lock, S. (1981). The influence of the media. In Cavalla, J. F. (ed.) *Risk-Benefit Analysis in Drug Research.* pp. 163–70. (Lancaster: MTP Press)

# 49
# Communications with the UK drug regulatory authorities

E. L. HARRIS

## INTRODUCTION

I will examine the requirements for good communication of the United Kingdom's Drug Regulatory Authority, henceforth referred to as the 'UK Centre'. This Centre comprises the staff of the Medicines Division of the Department of Health and Social Security who act on behalf of Health Ministers as the Licensing Authority as well as the various advisory bodies that have been established to assist with the implementation of the Medicines Act 1968. The total internal staff comprises some 230 and, surprisingly, the outside independent consultant advisers number almost 300.

The statutory advisory bodies are the Medicines Commission and four Section 4 committees – namely the Committee on Safety of Medicines, the Committee on the Review of Medicines, the British Pharmacopoeia Commission and the Committee on Dental and Surgical Materials. These committees have a total of 29 sub-committees as well as various *ad hoc* working parties. With such numbers of distinguished experts in particular fields there is a considerable problem in achieving a degree of consistency within the UK's overall philosophy on medicines' control. In order to achieve this staff spend a considerable amount of time on liaison between committees.

Figure 1 is a simplified diagram of the structure and main communication network of the UK Centre. It should be noted that the sub-committees dealing with anti-microbial substances, herbal products, anti-rheumatic agents and psychotropics have completed their tasks and have been disbanded. In 1982 the sub-committee on Toxicity, Clinical Trials and Therapeutic Efficacy and the sub-committee on Adverse Reactions to Drugs were amalgamated to form a new, enlarged Committee on Safety, Efficacy and Adverse Reactions (SEAR).

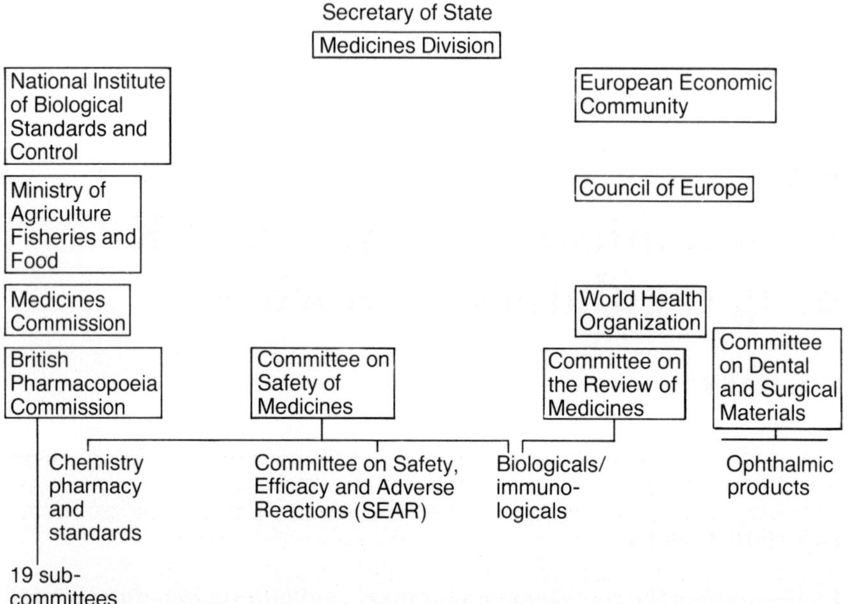


**Figure 1** Simplified advisory communication network of Medicines Division

When the officials and experts agree on the need for action, further steps are required. These may be simple or may involve consultation and preparation of a submission in order to secure Ministerial approval. In addition, the UK Centre must collaborate with other divisions of the DHSS, and other government departments such as the Home Office, the Department of Trade and Industry and the Department of Prices and Consumer Protection. As it is a UK Centre all the health departments, the Scottish, Welsh and Northern Ireland offices, must be consulted and kept informed. Similarly, when issues covering animal as well as human health are raised, the Ministry of Agriculture, Fisheries and Food are consulted.

Another element that has been added in recent years is membership of the European Community. Apart from adopted directives, two pharmaceutical directives came into effect in November 1976 with the aim of harmonizing the control of medicines in member states. Representation of the UK on the Pharmaceutical Committee and Committee on Proprietary Medicinal Products and of its working parties has required careful verbal and written communications. The interpretation of directives and translation of documents has presented problems.

Regular communication with international bodies such as the World Health Organization, the Council of Europe and other drug-regulatory authorities is maintained. The World Health Organization sponsors a biennial meeting of the Drug Regulatory Authorities (The International Conference of Drug Regulatory Authorities).

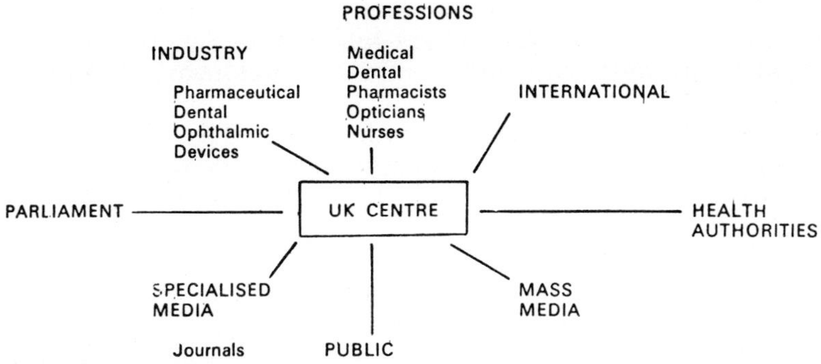


**Figure 2** UK Centre's main communications

The UK Centre communicates with a number of major groups. These are shown in Figure 2. They include Parliament; industry, in the form of trade associations; and over 800 individual companies which vary from small organizations producing one or two minor remedies to major multinationals; the professional groups – doctors, dentists, pharmacists, nurses, ophthalmic opticians, herbalists and many others. Contacts must also be maintained with the Royal Colleges and a wide variety of associations; the health authorities at all levels; specialized media such as scientific journals; the mass media; and last but certainly not least the general public. Communications with the public are often indirect, filtered through the professions or the media, but there is also direct contact through correspondence. Linked with the public interest is included Parliament, for Members of Parliament often take up individual cases or causes through correspondence with the UK Centre or in Parliamentary questions. Any of these consultations with the groups mentioned above can be arduous.

## OBJECTIVES

The Centre's prime objective in any communication is to project a message in such a way that it is understood and acted upon in the way intended. Secondary objectives include:

(a) To avoid premature disclosure by the mass media before the professions are informed.
(b) To avoid distortion and sensationalization of the message which would cause unneccessary public anxiety.
(c) To make appropriate use of its own information.
(d) To persuade the outside world to understand where the responsibility lies in any particular issue.

On a subject involving the public, for example child safety containers, the UK Centre may have to consult with several hundred companies, organizations and individuals before determining the final advice which is to be given to Ministers. This process often involves two or three rounds of consultation letters followed by lengthy correspondence and meetings with individuals and organizations who have specific queries or objections.

However, despite efforts to involve all interested parties, cases occur where aggrieved organizations or individuals claim that they have not been consulted. Every effort is made to identify those who should be consulted before regulations or any proposals are circulated, but because of the wide range of interests that may fall within the scope of the Medicines Act, some organizations may be left out inadvertently, because their interest in the particular subject, or even their existence, is not known to us. On one occasion, a copy of a consultation document went astray in the post and the organization concerned became convinced that there was some Machiavellian plot to exclude it from consultation. In fact, it is very much in the Centre's interests to ensure full consultation at the formative stage of policy; indeed in certain instances the need for consultation is written into the Medicines Act, and failure to do so may invalidate legislation.

## RELATIONS WITH THE MEDIA

Medicines are news; although on the whole co-operation by the media has been good and has been of great assistance in dealing with particular problems, difficulties have arisen. The UK Centre is fortunate in having professional advice from the DHSS Press Office; however, not all problems can be anticipated or forestalled. The main difficulty is that to make a 'good story' the media may sensationalize certain aspects and inject an unncessary sense of urgency into a situation. Their handling of the story on high-dose oestrogen contraceptives illustrates some of these points.

In the late 1960s there was some concern about the growing incidence of thromboembolism amongst women using oral contraceptives containing high levels of oestrogen. The Committee on Safety of Drugs (CSD) (predecessor of the present Committee on Safety of Medicines) had been alerted to this problem by its ADR reporting system, and decided to issue a warning to alert doctors to the possible hazard although it was not in a position to publish detailed findings for scientific scrutiny. Letters were posted to the profession, but unfortunately there was a 'leak' of information to the press before these had reached all doctors. Sensational newspaper stories told of a major new risk. In fact there was no new risk. The CSD was merely advising on how to reduce an already known small risk.

In the event hundreds of women were panicked into discontinuing the use of the pill, and doctors, confronted by a rush of anxious patients, reacted with justifiable anger. The CSD's secretariat had to deal with a stream of telephone calls and letters of complaint. Angry reactions also came from the pharmaceutical companies manufacturing oral contraceptives, who not unnaturally feared that the stories in the press would seriously damage their sales of oral contraceptives. This event demonstrates how the message became distorted leading to unnecessary anxiety, frustration, anger and – most important of all – the risk of unwanted pregnancies. This particular episode also suggests a general failure to appreciate the purpose of the UK Centre's early-warning system. The warning letter was issued prior to the publication of the full scientific data, indeed before the data had been fully analysed so that doctors would be aware of the hazard as early as possible. However, both the professions and industry demanded to see all the evidence, which at that stage was available only in preliminary form. Obviously early alerts can lead to the criticism that such action has been precipitate, but the alternative may be even less acceptable. In the case in point, many women would have continued to be at greater risk if they had remained on the high-dose oestrogen preparations.

Although one of the Centre's objectives is to avoid premature disclosure of information by the media before doctors have been informed, in some instances this is unavoidable. The drug 'Opren' (benoxaprofen) for example, posed a particular problem to the Regulatory Authority.

Early in 1981, the Committee on Safety of Medicines became increasingly concerned about the drug's safety because of the large number of reports of photosensitivity associated with it, and also reports of adverse gastrointestinal reactions. In 1982, the number of adverse reports increased significantly, this time with reports of fatal cases of liver and renal damage, both from the UK and abroad. By August 1982, the Committee had received over 3500 reports including 61 fatal cases. A decision to suspend the product licence was taken. At the time this decision was made, between one and two fatalities were reported each week. This incidence, together with the incidence of non-fatal but serious reactions, forced the decision to be made to issue through the media a statement about the suspension of the licence. This decision was taken with the knowledge that a number of medical practitioners would be aggrieved because they received the news of the withdrawal via the media rather than by a letter from the Chairman of the Committee on Safety of Medicines. His letter had to be printed and mailed, and in fact took up to 5 days to reach remotely situated practitioners.

## EXTERNAL COMMUNICATIONS

The main methods of external communication have been outlined in Chapter 1. Warnings in the Adverse Reactions Series are reserved for the most serious situations, in order to avoid diluting their impact. They are sent to all doctors and pharmacists individually, and also to the press to ensure wide coverage in the medical and professional journals. Where there is less urgency, papers may be published in medical journals and the relevant committee may issue a statement. This has the advantage of drawing attention to the published evidence. An example of this was the paper by Inman and Mushin (1974) on the hazards of repeated exposure to halothane. When this was published the CSM issued a statement drawing attention to its implications. Unexpected opposition came from a number of anaesthetists, but some of the most vocal critics subsequently published papers confirming the validity of the advice which had been given.

The UK Centre is constantly exploring new methods of communication, and in 1975 started an occasional series of leaflets called 'Current Problems' with the main object of giving early notice of potential problems for which no definite conclusion could be reached. In the second issue, for example, explanatory notes were given to help avoid confusion caused by the introduction of a number of new insulin preparations.

Another medium for disseminating information is through the Annual Report of the Medicines Commission and the various committees. Although the readership is limited it is a useful way of putting out a range of information on all the year's major activities.

A further method of communicating information to interested bodies is through *MAIL – the Medicines Act Information Letter* – which is distributed quarterly to all licence-holders and organizations which are normally consulted. Its function is to update and interpret the regulations, summarize new developments and give brief notes about any current consultation documents.

Finally, there is the series of 'Medicines Act Leaflets', commonly known as MALs. These give detailed information (mainly for the benefit of industry) on various aspects of the Act. One of them. 'MAL 99', explained the broad arrangements for the control of medicines in the UK, and this has been particularly popular. Other leaflets advise on how different types of licence applications should be set out and what accompanying data should be submitted, and give notes for guidance on labelling, data sheets and other requirements.

It is important to ensure that messages reach their target and that they are read, understood and acted upon. Mailing lists cannot always be kept up to date, and some doctors seek to keep their names off general lists in order to avoid being bombarded with advertising literature. Recently we conducted a small survey to see how many doctors received – or more importantly, remembered receiving – Current Problems; from a random sample of 500 practising doctors the figure was only 50%.

Communications must be geared to the knowledge, background and interest, and needs of the recipients. This was well illustrated when action had to be taken to prohibit the illegal importation and retail sale of a baby tonic containing lead. As this preparation was promoted to the Asian community it was necessary through their specialized press and through the broadcasts in Asian language programmes to alert mothers of the hazard.

Communication is not confined to the printed word. A great deal of time is spent by the staff in interviewing individuals from the professions and the industry. Radio or television interviews are given by chairmen of committees or by the staff, and all those involved regularly give lectures or participate at local, national and international meetings.

In November 1984 a viewdata pilot scheme commenced in which 500 general practitioners and 20 pharmaceutical companies who already have a computer terminal will be able to report adverse drug reactions to the Drug Regulatory Authority's central computer. These reports will be added to the Committee on Safety of Medicine's data base of reaction reports, and the reporting doctors will be able to receive a tabulated breakdown of reactions on generic drugs held in the computer. It will also be possible for the secretariat or the Committee on Safety of Medicines to send messages to the participating doctors and companies.

If this pilot scheme is successful then it is planned to be extended widely.

# 50 The pharmaceutical medical director

J. MARKS

## INTRODUCTION

Doctor or druggist, politician or patient, manufacturing mogul or media monger; all now accept the need for appropriate full communication of the truth about drugs. But this broad acceptance of the merit of full communication was not the situation a mere 25 years ago. It required a shattering tragedy like thalidomide to overcome all the prejudices and vested interests about the available information about drugs. There are, however, still differences of opinion about what constitutes 'the truth' – an aspect that will be considered later and to whom communications should be made.

The views expressed in this chapter are personal. Though based in part on my experience in a leading company in the pharmaceutical industry and broadly representing their views, no single person can represent the views of the industry in general. The pharmaceutical industry is not a uniform group. At one end of the scale there are the major multinational companies whose very existence is based upon a large annual research expenditure, the products derived from which are made available only through the medical profession – the so-called 'ethical' companies. At the other end of the scale there are the companies, the majority with an equally responsible attitude, who develop and sell special nostrums direct to the patient – the 'proprietary' section of the industry. Between these extremes are the companies, international or local, large or small, that undertake little or no research, but sell the standard preparations that represent the major share of total drug consumption through doctors, pharmacists, supermarkets and even 'street market mammies'.

But even if the industry were itself uniform, an internationally acceptable industry view could not be expressed, for there are major differences between national attitudes to drugs based both on differences in laws, governments and resources and on the personalities and customs of the people. The sophisticated interchange of information which is feasible in Manchester, Munich or Manhattan, is impossible for example in the mountains of Peru, Papua New Guinea or Puerto Rica.

This is, therefore, a personal view based on experience in practical therapeutics, in research, marketing and management in the pharmaceutical industry and in academia. Hopefully the views will stimulate thought and suggest fresh ideas about the subject.

## THE TRUTH, THE WHOLE TRUTH . . .

While there is a need for full communication of accurate drug information, it is often difficult to arrive at the 'truth' about adverse drug reactions (ADRs) as others in this book have also indicated. The prime information may be inaccurate, investigation may be slipshod and interpretation fallacious. In an unpublished study I conducted a few years ago I found a considerable measure of inaccuracy in coroner's verdicts on drug overdose cases even when autopsies had been performed. In several cases only one drug was quoted in the verdict where more than one had been taken simultaneously or large quantities of alcohol had been drunk; the wrong name of the drug was recorded; major concomitant pathology had been ignored.

Worry about the accuracy of information that is available puts a strain on all those connected with the problem. Not least is this true of the medical director of the company concerned, who has the duty of protecting the public, but at the same time should present the product in the most reasonable medical light, by providing valid information, both in favour of and against the substance. This problem becomes even more difficult when a possible adverse reaction is suspected but unproven. The medical director has to balance the importance of issuing an adequate warning against the commercial disadvantages to the company that result from a false and unnecessary warning. This dilemma can never be removed entirely, but the situation can be helped by careful and accurate investigation, as detailed elsewhere in this book. It can also be helped when it is possible to have good informal communication with the drug regulatory authority, a matter I shall consider later.

When a company records or reports ADRs it should differentiate between substantiated and unsubstantiated cases. To this end it is important for companies to encourage doctors to report any suspected reaction to them and then to follow them up diligently. A recent retrograde factor, at least in the United Kingdom, has been for doctors to refuse to discuss suspected reactions with the company. It is distressing to see that certain sections of WHO also appear to be unwilling to discuss adverse drug reaction information in an open and scientific fashion.

The most important single factor in good and useful communication however is to determine the true, factual information. Equally, however, there will be better appreciation of the validity of the information if it is recognized and accepted that drug benefits carry concomitant risks.

## COMMUNICATION WITH THE MEDICAL PROFESSION AND PARAMEDICALS

Surveys have shown that the medical profession relies heavily on the pharmaceutical industry for its information about drugs, and it behoves industry to maintain its record of providing accurate information that the profession respects.

Communication between the pharmaceutical industry and the medical profession, paramedicals and pharmacists is of two types: the on-going general advice about marketed drugs, and the occasional urgent warnings about proven or suspected adverse reactions.

Few would dissent from the view that in a free economy, the general information about their drugs should be provided by industry. The present restriction on expenditure imposed by the UK government is to be deprecated because it is bound to restrict the information which is supplied.

The regulatory authority must have a general responsibility for the accuracy of the material presented, but this should, in my opinion, be by statutory guidelines and not by state control of individual communications. Bureaucratic *executive* control slows down the whole process of communication, produces frustrations and increases costs. Moreover it is important to accept that industry has the responsibility for its own products. The executive responsibility for the accuracy of individual communication should be defined within statutory guidelines, and controlled either by the regulatory authority or by a powerful trade association. Of the two there are advantages in favour of administrative control from the regulatory authority. Within the company the executive responsibility will normally lie with the medical director. He must have access to all the relevant information collected by the company and by the health authorities, and all communications from the company should be passed at proof stage by him. He must be fully aware of his responsibility, but whether the medical director should be liable to criminal rather than civil charges in the event of negligence must be a matter of dispute. In most cases civil liability is probably an adequate safeguard.

The information disseminated by the company must always present a balanced view. The company, operating within a free economy, must sell its products to make a level of profit which is adequate to service the development of the company, maintain its research and provide adequate return on the invested capital. On the other hand there must be adequate safeguards to ensure that marketing enthusiasm does not lead to loss of balance in presentation. It is difficult to ensure that a balanced case is presented, and I believe that reasoned governmental persuasion is better than statutory regulation. Control by decree must, by its very nature, attempt to be all-embracing and can in consequence take little or no account of variation in need. Thus it often leads to a proliferation in warnings. These are not only wasteful but even positively dangerous, for the greater the mass of material the less is it likely to be read, and the greater the number of warnings the less are they likely to be heeded. I know of no evidence that the extensive regulations of the United States authorities have produced better practical therapeutics than the less rigid situation in most countries in Europe. Whether a sensible co-operative relationship can be achieved worldwide must remain a matter of conjecture. At present there are wide variations between different countries and little evidence of rationalization.

This ongoing information can be made available by mailings, by representatives and in package inserts in drug containers. The compendia issued either by the individual companies, by the pharmaceutical manufacturers association, or by the health authorities are important sources of information. The difficulty is to keep such publications sufficiently up-to-date.

While there is every need to ensure that all the published material is accurate, there remains the more difficult problem of trying to ensure that doctors consult the material. Examination of published official lists of ADRs reveals that the vast majority are well recognized and adequately described in the company's literature. Many ADRs might be avoided if the information was not ignored. It is difficult to see how a better level of readership can be achieved.

Several surveys have indicated that the pharmaceutical company's representatives are major sources of information for doctors. If representatives are such an important source of information and a large stimulus to drug usage, it is necessary to ensure that the information that they provide is reliable. Their great merit lies in the fact that their information should be current. Their great disadvantage is that it is almost impossible to make sure that they give a balanced and reliable presentation of the facts, rather than a biased view designed to sell the company's products. Control by legislation is virtually impossible and no satisfactory control system has yet been found. The current British rule, that at each interview the representative should make available on request the officially approved information sheet which the doctor may keep, may help to reduce abuse. However, the greatest measure of control lies with the medical profession itself. The industry realizes that the representatives are only cost-effective if they are accepted by the profession, and the profession should insist upon high standards of information.

I have made no comment about the place of journal advertising in the dissemination of information. In recent years the amount of information that must be given in journal advertisements has been increased, and this has perhaps been most marked in the United States. I have doubts about the wisdom of this requirement. Advertisements in journals should be regarded as reminders of the product names rather than as a source of prescribing information, and the presence of a mass of small-print information may be counterproductive. Journal advertisements are important to the medical profession not only because of the information that they contain, but from the fact that the revenue contributes substantially to the ability of the publishers of medical journals to make them available at an economic price, thus opening up an additional source of information to the profession. If the requirements become too irksome the revenue may well be reduced. The government restrictions on expenditure in the UK have already resulted in a substantial reduction in advertising and the demise of several medical journals that formed useful sources of information to practitioners.

All the above comments mainly apply to 'ethical' products. In the case of ongoing information on preparations that are sold direct to the public without prescription, it would be desirable in a Utopian society for the medical and paramedical professions to be informed of developments, but in our present less than ideal society this is not possible, and it is better that only urgent warnings are communicated to the profession in the hope that these will be heeded.

While I believe, as I have explained, that the dissemination of current information should largely rest with the industry, there is a different requirement in the case of urgent warnings about toxicity. The authorities have a greater responsibility here to ensure that the information is presented accurately, adequately and appropriately. Where a good relationship can be established between the industry and regulatory authority (see below), the form of the warning and the method of communication should be agreed between them. Where the danger lies with one product only, I believe that there are distinct advantages if the warning is actually transmitted by the company involved. On the other hand, when there is a problem that concerns a group of drugs, then communication can be made most appropriately by the regulatory authority jointly with industry.

I would stress again that the wording of such warnings and the form in which they are transmitted must be considered with great care. In a few instances the information may be adequate for dogmatic conclusions about a causal relationship at the time of the warning, but in most instances it is likely, and indeed correct, that an early warning be given when the information is suggestive but still inconclusive. It is important to ensure that the extent of the evidence is clearly stated, to avoid confusion, and that the phrasing be such that unnecessary worry is not occasioned to patients. The recent activity by the Health Authorities in the UK on the possible toxicity of the non-steroidal anti-inflammatory agents falls far short of this ideal. This is a great pity, for I previously had nothing but praise for the warning policy and practices of the United Kingdom's Drug Regulatory Authority. The practices in some other countries have in my opinion not reached a similar high standard.

One of the problems of information that occasions a lot of concern and still requires a solution is that of different therapeutic claims, dosages and warnings in different countries. There are logical reasons, such as different weights, metabolic patterns and dietary habits, why dosages may vary from one country to another, but there are no logical reasons why the therapeutic indications and warnings should so differ. This could theoretically be solved by the adoption of an international single drug regulatory authority which would cover such aspects for all countries. Unfortunately at the present time this would be a hopeless solution as anybody who has experienced the working of international bodies like the United Nations Organization or the World Health Organization will readily testify. Not only will political considerations weigh more heavily than medical or scientific but like a convoy, it will move at the speed of the slowest.

It is rational and realistic for a multinational pharmaceutical company to want to bring its information into line throughout all the countries in which the compound is available. This reduces both errors and costs. However, differences in therapeutic claims and warnings are usually the result of different demands from the different regulatory authorities, and until this can be solved such differences are likely to persist. It may perhaps be appropriate to stress that such differences are rarely the fault of the industry as many consumerists claim.

## COMMUNICATION WITH DRUG REGULATORY AUTHORITIES

Good communication between industry and the regulatory authority is a vital component of the successful monitoring of ADRs. This should be based on mutual respect for professional status and integrity, and informality in discussion of the medical problems involved. This implies that good communication is likely to exist when the maximum effort is placed on each side on professional competence and the minimum on bureaucracy and authoritarianism.

There must be ready acceptance that both sides have the same basic objectives, namely the availability of good pharmaceutical products, supported by adequate information and with an acceptably low level of adverse effects relative to the therapeutic target. This is stressed by Harris in Chapter 49. There must be mutual understanding about the problems that each has to solve, and a desire to reach the best solution in the minimum time. There may be advantages if there is a considerable known measure of independence between the medical officers of the regulatory authority who are concerned with the study of adverse effects and those concerned with legislative aspects.

Within this framework of mutual respect and confidence and indeed forming an integral part of it, there should be full, early and accurate interchange of information, which leads to discussion of the significance of the findings. I cannot stress too strongly that the informal professional exchange within the United Kingdom pioneered by Sir Derrick Dunlop in the days when the control of pharmaceutical marketing was based on a voluntary system and continued under Sir John Butterfield, has helped to produce a good communication system, which has not been achieved in some countries where a more formal system exists. Whether it is realistic to believe that such 'gentlemen's agreements' are feasible in other countries must be a matter of debate, but this in no way alters my opinion about the merits of such an arrangement, and it is sad that informality is reduced now in the UK.

It is clear that such mutual confidence does not currently exist in some countries. In some of these there are demands from the authorities for increasing data with no rational or scientific basis. One aspect of the communication process in these circumstances detailed by Cromie and Slater (Chapter 48) is that of educating the drug regulatory authority. I agree with the views that they express, and particularly that a reasoned challenge should be made against unreasonable extra work.

## COMMUNICATION WITH MEDICAL JOURNALS

Medical journals have a responsibility to try to provide accurate information and, in the case of drugs, to maintain a balance between the good and the bad aspects. To achieve this, good two-way flow of information is essential. In the past communication was not always good, and there was often mutual suspicion. The current situation appears to be better, but there is still room for further improvement.

The situation will be improved when every journal has a good, firm and independent editor backed by the editorial board. It must be accepted that major advertisers may unfortunately exert an influence on editorial boards in some countries and this must be accepted as a fact of life, however much it is deprecated.

Deliberate distortion luckily appears to be unusual, and a greater problem is the quotation of information, either inaccurately or out of context. This occurs all too commonly in the reporting of ADRs where, for example, one report is quoted with variable accuracy from one journal to another. It is often clear that the original report has not been read by successive authors. There is thus a need for the editorial staff to cross-check the information it proposes to publish, and consultation with the medical staff of the company and the medical staff of the drug regulatory authority should be aspects of this. The responsibility of the medical adviser of the company is never to try to suppress the information, but to try to ensure that the information given is accurate and presented in perspective, and a similar duty exists within the health authority. Hopefully journal editors, company medical officers and health authorities are now all acting with the same objectives.

## COMMUNICATION WITH THE LAY MEDIA

Whether we like it or not, we must accept that dramatic drug effects, good or bad, have news value and are, therefore, likely to be carried by the lay media – see also Chapters 44 and 45. The role of the media however, is not only to inform, but to present the information in such a way that it has news value, a result that is often achieved by dramatization. In the drug area they can act as a power for good or evil: for good, when the public is made aware of an important problem and appropriate action is taken: for bad, when an unnecessarily dramatic story about toxicity leads to considerable worry among those who are receiving therapy.

There is now a greater tendency for the media to contact manufacturers to check the story, but unfortunately in some cases a slanted version of the manufacturer's comment eventually appears. Since drugs are news, it is essential that pharmaceutical companies pay attention to their communication with the lay media, not only in terms of the method of communication, but also the material that is supplied. Co-operation with the lay press is more likely to lead to accurate reporting than is an 'ostrich-like' attitude. How far the industry should go out of its way to seek lay publicity is a matter of considerable dispute. Each case should be considered on its merits. Expert advice can be invaluable, and the services of a good public relations consultant or press adviser are very desirable, though the ultimate decision about the contact and its form should be made by the company on the basis of the advice that it receives.

So far as possible, information should not be given to the lay media unless and until it has been given to doctors and pharmacists. It is annoying for doctors to learn about therapy via their patients from the lay press rather than through the proper channels. It is rare that sudden and dramatic instances of ADRs occur, and for lay press comment to appear before doctors are notified is an admission of poor communication on the part of the company.

## COMMUNICATION WITH OTHER INTERESTED GROUPS

Among the groups that should be mentioned are politicians and consumer action groups. Each of these groups plays a role in the interaction that leads either to appropriate or inappropriate legislative action on drugs. It is, therefore, important that both should be furnished with accurate appropriate information about drug actions and reactions. For politicians, I believe that there are merits in the company establishing a good relationship with the local parliamentarian who represents the company's factory area, but there should also be good contact with Government and Opposition groups assigned the role of health-care interest. Such contact should, of course, be direct with the senior company management. It is also important that the relationship between the senior company management and government ministers should be good.

I find myself with less sympathy for many of the consumer action groups, though I accept that there are some who undertake a role that is to the benefit of both consumer and company. I have found, however, that many of the groups are biased and unreceptive to logical scientific argument, and I find this unattractive. Despite this, however, it is clear that nothing can be gained by not communicating accurate information to them. To do otherwise is to court suspicion. Hopefully, the better they are informed, the less inappropriate pressure they will exert.

## COMMUNICATION BETWEEN COMPANIES

Communication between companies, other than that defined within agreements, is still normally limited to matters of principle and to published material, although the situation has improved somewhat over the past 25 years. It is probably unrealistic to expect much more change due to the commercial pressures that are an integral part of marketing within a free economy. Moreover suspicion of cartel arrangements and restrictive practices will always make such contacts difficult.

There *might* be advantages in freer communication in certain circumstances (e.g. adverse reactions in one drug in a therapeutic group that is marketed by several companies). However, such problems can normally be solved by a professional and vigilant regulatory authority without any abuse of confidentiality.

## COMMUNICATION WITHIN THE THIRD WORLD

I have been mainly concerned with aspects of communication within industrially developed communities. The communication of pharmaceutical information within and to Third-World countries poses many additional problems, and their detailed consideration is not possible within the confines of this chapter.

The *per capita* sum available for health care is small, and in consequence sales to such countries are usually made at negligible profit and are even subsidized by the company or by external agencies. In consequence the money available for the provision of information is limited, even if appropriate communication channels exist.

Despite these circumstances it behoves companies to try to provide adequate current information on ADRs balanced with that on the beneficial effects. There is no justification for reduced medical or marketing ethics within the Third World. This philosophy is fully accepted by the major international pharmaceutical companies who are jealous of their reputation. A visit to a Third-World country shows that this ethic is not applied by all. In this respect it is often the indigenous industry that is the main offender.

## CONCLUSIONS

On the basis of this examination of the role of the pharmaceutical industry in the communication of information of drug effects and side-effects, there would appear to be three fundamental conclusions that should be drawn:

(1) Companies should ensure that the information is accurate and unbiased and directed to the right groups.

(2) It is essential that the company communicates all the relevant information that is available.

(3) It is important to realize that communication is a two-way interchange, and that it is most likely to take place in an effective form if there is mutual respect and understanding between the communicants.

# 51 Responsibility of the medical press

S. P. LOCK

## INTRODUCTION

In 1948 Bertrand Russell went to Norway to give a series of lectures. He chose to travel by air, though flying was a comparatively spartan form of travel 30 years ago compared with the luxurious conditions of today. One of the restrictions that irked Earl Russell was the ban on smoking, and on his way to Trondheim he complained to a pretty air hostess: 'I shall die unless I can smoke'. Since the aircraft was not full, and since the passenger was a distinguished guest of the Norwegian Government, the pilot suggested that she should put him at the back of the plane, where he could smoke his pipe in peace. So the journey itself was uneventful, but on coming in to land at Trondheim the plane undershot and crashed into the sea – from which Russell was rescued with a handful of other survivors.

For the rest of his life Bertrand Russell used this anecdote to prove that, in saying that he would die unless he could smoke, a philospher could sometimes state the truth. The pursuit of truth is certainly the medical journal's business, and in the case of both new and old drugs it has a special responsibility: to present the facts with speed, accuracy and balance. To this list should be added lucidity – for, however important its subject, the browser must be coaxed to read any article, and he must also be given space in the correspondence columns to comment on it.

Of course, this mixture of information, news, comment and entertainment is not peculiar to the medical journal. Nevertheless, where drugs are concerned the editor's problems are particularly difficult: the effects of an erroneous article are potentially far greater than those of most papers on other subjects. If a description of a so-called better method of measuring the serum-calcium concentration is found to be making false claims, it is unlikely to endanger patients' lives. Conversely, an article that recommends thalidomide as the ideal hypnotic during pregnancy, or that claims that penicillin is worthless in streptococcal cellulitis, could do great harm.

In this article I shall discuss how journals choose original articles for publication, commission editorials and teaching articles, assess letters to the editor, and monitor advertisements. Finally I shall deal with another recent development: the evaluation in medical journals of medical features in the public media (newspapers, radio and television).

## ORIGINAL ARTICLES

Every year between 4500 and 5000 original articles are submitted for publication to the *British Medical Journal*, and a similar number go to other general journals, such as the *Lancet* and the *Journal of the American Medical Association*. Something like 80% of the articles that come to the *BMJ* are rejected, and it is important that this is done quickly and fairly. I believe that an editor almost always needs expert advice in deciding whether to accept an article or not; true, he can probably eliminate about a fifth of all the articles without bothering an expert assessor, because these are obviously trivial, totally without originality, or so ultra-specialized that they would be unsuited to his general audience. Even so, before rejecting the article, he will invariably confirm this opinion with a medical editorial colleague, and if there is any doubt seek an external assessor's opinion.

All of the remaining articles must go to a referee, chosen individually after each article has been read by a medical editor. The referee is asked four main questions: is the article original (for the world or Britain), or does its importance outweigh this criterion; is it scientifically reliable (are the scientific methods, ethics, statistics and deductions sound); is it clinically important; and is it more suited to a general or a specialist journal?

With an assessor's opinion it is unfortunately all too easy to reject over half of all the articles submitted. There remains, however, the problem of deciding which to publish of the others – say, 20 out of every 100 submitted (because 20 of them have already been rejected on the editor's first reading). These 20 fulfil the journal's criteria, and yet it has space for only 12. At one time the final decision on which articles should be accepted and which rejected was taken entirely in the office. Seven years ago, feeling that this might be quixotic, unjust, or prejudiced, we introduced a 'hanging committee', a system already used by the *New England Journal of Medicine* and the *Annals of Internal Medicine*. Meeting weekly, this is composed of two medical editors and two outside consultant physicians, all of whom have read the article and the referee's comments. The committee discusses each article in turn and decides whether it should be accepted without revision, accepted with revision (either scientific or literary), or rejected; occasionally it decides to obtain the opinion of another referee – and, in any case, any article that is likely to be accepted and contains results based on statistical analysis is finally sent to an expert statistical adviser.

## Value of the referee

We aim at letting the author have a decision within a month – usually within 3 weeks, which is not easy given the postal delays and that most of our referees are busy people with many other commitments. Some have argued that the assessor is an unnecessary barrier, that decisions may be coloured by personal prejudice, and that the editor's decision is just as likely to be as correct as the referee's. I do not accept these views. Even specialists in one particular subject who are part-time editors of a journal devoted to it say that they can no longer keep abreast of the extremes – say, in the genetic, serological, and biochemical aspects of the subject. How much less is a full-time editor who has long ceased to practise able to give a definitive assessment of an article for its originality and scientific reliability.

Of course, mistakes are made with any system (and scope must be given in the correspondence columns to point these out), but I believe that these are more likely without the benefit of expert assessment than with it, particularly if the editor monitors his referees and checks their opinions with subsequent comments on the published article, and occasionally cross-checks these with another referee. Two other important functions of the referee are to educate the author (by sending an anonymous report on the article back with the rejection letter), and to improve the quality of accepted articles (by suggesting detailed changes in the original script). Finally, there is another serious hazard of not refereeing. The media are apt to believe that any paper published in a reputable journal is established truth rather than a contribution to a continuing scientific argument, so they are likely to highlight scare stories whose insubstantial basis any referee would have pointed out. That is not to say necessarily that such accounts should not be published – science thrives on hypothesis and speculation – merely that the editor should probably err on the side of arguments that have some reasoned basis (particularly where a general readership is concerned) and in any case should indicate by headings such as 'For Debate' or 'Hypothesis' that the ideas may be far from established.

## Extreme views

Articles which present extreme views which may have some validity deserve serious debate, but need expert appraisal, and are often better published in specialist journals, where the readership will have the necessary kind of critical sense. This is not to say that such ideas will get submerged: a general journal may well use them as the basis for a leading article in which they can be explained and discussed in the perspective of conventional views.

Medicine owes the large body of anonymous, often unpaid referees a debt of gratitude for maintaining standards of published articles. For the editor of a general journal the difficulty comes in knowing whether to send the referee's opinion to the author of a rejected article or not, largely for apparently trivial logistical reasons – the difficulty of coping with the load of typing entailed; the acrimonious arguments that result between an aggrieved author and an ignorant editor who is transmitting the opinion; and the tremendous and constant pressure on the space of a general journal. We have recently started routinely sending the referee's opinion and believe that this is a service a journal should offer young authors – even though it does take up virtually the whole time of one medical editor to do this.

## Articles on drugs

Although I have no figures, I suspect that we reject relatively more articles about drugs (either trials or side-effects) than on any other subject. The reasons for this would be apparent to anybody who saw a random sample of 100 such articles: lack of originality, poor design of trial or inadequately supported claims. With any new drug there is usually a rash of trials, and everyone comes to recognize that a company is out to push one of its wares. Often, unfortunately, many reports show features resulting from the poorly staffed and equipped peripheral centres where the trials have been carried out: small numbers, high drop-out rates, inadequate controls, and results that need every ounce of statistical braggadocio to make them mean anything.

Why cannot all drug firms co-ordinate such trials better, with the aim of producing one or two authoritative articles? Everyone knows the difficulties of organizing multi-centre trials – and medical research councils all over the world have been struggling with these since Bradford Hill introduced one of the most important concepts of twentieth-century medicine – the random controlled clinical trial – but the rewards far outweigh the trouble. Why should editors and referees have to waste their time in considering reports of trials in which the controls are grossly inadequate; in which the new agent has not been compared with the conventional drug or other method of treatment; in which an antibiotic has been used to treat a rag-bag of infections; and in which the results have no apparent application at all? Perhaps one of the results of the diminution in the number of drugs being developed and the stricter requirements by drug-releasing authorities all over the world will be better organized and more meaningful drug trials.

These veiws seem arrogant, but their converse is that every editor is likely to leap at accepting an article which fulfils all the journal's criteria: indeed, if the drug is in common use, a good large-scale study which defines its role may often be accepted for its importance despite the fact that the study is retrospective and unoriginal.

### Side-effects

One of the editor's main difficulties is in knowing what to do about reports of drug side-effects. On the one hand, the journal can play an important part in alerting doctors to a possibly important hazard; on the other hand, publishing an anecdotal account of apparently serious but uncorroborated side-effects might unjustly deprive patients of the benefits of a valuable drug as well as damaging the drug house which had developed it at great cost. Again, I believe that a pattern for reviewing these articles has to be established, particularly based on help from an expert referee.

In principle, articles about side-effects are little different from those about anything else: standards should not be lowered to accept inherently unlikely claims that are based on one case, or for which the evidence is unsatisfactory. For this reason the correspondence columns are not the place to publish such accounts: these are worth either a formal article, or nothing.

It might be objected that this attitude leaves little scope for the doctor in the periphery to give early warnings of possible drug hazards – that such an attitude, for example, would have suppressed the earliest warnings about thalidomide. Though the latter – a brief description of peripheral neuritis associated with taking thalidomide – was first made in a letter to the *BMJ*,[1] four patients were concerned and the suggested association was couched virtually as a question rather than as a statement. Today I believe that, after a referee's advice, we would have asked the writer to amplify his descriptions, and published them as a formal article: the right place for a single anecdotal report, however, is in a report to the Committee on Safety of Medicines.

If the report confirms and amplifies similar single-case reports, well and good, and action can be taken; if it does not, no harm will have been done – but after the furore over thalidomide harm was done by the publication of letters recording congenital defects purporting to have been caused by a variety of drugs taken by the mother during pregnancy. It needed a wide-scale and rigorous survey of the type carried out at Edinburgh to show that almost all of these anecdotes were without foundation.[2]

### Leading and other articles

Most readers will not obtain enough information about drugs from original articles: hence journals also have a responsibility to discuss the use of drugs in all aspects – not only their indications, side-effects, and contraindications, but also the latest views on their relative merits, particularly as compared with more established, and possibly better and cheaper, agents. To get the maximum amount of information across as many approaches as possible are needed.

Leading articles will often discuss one aspect of the use of a drug, or mention it briefly in an article primarily considering the treatment of a disease. For the *BMJ* we now believe that such editorials should be signed. So many decisions involving public policy are now being taken – some of them on the basis of such reviews – that it is important to know the standpoint of who is making the statements. Just as most journals abandoned anonymous book reviews several years ago, so the tendency has also been to sign leading articles, and I believe the process will continue so that eventually referees will be expected to sign their reports about the original articles on which they have been advising.

## Refresher articles

Inevitably, if only for reasons of space, a leading article is unlikely to present the full and rounded picture: refresher type, middle of the road features are the way to achieve this. Our weekly series 'Today's Treatment' is designed to bring the non-specialist doctor up-to-date on all important aspects of drug usage. Each unit aims at dealing with a particular system – for example, diseases of the skin or psychological disorders. It begins with an introduction to the anatomy and physiology of the system, and the pharmacology of the main drugs concerned, ending with a look at future possibilities in drug treatment. With the help of an expert adviser for each unit, the author of each individual article is carefully briefed – and, in particular, to answer the questions: what is the condition; what drug do you want; and, what is the place of other drugs (including corticosteroids) or other types of treatment (such as X-rays and surgery)? Two or three units are collected into a book, and the whole series takes about 5 years to run through all the major drugs and produces three or four books – which sell steadily and well.

By the time the last article in the series has finished enough changes have occurred in the treatment of diseases in the first unit for it to be time to start the whole cycle again. Practising doctors and medical students have told us how valuable they find such a series. Nevertheless, however well the individual articles are written, this system does have a certain lack of uniformity and the whole approach is inevitably that of a textbook.

## Other techniques

We have used other techniques. The first was to tape-record a series of undergraduate 'Therapeutic Conferences' at the Department of Therapeutics at Aberdeen; this ran over 3 years and from anecdotal reports we know that it was liked (at the Medical School at Mosul, in Northern Iraq, I found it being used as a class exercise, with students taking the roles of the various participants). Nevertheless, it entailed a lot of work for the department in transcribing the tape-recording, while the shortening inevitable in subediting made the dialogue slightly artificial and stilted. Another difficulty was the length of article needed to get the basic facts across – a problem solved better by a subsequent series 'Community Clinics in Clinical Pharmacology'. In this, based on an hour's seminar held weekly in a health centre, a general practitioner presents a case history, which is then discussed by the professor of clinical pharmacology who visits the practice once a week. He aims at making only two or three important practical points, and the whole article has rarely been longer than a page.

The initial run of 'Community Clinics' was so successful that the Department of Health ordered a large reprint for distribution to family doctors. Even so, we need as many ways as possible of getting across the important facts about drug usage, and at present are exploring the possibility of a much more visually orientated presentation, possibly on the lines of the successful ABC format used for other topics.

### Medical audit

Another approach which is becoming increasingly popular is to encourage good articles on medical audit, particularly of the use of drugs in hospitals and in general practice. To obtain worthwhile results, most doctors now agree that medical audit must be non-punitive, organized by those being audited, and designed to give an adequate answer to an important question. All these criteria were admirably shown in a study organized at Liverpool University. Based on a series of weekly discussions for general practitioners held by the Clinical Pharmacology department this study looked at the use of digitalis in general practice.[3,4] Among 391 patients an assessment of clinical, biochemical, and pharmacological data showed that digitalis treatment could be discontinued in 89 (23%); or the dose unchanged in 47 (12%), increased in 47 (12%) or decreased in 24 (6%).

In their discussion of these findings the authors emphasize that the motives were not economic – 'any savings on stopping digitalis were probably balanced by increasing the dose in other patients and paying for the study itself'. Nevertheless, publishing and encouraging such reports are another way of getting all doctors to review their own prescribing habits, and undoubtedly studies of process and outcome will become increasingly popular in the next few years.

## ADVERTISEMENT POLICY

It makes little sense for a journal to practise rational policy and critical evaluation of drug usage in its editorials and articles, only to refute these in the text of the advertisements it contains. For this reason at the *BMJ* we submit the text of new advertisements, or radically altered copy which makes new claims, to expert referees, asking them whether the claims made are supported by trustworthy evidence and whether the advertisement fulfils our code (see Table 1).

**Table 1 Code of advertisement policy**

(a) The publication of advertisements has become a recognized function of medical journals, but any advertisement may be refused without explanation.

(b) The advertisements in a journal, like the text, are sources of information for readers. This information is provided by the advertiser who is responsible for its accuracy; but care should be taken that no advertisement contravenes the principles set out below.

(c) Advertisements should not imply or promise benefit which, after due consideration and, if necessary, consultation with experts, appears highly improbable. Claims should be supported by trustworthy evidence.

(d) No therapeutic product should be advertised unless its essential constituents, and their quantity in each dose, are disclosed to the editor of the journal. Methods of manufacture need not be disclosed.

(e) Advertisements should not impugn the dignity of the medical profession or offend against good taste or recognized standards of medical practice.

(f) Advertisements of drugs or appliances should not contain testimonials, anonymous or otherwise. This does not exclude dated references to reputable medical journals, but such advertisements must not include misleading quotations from articles.

(g) Advertisements of books may contain quoted matter from reviews so long as a dated reference to the review is given, but not the name of the reviewer.

(h) Opinions expressed by contributors to medical journals must not be quoted in a way that makes them look like editorial opinions.

(i) The distinction between the advertisement columns and the text should be kept so clear that no ordinary reader can mistake one for the other.

(j) Publication of an advertisement means that in the Editor's judgement it does not contain misleading statements: but such publication does not necessarily mean that the journal endorses the claims made, and such endorsement must not be implied in advertisements of the same product in the lay press.

(k) Medical journals should not accept advertisements of products that are improperly advertised in the lay press or elsewhere.

(l) Advertisements should be considered on their own merits. An advertisement that is otherwise acceptable is not necessarily made unacceptable by the fact that the advertiser is putting forward improper claims for other products.

(m) Disparaging references: no advertisement should be published which appears to bring discredit on the products of other manufacturers.

If these conditions are fulfilled, however, we believe that the advertiser should be left alone. Save in gross breaches we are not arbiters of taste, and if companies want to use a picture of a blonde to advertise their wares that is their business. The number of advertisements opposite the text pages is limited, and their relation to individual articles is entirely fortuitous. This point can hardly be overemphasized, or that we enjoy excellent relations with our advertisers, none of whom has ever tried to influence editorial policy on any matter in any way.

## MEDICINE AND THE MEDIA

Not only has medicine recently become more prominent in the newspapers, and on radio and television: attitudes to it have also changed. The rise of consumerism has meant that traditional practices in all professions are being questioned and debated in a way that would have been unthinkable even 25 years ago. Although inevitably they sometimes feel threatened, most doctors welcome this trend: dealing with informed patients must be better for patients, doctors and medicine, *provided* that the information is true – and, since truth is not an absolute, this means that the media should give both sides of the case, together with some sort of reasoned conclusion.

Many journalists dealing with medicine do this job well, and make an important contribution to the public's knowledge. The difficulty comes perhaps in 10% of cases, where the article or feature is on a crusading course – to uncover a scandal that has been concealed by a professional conspiracy. True, a very few scandals do exist (as in all professions), but invariably these are never the ones featured in the papers or on televison. It is here that the comparative ignorance of some non-medical communicators becomes so obvious to the health professional. They may start out with blinkered ideas, perhaps reinforced by talking to one or two sincere medical eccentrics who agree with them; they will probably be tempted not to talk to reasonable people holding middle-of-the-road views, because these tend not to crystallize any argument enough, and programmes or articles aimed at the masses tend to be couched in black and white. Laudably, they will certainly want to make their contributions good entertainment – and, in their minds, this means sharp polarization of attitudes.

### Unbalanced contributions

All this results in unbalanced contributions, particularly in television, where any harm done by programmes cannot be corrected in the correspondence columns two days later. Occasionally programmes are so distorted that they harm the doctor-patient relationship; ordinary doctors become angry at the one-sided presentation and erroneous conclusions, and refuse to take part in future programmes; those holding minority views are the only ones who will agree to appear, and hence a vicious circle is created, in which all concerned are the losers – and none more so than the public.

It would be foolish to pretend that this problem has occurred frequently: most newspaper articles and television programmes are first-class, being accurate and balanced and written by professionals who are expert in communicating to a lay audience. Nevertheless, some features – particularly, for example, the 'trial by television' of both practolol and electroconvulsive therapy – have been so seriously unbalanced and out of step with current medical opinion that they have definitely disturbed medical confidence in television. Even worse was the *Panorama* programme on brain death, which despite its being shown to be based on false data (with an obvious fall in the donor rate of kidneys for transplantation) was never the subject of an apology.

I believe that several new measures are needed: more journalists specializing in health matters; greater use of outside medical advisers (which in television should apply to all programmes featuring medicine); and the creation of an independent National Television Council, analogous to the Press Council, to hear and pass judgement on major complaints – thereby placing on television the same emphasis on using its power with its responsibility as is done on the rest of the media and the professions.

### Positive role

Finally, journals also have a positive role in raising standards of the media: by providing the feedback on individual items that their creators often complain that they lack, journals can educate the educators. For example, most lay writers on medicine are only just beginning to emphasize that the use of powerful drugs almost inevitably carries some risk – and this may be a reflection that doctors themselves have been uncritical in their attitude to 'wonder' drugs.

To give journalists some sort of feedback 7 years ago we started a weekly column called 'Medicine and the Media', which aims at reviewing anything relating to medicine that is intended for the general public, whether in newspapers, magazines, or books, or on radio or television. It is too early to say whether this will achieve our aims, but the media could be such useful allies in telling the public about their own bodies and illnesses and the prescription for a balanced life that it would be a tragedy for them not to be used as colleagues rather than opponents.

## CONCLUSIONS

To sum up, I believe that the general medical journal has two main responsibilities. First, to the profession to keep doctors informed about new developments and to review existing knowledge. Secondly, to the public (through the medical journalist) to tell them of the risks and benefits of adopting various life styles and of using various forms of medical treatment, as well as emphasizing their vital role in public decision-making on important general matters such as the allocation of resources to health and within the Health Service itself.

For both groups it is particularly important to promote the concept of balance – that some medical problems are major and some relatively minor; that a totally avoidable habit, cigarette-smoking, is now killing as many people as tuberculosis did only a few generations ago; that there is little evidence that immunization against pertussis has harmed more than a handful of children while it has benefited millions; and that the solutions to the vast problems of the Third World are known, being those developed by the advanced countries many years ago.

The journal should carry out these tasks responsibly, leaning heavily on expert advisers, but without silencing the unconventional view. Above all, it should have a large section for correspondence, open to all, where virtually anything can be challenged or debated.

If it can fulfil these roles then, so far as drugs are concerned, both doctors and public may develop a more informed attitude to them – somewhere in between the lethal bullets which the Devil sells the hero of Weber's opera *Der Freischütz* and the magic bullets envisaged by Ehrlich which would kill a parasite but not harm the patient.

## References


1. Florence, A. L. (1960). Is thalidomide to blame? *Br. Med. J.*, **2,** 1954
2. Nelson, M. M. and Forfar, J. O. (1971). Associations between drugs administered during pregnancy and congenital abnormalities. *Br. Med. J.*, **1,** 523
3. Breckenridge, A., Orme, M., Serline, M. J., Davidson, A. S. and Lowe, J. F. (1978). Postgraduate education in therapeutics: experience in Merseyside. *Br. Med. J.*, **2,** 671
4. Liverpool Therapeutics Group (1978). Use of digitalis in general practice. *Br. Med. J.*, **2,** 673

# Index